Understanding

NURSING
RESEARCH

Understanding

NURSING RESEARCH

RESEARCH

THIRD EDITION

Nancy Burns, PhD, RN, FAAN

Jenkins Garrett Professor
School of Nursing
The University of Texas at Arlington
Arlington, Texas

Susan K. Grove, PhD, RN, ANP, GNP, APRN, BC

Professor of Nursing
Assistant Dean, Graduate Nursing Program
School of Nursing
The University of Texas at Arlington
Arlington, Texas

SAUNDERS

An Imprint of Elsevier Science
Philadelphia London New York St. Louis Sydney Toronto

SAUNDERS

An Imprint of Elsevier Science

The Curtis Center
Independence Square West
Philadelphia, Pennsylvania 19106

UNDERSTANDING NURSING RESEARCH, 3rd edition   ISBN 0-7216-0011-5

Vice President and Publishing Director, Nursing: Sally Schrefer
Executive Publisher: Barbara Nelson Cullen
Developmental Editor: Victoria Bruno
Publishing Services Manager: Linda McKinley
Cover Designer: Julia Dummitt

QWF/GC

Printed in the United States of America

Last digit is the print number: 9 8 7 6 5 4 3 2 1

To Helen Hough, librarian extraordinaire, who always goes beyond the norm to assist faculty and students and who knows all the intricacies of getting the sources I need for my writing in the current world of electronic library sources. Her commitment to nursing students and her pleasure at seeing them discover new knowledge is a wonderful gift to students.

Nancy

To Sheryl Grove, my sister and my best friend. She has touched my life in so many wonderful ways.

Susan

To Helen Hough, librarian extraordinaire, who always goes beyond the norm to assist faculty and students and who knows all the intricacies of getting the sources I need for my writing in the current world of electronic library sources. Her commitment to nursing students and her pleasure at seeing them discover new knowledge is a wonderful gift to students.

Nancy

To Sheryl Grove, my sister and my best friend. She has touched my life in so many wonderful ways.

Susan

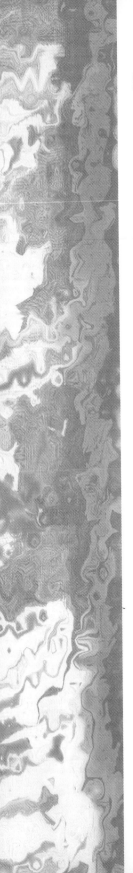

REVIEWERS

Patricia Lee Ackerman, PhD, RN, CPND
Division of Nursing
California State University
Sacramento, California

Wendy C. Budin, PhD, RNC
Associate Professor of Nursing
Seton Hall University
South Orange, New Jersey

Ann Harley, EdD, RN
Dean and Professor of Nursing
Chair of Graduate Studies in Nursing
Carson-Newman College
Jefferson City, Tennessee

Kathleen Collins Insel, PhD, RN
University of Texas Health Science Center at San Antonio
San Antonio, Texas

Erika Madrid, DNSc, RN, CS
School of Nursing
University of California, San Francisco
San Francisco, California

Cora Newell-Withrow, DSN, RN, MPH, FAAN
Professor
College of Health Sciences
Eastern Kentucky University
Richmond, Kentucky

Karen E. Pugsley, MN, RN
Shepherd College
Shepherdstown, West Virginia

PREFACE

Research is a major force in nursing, and the knowledge generated from research is changing practice, education, and health policy. Our aim in developing this essentials research text, *Understanding Nursing Research,* is to create an excitement about research in undergraduate students. The text emphasizes the importance of baccalaureate-educated nurses being able to critique research and use the findings in practice with the ultimate goal of developing an evidence-based practice for nursing. Thus a major strand throughout the text is critiquing the steps of the research process with the goal of using research findings in clinical practice. By making nursing research an integral part of baccalaureate education, we hope to facilitate the movement of research into the mainstream of nursing. We also hope this text increases student awareness of the knowledge that has been generated through nursing research and the knowledge that is relevant to their practice, as well as the importance of having a practice based on research evidence. Only through research can nursing truly be recognized as a profession with documented effective outcomes for the patient, family, nurse provider, and health care system.

Developing a third edition of *Understanding Nursing Research* has provided us with an opportunity to clarify and refine the essential content for an undergraduate text. The text is designed to assist undergraduate students in overcoming the barriers they frequently encounter to understanding the language used in nursing research. The revisions in the third edition are based on our own experiences with the text and input from dedicated reviewers and inquisitive students who provided us with many helpful suggestions.

Chapter 1, "Discovering Nursing Research," introduces the reader to nursing research, the history of research, and the significance of research for nursing practice. The discussion of research methodologies and their importance in generating an evidence-based practice for nursing is expanded. The historical information regarding nursing research is updated to reflect current trends and events in the profession. Chapter 2, "Introduction to the Quantitative Research Process," presents the steps of the quantitative research process in a concise manner and introduces students to the focus and findings of quantitative research. Extensive, recent examples of descriptive, correlational, quasi-experimental, and experimental studies are provided, which reflect the quality of current nursing research. Chapter 3, "Research Problems, Purposes, and Hypotheses," includes a refined definition of the research problem and clarifies the difference between a problem and a purpose. Example problem and purpose statements are included from current qualitative, quantitative, and outcome studies. Chapter 4, "Review of Literature," provides a background for reading, critiquing, and summarizing research literature to determine the current knowledge in a selected area for use in nursing practice. This chapter is significantly revised to include the process for accessing online sources and relevant practice information from the Internet. Chapter 5, "Understanding Theory and Research Frameworks," stresses the importance of frameworks in research and provides guidelines for critiquing frameworks in published studies. Chapter 6, "Examining Ethics in Nursing Research," includes a detailed discussion of the use of ethics in research. In this edition, the ethics of qualitative and outcomes research is expanded and clarified with examples from current studies. The content on scientific misconduct is updated to reflect current regulations. Chapter 7, "Clarifying Research Designs," is expanded to include designs of clinical trials in nursing and intervention research. In addition, the difference between quasi-experimental and experimental designs is clarified. Chapter 8, "Populations and Samples," now includes a section on the use of sampling in qualitative research and offers supportive examples from current studies. Chapter 9, "Measurement and Data Collection in Research," is updated to reflect current knowledge in the literature. Chapter 10, "Understanding Statistics in Research," is significantly revised to include the following essential topics: processing data analysis; understanding the reasoning behind statistics; describing, predicting, and testing hypotheses using statistics; examining relationships using statistics, interpreting statistical outcomes, and judging statistical suitability. In Chapter 11, "Introduction to Qualitative Research," the qualitative research methodologies are expanded to include storytelling and narrative analysis. Opportunities for students to have simple group experiences in collecting and analyzing qualitative data are suggested in this chapter. Chapter 12, "Critiquing Nursing Studies," summarizes and builds on the critique content provided in previous chapters and offers direction for conducting critiques of quantitative and qualitative studies. Chapter 13, "Using Research in Nursing Practice with a Goal of Evidence-Based Practice," is refined to include a variety of traditional and electronic approaches for communicating and using research findings in practice. This chapter includes a discussion of evidence-based practice, best practices, and clinical practice guidelines as a basis for building evidence-based practice in nursing. A model is provided to facilitate the use of research findings in practice and to move nurses toward providing an evidence-based practice.

A variety of changes are made throughout the third edition of this text. Strategies designed to assist the reader in linking research findings to practice are increased; an example of such strategies is selecting study examples with which students as beginning clinicians can easily relate. Research examples are updated to include recently published quantitative, qualitative, and outcomes nursing studies.

The third edition of *Understanding Nursing Research* is appropriate for use in a variety of undergraduate research courses for generic and RN students because it provides an introduction to a variety of research methodologies, such as quantitative, qualitative, and outcomes research. We believe this text will assist students in reading research literature, critiquing published studies, and summarizing research findings for use in practice. We also believe this text will be a valuable resource for practicing nurses in critiquing and using research findings in their clinical settings.

Learning Resources to Accompany Understanding Nursing Research, third edition

A major change to this edition is the transition to a web-enhanced text in which students are prompted to visit the Internet for further practice. As students log onto the text's web site, they will find "open book quizzes" that include cross-word puzzles, multiple-choice questions, matching questions, and fill-in-the-blank questions.

Instructor's Resource to Accompany Understanding Nursing Research, third edition

The entire instructor's ancillary is available both online and on CD-ROM. The Instructor's Resource will consist of an *Instructor's Manual*, test bank, PowerPoint presentation, electronic image collection, and WebLinks.

Instructor's Manual

The *Instructor's Manual* presents chapter purpose, objectives, learning activities, and evaluation strategies for each chapter in the text. The chapter purpose states the concepts to which the reader will be introduced when reading the chapter. Relevant objectives are developed for undergraduate students. Instructors can select the objectives that are most appropriate for their particular curricula and courses. The learning activities are student assignments provided for use in or out of class to facilitate the learning of research content. Evaluation strategies include essay questions for each chapter. Answers or page references are provided for these questions. Example course syllabi are also included in the *Instructor's Manual* to assist you in developing a syllabus for your research course. The *Instructor's Manual* can be saved, revised, and printed to custom fit your classes and teaching style.

Test Bank

The test bank is a completely new component to this edition. It is made up of approximately 300 multiple-choice questions, including the topic, objective, cognitive level, correct answer, rationale, and text reference. It, too, can be saved, revised, and printed to custom fit your needs.

PowerPoint Presentation

The PowerPoint presentation contains over 700 slides. You can customize your slide presentations by revising or changing the order of existing slides. This teaching aid is provided to facilitate lecture preparation and presentation.

Electronic Image Collection

The electronic image collection consists of approximately 26 images from the text. This collection can be used in classroom lectures to reinforce student learning.

WebLinks

WebLinks is the final component of the instructor's resource. Here you will find links organized according to the chapters of the text and to various related web sites for each chapter.

Study Guide

The *Study Guide,* available as a companion to the text, includes three recently published nursing studies that can be used in classroom discussions, as well as to address the study guide questions. The *Study Guide* provides exercises that target comprehension of the meaning of concepts used in each chapter. Exercises, including fill-in-the-blank, matching, and multiple-choice questions, encourage students to validate their understanding of the chapter content. Critique activities provide student opportunities to apply their new research knowledge to evaluate the studies provided in the back of the *Study Guide.* For students who enjoy a little fun with their learning, crossword puzzles related to chapter content are provided.

Online Learning Resources to Accompany the Study Guide for Understanding Nursing Research, third edition

The questions that were available in the last edition are revised, and new questions are added to increase the total number of 20 to 25 questions per chapter. As students use the *Study Guide,* they are prompted to visit the Internet and access these questions.

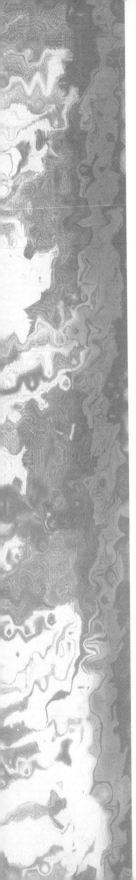

ACKNOWLEDGMENTS

Developing this essentials research text was a 2-year project, and there are many people we would like to thank. We express our appreciation to Dean Elizabeth Poster, Associate Dean Carolyn Cason, and Assistant Dean Josie L. O'Quinn, as well as to the faculty of the School of Nursing at the University of Texas at Arlington, for their endless support and encouragement. We also would like to thank other nursing faculty across the country who have used our book to teach research and have spent valuable time to send us ideas and to identify errors in the text. Special thanks to the students who have read our book and provided honest feedback on its clarity and usefulness to them. We would also like to recognize the excellent reviews of colleagues who helped us make important revisions in the text.

In conclusion, we would like to thank the people at Elsevier Science who helped produce this book. We would like to thank the following individuals who have devoted extensive time to the development of the third edition, the instructor's ancillary, student study guide, and all the web-based components. These individuals include Barbara Nelson Cullen, Executive Publisher; Victoria Bruno, Developmental Editor; Linda McKinley, Publishing Services Manager; Julia Dummitt, Senior Designer; and Michele Trope, Managing Editor, Electronic Publishing.

Nancy Burns, PhD, RN, FAAN
Susan K. Grove, PhD, RN, ANP, GNP, APRN, BC

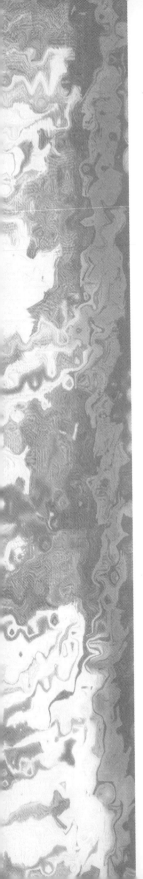

CONTENTS

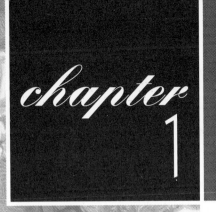

chapter 1

Discovering Nursing Research

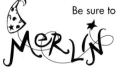

Be sure to check out the free exercises on-line at
www.wbsaunders.com/MERLIN/Burns/
understanding

OBJECTIVES

Completing this chapter should enable you to:
1. Define research and nursing research.
2. Discuss the importance of research in developing an evidence-based practice for the nursing profession.
3. Identify your role in research as a professional nurse.
4. Describe the development of nursing research from the time of Florence Nightingale into the twenty-first century.
5. Describe the ways of acquiring nursing knowledge (tradition, authority, borrowing, trial and error, personal experience, role modeling, intuition, reasoning, and research) that you use in your practice.
6. Identify the different types of quantitative and qualitative research conducted in nursing.
7. Discuss the contribution of quantitative, qualitative, and outcomes research to the development of nursing knowledge.

RELEVANT TERMS

Authority	Nursing research
Borrowing	Outcomes research
Case study	Personal experience
Control	Prediction
Critique	Premise
Deductive reasoning	Qualitative research
Description	Quantitative research
Evidence-based practice	Reasoning
Explanation	Research
Inductive reasoning	Role modeling
Intuition	Traditions
Knowledge	Trial and error
Mentorship	

Welcome to the world of nursing research. You may think it strange to consider research a "world," but it is truly a new way of experiencing reality. Entering a new world requires learning a unique language, incorporating new rules, and using new experiences to learn how to interact effectively within that world. As you become a part of this new world, your perceptions and methods of reasoning will be modified and expanded. For example, research involves questioning, and you will be encouraged to ask such questions as these: Why is this nursing intervention being used? What is the effect of this intervention? Would another intervention be more effective? What research has been conducted in this area? What is the quality of the studies conducted to determine the effectiveness of this intervention? Do the findings from the studies conducted on this nursing intervention provide sound evidence for use in practice? How can you use these research findings in your practice?

Because research is a new world to many of you, we have developed this text to facilitate your entry into and understanding of this world and its contribution to the delivery of quality nursing care. The purpose of this chapter is to explain broadly the world of nursing research. The importance of nursing research in developing an evidence-based practice and your role in research are addressed. The past, present, and future of nursing research are explored, including the scientific accomplishments in the profession over the last 150 years. The ways of acquiring knowledge in nursing are discussed, including the significance of research in developing nursing knowledge. The chapter concludes with a discussion of the common research methodologies used in generating nursing knowledge: quantitative, qualitative, and outcomes research.

WHAT IS NURSING RESEARCH?

The word *research* means "to search again" or "to examine carefully." More specifically, research is a diligent, systemic inquiry or study that validates and refines existing knowledge and develops new knowledge. Diligent, systematic study indicates planning, organization, and persistence. The ultimate goal of research is the development of an empirical body of knowledge for a discipline or profession, such as nursing.

Defining nursing research requires determining what is relevant knowledge for nurses. Because nursing is a practice profession, research is essential to develop and refine knowledge that can be used to improve clinical practice. Practicing nurses, such as yourself, need to be able to read research reports, identify effective interventions for practice, and implement these interventions to promote positive outcomes for patients and families. For example, extensive research has been done to determine the most effective technique for administering medications through an intramuscular (IM) injection. Beyea and Nicoll (1995) summarized this research and developed guidelines for administering IM injections. Summarizing research involves critiquing studies on a selected topic or practice problem, such as safe administration of IM injections, and synthesizing the findings from these studies to describe what is known and not known on the selected topic. This summary of current research knowledge is used to generate guidelines for practice. Beyea and Nicoll's (1995) guidelines identify the best needle size and length to use for administering different types of medications; the safest injection site (ventrogluteal site) for many medications; and the best injection technique to deliver a medication, minimize patient discomfort, and prevent physical damage. This information is essential for you to know in giving IM injections to ensure that the outcomes are accurate delivery of medication, minimal discomfort for the patient, and no physical damage to the patient. (These guidelines for administration of IM injections are presented in Chapter 13.)

Nursing research is also needed to generate knowledge about nursing education, nursing administration, health care services, characteristics of nurses, and nursing roles. The findings from these studies indirectly influence nursing practice and thus add to nursing's body of knowledge. Educational research is needed to provide high-quality learning experiences for nursing students. Nursing administration and health services studies are needed to improve the quality and cost-effectiveness of the health care delivery system. Studies of nurses and nursing roles can influence nurses' productivity, job satisfaction, and retention. In this era of nursing shortage, additional research is needed to determine effective ways to recruit individuals into and retain them in the profession of nursing. This type of research could have a major impact on the quality and number of nurses providing care to patients and families in the future.

The ultimate goal of nursing research is the generation of an empirical knowledge base to guide practice. Extensive research is needed to develop sound empirical knowledge that can be synthesized into evidence for use in nursing practice. This research evidence might be synthesized to develop guidelines, standards, protocols, or policies to direct the implementation of a variety of nursing interventions. The ultimate goal of nursing is providing evidence-based care that promotes quality outcomes for patients, families, health care providers, and the health care system (Brown, 1999; Omery & Williams, 1999). *Evidence-based practice* involves the use of collective qualitative, quantitative, and outcomes research findings in (1) promoting the understanding of patients' and families' experiences with health and illness (a common focus of qualitative research); (2) implementing effective nursing interventions to promote patient health (a common focus of quantitative research); and (3) providing quality, cost-effective care within the health care system (a common focus of outcomes research). For example, research related to the administration of IM injections has been critiqued, summarized, and developed into guidelines to direct the administration of medications by an IM route to infants, children, and adults in a variety of practice settings. The outcomes from using these research-based guidelines in practice include (1) adequate administration of medication to promote patient health, (2) minimal patient discomfort, and (3) no physical damage to the patient, which promotes high-quality, cost-effective care. Using research-based guidelines in practice increases the likelihood of achieving these positive outcomes.

In summary, nursing research is needed to generate knowledge that will directly and indirectly influence nursing practice. In this text, *nursing research* is defined as a scientific process that validates and refines existing knowledge and generates new knowledge that directly and indirectly influences nursing practice.

WHY IS RESEARCH IMPORTANT IN GENERATING AN EVIDENCE-BASED PRACTICE FOR NURSING?

Nursing research is essential for the development of scientific knowledge that enables nurses to provide evidence-based nursing care (Brown, 1999; Omery & Williams, 1999). Broadly, the nursing profession is accountable to society for providing high-quality, cost-effective care for patients and families. Thus the care provided by nurses must be constantly evaluated and improved based on new and refined knowledge. Through nursing research, scientific knowledge can be developed to improve nursing care, patient outcomes, and the health care delivery system. For example, nurses need scientific knowledge to improve their decision making in prioritizing and organizing their nursing care. A solid research base is needed to document the effectiveness of selected nursing interventions in treating particular patient problems and promoting positive patient and family outcomes. In addition, nurses need to use research findings to determine the best way to deliver health care services to ensure that the greatest number of people receives care. Accomplishing these goals will require you to critique, summarize, and use research evidence that provides description, explanation, prediction, and control of phenomena in your clinical practice.

Description

Description involves identifying and understanding the nature of nursing phenomena and sometimes the relationships among these phenomena (Chinn & Kramer, 1998). Through research, nurses are able to (1) describe what exists in nursing practice, (2) discover new information, (3) promote understanding of situations, and (4) classify information for use in the discipline. For example, Jacobs (2000) conducted a study to describe the informational needs of surgical patients following discharge. The findings from this study could be used to develop discharge instruction guidelines for surgical patients. This study concludes that discharge instructions need to include content on activity levels, pain management techniques, and strategies to prevent complications (Jacobs, 2000). This research information might be used to develop discharge instruction guidelines or to revise existing guidelines in your clinical agency. Research focused on description provides essential groundwork for studies focused on explanation, prediction, and control of nursing phenomena.

Explanation

Explanation clarifies the relationships among phenomena and identifies the reasons why certain events occur. For example, Pronk, Goodman, O'Connor, and Martinson (1999) studied the relationships between modifiable health risks (physical inactivity, obesity, and smoking) and health care charges and found that adverse health risks translate into significantly higher health care charges. Thus managed health care plans and nursing care providers seeking to reduce health care charges will need to identify and implement interventions that will effectively modify adverse health risks of inactivity, obesity, and smoking. This study provides an example of how explanatory research is useful in identifying relationships among variables, such as health risks, interventions, patient outcomes, and costs. Identifying relationships among nursing phenomena provides a basis for research focused on prediction and control.

Prediction

Through *prediction*, the probability of a specific outcome can be estimated in a given situation (Chinn & Kramer, 1998). However, predicting an outcome does not necessarily enable the nurse to modify or control the outcome. With predictive knowledge, nurses could anticipate the effects that nursing interventions would have on patients and families. For example, Defloor (2000) conducted a study to determine the effects of position and type of mattress on skin pressure of persons lying in bed. The researcher found that the 30-degree semi-Fowler position and polyethylene-urethane mattress produced a significant reduction in interface pressure between the mattress and skin. However, this type of study does not determine whether reducing interface pressure will decrease the incidence of pressure ulcers. Further research is needed to determine whether controlling the position and type of mattress will decrease the incidence of pressure ulcer development in patients on bed rest. Predictive studies isolate independent variables that require additional research to ensure their manipulation results in successful outcomes, as measured by designated dependent variables (Omery, Kasper, & Page, 1995).

Control

If the outcome of a situation can be predicted, the next step is to control or manipulate the situation to produce the desired outcome. *Control* can be described as the ability to write a prescription to produce the desired outcome. Currently, nurses prescribe specific interventions in their care plans to assist patients and families in achieving their health goals. These care plans need to reflect the most current evidence-based interventions to produce high-quality, cost-effective outcomes for patients and their families. For example, Parker, McFarlane, Soeken, Silva, and Reel (1999) conducted a study that implemented a prescribed intervention to prevent further abuse to pregnant women. They found significantly less violence and abuse was reported by women in the intervention group than by women in the comparison group. Thus implementing this intervention manipulated or controlled the situation to produce the positive outcome of reduced abuse and violence toward pregnant women.

In summary, studies that document the effectiveness of specific nursing interventions make it possible to implement evidence-based care that will produce the best outcomes for patients and their families. The quality of research conducted in nursing affects not only the quality of care delivered but also the power of nurses in making decisions about the health care delivery system. A limited number of studies have developed knowledge that is useful for prediction and control in nursing practice. However, the extensive number of nursing studies conducted in the last two decades has greatly expanded the scientific knowledge for you to use in describing, explaining, predicting, and controlling phenomena within your nursing practice.

WHAT IS YOUR ROLE IN NURSING RESEARCH?

Now that you have been introduced to the world of nursing research, what do you think will be your research role? You may believe that you have no role in research, that research is the responsibility of other nurses. However, generating a scientific knowledge base and using this research evidence in practice requires the participation of all nurses in a variety of research activities. Some nurses are producers of research and conduct studies to generate and refine the knowledge needed for nursing practice. Others are consumers of research and use research findings to improve their nursing practice.

Professional nursing organizations, such as American Nurses Association (ANA) (1989) and the American Association of Colleges of Nursing (AACN) (1999), have published position statements that identify the participation of nurses in research based on their educational preparation. Nurses with an associate degree in nursing (ADN), a bachelor of science degree in nursing (BSN), a master of science degree in nursing (MSN), a doctorate degree, and postdoctorate education each have a clearly designated role in research (ANA, 1989) (Fig. 1-1). The researcher role a nurse assumes expands with his or her advanced education and expertise. Thus the nurse with a BSN has a significant role in critiquing and synthesizing research findings from the nursing profession and other disciplines for use in practice. These nurses are also important members of the health care teams that plan and implement changes in nursing care and in the health care system based on research (AACN, 1999). In addition, nurses with a BSN also provide valuable assistance in identifying research problems and collecting data for studies.

Nurses with an MSN are provided the educational preparation to lead health care teams in making essential changes in nursing practice and in the health care system based on research. MSN-prepared nurses also conduct focused, initial studies in collaboration with other nurse scientists (ANA, 1989). Doctorally prepared nurses assume a major role in the conduct of research and in the generation of nursing knowledge in a selected area of interest. These nurse scientists often coordinate research teams that include MSN- and BSN-prepared nurses to facilitate the conduct of quality studies in a variety of health care agencies. The postdoctorally prepared nurse usually assumes a researcher role fully and has a funded program of research. These scientists are often identified as experts in selected areas and provide mentoring of new nurse researchers. The maximum preparation of postdoctorate education provides a background for doing all the research activities identified for the other levels of educational preparation (see Fig. 1-1).

This text was developed to encourage you to be a consumer of research. It provides content to assist you in reading research reports, critiquing these reports, and summarizing the findings for use in practice. Nursing's scientific knowledge base is rapidly expanding with the generation of new findings by nurses and other health pro-

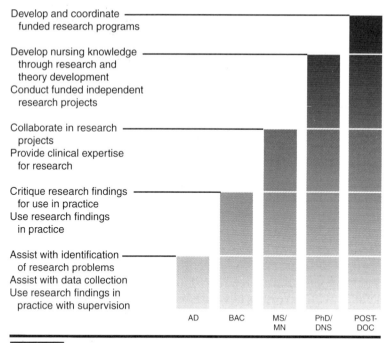

Develop and coordinate
   funded research programs

Develop nursing knowledge
   through research and
   theory development
Conduct funded independent
   research projects

Collaborate in research
   projects
Provide clinical expertise
   for research

Critique research findings
   for use in practice
Use research findings
   in practice

Assist with identification
   of research problems
Assist with data collection
Use research findings in
   practice with supervision

AD   BAC   MS/   PhD/   POST-
             MN   DNS   DOC

Fig. 1-1   RESEARCH PARTICIPATION at various levels of education preparation. *(American Nurses Association [1989].* Education for participation in nursing research. *Kansas City, MO: American Nurses Association. Reprinted with permission.)*

fessionals using a variety of research methods. You can learn about these relevant research findings by reading research in clinical journals; attending professional conferences and meetings; and examining the extensive health care studies, evidence-based guidelines, and protocols that are provided on the Internet. Reading research reports requires an understanding of the research process, which is detailed throughout this text. A *critique* of research involves careful examination of all aspects of a study to judge its strengths, limitations, meaning, and significance. Conducting critiques of studies is a major focus of this text, with critique activities highlighted in each chapter. The findings from multiple studies on a specific topic need to be summarized to determine their potential use in practice. This text provides direction for reading, critiquing, and summarizing the research literature as a basis for making changes in your practice. We hope that this text will increase your understanding of research and facilitate your implementation of an evidence-based practice.

NURSING'S PARTICIPATION IN RESEARCH: PAST TO PRESENT

Nursing's participation in research has changed drastically over the last 150 years and holds great promise for the twenty-first century. Initially, nursing research evolved slowly, from the investigations of Nightingale in the nineteenth century to the studies of nursing education in the 1930s and 1940s and the research of nurses and nursing roles in the 1950s and 1960s. In the 1970s through the 1990s, an increasing number of nursing studies focused on clinical problems and produced findings that had a direct impact on practice. Clinical research continues to be a major focus for the twenty-first century, with the goal of developing an evidence-based practice for nursing. Reviewing the history of nursing research enables you to identify the accomplishments and understand the need for further research. Table 1-1 outlines the key historical events that have influenced the development of research in nursing.

Florence Nightingale

Nightingale's (1859) initial research focused on the importance of a healthy environment in promoting patients' physical and mental well being. She studied aspects of the environment such as ventilation, cleanliness, purity of water, and diet to determine the influence on patients' health (Herbert, 1981). However, Nightingale is most noted for her collection and analysis of soldier morbidity and mortality data during the Crimean War. This research enabled her to change the attitudes of the military and society toward the care of the sick. The military began to view the sick as having the right to adequate food, suitable quarters, and appropriate medical treatment. These interventions drastically reduced mortality from 43% to 2% in the Crimean War (Cook, 1913). Nightingale also used research knowledge to make significant changes in society, such as testing public water, improving sanitation, preventing starvation, and decreasing morbidity and mortality (Palmer, 1977).

Nursing Research: 1900s through 1970s

The *American Journal of Nursing* was first published in 1900, and late in the 1920s and 1930s, case studies began appearing in this journal. A *case study* involves an in-depth analysis and a systematic description of one patient or a group of similar patients to promote understanding of nursing interventions. Case studies are one example of the practice-related research that has been conducted in nursing over the last century.

Nursing educational opportunities expanded with Teacher's College at Columbia offering the first educational doctoral program for nurses in 1923 and Yale University offering the first masters in nursing degree in 1929. In 1950 the American Nurses Association (ANA) initiated a 5-year study on nursing functions and activities. In 1959 the findings from this study were used to develop statements on functions, standards, and qualifications for professional nurses. During this time, clinical research began expanding as nursing specialty groups, such as community health, psychiatric–mental health, medical-surgical, pediatrics, and obstetrics, developed standards of care. The research conducted by the ANA and specialty groups provided the basis for the nursing practice standards that currently guide professional practice (Gortner & Nahm, 1977). The increase in research activity during the 1940s prompted the publication of the first research journal, *Nursing Research,* in 1952.

TABLE 1-1

HISTORICAL EVENTS INFLUENCING RESEARCH IN NURSING

YEAR	HISTORICAL EVENT
1850	Nightingale, first nurse researcher
1900	*American Journal of Nursing* first published
1923	Teacher's College at Columbia offers the first educational doctoral program for nurses
1929	First Masters in Nursing Degree is offered at Yale University
1932	The Association of Collegiate Schools of Nursing is organized
1950	American Nurses' Association study of nursing functions and activities
1952	*Nursing Research* first published
1953	Institute of Research and Service in Nursing Education established
1955	American Nurses Foundation established to fund nursing research
1963	*International Journal of Nursing Studies* first published
1965	ANA sponsored first nursing research conferences
1967	*Image* (Sigma Theta Tau Journal) first published, now entitled *Journal of Nursing Scholarship*
1970	ANA Commission on Nursing Research established
1972	ANA Council of Nurse Researchers established
1973	First Nursing Diagnosis Conference was held
1978	*Research in Nursing & Health* first published *Advances in Nursing Science* first published
1979	*Western Journal of Nursing Research* first published
1982-83	Conduct and Utilization of Research in Nursing (CURN) Project (published)
1983	*Annual Review of Nursing Research* first published
1985	National Center for Nursing Research (NCNR) was established within the National Institutes of Health
1987	*Scholarly Inquiry for Nursing Practice* first published
1988	*Applied Nursing Research* first published
1989	Agency for Health Care Policy and Research (AHCPR) was established Clinical practice guidelines were first published by the AHCPR
1992	*Healthy People 2000* was published by Department of Health and Human Services
1993	NCNR was renamed the National Institute of Nursing Research (NINR)
1994	*Qualitative Nursing Research* first published
1999	AHCPR renamed Agency for Healthcare Research and Quality (AHRQ)
1999	American Association of Colleges of Nursing position statement on nursing research
2000	NINR identified mission and funding priorities for 2000-2004; http://www.nih/gov/ninr
2000	AHRQ identified mission and funding priorities; http://www.ahrq.gov
2000	*Healthy People 2010* was published by Department of Health and Human Services

In the 1950s and 1960s, nursing schools began introducing research and the steps of the research process at the baccalaureate level, and MSN-level nurses were provided a background for conducting research. In 1953 the Institute for Research and Service in Nursing Education was established at Teacher's College, Columbia University, New York, which provided learning experiences in research for doctoral students (Gortner & Nahm, 1977).

In the 1960s an increasing number of clinical studies focused on quality care and the development of criteria to measure patient outcomes. Intensive care units were developed, which promoted the investigation of nursing interventions, staffing patterns, and cost effectiveness of care (Gortner & Nahm, 1977). An additional research journal, the *International Journal of Nursing Studies,* was published in 1963. In 1965 the ANA sponsored the first of a series of nursing research conferences to promote the communication of research findings and the use of these findings in practice.

In the late 1960s and 1970s, nurses were involved in the development of models, conceptual frameworks, and theories to guide nursing practice. The nursing theorists' works provided direction for future nursing research. In 1978, Chinn began publishing the journal *Advances in Nursing Science,* which included nursing theorists' works and related research. Another event influencing research during the 1970s was the establishment of the ANA Commission on Nursing Research in 1970. In 1972 the commission established the Council of Nurse Researchers to advance research activities, provide an exchange of ideas, and recognize excellence in research. The commission also influenced the development of federal guidelines concerning research with human subjects and sponsored research programs nationally and internationally (See, 1977).

The communication of research findings was a major issue in the 1970s (Barnard, 1980). Sigma Theta Tau, the international honor society for nursing, sponsored national and international research conferences; the chapters of this organization sponsored many local conferences to communicate research findings. *Image,* now entitled *Journal of Nursing Scholarship*, was first published in 1967 by Sigma Theta Tau and includes research articles and summaries of research conducted on selected topics. Two additional research journals were first published in the 1970s: *Research in Nursing & Health* in 1978 and *Western Journal of Nursing Research* in 1979.

Nursing Research: 1980s and 1990s

The conduct of clinical research was the focus of the 1980s, and clinical journals began publishing more studies. One new research journal was published in 1987, *Scholarly Inquiry for Nursing Practice,* and two in 1988, *Applied Nursing Research* and *Nursing Science Quarterly.* Although the body of empirical knowledge generated through clinical research increased rapidly in the 1980s, little of this knowledge was used in practice. During 1982 and 1983 the materials from a federally funded project, Conduct and Utilization of Research in Nursing (CURN), were published to facilitate the use of research to improve nursing practice (Horsley, Crane, Crabtree, & Wood, 1983). In 1983 the first volume of the *Annual Review of Nursing Research* was published (Werley & Fitzpatrick,

1983). These volumes include experts' reviews of research organized into four areas: nursing practice, nursing care delivery, nursing education, and the nursing profession. These summaries of current research knowledge encourage the use of research findings in practice and provide direction for future research. The *Annual Review of Nursing Research* is a publication that continues today, with leading expert nurse scientists providing summaries of research in their areas of expertise.

Qualitative research was introduced in the late 1970s, but the first studies began appearing in nursing journals in the 1980s. The focus of qualitative research was holistic with intent to discover meaning and gain new insights and understanding of phenomena relevant to nursing. The number of qualitative researchers and studies expanded greatly in the 1990s, with qualitative studies appearing in most of the nursing research and clinical journals. In 1994 a journal focused on disseminating qualitative research, *Qualitative Nursing Research*, was published. However, quantitative research has been and continues to be the most frequently used research methodology in conducing nursing research.

Another priority of the 1980s was to obtain increased funding for nursing research. Most of the federal funds in the 1980s were designated for medical studies involving the diagnosis and cure of diseases. However, the ANA achieved a major political victory for nursing research with the creation of the National Center for Nursing Research (NCNR) in 1985. The purpose of this center is to support the conduct and dissemination of knowledge developed through basic and clinical nursing research, training, and other programs in patient care research (Bauknecht, 1985). Under the direction of Dr. Ada Sue Hinshaw, the NCNR became the National Institute of Nursing Research (NINR) in 1993. During the 1990s the NINR (1993) focused its support on five research priorities: community-based nursing models, effectiveness of nursing interventions in human immunodeficiency virus and acquired immunodeficiency syndrome (HIV/AIDS), cognitive impairment, living with chronic illness, and biobehavioral factors related to immunocompetence. The NINR web site provides the most current information on the institute's research priorities and activities (see Table 1-1).

Outcomes research emerged as an important methodology for documenting the effectiveness of health care services in the 1980s and 1990s. This effectiveness research evolved from the quality assessment and quality assurance functions that originated with the professional standards review organizations (the PSROs) in 1972. William Roper, director of the Health Care Finance Administration (HCFA), promoted outcomes research during the 1980s to determine quality and cost-effectiveness of patient care. In 1989 the Agency for Health Care Policy and Research (AHCPR) was established to facilitate the conduct of outcomes research (Rettig, 1991). AHCPR also had an active role in communicating research findings to health care practitioners and was responsible for publishing the first clinical practice guidelines in 1989. These guidelines included a synthesis of the latest research findings with directives for practice developed by health care experts in a variety of areas. Several of these evidence-based guidelines were published in the 1990s and provided standards for practice in nursing and medicine. The Healthcare Research and Quality Act of 1999 reauthorized the AHCPR, changing its name to the Agency for Healthcare Research and Quality (AHRQ). This significant change positioned the AHRQ as a scientific partner with the public and private sectors to improve the quality and safety of patient care. The AHRQ web site provides the most current information on this agency and includes current guidelines for clinical practice (see Table 1-1).

Nursing Research: Twenty-First Century

The vision for nursing in the twenty-first century is the development of a scientific knowledge base that enables nurses to implement an evidence-based practice (EBP) (Brown, 1999; Omery & Williams, 1999). This vision is consistent with the mission of NINR, which is to "support clinical and basic research to establish a scientific basis for the care of individuals across the lifespan—from management of patients during illness and recovery to the reduction of risks for disease and disability, the promotion of healthy lifestyles, promoting quality of life in those with chronic illness, and care for the individuals at the end of life."* NINR is seeking expanded funding for nursing research and is encouraging a variety of methodologies (quantitative, qualitative, and outcomes research) to be used to generate essential knowledge for nursing practice.

The AHRQ has been designated as the lead agency supporting research designed to improve the quality of health care, reduce its cost, improve patient safety, decrease medical errors, and broaden access to essential services. AHRQ conducts and sponsors research that provides evidence-based information on health care outcomes, quality, cost, use, and access. This research information is needed to promote effective health care decision making by patients, clinicians, health system executives, and policy makers.

The focus of health care research and funding is expanding from the treatment of illness to include health promotion and illness prevention interventions. *Healthy People 2010,* published by the Department of Health and Human Services, increases the visibility of and identified priorities for health promotion research. In the twenty-first century, nurses could play a major role in the development of interventions to promote health and prevent illness in individuals, families, and communities. To ensure an effective research enterprise in nursing, the discipline must (1) create a research culture; (2) provide quality educational programs (baccalaureate, masters, doctorate, and postdoctorate) to prepare a workforce of nurse scientists; (3) develop a sound research infrastructure; and (4) obtain sufficient funding for essential research (AACN, 1999).

ACQUIRING KNOWLEDGE IN NURSING

Some key questions that might be asked about knowledge include the following: What is knowledge? How is knowledge acquired in nursing? Is most of nursing's knowledge based on research? *Knowledge* is essential information acquired in a variety of ways,

*http://www.nih.gov/ninr.

expected to be an accurate reflection of reality, and incorporated and used to direct a person's actions (Kaplan, 1964). During nursing education, an extensive amount of knowledge is acquired from classroom and clinical experiences. You had to learn, synthesize, incorporate, and apply this knowledge so that you could practice as a nurse.

The quality of your nursing practice depends on the quality of the knowledge that you learned. Thus you need to question the quality and credibility of new information that you hear or read. For example, what were the sources of the knowledge that you acquired during your nursing education? Were the nursing interventions taught based on research or tradition? Which interventions were based on research, and which need further study to determine their effectiveness? Nursing has historically acquired knowledge through traditions, authority, borrowing, trial and error, personal experience, role modeling, intuition, and reasoning. Only in the last decade have many of the research findings been included in nursing textbooks or instructors' lectures. This section introduces different ways of acquiring knowledge in nursing. Some nursing actions are based on sound scientific knowledge, but others need to be questioned, studied, and revised to reflect current research findings.

Traditions

Traditions include "truths" or beliefs that are based on customs and trends. Nursing traditions from the past have been transferred to the present by written and oral communication and role modeling, and they continue to influence the practice of nursing. For example, many of the policy and procedure manuals in hospitals contain traditional ideas. Traditions can positively influence nursing practice because they were developed from effective past experiences.

However, traditions can also narrow and limit the knowledge sought for nursing practice. For example, nursing units are frequently organized and run according to set rules or traditions that may not be efficient or effective. Often these traditions are neither questioned nor changed because they have existed for years and are frequently supported by people with power and authority. Many traditions have not been tested for accuracy or efficiency through research, and even those not supported through research tend to persist. For example, many patients with cardiac conditions are required to take basin baths throughout their hospitalization despite findings from nursing research that "the physiologic costs of the three types of baths (basin, tub, and shower) are similar; differences in responses to bathing seem more a function of subject variability than bath types; and many cardiac patients can take a tub bath or shower earlier in their hospitalization" (Winslow, Lane, & Gaffney, 1985, p. 164). Nursing's body of knowledge needs to have an empirical rather than a traditional base if nurses are to have a powerful impact on health care and patient outcomes.

Authority

An *authority* is a person with expertise and power who is able to influence opinion and behavior. A person is given authority because it is thought that she or he knows more in a given area than others do. Knowledge acquired from an authority is illustrated when one person credits another as the source of information. Nurses who publish articles and books or develop theories are frequently considered authorities. Students usually view their instructors as authorities, and clinical nursing experts are considered authorities within their clinical settings. Authorities maintain many customs or traditional ways of knowing; however, like tradition, much of the knowledge acquired from authorities has not been validated by research. Although the knowledge may be useful, it needs to be questioned and verified through research.

Borrowing

Some nursing leaders have described part of nursing's knowledge as information borrowed from disciplines such as medicine, sociology, psychology, physiology, and education (McMurrey, 1982). *Borrowing* in nursing involves the appropriation and use of knowledge from other fields or disciplines to guide nursing practice. Nursing has borrowed in two ways. For years, some nurses have taken information from other disciplines and applied it directly to nursing practice. This information was not integrated within the unique focus of nursing. For example, some nurses have used the medical model to guide their nursing practice, thus focusing on the diagnosis and treatment of disease. This type of borrowing continues today as nurses use advances in technology to become highly specialized and focused on the detection and treatment of disease.

The second way of borrowing, which is more useful in nursing, involves integrating information from other disciplines within the focus of nursing. Because disciplines share knowledge, it is sometimes difficult to know where the boundaries exist between nursing's knowledge base and that of other disciplines. However, borrowed knowledge has been inadequate for answering many questions generated in nursing practice.

Trial and Error

Trial and error is an approach with unknown outcomes that is used in a situation of uncertainty in which other sources of knowledge are unavailable. Because each patient responds uniquely to a situation, there is uncertainty in nursing practice. Hence, nurses must use trial and error in providing nursing care. However, trial and error frequently involves no formal documentation of effective and ineffective nursing actions. With this strategy, knowledge is gained from experience, but often it is not shared with others. The trial-and-error approach to acquiring knowledge can also be time consuming because multiple interventions may be implemented before one is found to be effective. There is also a risk of implementing nursing actions that are detrimental to patients' health. If studies were conducted on nursing interventions, selection and implementation of interventions could be based on scientific knowledge rather than chance.

Personal Experience

Personal experience involves gaining knowledge by being personally involved in an event, a situation, or a circumstance. Personal experience enables the nurse to gain skills and expertise by providing care to patients and families in clinical settings. Learning that occurs from personal experience enables the nurse to cluster ideas into a meaningful whole. For example, you may read about giving an injection or be told how to give an injection in a classroom setting, but you do not "know" how to give an injection until you observe other nurses giving injections to patients and actually give several injections yourself.

The amount of personal experience affects the complexity of a nurse's knowledge base. Benner (1984) described five levels of experience in the development of clinical knowledge and expertise: (1) novice, (2) advanced beginner, (3) competent, (4) proficient, and (5) expert. Novice nurses have no personal experience in the work they are to perform, but they have preconceived notions and expectations about clinical practice that they obtained during their education. These notions and expectations are challenged, refined, confirmed, or refuted by personal experience in a clinical setting. The advanced beginner nurse has just enough experience to recognize and intervene in recurrent situations. For example, the advanced beginner is able to recognize and intervene in managing patients' pain. Competent nurses are able to generate and achieve long-range goals and plans because of years of personal experience. The competent nurse is also able to use personal knowledge to take conscious, deliberate actions that are efficient and organized. From a more complex knowledge base, the proficient nurse views the patient as a whole and as a member of a family and community. The proficient nurse recognizes that each patient and family responds differently to illness and health. The expert nurse has an extensive background of experience and is able to identify accurately and intervene skillfully in a situation. Personal experience increases the ability of the expert nurse to grasp a situation intuitively with accuracy and speed. Benner's (1984) qualitative research provides an increased understanding of how knowledge is acquired through personal experience. Additional research is needed to clarify the dynamics of expert nursing practice and to determine methods that will facilitate meaningful personal experiences for nursing students and new graduates.

Role Modeling

Role modeling is learning by imitating the behaviors of an expert. In nursing, role modeling enables the novice nurse to learn through interactions with or examples set by highly competent, expert nurses. Role models include admired teachers, expert clinicians, researchers, or individuals who inspire others through their examples (Rempusheski, 1992). An intense form of role modeling is *mentorship,* in which the expert nurse serves as a teacher, sponsor, guide, and counselor for the novice nurse. The knowledge gained through personal experience is greatly enhanced by a high-quality relationship with a role model or mentor. Some new graduates enter internship programs provided by clinical agencies so that expert nurses can mentor them during the novices' first few months of employment.

Intuition

Intuition is an insight or understanding of a situation or event as a whole that usually cannot be explained logically (Rew & Barrow, 1987). Because intuition is a type of knowing that seems to come unbidden, it may also be described as a "gut feeling" or a "hunch." Because intuition cannot be explained scientifically with ease, many people are uncomfortable with it. Some even believe that it does not exist. However, intuition is not the lack of knowing; rather, it is a result of "deep" knowledge (Benner, 1984). The knowledge is so deeply incorporated that it is difficult to bring it to the surface consciously and express it in a logical manner. Some nurses can intuitively recognize when a patient is experiencing a health crisis. Using this intuitive knowledge, they can assess the patient's condition and contact the physician for medical intervention.

Reasoning

Reasoning is the processing and organizing of ideas in order to reach conclusions. Through reasoning, people are able to make sense of both their thoughts and experiences. This type of logical thinking is often evident in the oral presentation of an argument in which each part is linked to reach a logical conclusion. The science of logic includes inductive and deductive reasoning. *Inductive reasoning* moves from the specific to the general; particular instances are observed and then combined into a larger whole or a general statement (Chinn & Kramer, 1998). An example of inductive reasoning follows:

Particular Instances

A headache is an altered level of health that is stressful.
A terminal illness is an altered level of health that is stressful.

General Statement

Therefore it can be induced that all altered levels of health are stressful.

Deductive reasoning moves from the general to the specific or from a general premise to a particular situation or conclusion (Chinn & Kramer, 1998). A *premise* or proposition is a statement of the proposed relationship between two or more concepts. An example of deductive reasoning follows:

Premises

All human beings experience loss.
All adolescents are human beings.

Conclusion

Therefore it can be deduced that all adolescents experience loss.

In this example, deductive reasoning is used to move from the two general premises about human beings and adolescents to the conclusion that "All adolescents experience loss." However, the conclusions generated from deductive reasoning are valid only if they are based on valid premises. Research is a means to test and confirm or refute a premise so that valid premises can be used as a basis for reasoning in nursing practice.

ACQUIRING KNOWLEDGE THROUGH NURSING RESEARCH

Acquiring knowledge through traditions, authority, borrowing, trial and error, personal experience, role modeling, intuition, and reasoning is important in nursing. However, these ways of acquiring knowledge are inadequate in providing a scientific knowledge base for nursing practice. The knowledge needed for practice is both specific and holistic, as well as process oriented and outcomes focused; thus a variety of research methods are needed to generate this knowledge. This section introduces quantitative, qualitative, and outcomes research methods that have been used to generate knowledge for nursing practice.

Introduction to Quantitative and Qualitative Research

Quantitative and qualitative research complement each other because they generate different kinds of knowledge that are useful in nursing practice. Knowing about these two types of research will help you identify, understand, and critique these studies in journals and books. Quantitative and qualitative research methodologies have some similarities; both require researcher expertise, involve rigor in implementation, and generate scientific knowledge for nursing practice. Some of the differences between the two methodologies are presented in Table 1-2.

The majority of the studies conducted in nursing have used quantitative research methods. *Quantitative research* is a formal, objective, systematic process in which numerical data are used to obtain information about the world. The quantitative

TABLE 1-2

QUANTITATIVE AND QUALITATIVE RESEARCH CHARACTERISTICS

CHARACTERISTIC	QUANTITATIVE RESEARCH	QUALITATIVE RESEARCH
Philosophical origin	Logical positivism	Naturalistic, interpretive, humanistic
Focus	Concise, objective, reductionistic	Broad, subjective, holistic
Reasoning	Logistic, deductive	Dialectic, inductive
Basis of knowing	Cause-and-effect relationships	Meaning, discovery, understanding
Theoretical focus	Tests theory	Theory development

approach toward scientific inquiry emerged from a branch of philosophy called logical positivism, which operates on strict rules of logic, truth, laws, and predictions. Quantitative researchers hold the position that "truth" is absolute and that a single reality can be defined by careful measurement. To find truth, the researcher must be objective, which means that values, feelings, and personal perceptions cannot enter into the measurement of reality. Quantitative research is conducted to test theory by describing variables, examining relationships among variables, and determining cause-and-effect interactions between variables (Burns & Grove, 2001).

Qualitative research is a systematic, subjective approach used to describe life experiences and situations and to give them meaning (Munhall, 2001). This research methodology evolved from the behavioral and social sciences as a method of understanding the unique, dynamic, holistic nature of human beings. The philosophical base of qualitative research is interpretive, humanistic, and naturalistic and is concerned with understanding the meaning of social interactions by those involved. Qualitative researchers believe that "truth" is both complex and dynamic and can be found only by studying individuals as they interact with and in their sociohistorical settings (Munhall, 1989; 2001). Nurses' interest in conducting qualitative research began in the late 1970s; currently, an extensive number of qualitative studies are conducted using a variety of qualitative research methods. Qualitative research is conducted to promote understanding of human experiences and situations and to develop theories that describe these experiences and situations. Because human emotions are difficult to quantify (i.e., assign a numerical value), qualitative research seems to be a more effective method of investigating emotional responses than quantitative research (see Table 1-2).

Several types of quantitative and qualitative research have been conducted to generate nursing knowledge for practice. These types of research can be classified in a variety of ways. The classification system for this text (Table 1-3) includes the most

---

TABLE 1-3

CLASSIFICATION SYSTEM FOR NURSING RESEARCH METHODS

I. TYPES OF QUANTITATIVE RESEARCH
Descriptive research
Correlational research
Quasi-experimental research
Experimental research

II. TYPES OF QUALITATIVE RESEARCH
Phenomenological research
Grounded theory research
Ethnographical research
Historical research

III. OUTCOMES RESEARCH

common types of quantitative and qualitative research conducted in nursing. The quantitative research methods are classified into four categories: descriptive, correlational, quasi-experimental, and experimental. Descriptive research is conducted to explore new areas of research and to describe situations as they exist in the world. Correlational research is conducted to examine relationships and to develop and refine explanatory knowledge for nursing practice. Quasi-experimental and experimental studies are conducted to determine the effectiveness of nursing interventions in producing positive outcomes for patients and families. (These types of research are discussed in detail in Chapter 2.)

The qualitative research methods included in this text are phenomenological, grounded theory, ethnographical, and historical research (see Table 1-3). Phenomenological research is an inductive descriptive approach used to describe an experience as it is lived by an individual, such as the lived experience of chronic pain. Grounded theory is an inductive research technique that is used to formulate, test, and refine a theory about a particular phenomenon. Grounded theory was initially developed by Glaser and Strauss (1967) and was used to formulate a theory about the grieving process. Ethnographical research was developed by the discipline of anthropology for investigating cultures through an in-depth study of the members of the culture. Health practices vary among cultures, and these practices need to be recognized in delivering care to patients, families, and communities. Historical research is a narrative description or analysis of events that occurred in the remote or recent past. Through historical research, past mistakes are examined to facilitate an understanding of and an effective response to present situations (Munhall, 2001). (Qualitative research methods are the focus of Chapter 11.)

Introduction to Outcomes Research

The spiraling cost of health care has generated many questions about the quality and effectiveness of health care services and the patient's outcomes related to these services. Consumers want to know what services they are purchasing and if these services will improve their health. Health care policymakers want to know whether the care is cost effective and high in quality. These concerns have promoted the conduct of *outcomes research* that focuses on examining the result of care or determining the changes in health status for the patient (Rettig, 1991). Four essential areas that require examination through outcomes research are the following: (1) patient responses to medical and nursing interventions; (2) functional maintenance or improvement of physical functioning for the patient; (3) financial outcomes achieved with the provision of health care services; and (4) patient satisfaction with the health outcomes, care received, and health care providers (Jones, 1993). Nurses are playing an active role in conducting outcomes research by participating in multidisciplinary research teams that examine the outcomes of health care services. This knowledge provides a basis for improving the quality of care nurses deliver in practice.

SUMMARY

The purpose of this chapter is to introduce you to the world of nursing research. Research is defined as diligent, systematic inquiry to validate and refine existing knowledge and generate new knowledge. Nursing research is defined as a scientific process that validates and refines existing knowledge and generates new knowledge that directly and indirectly influences nursing practice. The ultimate goal of nursing research is the generation of an empirical knowledge base to guide practice. Extensive research is needed to develop sound empirical knowledge that can be synthesized into evidence for use in nursing practice. This research evidence may be synthesized to develop guidelines, standards, protocols, or policies to direct the implementation of a variety of nursing interventions. The ultimate goal of nursing is providing evidence-based care that promotes quality outcomes for patients, families, health care providers, and the health care system. Evidence-based practice involves the use of collective qualitative, quantitative, and outcomes research findings in (1) promoting the understanding of patient and family experiences with health and illness (a common focus of qualitative research); (2) implementing effective nursing interventions to promote patient health (a common focus of quantitative research); and (3) providing high-quality, cost-effective care within the health care system (a common focus of outcomes research). Accomplishing these goals will require you to critique, synthesize, and use research evidence that provides description, explanation, prediction, and control of phenomena in your clinical practice.

Nurses' participation in research over the past 150 years has changed drastically. Initially, research evolved slowly from the investiga-tions of Nightingale in the nineteenth century to the studies of nursing education in the 1930s and 1940s and the research of nurses and nursing roles in the 1950s and 1960s. However, from the 1970s through the 1990s, an increasing number of nursing studies focused on clinical problems. The conduct of clinical research continues to be a major focus in the twenty-first century, with the goal of developing a research or evidence-based practice for nursing. A significant accomplishment for nursing was the development of the NINR, which provides essential funding to further nursing research. The historical review of nursing research activities clearly indicates the gains that have been made in developing nursing knowledge.

Nursing has historically acquired knowledge primarily through traditions, authority, borrowing, trial and error, personal experience, role modeling, intuition, and reasoning. However, these ways of acquiring knowledge are inadequate in providing a scientific knowledge base for nursing. Research is needed to develop and refine scientific knowledge for use in practice. The knowledge nurses need is not only narrow and specific, but it is also broad and holistic. Thus a variety of research methods are needed to generate nursing knowledge. Nurses conduct both quantitative and qualitative research to address nursing problems. Quantitative research is a formal, objective, systematic process using numerical data to obtain information about the world. This research method is used to describe, examine relationships, and determine cause and effect. Qualitative research is a systematic, subjective approach used to describe life experiences and give them meaning. Knowledge generated from qualitative research will provide meaning and understanding of specific emotions, values, and life experiences. Quantitative and qualitative research complement each other because they generate different kinds of knowledge that are useful in nursing practice.

Different research methods can be classified in a variety of ways. In this text, quantitative research is classified into four types: descriptive, correlational, quasi-experimental, and experimental. Four types of qualitative research included are phenomenological, grounded theory, ethnographical, and historical. A third research method presented in this text is outcomes research, which focuses on examining the result of care or in determining the changes in health status for the patient. The spiraling cost of health care has generated many questions about the quality and effectiveness of health care services and the patient's outcomes related to these services; these questions are often best addressed by conducting outcomes research.

In conclusion, this text was developed to encourage you to be a consumer of research. You are provided content to assist you in reading research reports, critiquing the reports, and summarizing the findings for use in practice. We hope you will come to value research and to recognize the impact it can have on your practice, the nursing profession, and the health care system.

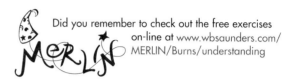

Did you remember to check out the free exercises on-line at www.wbsaunders.com/ MERLIN/Burns/understanding

REFERENCES

American Association of Colleges of Nursing. (1999). Position statement: Nursing research. *Journal of Professional Nursing, 15*(4), 253–257.

American Nurses Association (ANA). (1989). *Education for participation in nursing research.* Kansas City, MO: American Nurses Association.

Barnard, K. E. (1980). Knowledge for practice: Directions for the future. *Nursing Research, 29*(4), 208–212.

Bauknecht, V. L. (1985). Capital commentary: NIH bill passes, includes nursing research center. *American Nurse, 17*(10), 2.

Benner, P. (1984). *From novice to expert: Excellence and power in clinical nursing practice.* Menlo Park, CA: Addison-Wesley.

Beyea, S. C., & Nicoll, L. H. (1995). Administration of medications via the intramuscular route: An integrative review of the literature and research-based protocol for the procedure. *Applied Nursing Research, 8*(1), 23–33.

Brown, S. J. (1999). *Knowledge for healthcare practice: A guide to using research evidence.* Philadelphia: Saunders.

Burns, N., & Grove, S. K. (2001). *The practice of nursing research: Conduct, critique, and utilization* (4th ed.). Philadelphia: Saunders.

Chinn, P. L., & Kramer, M. K. (1998). *Theory and nursing: A systematic approach* (5th ed.). St. Louis: Mosby.

Cook, E. (1913). *The life of Florence Nightingale* (Vol. 1). London: Macmillan.

Defloor, T. (2000). The effect of position and mattress on interface pressure. *Applied Nursing Research, 13*(1), 2–11.

Glaser, B. G., & Strauss, A. L. (1967). *The discovery of grounded theory: Strategies for qualitative research.* Chicago: Aldine.

Gortner, S. R., & Nahm, H. (1977). An overview of nursing research in the United States. *Nursing Research, 26*(1), 10–33.

Herbert, R. G. (1981). *Florence Nightingale: Saint, reformer or rebel?* Malabar, FL: Robert E. Krieger.

Horsley, J. A., Crane, J., Crabtree, M. K., & Wood, D. J. (1983). *Using research to improve nursing practice: A guide, CURN Project.* New York: Grune & Stratton.

Jacobs, V. (2000). Informational needs of surgical patients following discharge. *Applied Nursing Research, 13*(1), 12–18.

Jones, K. R. (1993). Outcomes analysis: Methods and issues. *Nursing Economics, 11*(3), 145–152.

Kaplan, A. (1964). *The conduct of inquiry.* New York: Harper & Row.

McMurrey, P. H. (1982). *Toward a unique knowledge base in nursing. Image, 14*(1), 12–15.

Munhall, P. L. (1989). Philosophical ponderings on qualitative research methods in nursing. *Nursing Science Quarterly, 2*(1), 20–28.

Munhall, P. L. (2001). *Nursing Research: A qualitative perspective* (3rd ed.). Boston: Jones and Bartlett Publishers.

National Institute of Nursing Research (NINR) (September 23, 1993). *National nursing research agenda: Setting nursing research priorities.* Bethesda, MD: National Institutes of Health.

Nightingale, F. (1859). *Notes on Nursing: What it is, and what it is not.* Philadelphia: Lippincott.

Omery, A., Kasper, C. E., & Page, G. G. (1995). *In search of nursing science.* Thousand Oaks: Sage Publications.

Omery, A., & Williams, R. P. (1999). An appraisal of research utilization across the United States. *Journal of Nursing Administration, 29*(12), 50–56.

Palmer, I. S. (1977). Florence Nightingale: Reformer, reactionary, researcher. *Nursing Research, 26*(2), 84–89.

Parker, B., McFarlane, J., Soeken, K., Silva, C., & Reel, S. (1999). Testing an intervention to prevent further abuse to pregnant women. *Research in Nursing & Health, 22*(1), 59–66.

Pronk, N. P., Goodman, M. J., O'Connor, P. J., & Martinson, B. C. (1999). Relationship between modifiable health risks and short-term healthcare charges. *Journal of the American Medical Association, 282*(23), 2235–2239.

Rempusheski, V. F. (1992). A researcher as resource, mentor, and preceptor. *Applied Nursing Research, 5*(2), 105–107.

Rettig, R. (1991). History, development, and importance to nursing of outcomes research. *Journal of Nursing Quality Assurance, 5*(2), 13–17.

Rew, L., & Barrow, E. M. (1987). Intuition: A neglected hallmark of nursing knowledge. *Advances in Nursing Science, 10*(1), 49–62.

See, E. M. (1977). The ANA and research in nursing. *Nursing Research, 26*(3), 165–171.

Werley, H. H., & Fitzpatrick, J. J. (1983). *Annual review of nursing research* (Vol. 1). New York: Springer.

Winslow, E. H., Lane, L. D., & Gaffney, F. A. (1985). Oxygen uptake and cardiovascular responses in control adults and acute myocardial infarction patients during bathing. *Nursing Research, 34*(3), 164–169.

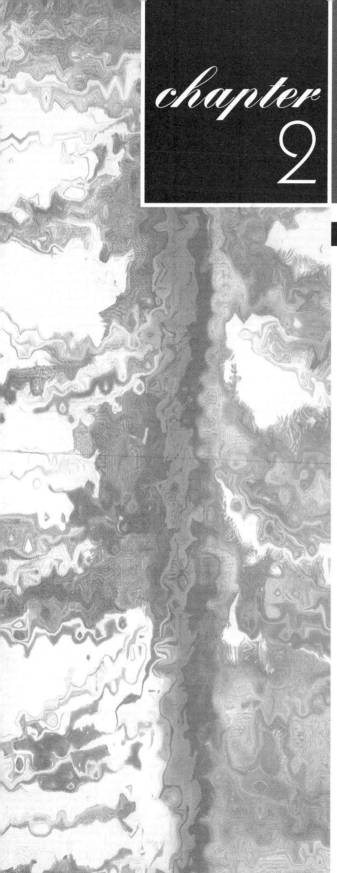

chapter 2

Introduction to the Quantitative Research Process

OUTLINE

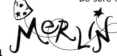

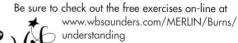

Be sure to check out the free exercises on-line at
www.wbsaunders.com/MERLIN/Burns/
understanding

OBJECTIVES

Completing this chapter should enable you to:

1. Define quantitative research and discuss its importance in generating knowledge for nursing practice.
2. Define terms relevant to the quantitative research process: basic research, applied research, rigor, and control.
3. Compare and contrast the use of control in quantitative research.
4. Describe the natural, partially controlled, and highly controlled settings in which quantitative research is conducted.
5. Compare and contrast the problem-solving process, nursing process, and research process.
6. Describe the steps of the quantitative research process.
7. Explain the purposes of a pilot study.
8. Identify sources that publish nursing research reports.
9. Read research reports.
10. Identify the steps of the quantitative research process in a research article.
11. Conduct an initial critique of a research report.
12. Examine the different types of quantitative research reports: descriptive, correlational, quasi-experimental, and experimental.

RELEVANT TERMS

Abstract
Applied (practical) research
Assumptions
Basic (pure) research
Concepts
Control
Correlational research
Data analysis
Data collection
Descriptive research
Design
Experiment
Experimental research
Framework
Generalization
Interpretation of research outcomes
Limitations
    Methodological limitations
    Theoretical limitations
Literature review
Measurement
Nursing process
Pilot study
Population
Problem-solving process

Process
Quantitative research
Quantitative research process
Quasi-experimental research
Reading research reports
    Analyzing research reports
    Comprehending research reports
    Skimming research reports
Research outcomes
Research problem
Research process
Research purpose
Research report
Rigor
Sample
Sampling
Setting
    Highly controlled setting
    Natural (field) setting
    Partially controlled setting
Theory
Variables
    Conceptual definition
    Operational definition

What do you think of when you hear the word *research?* Frequently, the word *experiment* comes to mind. Experimentation may be equated with randomizing subjects into groups, collecting data, and conducting statistical analyses. Frequently, an experiment is thought to be conducted to "prove" something, such as proving that a drug is an effective treatment for an illness. These ideas are associated with quantitative research. Quantitative research includes specific steps that are detailed in research reports. Reading and critiquing quantitative studies require learning new terms, understanding the steps of quantitative research, and applying a variety of analytical skills.

This chapter provides an introduction to quantitative research and a background for reading a research report. Relevant terms are defined, and the problem solving and nursing processes are presented to provide a basis for understanding the quantitative research process. The steps of the quantitative research process are introduced, and a descriptive correlational study is presented as an example to promote understanding of the process. The chapter concludes with a discussion of the critical thinking skills needed for reading research reports and guidelines for conducting an initial critique of these reports. The appendix to this chapter identifies the steps of the research process from a published quasi-experimental study and an experimental study.

WHAT IS QUANTITATIVE RESEARCH?

Quantitative research is a formal, objective, rigorous, systematic process for generating information about the world. Quantitative research is conducted to describe new situations, events, or concepts in the world, such as describing cloning and its potential influence on health care; to examine relationships among concepts or ideas, such as the relationship between red wine consumption and cholesterol level; and to determine the effectiveness of treatments such as herbal medicines on the health of patients and families. The classic experimental designs to test the effectiveness of treatments were originated by Sir Ronald Fisher (1935). He is noted for adding structure to the steps of the research process with such ideas as the hypothesis, research design, and statistical analysis. Fisher's studies provided the groundwork for what is now known as experimental research.

Throughout the years, a number of other quantitative approaches have been developed. Campbell and Stanley (1963) developed quasi-experimental approaches to study the effects of treatments under less controlled conditions. Karl Pearson developed statistical approaches for examining relationships between variables, which increased the conduct of correlational research. The fields of sociology, education, and psychology are noted for their development and expansion of strategies for conducting descriptive research. A broad range of quantitative research approaches is needed to develop knowledge for nursing practice. This section introduces the different types of quantitative research and provides definitions of terms relevant to the quantitative research process.

Types of Quantitative Research

Four types of quantitative research are included in this text: (1) descriptive, (2) correlational, (3) quasi-experimental, and (4) experimental. The type of research conducted is influenced by the current knowledge of a research problem. When little knowledge is available, descriptive studies often are conducted. As the knowledge level increases, correlational, quasi-experimental, and experimental studies are conducted.

Descriptive Research

Descriptive research is the exploration and description of phenomena in real-life situations; it provides an accurate account of characteristics of particular individuals, situations, or groups (Kerlinger & Lee, 1999). Through descriptive studies, researchers discover new meaning, describe what exists, determine the frequency with which something occurs, and categorize information. The outcomes of descriptive research include the description of concepts, identification of relationships, and development of hypotheses that provide a basis for future quantitative research.

Correlational Research

Correlational research involves the systematic investigation of relationships between or among two or more variables. To do this, the researcher measures the selected variables in a sample and then uses correlational statistics to determine the relationships among the variables. Using correlational analysis, the researcher is able to determine the degree or strength and type (positive or negative) of a relationship between two variables. The strength of a relationship varies from −1 (perfect negative correlation) to +1 (perfect positive correlation), with 0 indicating no relationship. The positive relationship indicates that the variables vary together, that is, both variables either increase or decrease together. For example, research has shown that the more people smoke, the more lung damage they experience. The negative relationship indicates that the variables vary in opposite directions; thus as one variable increases, the other will decrease. For example, research has shown that an increase in the number of years of smoking is correlated with a decrease in life span. The primary intent of correlational studies is to explain the nature of relationships in the real world, not to determine cause and effect. However, correlational studies are the means for generating hypotheses to guide quasi-experimental and experimental studies that do focus on examining cause-and-effect relationships.

Quasi-Experimental Research

The purpose of *quasi-experimental research* is to examine causal relationships or to determine the effect of one variable on another. Quasi-experimental studies involve implementing a treatment and examining the effects of this treatment using selected methods of measurement (Cook & Campbell, 1979). Quasi-experimental studies differ from experimental studies by the level of control achieved by the researcher. Quasi-experimental studies usually lack a certain amount of control over the manipulation of the treatment, management of the setting, or selection of the subjects. When studying human behavior, especially in clinical settings, researchers are frequently unable to randomly select the subjects or to manipulate or control certain variables related to the subjects or the setting. Thus nurse researchers conduct more quasi-experimental studies than experimental studies.

Experimental Research

Experimental research is an objective, systematic, highly controlled investigation for the purpose of predicting and controlling phenomena in nursing practice. In an experimental study, causality between the independent and dependent variables is examined under highly controlled conditions (Kerlinger & Lee, 1999). Experimental research is considered the most powerful quantitative method because of the rigorous control of variables. The three main characteristics of experimental studies are (1) controlled manipulation of at least one treatment variable (independent variable); (2) exposure of some of the subjects to the treatment (experimental group), and no exposure of the remaining subjects (control group); and (3) random assignment of subjects to either the control or experimental group. Control in an experimental study is strengthened by random selection of subjects. The degree of control achieved in experimental studies varies based on the population studied and the variables examined.

Defining Terms Relevant to Quantitative Research

Understanding quantitative research requires an introduction to the terms *basic research, applied research, rigor,* and *control.* In this section, these terms are defined and examples are provided from quantitative studies.

Basic Research

Basic research (or *pure research*) is scientific investigation that involves the pursuit of "knowledge for knowledge's sake" or for the pleasure of learning and finding truth (Miller, 1991). Basic scientific investigation seeks new knowledge about health phenomena with the hope of establishing general principles. The purpose of basic research is to generate and refine theory; thus the findings are frequently not directly useful in practice (Wysocki, 1983). Basic nursing research on physiological variables might include laboratory investigations of animals or humans to develop principles about physiological functioning, pathology, or the effects of treatments on physiological and pathological functioning. These studies might focus on increasing our understanding of oxygenation, perfusion, fluid and electrolyte balance, acid-base status, eating and sleeping patterns, and comfort status, as well as pathophysiology of the immune system (Bond & Heitkemper, 1987).

The study by McCarthy, Lo, Nguyen, and Ney (1997) is an example of basic research. This laboratory study was conducted to determine if increasing the protein density of food would positively influence total protein and food intake of tumor-bearing rats. The findings indicated that increasing the protein density of the food consumed resulted in an increase in net protein intake but also in a decrease in food intake of both the healthy and tumor-bearing animals. Thus the increased protein intake did not affect the nutritional status of the tumor-bearing rats, as indicated by their body weight and serum level of total protein, insulin, or insulin-like growth factor-1. Basic research usually precedes or is the basis for applied research. There is little research to support the hypothesis that increased nutritional intake affects the morbidity and mortality of cancer patients. McCarthy et al.'s (1997) basic study provides a basis for studying the effects of nutritional interventions on appetite and food intake of cancer patients.

Applied Research

Applied research (or *practical research*) is scientific investigation conducted to generate knowledge that will directly influence or improve clinical practice. The purpose of applied research is to solve problems, make decisions, or predict or control outcomes in real-life practice situations. The findings from applied studies can also be invaluable to policymakers as a basis for making changes to address social problems (Miller, 1991). Many of the studies conducted in nursing are applied because researchers have chosen to focus on clinical problems and the testing of the effect of nursing interventions on patient outcomes in clinical settings. Applied research is also used to test theory and validate its usefulness in clinical practice. Often the new knowledge discovered through basic research is examined for usefulness in practice by applied research, making these approaches complementary (Wysocki, 1983).

Neuberger et al. (1997) conducted an applied study to determine the effects of exercise on fatigue, aerobic fitness, and disease activity in persons with rheumatoid arthritis (RA). The subjects participated in a 12-week program of low-impact aerobic exercise (treatment or independent variable), and the dependent or outcome variables of fatigue, aerobic fitness, and disease activity level were measured three times during the study. Study findings indicated that the fatigue level decreased for moderate-to-high frequency exercisers and increased for low-frequency exercisers. All subjects participating in the exercise program experienced increased aerobic fitness and increased grip strength, decreased walk time, and decreased pain. These improvements in fatigue level and aerobic fitness occurred without significant changes in the subjects' RA disease, as measured by joint count and sedimentation rate.

Neuberger et al.'s (1997) study addressed the problem in clinical practice of maintaining the mobility, strength, and independence of individuals with RA. The findings from this study can be applied directly to practice. Nurses can use this research information to develop low-impact aerobic exercise programs for persons with RA to decrease their fatigue and increase their aerobic fitness without worsening the symptoms and signs from their arthritis.

Rigor in Quantitative Research

Rigor is the striving for excellence in research, and it requires discipline, adherence to detail, and strict accuracy. A rigorously conducted quantitative study has precise measuring tools, a representative sample, and a tightly controlled study design. To critique the rigor of a study, the reasoning and precision used in conducting the study must be examined. Logical reasoning, including deductive and inductive reasoning, is essential to the development of quantitative studies. The research process includes specific steps that are developed with meticulous detail and are logically linked. These steps, such as design, measurement, sample, data collection, and statistical analysis, need to be examined for errors and weaknesses.

Another aspect of rigor is precision, which encompasses accuracy, detail, and order. Precision is evident in the concise statement of the research purpose and detailed development of the study design. But the most explicit example of precision is the measurement or quantification of the study variables. For example, a researcher might use a cardiac monitor to measure and record the heart rate of subjects during an exercise program, rather than palpating a radial pulse for 30 seconds and recording it on a data collection sheet.

Control in Quantitative Research

Control involves the imposing of rules by the researcher to decrease the possibility of error, and thus increase the probability that the study's findings are an accurate reflection of reality. The rules used to achieve control in research are referred to as *design*. Thus quantitative research includes varying degrees of control, ranging from uncontrolled to highly controlled, depending on the type of study (Table 2-1). Descriptive studies are designed with little or no researcher control because subjects are examined as they exist in their natural setting, such as home, work, or school.

TABLE 2-1

CONTROL IN QUANTITATIVE RESEARCH

TYPE OF QUANTITATIVE RESEARCH	RESEARCHER CONTROL	RESEARCH SETTING
Descriptive	Uncontrolled	Natural setting; partially controlled
Correlational	Uncontrolled/partially controlled	Natural setting; partially controlled
Quasi-experimental	Partially controlled/highly controlled	Partially controlled
Experimental	Highly controlled	Highly controlled; laboratory

Experimental studies focus on determining the effectiveness of a treatment (independent variable) in producing a desired outcome (dependent variable) in a controlled setting. Thus experimental studies are often conducted on subjects in experimental units in health care agencies, or on animals in laboratory settings.

Extraneous variables. Through control, the researcher can reduce the influence of extraneous variables. Extraneous variables exist in all studies and can interfere with obtaining a clear understanding of the relationships among the study variables. For example, if a study focused on the effect of relaxation therapy on perception of incisional pain, the extraneous variables, such as type of surgical incision and time, amount, and type of pain medication administered following surgery, would have to be controlled to prevent their influence on the patient's perception of pain. Selecting only patients with abdominal incisions, who are hospitalized and intravenously receiving only one type of pain medication after surgery, might control some of these extraneous variables. Thus a study can be designed to decrease the influence of extraneous variables through the selection of subjects (sampling) and the research settings. Controlling extraneous variables enables the researcher to accurately determine the effect of an independent or treatment variable on a dependent or outcome variable.

Sampling. *Sampling* is a process of selecting subjects who are representative of the population being studied. Random sampling usually provides a sample that is representative of a population because each member of the population is selected independently and has an equal chance or probability of being included in the study. In quantitative research, both random and nonrandom samples are used. Descriptive studies are often conducted with nonrandom or nonprobability samples, in which the subjects are selected based on convenience. Correlation and quasi-experimental studies include either nonrandom or random sampling methods, but having a randomly selected sample strengthens highly controlled experimental studies. A randomly selected sample is very difficult to obtain in nursing research, so quantitative studies are often conducted with convenience samples. To increase the control and rigor of a study and to decrease the potential for bias, the subjects who are part of a convenience sample are randomly assigned to a treatment or control group.

Research settings. The *setting* is the location where a study is conducted. There are three common settings for conducting research: natural, partially controlled, and highly controlled (see Table 2-1). A *natural setting,* or *field setting,* is an uncontrolled, real-life situation or environment (Miller, 1991). Conducting a study in a natural setting means that the researcher does not manipulate or change the environment for the study. Descriptive and correlational studies are often conducted in natural settings. For example, Kelly (2001) conducted a descriptive study to assess the dietary intake of preschool children living in a homeless shelter. The sample of convenience included 75 children, of whom 75% were African American, 16% were Hispanic, and 9% were Caucasian. Nursing students and faculty conducted the study in a homeless shelter, a natural setting described as follows.

> **Setting**
>
> "The shelter is located in an industrial section of a large city in Southwestern United States. It has 70 rooms, with four adult-sized beds in each. Cribs are available for infants and children younger than one year of age. The eating area, which also serves as the general meeting area, is located in the center of the two-story building. All the rooms are on either floor and open into this area. The kitchen is located on one edge of the building and food is served from the kitchen cafeteria-style." (Kelly, 2001, p. 149)

The data on the children's dietary intake were collected from their mothers during their stay in the shelter. No attempts were made during the study to manipulate, change, or control the environment of the shelters. Thus the researcher's intent was to study these homeless children's diet in a natural, real-life environment of the shelter. As a result of this study, the shelter staff started planning more frequent meals for the children and providing food servings more appropriate to their age.

A *partially controlled setting* is an environment that is manipulated or modified in some way by the researcher. An increasing number of nursing studies are being conducted in partially controlled settings. Neuberger et al. (1997) conducted a quasi-experimental study to examine the effects of exercise on fatigue, aerobic fitness, and the disease process of persons with RA in a partially controlled setting. The study involved implementing an exercise regimen that was

> "designed by two physical therapists, an aerobic instructor hired to teach the class, and the principle investigator. The class consisted of four phases: warm-up exercises, strengthening exercises, low-impact aerobic exercises, and cool-down exercises.... The exercise class was held in a room in the exercise facility on the medical center campus." (p. 199)

The researchers controlled the development of the exercise class treatment and the implementation of the treatment by a specific instructor in a selected room of the exercise facility. However, the researcher did not control other aspects of the environment, such as the interactions of the subjects during the class, the physical activities of the subjects outside of the class, the family support for the exercise program, and the subjects' interactions with other health professionals during the program. The personal characteristics of the subjects, such as their motivational level and physical fitness status, were not controlled. These factors could have influenced the fatigue, aerobic fitness, and disease status of the subjects during the study.

A *highly controlled setting* is an artificially constructed environment developed for the sole purpose of conducting research. Laboratories, research or experimental centers, and test units in hospitals or other health care agencies are highly controlled settings where experimental studies are often conducted. This type of setting reduces the influence of extraneous variables, which enables the researcher to examine accurately the effect of one variable on another. McCarthy et al. (1997) conducted their study on the effect of protein density of food on food intake and nutritional status of tumor-bearing rats in a laboratory setting. The environment of the rats was highly controlled by the researcher, with each rat being

> "housed individually and maintained on a 12-hour light-dark cycle commencing at 6:00 AM. Food and water were freely available. The animals were conditioned to the housing for 5 days before the start of the experiment and were treated at all times in a manner consistent with Department of Health, Education, and Welfare *Guidelines for the Care and Use of Laboratory Animals....* The animals were matched according to weight and a total of 30 were randomly selected for tumor implant, leaving 30 healthy animals as controls." (pp. 132-133)

The study clearly indicates the use of a highly controlled setting, random selection of subjects for the treatment and control groups, and the controlled implementation of study procedures that are essential in the conduct of experimental research.

PROBLEM-SOLVING AND NURSING PROCESSES: BASIS FOR UNDERSTANDING THE QUANTITATIVE RESEARCH PROCESS

Research is a process, and it is similar in some ways to other processes. Therefore the background acquired early in a nursing education in problem solving and the nursing process are also useful in research. A *process* includes a purpose, a series of actions, and a goal. The purpose provides direction for the implementation of a series of actions to achieve an identified goal. The specific steps of the process can be revised and reimplemented in order to reach the endpoint or goal. The problem-solving process, nursing process, and research process are presented in Table 2-2. Relating the research process to problem solving and the nursing process may be helpful in understanding the steps of the quantitative research process.

TABLE 2-2

COMPARISON OF THE PROBLEM-SOLVING PROCESS, NURSING PROCESS, AND RESEARCH PROCESS

PROBLEM-SOLVING PROCESS	NURSING PROCESS	RESEARCH PROCESS

Data Collection	Assessment
	  Data collection
	  Data interpretation
		Knowledge of the world of
		  nursing
		Clinical experiences
		Literature review

Problem definition	Nursing diagnosis	Problem and purpose identification

Plan
  Setting goals
  Identifying solutions
	Plan
	  Setting goals
	  Planned interventions
		Methodology plan
		  Design
		  Sample
		  Methods of measurement
		  Data collection
		  Data analysis

Implementation	Implementation	Implementation

Evaluation and revision	Evaluation and
	  modification
		Outcomes, communication
		  of findings, and use of
		  findings in practice

Comparing Problem Solving with the Nursing Process

The *problem-solving process* involves the systematic identification of a problem, determination of goals related to the problem, identification of possible approaches to achieve those goals (planning), implementation of selected approaches, and evaluation of goal achievement. Problem solving is frequently used in daily activities and in nursing practice. For example, you use problem solving when you select your clothing, decide where to live, and turn a patient with a fractured hip.

The *nursing process* is a subset of the problem-solving process. The steps of the nursing process are assessment, diagnosis, plan, implementation, evaluation, and modification (see Table 2-2). Assessment involves the collection and interpretation of data for the development of nursing diagnoses. These diagnoses guide the remaining steps of the nursing process, just as the step of identifying the problem directs the remaining steps of the problem-solving process. The planning step in the nursing process is the same as in the problem-solving process. Both processes involve implementation (putting the plan into action) and evaluation (determining the effectiveness of the process). If the process is ineffective, all steps are reviewed and revised (modified) as necessary. The process is implemented until the problems/diagnoses are resolved and the identified goals are achieved.

Comparing the Nursing Process with the Research Process

The nursing process and the research process have important similarities and differences. The two processes are similar because they both involve abstract, critical thinking and complex reasoning (Miller & Babcock, 1996). Using these processes, new information can be identified, relationships can be discovered, and predictions can be made about phenomena. In both processes, information is gathered, observations are made, problems are identified, plans are developed (methodology), and actions are taken (data collection and analysis) (Whitney, 1986). Both processes are reviewed for effectiveness and efficiency; the nursing process is evaluated, and outcomes are determined in the research process (see Table 2-2). Implementing the two processes expands and refines the user's knowledge. With this growth in knowledge and critical thinking, the user is able to implement increasingly complex nursing processes and studies.

The research and nursing processes also have definite differences. Knowledge of the nursing process will assist you in understanding the research process. However, the *research process* is more complex than the nursing process. It requires an understanding of a unique language and involves the rigorous application of a variety of research methods (Burns, 1989; Burns & Grove, 2001). The research process also has a broader focus than the nursing process, in which the nurse focuses on a specific patient and family. During the research process, the researcher focuses on groups of patients and their families. In addition, researchers must be knowledgeable about the world of nursing to identify problems that require study. This knowledge is obtained from clinical and other personal experiences and by conducting a review of the literature.

The theoretical underpinnings of the research process are much stronger than those of the nursing process. All steps of the research process are logically linked to each other, as well as to the theoretical foundations of the study. The conduct of research requires greater precision, rigor, and control than the implementation of the nursing process. The outcomes from research are frequently shared with a large number of nurses and other health professionals through presentations and publications. In addition, the outcomes from several studies can be synthesized to provide sound evidence for nursing practice (Brown, 1999).

IDENTIFYING THE STEPS OF THE QUANTITATIVE RESEARCH PROCESS

The *quantitative research process* involves conceptualizing a research project, planning and implementing that project, and communicating the findings. Fig. 2-1 identifies the steps of the quantitative research process that are usually included in a research report. This figure indicates the logical flow of the process as one step builds progressively on another. The steps of the quantitative research process are briefly introduced in this chapter and are presented in detail in Chapters 3 through 10. The descriptive correlational study conducted by Hulme and Grove (1994) on the symptoms of female survivors of child sexual abuse is used as an example to introduce the steps of the quantitative research process.

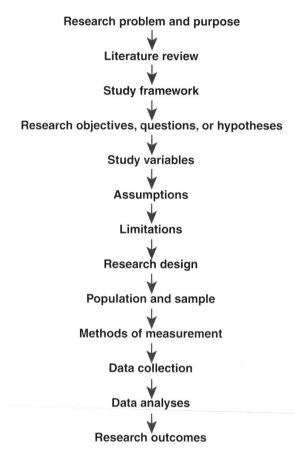

Research problem and purpose
↓
Literature review
↓
Study framework
↓
Research objectives, questions, or hypotheses
↓
Study variables
↓
Assumptions
↓
Limitations
↓
Research design
↓
Population and sample
↓
Methods of measurement
↓
Data collection
↓
Data analyses
↓
Research outcomes

Fig. 2-1 Steps of the quantitative research process.

Research Problem and Purpose

A *research problem* is an area of concern in which there is a gap in the knowledge base needed for nursing practice. The problem statement in a study usually identifies an area of concern for a particular population that requires investigation. Research is then conducted to generate essential knowledge that addresses the practice concern, with the ultimate goal of providing evidence-based practice. The *research purpose* is generated from the problem and identifies the specific goal or aim of the study. The goal of a study might be to identify, describe, or explain a situation; predict a solution to a situation; or control a situation to produce positive outcomes in practice. The purpose includes the variables, population, and often the setting for the study. A detailed discussion of the research problem and purpose is presented in Chapter 3. Hulme and Grove (1994) identified the following problem and purpose for their study of female survivors of child sexual abuse.

Research Problem

"The actual prevalence of child sexual abuse is unknown but is thought to be high. Bagley and King (1990) were able to generalize from compiled research that at least 20% of all women in the samples surveyed had been victims of serious sexual abuse involving unwanted or coerced sexual contact up to the age of 17 years. Evidence indicates that the prevalence is greater for women born after 1960 than before (Bagley, 1990).

The impact of child sexual abuse on the lives of the girl victims and the women they become has only lately received the attention it deserves…the knowledge generated from research and theory has slowly forced the recognition of the long-term effects of child sexual abuse on both the survivors and society as a whole…. Recently, Brown and Garrison (1990) developed the Adult Survivors of Incest (ASI) Questionnaire to identify the patterns of symptoms and the factors contributing to the severity of these symptoms in survivors of childhood sexual abuse. This tool requires additional testing to determine its usefulness in identifying symptoms and contributing factors of adult survivors of incest and other types of child sexual abuse." (pp. 519-520)

Research Purpose

"Thus, the purpose of this study was twofold: (a) to describe the patterns of physical and psychosocial symptoms in female sexual abuse survivors using the ASI Questionnaire, and (b) to examine relationships among the symptoms and identified contributing factors." (p. 520)

Literature Review

Researchers conduct a *literature review* to generate a picture of what is known and not known about a particular problem. Relevant literature is only those sources that are pertinent or highly important in providing the in-depth knowledge needed to study a selected problem. The literature review indicates whether adequate knowledge exists to make changes in practice or whether additional research is needed. The process for reviewing the literature is described in Chapter 4. Hulme and Grove's (1994) review of the literature covered relevant theories and studies related to child sexual abuse and its contributing factors and long-term effects.

"Theorists indicated that…the act of child sexual abuse can be explained as an abuse of power by a trusted parent figure, usually male, on a dependent child, violating the child's body, mind, and spirit. The family, which normally functions to nurture and protect the child from harm, is viewed as not fulfilling this function, leaving the child to feel further betrayed and powerless. Acceptance of the immediate psychological trauma of child sexual abuse has given impetus for acknowledging the long-term effects.

Studies of both nonclinical and clinical populations have lent support to these theoretical developments. When compared with control groups consisting of

Continued

women who had not been sexually abused as children, survivors of child sexual abuse consistently have higher incidence of depression and lower self-esteem. Other psychosocial long-term effects encountered include suicidal plans, anxiety, distorted body image, decreased sexual satisfaction, poor general social adjustment, lower positive affect, negative personality characteristics, and feeling different from significant others…. The physical long-term effects suggested by research include gastrointestinal problems such as ulcers, spastic colitis, irritable bowel syndrome, and chronic abdominal pain; gynecological disorders; chronic headache; obesity; and increased lifetime surgeries.

Studies of contributing factors that may affect the traumatic impact of child sexual abuse are less in number and less conclusive than those that identify long-term effects. However, poor family functioning, increased age difference between the victim and perpetrator, threat or use of force or violence, multiple abusers, parent or primary caretaker as perpetrator, prolonged or intrusive abuse, and strong emotional bond to the perpetrator with betrayal of trust may all contribute to the increased severity of the long-term effects." (pp. 521-522)

Study Framework

A *framework* is the abstract, theoretical basis for a study that enables the researcher to link the findings to nursing's body of knowledge. In quantitative research, the framework is a testable theory that has been developed in nursing or in another discipline, such as psychology, physiology, or sociology. A *theory* consists of an integrated set of defined concepts and relational statements that present a view of a phenomenon and can be used to describe, explain, predict, or control the phenomenon. The relational statements of the theory, not the theory itself, are tested through research. A study framework can be expressed as a map or a diagram of the relationships that provide the basis for a study, or the framework can be presented in narrative format. Chapter 5 provides a background for understanding and critiquing study frameworks. The framework for Hulme and Grove's (1994) study is based on Browne and Finkelhor's (1986) theory of Traumagenic Dynamics in the Impact of Child Sexual Abuse and is expressed in a map.

"…As shown in Fig. 2-2, child sexual abuse is at the center of the adult survivor's existence. Arising from the abuse are four trauma-causing dynamics: traumatic sexualization, betrayal, powerlessness, and stigmatization. These traumagenic dynamics lead to behavioral manifestations and collectively indicate a history of child sexual abuse. The behavioral manifestations were operationalized as physical and psychosocial symptoms for the purposes of this study. Penetrating the core of the adult survivors are the contributing factors, including the characteristics of the child sexual abuse and other factors occurring later in the survivor's life, that affect the severity of behavioral manifestations (Follette, Alexander, & Follette, 1991). The contributing factors examined in this study were age when the abuse began, duration of the abuse, and other victimizations. Other victimizations included past or present physical and emotional abuse, rape, control by others, and prostitution." (pp. 522-523)

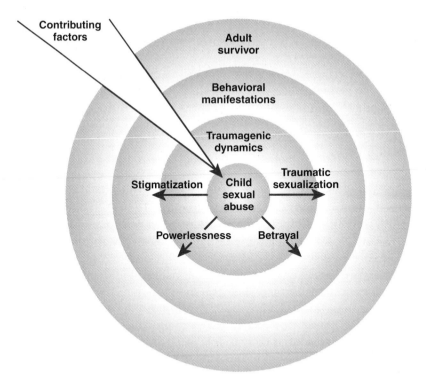

Research Objectives, Questions, and Hypotheses

Research objectives, questions, or hypotheses are formulated to bridge the gap between the more abstractly stated research problem and purpose and the study design and plan for data collection and analysis. Objectives, questions, and hypotheses are narrower in focus than the purpose and often specify only one or two research variables, identify the relationship between the variables, and indicate the population to be studied. Some descriptive studies include only a research purpose, whereas others include a purpose and either objectives or questions to direct the study. Some correlational studies include a purpose and specific questions or hypotheses. Quasi-experimental and experimental studies need to include hypotheses to direct the conduct of the studies and the interpretation of findings. Chapter 3 provides guidelines for critiquing objectives, questions, and hypotheses in research reports. Hulme and Grove (1994) developed the following research questions to direct their study.

Research Questions

"1. What patterns of physical and psychosocial symptoms are present in women 18 to 40 years of age who have experienced child sexual abuse?
2. Are there relationships among the number of physical and psychosocial symptoms, the age when the abuse began, the duration of abuse, and [the] number of other victimizations?" (p. 523)

Study Variables

The research purpose and the objectives, questions, or hypotheses identify the variables to be examined in a study. *Variables* are concepts at various levels of abstraction that are measured, manipulated, or controlled in a study. The more concrete concepts like temperature, weight, or blood pressure are referred to as variables in a study. The more abstract concepts like creativity, empathy, or social support are sometimes referred to as research *concepts*.

The variables or concepts in a study are operationalized by identifying conceptual and operational definitions. A *conceptual definition* provides a variable or concept with theoretical meaning (Burns & Grove, 2001), and it is either derived from a theorist's definition of the concept or developed through concept analysis. An *operational definition* is developed so that the variable can be measured or manipulated in a study. The knowledge gained from studying the variable will increase understanding of the theoretical concept that the variable represents. A more extensive discussion of variables is provided in Chapter 3. Hulme and Grove (1994) provided conceptual and operational definitions of the study variables, physical and psychosocial symptoms, age when the abuse began, duration of abuse, and victimizations, identified in their purpose and/or research questions. Only the definitions for physical symptoms and victimizations are presented as examples.

Physical Symptoms

CONCEPTUAL DEFINITION. Physical symptoms are "behavioral manifestations that result directly from the traumagenic dynamics of child sexual abuse" (Hulme & Grove, 1994, p. 522).
OPERATIONAL DEFINITION. ASI Questionnaire was used to measure physical symptoms.

Victimizations

CONCEPTUAL DEFINITION. Adult survivor who has experienced multiple forms of abuse, including "past and present physical and emotional abuse, rape, control by others, and prostitution" (p. 523).
OPERATIONAL DEFINITION. ASI Questionnaire was used to measure victimizations.

Assumptions

Assumptions are statements that are taken for granted or are considered true, even though they have not been scientifically tested. Assumptions are often embedded (unrecognized) in thinking and behavior, and uncovering these assumptions requires introspection and a strong knowledge base in a research area. Sources of assumptions are universally accepted truths (e.g., "all humans are rational beings"), theories, previous research, and nursing practice (Myers, 1982).

In studies, assumptions are embedded in the philosophical base of the framework, study design, and interpretation of findings. Theories and research instruments are developed based on assumptions that may or may not be recognized by the researcher. These assumptions influence the development and implementation of the research process. The recognition of assumptions by the researcher is a strength, not a weakness. Assumptions influence the logic of the study, and their recognition leads to more rigorous study development. Williams (1980) reviewed published nursing studies and other health care literature to identify 13 commonly embedded assumptions:

"1. People want to assume control of their own health problems.
2. Stress should be avoided.
3. People are aware of the experiences that most affect their life choices.
4. Health is a priority for most people.
5. People in undeserved areas feel undeserved.
6. Most measurable attitudes are held strongly enough to direct behavior.
7. Health professionals view health care in a different manner than do lay persons.
8. Human biological and chemical factors show less variation than do cultural and social factors.
9. The nursing process is the best way of conceptualizing nursing practice.
10. Statistically significant differences relate to the variable or variables under consideration.
11. People operate on the basis of cognitive information.
12. Increased knowledge about an event lowers anxiety about the event.
13. Receipt of health care at home is preferable to receipt of care in an institution" (p. 48).

Hulme and Grove (1994) did not identify assumptions for their study, but the following assumptions seem to provide a basis for this study: (1) the child victim bears no responsibility for the sexual contact, (2) survivors can remember and are willing to report their past child sexual abuse, and (3) behavioral manifestations (physical and psychological symptoms) indicate altered health and functioning.

Limitations

Limitations are restrictions in a study that may decrease the credibility and generalizability of the findings. *Generalization* is the extension of the implications of the research findings from the sample to a larger population. For example, the findings from studying adult female survivors of child sexual abuse might be extended from this sample studied to all females who have survived child sexual abuse. The two types of limitations are theoretical and methodological. *Theoretical limitations* restrict the abstract generalization of the findings and are reflected in the study framework and the conceptual and operational definitions of the variables. Theoretical limitations might include (1) a concept that lacks clarity of definition in the theory used to develop the study framework; (2) the unclear relationships among some concepts in the theorist's work; (3) a study variable that lacks a clear link to a concept in the framework; and (4) an objective, question, or hypothesis that lacks a clear link to a relationship (or proposition) expressed in the study framework.

Methodological limitations can limit the credibility of the findings and restrict the population to which the findings can be generalized. Methodological limitations result from such factors as unrepresentative sample, weak design, single setting, limited control over treatment implementation, instruments with limited reliability and validity, limited control over data collection, and improper use of statistical analyses. Hulme and Grove (1994) identified the following methodological limitation.

Methodological Limitation

"...[T]his study has limited generalizability due to the relatively small non-probability sample..." (p. 528).

"Additional replications drawing from various social classes and age groups are needed to improve the generalizability of Brown and Garrison's (1990) findings and establish reliability and validity of their tool" (p. 529).

Research Design

Research *design* is a blueprint for the conduct of a study that maximizes control over factors that could interfere with the study's desired outcome. The type of design directs the selection of a population, procedures for sampling, methods of measurement, and plans for data collection and analysis. The choice of research design depends on the researcher's expertise, the problem and purpose of the study, and the desire to generalize the findings. Sometimes the design of a study indicates that a pilot study was conducted. A *pilot study* is frequently defined as a smaller version of a proposed study, and it is conducted to refine the methodology. The pilot study is often developed similarly to the proposed study, using similar subjects, the same setting, the same treatment, and the same data collection and analysis techniques. Prescott and Soeken (1989), however, believe a pilot study can be conducted to develop and refine any of the steps in the research process. The reasons for conducting pilot studies are to:

1. Determine whether the proposed study is feasible (e.g., Are the subjects ... ne and money to do the study?)

... of a treatment.

... ative of the population or whether

... research instruments.

...nts.

...ns.

...bjects, setting, methodology, and

...ott & Soeken, 1989; Van Ort, 1981)

Prospective

Longitudinal

correlational
(statistically significant
links)

... research needs as they emerge; thus ... rimental, and experimental designs ... correlational studies, no treatment is administered, so the purpose of the study design is to improve the precision of measurement. Quasi-experimental and experimental study designs usually involve treatment and control groups, and focus on achieving high levels of control as well as precision in measurement. A study's design is usually described in the methodology section of a research report. In the study by Hulme and Grove (1994), a descriptive correlational design was used to direct the study. A diagram of the design is presented in Fig. 2-3 and indicates the variables described and the relationships examined. The findings generated from correlational research provide a basis for generating hypotheses for testing in future research.

Population and Sample

The *population* is all elements (individuals, objects, or substances) that meet certain criteria for inclusion in a study (Kerlinger & Lee, 1999). A *sample* is a subset of the population that is selected for a particular study, and the members of a sample are the subjects. *Sampling* defines the process of selecting a group of people, events, behaviors, or other elements with which to conduct a study. Chapter 8 provides a background for critiquing populations and samples in research reports. The following quote identifies the sampling method, setting, sample size, population, sample criteria, and sample characteristics for the study conducted by Hulme and Grove (1994).

"The convenience sample [sampling method] was obtained by advertising for subjects at three state universities in the southwest [setting]. Despite the sensitive nature of the study, 22 [sample size] usable interviews were obtained. The sample included women between the ages of 18 and 39 years ($\overline{X}$ = 28 years, SD = 6.5 years) who were identified as survivors of child sexual abuse [population]

Continued

[sample criteria]. The majority of these women were white (91%) and students (82%). A little more than half (54%) were single, seven (32%) were divorced, and three (14%) were married. Most (64%) had no children. A small percentage (14%) were on some form of public assistance and only 14% had been arrested. Although 27% of the subjects had step family members, the parents of 14 subjects (64%) were still married. Half the fathers were working class or self-employed; the rest were professionals. Mothers were either working class or self-employed (50%), homemakers (27%), or professionals (11%). Most subjects (95%) had siblings, and 36% knew or suspected their siblings also had been abused" [sample characteristics]. (pp. 523-524)

MEASUREMENT OF VARIABLES

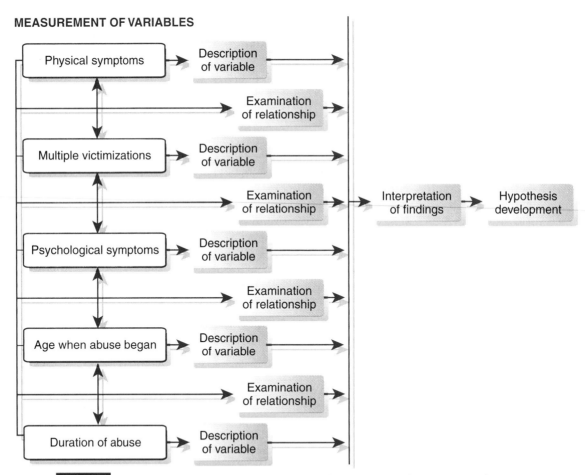

Fig. 2-3 Proposed descriptive correlational design for Hulme and Grove's study of symptoms of female survivors of child sexual abuse. *(From Hulme, P. A. & Grove, S. K. [1994]. Physical and psychosocial symptomatology of female survivors of child sexual abuse, 55. Reproduced with permission.)*

Methods of Measurement

Measurement is the process of assigning "numbers to objects (or events or situations) in accord with some rule" (Kaplan, 1964, p. 177). A component of measurement is instrumentation, which is the application of specific rules to the development of a measurement device or instrument. An instrument is selected to examine a specific variable in a study. Data generated with an instrument are at the nominal, ordinal, interval, or ratio level of measurement. The level of measurement, with nominal being the lowest form of measurement and ratio being the highest, determines the type of statistical analysis that can be performed on the data.

Critiquing a method of measurement in a study requires examining its reliability and validity. Reliability is concerned with how consistently the measurement technique measures a variable or concept. Validity is the extent to which the instrument actually reflects or measures what it is supposed to measure. For example, if an instrument was developed to measure chronic pain, the validity is the extent to which the instrument actually measures chronic pain and the reliability is how consistently it measures chronic pain. Chapter 9 introduces the concept of measurement and explains the different types of reliability and validity. Hulme and Grove (1994) used the ASI Questionnaire to measure the study variables.

> "The ASI Questionnaire contains 10 sections: demographics; family origin; educational history, occupational history and public assistance; legal history; characteristics of the child sexual abuse (duration, perpetrator, pregnancy, type, and threats); past and present other victimizations; past and present physical symptoms; past and present psychosocial symptoms; and relationship with own children. Each section is followed by a response set that includes space for 'other.' Content validity was established by Brown and Garrison (1990) using an in-depth review of 132 clinical records.... For this descriptive correlational study...content validity of the tool was examined by asking an open-ended question: 'Is there additional information you would like to share?'" (p. 524)

Data Collection

Data collection is the precise, systematic gathering of information relevant to the research purpose or the specific objectives, questions, or hypotheses of a study. In order to collect data, the researcher must obtain permission from the setting or agency where the study is to be conducted. Consent must also be obtained from the research subjects to indicate their willingness to participate in the study. Frequently, the subjects are asked to sign a consent form, which describes the study, promises the subjects confidentiality, and indicates that the subjects can withdraw from the study at any time. Obtaining permission from an agency to conduct a study and consent from the subjects to participate in the study should be documented in the research report (see Chapter 6).

During data collection, the study variables are measured using a variety of techniques, such as observation, interview, questionnaires, or scales. In an increasing number of studies, nurses are measuring physiological variables with high-technology equipment. The data are collected and recorded systematically on each subject and are organized in a way that facilitates computer entry. Data collection is usually described in the methodology section of a research report under the subheading of "Procedures." Hulme and Grove (1994) identified the following procedure for data collection.

> "Although the tool can be self-reporting, it was administered by personal interview to allow for elaboration of 'other' responses. The interviews lasted about one hour and were conducted in a private room provided by The University of Texas at Arlington. Each interview started with a discussion of the study benefits and risks and included signing a consent form. Risks included possible painful memories, anger, and sadness during the interview as well as emotional and physical discomfort after the interview. Sources of public and private counseling were provided to assist subjects with any difficulties experienced related to the study." (pp. 524-525)

Data Analysis

Data analysis is conducted to reduce, organize, and give meaning to the data. Analysis techniques conducted in quantitative research include descriptive and inferential analyses (see Chapter 10) and some sophisticated, advanced analyses (Burns & Grove, 2001). The analysis techniques implemented are determined primarily by the research objectives, questions, or hypotheses, and the level of measurement achieved by the research instruments. The data analysis process is described in the results section of the research report and this section is usually organized by the research objectives, questions, or hypotheses. Hulme and Grove (1994) conducted frequencies, percents, means, standard deviations, and Pearson correlations to answer their research questions.

> ### Results
>
> "The first research question focused on patterns of physical and psychosocial symptoms. Six physical symptoms occurred in 50% or more of the subjects: insomnia, sexual dysfunction, overeating, drug abuse, severe headache, and two or more major surgeries.... Eleven psychosocial symptoms occurred in 75% or more of the subjects: depression, guilt, low self-esteem, inability to trust others, mood swings, suicidal thoughts, difficulty in relationships, confusion, flashbacks of the abuse, extreme anger, and memory lapse.... Self-injurious behavior was reported by eight subjects (33%)." (pp. 527-528)

"The second research question focused on the relationships among the number of physical and psychosocial symptoms and three contributing factors (age abuse began, duration of abuse, and other victimizations). There were five significant correlations among study variables: physical symptoms with other victimizations ($r = .59, p = .002$), physical symptoms with psychosocial symptoms ($r = .56, p = .003$), age abuse began with duration of abuse ($r = -.50, p = .009$), psychosocial symptoms with other victimizations ($r = .40, p = .033$), and duration of abuse with psychosocial symptoms ($r = .40, p = .034$)." (p. 528)

Research Outcomes

The results obtained from data analyses require interpretation to be meaningful. *Interpretation of research outcomes* involves examining the results from data analysis, forming conclusions, considering the implications for nursing, exploring the significance of the findings, generalizing the findings, and suggesting further studies. The research outcomes are presented in the discussion section of a research report. Hulme and Grove (1994) provided the following discussion of their findings, with implications for nursing and suggestions for further study.

Discussion

"While this study may have limited generalizability due to the relatively small nonprobability sample, the findings do support previous research.... In addition, the findings support Browne and Finkelhor's (1986) framework that a wide range of behavioral manifestations (physical and psychosocial symptoms) comprise the long-term effects of child sexual abuse." (p. 528)

"Brown and Garrison's (1990) ASI Questionnaire was effective in identifying patterns of physical and psychosocial symptoms in women with a history of child sexual abuse.... As data on the behavioral manifestations (physical and psychosocial symptoms) and the effect of each of the contributing factors accumulate, hypotheses need to be formulated to further test Browne and Finkelhor's (1986) framework explaining the long-term effects of child sexual abuse.... With additional research, the ASI Questionnaire might be adapted for use in clinical situations. This questionnaire might facilitate identification and delivery of appropriate treatment to female survivors of child sexual abuse in clinical settings." (pp. 529-530)

READING RESEARCH REPORTS

Understanding the steps of the research process and learning new terms related to those steps will assist you in reading research reports. A *research report* summarizes the major elements of a study and identifies the contributions of that study to nursing knowledge. Research reports are presented at professional meetings and conferences and are published in journals and books. These reports are often overwhelming to nursing students and new graduates. Maybe you have had difficulty locating research articles or understanding the content of these articles. Research reports are usually written to communicate with other researchers, not with clinicians. Thus the style of the report is often technical and sometimes filled with jargon, which is very confusing to students and practicing nurses. We would like to help you overcome some of these barriers and assist you in understanding the research literature by (1) identifying sources that publish research reports, (2) describing the content of a research report, and (3) providing tips for reading the research literature.

Sources of Research Reports

The most common sources for nursing research reports are professional journals. Research reports are the major focus of the following nursing research journals: *Advances in Nursing Science, Applied Nursing Research, Clinical Nursing Research: An International Journal, Journal of Nursing Scholarship, Nursing Research, Qualitative Nursing Research, Research in Nursing & Health, Scholarly Inquiry for Nursing Practice: An International Journal,* and *Western Journal of Nursing Research.* Two of these journals, *Applied Nursing Research* and *Clinical Nursing Research,* have focused on communicating research findings to practicing nurses. Thus the journals include less detail on the framework, methodology, and the statistical results of a study and more on discussion of the findings and the implications for practice. Many of the nursing clinical specialty journals also place a high priority on publishing research findings. Table 2-3 identifies the clinical journals in which research reports compose 50% or more of the journal content. More than 95 nursing journals are published in the United States, and many of them include research articles (Swanson, McCloskey, & Bodensteiner, 1991).

Some research reports, such as those for complex qualitative studies, are lengthy and might be published as books or as chapters in books. Research reports of master's degree students are presented as theses, and doctoral students produce dissertations summarizing their research projects. Before publication, many research reports are presented at local, national, and international nursing and health care conferences. Often, brochures for conferences will indicate whether research reports are part of the program. The findings from many studies are now communicated through the Internet as journals are placed on-line, and selected Web sites include the most current health research.

Content of Research Reports

At this point, you are probably overwhelmed by the appearance of a research report. You might find it easier to read and comprehend these reports if you understand each of the component parts. A research report often includes six parts: (1) abstract, (2) introduction, (3) methods, (4) results, (5) discussion, and (6) reference list. These parts are described in this section, and the study by Neuberger et al. (1997) that examined the effects of exercise on the health status of persons with RA is presented as an example.

TABLE 2-3	

JOURNALS THAT FOCUS ON RESEARCH ARTICLES

JOURNAL TITLE	PERCENTAGE OF JOURNAL FOCUSED ON RESEARCH
RESEARCH JOURNALS	
Applied Nursing Research	100
Image: Journal of Nursing Scholarship	70
Nursing Research	80
Research in Nursing & Health	100
Scholarly Inquiry for Nursing Practice	60
Western Journal of Nursing Research	90
CLINICAL JOURNALS	
American Journal of Alzheimer's Care & Related Disorders and Research	60
Birth	70
Cardiovascular Nursing	60
Computers in Nursing	70
Heart & Lung: Journal of Critical Care	50
Issues in Comprehensive Pediatric Nursing	100
Issues in Mental Health Nursing	67
Journal of Child and Adolescent Psychiatric and Mental Health Nursing	75
Journal of Continuing Education in Nursing	50
Journal of Holistic Nursing	50
Journal of National Black Nurses' Association	75
Journal of Nursing Education	80
Journal of Pediatric Nursing: Nursing Care of Children and Families	50
Journal of Transcultural Nursing	87
Maternal-Child Nursing Journal	75
Nursing Diagnosis	80
Public Health Nursing	75
Rehabilitation Nursing	50
The Diabetes Educator	75

Data from Swanson, E. A., McCloskey, J. C., & Bodensteiner, A. (1991). Publishing opportunities for nurses: A comparison of 92 U.S. journals. *Image: Journal of Nursing Scholarship, 23*(1), 33–38.

Abstract

The report usually begins with an *abstract*, which is a clear, concise summary of a study (Crosby, 1990). Abstracts range from 100 to 250 words and usually include the study purpose, design, setting, sample size, major results, and conclusions. Researchers hope their abstracts will concisely convey the findings from their study and capture your attention so you will read the entire report. Neuberger et al. (1997) developed the following clear, concise abstract, which conveys the critical information about their study.

Abstract

"The effects of 12 weeks of low-impact aerobic exercise on fatigue, aerobic fitness, and disease activity were examined in a quasi-experimental time series study of 25 adults with rheumatoid arthritis (RA). Measures were obtained preintervention, midtreatment (after 6 weeks of exercise), end of treatment (after 12 weeks of exercise), and at a 15-week follow-up. ANOVAs (analysis of variances) for repeated measures showed that those subjects who participated more frequently reported decreased fatigue, while those who participated less frequently reported an increase in fatigue. All subjects, on average, showed increased aerobic fitness and increased right and left hand grip strength, decreased pain, and decreased walk time. There were no significant increases in joint count or sedimentation rate. Significant improvement measures at 15-week follow-up also were found. Findings indicate that persons with RA who participate in appropriate exercises may lessen fatigue levels, and experience other positive effects without worsening their arthritis." (p. 195)

Usually, four major content sections of a research report follow the abstract: introduction, methods, results, and discussion. The content covered in each of these sections is outlined in Table 2-4 and is briefly discussed in the following sections.

TABLE 2-4

ABSTRACT

Introduction
Statement of the problem, with background and significance
Statement of the purpose
Brief literature review
Identification of the framework
Identification of the research objectives, questions, or hypotheses (if applicable)

Methods
Identification of the research design
Description of the treatment or intervention (if applicable)
Description of the sample and setting
Description of the methods of measurement (including reliability and validity)
Discussion of the data collection process

Results
Description of the data analysis procedures
Presentation of results in tables, figures, or narrative organized by the purpose and/or objectives, questions, or hypotheses

Discussion
Discussion of major findings
Identification of the limitations
Presentation of conclusions
Implications of the findings for nursing practice
Recommendations for further research

Introduction

The introduction section of a research report identifies the nature and scope of the problem being investigated and provides a case for the conduct of the study. You should be able to clearly identify the significance of conducting the study to generate knowledge for nursing practice. Neuberger et al.'s (1997) study was significant because it generated knowledge to assist individuals with chronic illnesses to promote their health and maintain their independence. The purpose of their study was clearly stated in the first sentence of the abstract.

Depending on the type of research report, the literature review and the framework may be separate sections or part of the introduction. The literature review documents the current knowledge of the problem investigated and includes the sources that were used to develop the study and interpret the findings. For example, Neuberger et al. (1997) summarized literature that focused on the concepts of fatigue, exercise, and RA. A research report also needs to include a framework, but only about half of the published studies identify one (Moody et al., 1988). Neuberger et al. (1997) clearly identified their framework as a biobehavioral framework that was "based on concepts of self-regulation and self-monitoring which refer to unconscious as well as conscious mechanisms used by individuals to maintain homeostasis and prevent fatigue. The four concepts of this framework are resources, utilization, activity, and restoration" (p. 197). The framework concepts were clearly defined and interrelated to provide a theoretical basis for the study. A model or map is sometimes developed to clarify the logic within the framework, but one was not included in this study.

The literature review and framework are presented in such a way as to stress the importance of and to provide support for the study being reported. Often the introduction ends with an identification of the objectives, questions, or hypotheses that were used to direct the study. Since this was a quasi-experimental study, Neuberger et al. (1997) identified the following hypotheses: "Participation in a low-impact aerobic exercise program (a) will decrease fatigue in outpatients with RA; (b) will increase aerobic fitness levels of subjects; and (c) will not increase measures of disease activity" (p. 197).

Methods

The methods section of a research report describes how the study was conducted and usually includes the study design, treatment (if appropriate), sample, setting, methods of measurement, and data collection process. This section of the report needs to be presented in enough detail so that the reader can critique the adequacy of the study methods to produce reliable findings (Tornquist, Funk, Champagne, & Wiese, 1993). Neuberger et al. (1997) identified their design as quasi-experimental time series. They included the subsection "Sample," which described the population, sampling method, sample size, sample characteristics, and setting. "Measurement," a subsection under "Methods," detailed the instruments used to measure the independent variables of fatigue, aerobic fitness, and disease activity. The validity and reliability of the instruments were examined for previous studies and for this study. The subsection "Procedure" detailed the exercise intervention (treatment) and the implementation of the study, including who implemented the treatment, who collected the data, the procedure for collecting data, and the type and frequency of measurements obtained. The effectiveness of the treatment needs to be determined, as well as the feasibility of using the treatment in the real world of clinical practice. The protection of subjects' rights and the informed consent process were also covered in the "Procedure" subsection.

Results

The results section presents the outcomes of the statistical tests used to analyze the study data and the significance of these outcomes. The research purpose or objectives, questions, and hypotheses formulated for the study are used to organize this section. The statistical analyses conducted to address the purpose or each objective, question, or hypothesis are identified, and the specific results obtained from the analyses are presented in tables, figures, or narrative of the report (Burns & Grove, 2001). Focusing more on the summary of the study results and their significance than on the statistical results will hopefully reduce the confusion that may be caused by the numbers. Neuberger et al. (1997) conducted statistical analyses to address their study hypotheses. The analyses were comprehensive and clearly presented using tables and narrative. Analysis of variance (ANOVA) for repeated measures was used to test differences among the three measurement points (6, 12, and 15 weeks). Results indicated a significant decrease in fatigue and an increase in aerobic fitness without a worsening of the disease status. Thus the study results provided support for the three hypotheses stated to direct the study.

Discussion

The discussion section ties the other sections of the research report together and gives them meaning. This section includes the major findings, limitations of the study, conclusions drawn from the findings, implications of the findings for nursing, and recommendations for further research. Neuberger et al. (1997) discussed their findings in detail, and compared and contrasted them with the findings of previous research. They also linked their findings to their framework with the statement: "The findings suggest that improvements in aerobic fitness, hand grip strength, walk time, and pain levels after the exercise intervention may have contributed to increased energy resources and decreased levels of fatigue" (p. 203). The limitations of the study were small sample size, lack of a separate control group, and lack of completely blinded observers. Directions for further research followed these limitations. Implications of the study findings for practice were addressed with a discussion of the importance of low-impact exercise for individuals with RA.

The conclusions drawn from a research project can be useful in at least three different ways. First, the intervention or treatment tested in a study can be used with patients to improve their care and promote a positive health outcome. Second, reading research reports might change your view of a patient's situation or give you greater insight into the situation. Lastly, studies heighten your awareness of the problems experienced by patients and assist you in assessing and working toward solutions for these problems.

References

A reference list that includes all sources cited in the research report follows the discussion section. The reference list includes the studies and theories that provide a basis for the conduct of the study. These sources provide an opportunity to read about the research problem in greater depth. The authors strongly encourage you to read the Neuberger et al. (1997) article to identify the sections of a research report and to examine the content in each of these sections. Neuberger et al. (1997) detail a rigorously conducted quasi-experimental study, provide findings that are supportive of previous research, and identify conclusions that provide sound evidence to direct the care of patients with RA.

Tips for Reading Research Reports

When you start reading research reports, you will probably be overwhelmed by the new terms and complex information presented. Hopefully, you will not be discouraged but will see the challenge of examining new knowledge generated through research. You will probably need to read the report slowly two or three times and will need to use the glossary at the end of this textbook to review the definitions of unfamiliar terms. We recommend that you read the abstract first and then the discussion section of the report. Hopefully, this approach will enable you to determine the relevance of the findings to you personally and to your practice. Initially, your focus should be on research reports you believe can provide relevant knowledge for your practice.

Reading a research report requires the use of a variety of critical thinking skills, such as skimming, comprehending, and analyzing to facilitate an understanding of the study (Miller & Babcock, 1996). *Skimming a research report* involves quickly reviewing the source to gain a broad overview of the content. You would probably read the title, the author's name, the abstract or introduction, and the discussion section. Knowing the findings of the study provides you with a standard for evaluating the rest of the article (Tornquist et al., 1993). Then you might read the major headings and sometimes one or two sentences under each heading. Lastly, you might reexamine the conclusions and implications for practices from the study. Skimming enables you to make a preliminary judgment about the value of a source and a determination about reading the report in depth.

Comprehending a research report requires that the entire study be read carefully. You need to focus on understanding major concepts and the logical flow of ideas within the study. You might highlight information about the researchers, such as their education, their current positions, and any funding they received for the study. As you read the study, steps of the research process might also be highlighted. You might record notes in the margin so that you can easily identify the problem, purpose, framework, major variables, study design, treatment, sample, measuring methods, data collection process, analysis techniques, results, and study outcomes. You might also record creative ideas or questions you have in the margin of the report.

We encourage you to highlight the parts of the article that you do not understand and ask your instructor or other nurse researchers for clarification. Your greatest difficulty in reading the research report will probably be in understanding the statistical analyses. Information in Chapter 10 should help you comprehend the analyses. Basically, you need to identify the particular statistics used, the results from each statistical analysis, and the meaning of the results. Statistical analyses are conducted to describe variables, examine relationships among variables, or determine differences among groups (see Chapter 10). The study purpose or specific objectives, questions, or hypotheses indicate whether the focus is description, relationships, or differences. Therefore you need to link each analysis technique to its results and then to the study purpose or objectives, questions, or hypotheses presented in the study.

The final reading skill, *analyzing a research report,* involves determining the value of the report's content. The content of the report should be broken into parts, and the parts should be examined in depth for accuracy, completeness, uniqueness of information, and organization. It should be noted whether the steps of the research process build logically on each other or whether steps are missing or incomplete. The discussion section of the report should be examined and it should be determined whether the researchers have provided a critical argument for using the study findings in practice. Using the skills of skimming, comprehending, and analyzing while reading research reports will increase your comfort with studies, allow you to become an informed consumer of research, and expand your knowledge for making changes in practice. These skills for reading research reports are critical for conducting a comprehensive research critique. The guidelines for critiquing quantitative and qualitative studies are the focus of Chapter 12.

CONDUCTING AN INITIAL CRITIQUE OF A RESEARCH REPORT

Being able to read research reports and identify the steps of the research process should enable you to conduct an initial critique of a report.

 The following questions are important in conducting an initial critique of a quantitative research report.

1. Was a quantitative or a qualitative study conducted?
2. If the research was quantitative, was the study descriptive, correlational, quasi-experimental, or experimental?
3. Was the setting for the study natural, partially controlled, or highly controlled?
4. Were the steps of the study clearly identified?
5. Can you identify the following sections in the research report: problem, purpose, literature review, framework, variables, definitions of variables, design, treatment (if appropriate), sample, measuring methods, data collection, data analyses, and outcomes?
6. Were any of the steps of the research process missing?
7. Were the steps of the study logically linked? Thus the study problem and purpose need to provide a basis for the literature review and the framework presented. The purpose and framework provide a basis for the objectives, questions, or hypotheses identified. The objectives, questions, or hypotheses provide a basis for the study design, measurement, data collection, and data analyses. The findings from the study need to be linked to the framework and to previous studies cited in the literature review.

SUMMARY

Quantitative research is the traditional research approach in nursing. Nurses use a broad range of quantitative approaches, including descriptive, correlational, quasi-experimental, and experimental, to develop nursing knowledge. Some of the terms relevant to quantitative research include basic and applied research, rigor, and control. Basic, or pure, research is a scientific investigation that involves the pursuit of "knowledge for knowledge's sake," or for the pleasure of learning and finding truth. Applied, or practical, research is a scientific investigation conducted to generate knowledge that will directly influence or improve clinical practice.

Conducting quantitative research requires rigor, which is the striving for excellence in research. Rigor requires discipline, adherence to detail, and strict accuracy. A rigorous quantitative researcher constantly strives for more tightly controlled study designs that include precise measuring tools, protocol-based treatments, and representative samples. Control involves the imposing of rules by the researcher to decrease the influence of extraneous variables and the possibility of error, and thus increase the probability that the study's findings are an accurate reflection of reality. Some of the mechanisms for control within quantitative research include the selection of subjects and the setting. Sampling is a process of selecting subjects who are representative of the population being studied. The three settings for conducting research are natural, partially controlled, and highly controlled.

Research is a process that is similar in some ways to other processes. Therefore the background you acquired early in your nursing education in problem solving and the nursing process is also useful in research. A comparison of the problem-solving process, the nursing process, and the research process shows the similarities and differences in these processes and provides a basis for understanding the research process.

The quantitative research process involves conceptualizing a research project, planning and implementing that project, and communicating the findings. The following steps of the quantitative research process are briefly introduced in this chapter and are presented in detail in Chapters 3 through 10.

1. *Research problem and purpose.* The research problem is an area of concern in which there is a gap in the knowledge needed for nursing practice. The research purpose is generated from the problem and identifies the specific goal or aim of the study.
2. *Literature review.* The review of relevant literature is conducted to generate a picture of what is known and unknown about a particular topic.
3. *Study framework.* The framework is the theoretical basis for a study that guides the development of the study and enables the researcher to link the findings to nursing's body of knowledge.
4. *Research objectives, questions, or hypotheses.* Research objectives, questions, or hypotheses are formulated to bridge the gap between the more abstractly stated research problem and purpose and the study design and plan for data collection and analysis. The objectives, questions, and hypotheses direct the development of the design, analysis of the study data, and the interpretation of the findings.
5. *Study variables.* Variables are concepts, at various levels of abstraction, that are measured, manipulated, or controlled in a study.
6. *Assumptions.* Assumptions are statements that are taken for granted or are considered true even though they have not been scientifically tested.

7. *Limitations.* Limitations are theoretical or methodological restrictions in a study that may decrease the generalizability of the findings.
8. *Research design.* Research design is a blueprint for conducting a study that maximizes control over factors that could interfere with the study's desired outcomes.
9. *Population and sample.* The population is all the elements that meet certain criteria for inclusion in a study. A sample is a subset of the population that is selected for a particular study; the members of a sample are the subjects.
10. *Methods of measurement.* Measurement is the process of assigning numbers to objects, events, or situations in accord with some rule. Methods of measurement are identified to measure each of the variables in a study.
11. *Data collection.* The data collection process involves the precise, systematic gathering of information relevant to the research purpose or the objectives, questions, or hypotheses of a study.

12. *Data analyses.* Data analyses are conducted to reduce, organize, and give meaning to the data and to address the research purpose and/or objectives, questions, and hypotheses.
13. *Research outcomes.* Research outcomes include the conclusions or findings, generalization of findings, implications for nursing, and suggestions for further research.

Understanding the steps of the quantitative research process provides a background for reading research reports. To assist you in reading the research literature, sources of research reports are identified, the content of a research report is described, and the critical skills for reading the report are detailed. The chapter concludes with guidelines for conducting an initial critique of a quantitative study. In the appendix of this chapter are examples of the steps of the research process excerpted from quasi-experimental and experimental published studies.

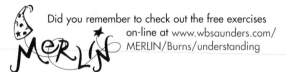

Did you remember to check out the free exercises on-line at www.wbsaunders.com/ MERLIN/Burns/understanding

REFERENCES

Bagley, C. (1990). Development of a measure of unwanted sexual contact in childhood, for use in community health surveys. *Psychology Reports, 66*(2), 401–402.

Bagley, C. & King, K. K. (1990). *Child sexual abuse. The search for healing.* New York: Travistock/Routledge.

Bond, E. F., & Heitkemper, M. M. (1987). Importance of basic physiologic research in nursing science. *Heart & Lung, 16*(4), 347–349.

Brown, B. E., & Garrison, C. J. (1990). Patterns of symptomatology of adult women incest survivors. *Western Journal of Nursing Research, 12*(5), 587–600.

Brown, S. J. (1999). *Knowledge for health care practice: A guide to using research evidence.* Philadelphia: Saunders.

Browne, A., & Finkelhor, D. (1986). Initial and long-term effects: A review of the research. In D. Finkelhor (Ed.), *A source book on child sexual abuse* (pp. 143–179). Beverly Hills, CA: Sage.

Burns, N. (1989). The research process and the nursing process: Distinctly different. *Nursing Science Quarterly, 2*(4), 157–158.

Burns, N., & Grove, S. K. (2001). *The practice of nursing research: Conduct, critique, and utilization* (4th ed.). Philadelphia: Saunders.

Campbell, D. T., & Stanley, J. C. (1963). *Experimental and quasi-experimental designs for research.* Chicago: Rand McNally.

Cook, T. D., & Campbell, D. T. (1979). *Quasi-experimentation: Design and analysis issues for field settings.* Chicago: Rand McNally.

Crosby, L. J. (1990). The abstract: An important first impression. *Journal of Neuroscience Nursing, 22*(3), 192–194.

Fisher, Sir R. A. (1935). *The designs of experiments.* New York: Hafner.

Follette, N. M., Alexander, P. C., & Follette, W. C. (1991). Individual predictors of outcome in group treatment for incest survivors. *Journal of Consulting and Clinical Psychology, 59*(1), 150–155.

Hastings-Tolsma, M. T., Yucha, C. B., Tompkins, J., Robson, L., & Szeverenyi, N. (1993). Effect of warm and cold applications on the resolution of IV infiltrations. *Research in Nursing & Health, 16*(3), 171–178.

Hulme, P. A., & Grove, S. K. (1994). Symptoms of female survivors of child sexual abuse. *Issues in Mental Health Nursing, 15*(5), 519–532.

Kaplan, A. (1964). *The conduct of inquiry: Methodology for behavioral science.* New York: Chandler.

Kelly, E. (2001). Assessment of dietary intake of preschool children living in a homeless shelter. *Applied Nursing Research, 14*(3), 146–154.

Kerlinger, F. N., & Lee, H. B. (1999). *Foundations of behavioral research.* New York: Harcourt Brace.

Lewis, G. B. H., & Hecker, J. F. (1991). Radiological examination of failure of intravenous infusions. *British Journal of Surgery, 78*(4), 500–501.

MacCara, M. E. (1983). Extravasation: A hazard of intravenous therapy. *Drug Intelligence and Clinical Pharmacy, 17*(10), 713–717.

McCarthy, D. O., Lo, C., Nguyen, H., & Ney, D. M. (1997). The effect of protein density of food on food intake and nutritional status of tumor-bearing rats. *Research in Nursing & Health, 20*(2), 131–138.

Millam, D. A. (1988). Managing complications of I.V. therapy. *Nursing 88, 18*(3), 34–42.

Miller, D. C. (1991). *Handbook of research design and social measurement* (5th ed.). Newbury Park, CA: Sage.

Miller, M. A., & Babcock, D. E. (1996). *Critical thinking applied to nursing.* St. Louis: Mosby.

Moody, L. E., Wilson, M. E., Smyth, K., Schwartz, R., Tittle, M., & Van Cott, M. L. (1988). Analysis of a decade of nursing practice research: 1977–1986. *Nursing Research, 42*(4), 197–203.

Myers, S. T. (1982). The search for assumptions. *Western Journal of Nursing Research, 4*(1), 91–98.

Neuberger, G. B., Press, A. N., Lindsley, H. B., Hinton, R., Cagle, P. E., Carlson, K., et al. (1997). Effects of exercise on fatigue, aerobic fitness, and disease activity measures in persons with rheumatoid arthritis. *Research in Nursing & Health, 20*(3), 195–204.

Prescott, P. A., & Soeken, K. L. (1989). Methodology corner: The potential uses of pilot work. *Nursing Research, 38*(1), 60–62.

Swanson, E. A., McCloskey, J. C., & Bodensteiner, A. (1991). Publishing opportunities for nurses: A comparison of 92 U.S. journals. *Image: Journal of Nursing Scholarship, 23*(1), 33–38.

Tornquist, E. M., Funk, S. G., Champagne, M. T., & Wiese, R. A. (1993). Advice on reading research: Overcoming the barriers. *Applied Nursing Research, 6*(4), 177–183.

Van Ort, S. (1981). Research design: Pilot study. In S. D. Krampitz & N. Pavlovich (Eds.), *Readings for nursing research* (pp. 49–53). St. Louis: Mosby.

Whitney, F. W. (1986). Turning clinical problems into research. *Heart & Lung, 15*(1), 57–59.

Williams, M. A. (1980). Editorial: Assumptions in research. *Research in Nursing & Health, 3*(2), 47–48.

Wysocki, A. B. (1983). Basic versus applied research: Intrinsic and extrinsic considerations. *Western Journal of Nursing Research, 5*(3), 217–224.

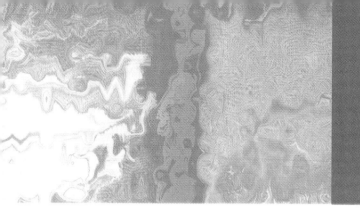

Appendix

QUASI-EXPERIMENTAL STUDY

Quasi-experimental studies are conducted to determine the effect of a treatment or intervention on dependent or outcome variables. Quasi-experimental studies lack the control of the design, sample, or setting that might be used in an experimental study. Hastings-Tolsma, Yucha, Tompkins, Robson, and Szeverenyi (1993) conducted a quasi-experimental study of the "effect of warm and cold applications on the resolution of IV infiltrations" (p. 171). The steps of this study are outlined in the following text:

Steps of the Research Process

1. **Research problem.** "It has been estimated that as many as 80% of hospitalized patients receive intravenous (IV) therapy each day (Millam, 1988). IV infiltration, or extravasation, occurs in as many as 23% of all IV infusion failures (MacCara, 1983) and is second only to phlebitis as a cause of IV morbidity (Lewis & Hecker, 1991). The resulting tissue injury depends on the clinical condition of the patient, the nature of the infusate, and the volume infiltrated, and may range from little apparent injury to serious damage. In addition, considerable patient suffering, prolonged hospitalization, and significant costs may be incurred. Despite the frequency and potential severity of injury, little is known about how to treat IV infiltration effectively once it is identified." (Hastings-Tolsma et al., 1993, p. 171)
2. **Research purpose.** "The purpose of this research was to determine the effect of warm versus cold applications on the pain intensity and the speed of resolution of the extravasation of a variety of commonly used intravenous solutions." (p. 172)
3. **Review of literature.** The literature review included relevant, current sources that ranged from 1976 to 1991. The journal article was received in April 1992 and was accepted for publication in January 1993. The signs and symptoms of IV infiltration were identified, and the tissue damage that occurs with IV infiltration was described. The effects of the pH and osmolarity of different types of IV solutions on IV infiltration were also discussed. The literature review concluded with a

description of the effects of a variety of treatments, including warm and cold applications, on the resolution of IV infiltrations. Hastings-Tolsma et al. (1993, p. 172) concluded that "examination of warm and cold application with less toxic infiltrates has not been studied carefully under controlled conditions."

4. **Framework.** Hastings-Tolsma and colleagues (1993) did not identify a framework for their study. They did identify relevant concepts (IV therapy, nature of infusate, vessel damage, extravasation, tissue damage, treatment, and resolution) and discuss the relationships among these concepts in their literature review. A possible map for their study framework is presented in Fig. 2A-1. The map indicates that the more IV therapy patients receive, the more likely they are to experience vessel damage that leads to extravasation or IV infiltration. The nature of the IV infusate (solution) also affects the severity of the vessel damage and extravasation. Extravasation leads to tissue damage, and the greater the extravasation, the greater the tissue damage. The treatment with warm and cold applications has an unknown effect on the extravasation and tissue damage. If the extravasation and tissue damage are decreased by either the cold or the warm treatment, then the patient experiences resolution of the extravasation.

5. **Research questions.** "(a) What are the differences in tissue response as measured by pain, erythema, induration, and interstitial fluid volume between warm versus cold applications to infiltrated IV sites? (b) What is the effect of warm versus cold applications in the resolution of infiltrated solutions of varying osmolarity when pH is held constant?" (Hastings-Tolsma et al., 1993, pp. 172-173). Hypotheses might have been more appropriate to direct this quasi-experimental study.

6. **Variables.** The independent variables were temperature applications (warm and cold) and osmolarity of the IV solution. The dependent variables were pain, erythema, induration, and interstitial fluid volume.

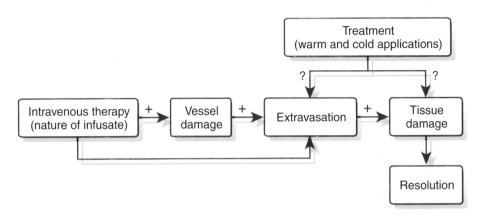

Fig. 2A-1 Proposed framework map for Hastings-Tolsma, Yucha, Tompkins, Robson, and Szeverenyi's (1993) study of the effect of warm and cold applications on the resolution of intravenous infiltrations.

Temperature applications

Conceptual definition. Topical warm and cold applications to the sites of extravasation to promote reabsorption of infusate and resolution of the infiltration.

Operational definition. Warm (43° C) or cold (0° C) topical applications using a thermostatic pad to the sites of IV infiltration.

Osmolarity of the IV solution

Conceptual definition. Osmolar concentration expressing osmoles per liter of solution.

Operational definition. IV solutions of 50% saline (154 mOsm), normal saline (308 mOsm), or 3% saline (1027 mOsm) infiltrated at subject's IV site.

Pain

Conceptual definition. Sensation of discomfort caused by tissue damage and inflammatory response.

Operational definition. Pain measured with the Analogue Chromatic Continuous Scale (ACCS), a self-report, one-dimensional visual analogue scale for quantifying pain intensity.

Erythema

Conceptual definition. Redness at the IV infiltration site as a result of inflammatory response.

Operational definition. Indelible ink used to mark the borders of erythema; then a centimeter ruler used to measure the widest perpendicular widths, and the two widths multiplied to estimate surface area of erythema.

Induration

Conceptual definition. Swelling at the IV infiltration site created by the IV solution, tissue damage, and inflammatory response.

Operational definition. Indelible ink used to mark the borders of induration; then a centimeter ruler used to measure the widest perpendicular widths, and the two widths multiplied to estimate the surface area of induration.

Interstitial fluid volume

Conceptual definition. Amount of fluid that leaks from the damaged blood vessel into the surrounding tissues.

Operational definition. Magnetic resonance imaging (MRI) used to quantify the amount of infiltrate remaining at the IV site.

7. **Design.** The design most closely resembled an interrupted time series, with each subject receiving both the warm and cold applications (treatment) to an IV site infiltrated by one of three types of solutions (50% saline, normal saline, or 3% saline) (treatment). The dependent variables were pain, erythema, induration, and interstitial fluid volume. They were measured at various times before and after the infiltration of the three IV solutions and the warm and cold applications.

8. **Sample.** "The sample was composed of 18 healthy adult volunteers. All participants were nonpregnant and taking no medications.... Of the 18 participants studied, 78% were female ($n = 14$) and 22% were male ($n = 4$), and they ranged in age from 20 to 45 years with a mean age of 35 years (SD = 7). All subjects were Caucasian. The Health Science Center Institutional Review Board for the Protection of Human Subjects approved the research. After the study was explained to interested individuals, written informed consent was obtained from volunteers. All individuals were offered financial compensation for their participation." (Hastings-Tolsma et al., 1993, p. 173)

9. **Procedures.** "All measurements were taken in the Health Science Center's Department of Radiology NMR Laboratory. After obtaining written informed consent, participants were taken to the MR imaging suite where infiltrations and subsequent measurements were made.... Total data collection time was approximately 32 hours. One of three solutions was infiltrated into the cephalic vein of the forearm: $1/2$ saline (154 mOsm), normal saline (308 mOsm), or 3% saline (1027 mOsm). These solutions were selected because of the varying osmolarity range, as well as relatively common clinical use. Solutions were infiltrated sequentially so that each participant was given a different solution in the order of recruitment into the study. Randomization was used to determine right or left arm, as well as which application, warm or cold, would be used." (p. 174)

10. **Results.** "Warm and cold treatments to the infiltrated IV sites using three solutions revealed significant differences in tissue response as measured by the interstitial fluid volume.... For all three solutions, the volume remaining was always less with warm than with cold application, $F_{(1,15)} = 46.69, p < .001$. There was no difference in pain with warm or cold applications.... Surface area measurement failed to demonstrate the presence of erythema with any of the solutions.... Surface induration reflected a significant decrease over time, $F_{(2,16)} = 14.38, p = .001$, although accurate measurement of the infiltrate was nearly impossible after the first or second imaging period as the borders were so poorly defined.... There was no significant effect of warmth or cold on surface area." (p. 175)

11. **Discussion.** This section includes the study conclusions, recommendations for further research, and implications of the findings for nursing practice. "These findings demonstrate that the application of warmth to sites of IV infiltration produces faster resolution of the extravasation than does cold, as monitored over 1 hour.... It is interesting to note that cold appeared to have a more immediate dramatic effect on the increase in interstitial edema than warmth when applied to the hyperosmolar infiltrate. Presumably this is due to osmosis of fluid from the plasma and surrounding tissues into the area of infiltration....

Other factors that might influence accurate assessment and treatment of infiltrations need to be examined. These should include the use of larger amounts of extravasate and other more varied and caustic solutions, as well as other treatments such as elevation, differing IV site placement, differing gauge needles, and the study of patients of varying ages and clinical conditions...." (p. 176)

"The nurse generally has responsibility for IV therapy and criteria for accurate assessment and appropriate intervention clearly are needed. Findings from this research support the use of warm application to sites of infiltration of non-caustic solutions of varying osmolarity, but raise questions about the adequacy of currently used indicators of IV infiltrations. Continued scientific scrutiny should contribute to the development of standards useful in the assessment and treatment of IV extravasation." (p. 177)

EXPERIMENTAL STUDY

The purpose of experimental research is to examine cause-and-effect relationships between independent and dependent variables under highly controlled conditions. The planning and implementation of experimental studies are highly controlled by the researcher, and often these studies are conducted in a laboratory setting on animals or objects. Few nursing studies are "purely" experimental. McCarthy, Lo, Nguyen and Ney (1997) conducted an experimental study of "the effect of protein density of food on food intake and nutritional status of tumor-bearing rats" (pp. 74-81).

Steps of the Research Process

1. **Research problem.** "Anorexia and weight loss are significant concerns to cancer patients and their loved ones.... The progressive decline[s] in food intake and body weight are powerful negative prognostic indicators of survival in cancer patients.... The loss of lean body mass is a major aspect of the nutritional decline of cancer patients. The literature presents a uniform emphasis on increasing dietary protein intake with the expectation of preserving lean body mass of cancer patients.... However, it has been shown that healthy animals will reduce their food intake when protein density of their food is increased.... It is not known if this response to increased protein density of food will occur in hypophagic tumor-bearing rats.

   It also should be noted that tumor growth is associated with depressed serum levels of insulin associated with depressed serum levels of insulin-like growth factor 1(IGF-1).... It is not known if serum levels of insulin or IGF-1 will improve in hypophagic tumor-bearing rats fed a diet of increased protein density." (pp. 130-132)

2. **Research purpose.** The purpose of this laboratory study "was to determine (a) if increasing the protein density of food would affect food and total protein intake of tumor-bearing rats and (b) if increased protein intake would alter serum levels of insulin and IGF-1, two hormones requisite to protein synthesis and tissue anabolism." (p. 132)

3. **Review of literature.** The literature review included current sources that ranged from 1975 to 1995, with 31 (80%) of the 39 sources published in the last 5 years (1991-1996). This article was submitted for publication in 1996, accepted for publication in October 1996, and published in April of 1997. The literature review included mainly studies focused on causes of tumor-induced anorexia and

weight loss in cancer patients, impact of high calorie and high-density protein diets on healthy animals, and the link between tumor growth and serum levels of insulin and IGF-1.

4. **Framework.** This study has an implied framework that is a combination of physiological and pathological theories about nutrient utilization, tumor development, body response to tumor development, anorexia, nutritional treatment of anorexia, and body response to nutritional supplement.

5. **Variables.** The independent variable was high-density protein diet. The dependent variables were serum insulin, serum IGF-1, food intake, protein intake, and body weight.

Independent variable—high-density protein diet

Conceptual definition. Nutritional supplement to promote increased intake, nutrient utilization, and weight stabilization with cancerous conditions.

Operational definition. Isocaloric diet containing 40% casein protein (TD#93331, Harlan Tecklad, Madison, WI). (The specific ingredients of this diet are provided in a table in the article.)

Dependent variables—serum insulin and IGF-1

Conceptual definition. Sensitive markers indicating nutritional status and playing an important role in protein metabolism and tissue anabolism.

Operational definitions. "Analysis of serum insulin was done using a radioimmunoassay (RIA).... Serum IGF-1 was determined by RIA after the IGF binding proteins were removed by high-performance chromatography under acid conditions." (McCarthy et al., 1997, p. 133)

Dependent variables—food intake and protein intake

Conceptual definition. Nutrients consumed by healthy and tumor-bearing animals.

Operational definitions. Food intake operationalized as the number of grams of food eaten by both the healthy and the tumor-bearing rats. Protein intake was operationalized as the number of milligrams of protein consumed by the healthy and tumor-bearing rats.

Dependent variables—body weight

Conceptual definition. Body mass of healthy and tumor-bearing rats.

Operational definitions. Body weight in grams of healthy and tumor-bearing rats at days 0, 15, 18, 24, and 27 of the experiment.

6. **Design.** This study has an experimental design that included four groups: (1) 15 healthy rats in the control group on a regular diet, (2) 15 healthy rats in a group on 40% protein diet, (3) 15 tumor-bearing rats on a regular diet, and (4) 15 tumor-bearing rats on 40% protein diet, with repeated measures of three of the five dependent variables. "The experimental period lasted for 27 days. For the first 15

days, all animals were maintained on a semipurified rodent diet containing 20% casein protein.... After day 15 of tumor growth, one half of the tumor-bearing and one half of the healthy controls were switched to an isocaloric diet containing 40% casein protein. The dependent variables of serum insulin and serum IGF-1 were measured on day 27, and the other dependent variables of food intake, protein intake, and body weight were measured at day 0, 15, 18, 24, and 27." (p. 133)

7. **Sample and setting.** "A total of 60 randomly selected male Buffalo rats, weighing between 100 and 120 grams were housed individually and maintained on a 12-hour light-dark cycle commencing at 6:00 AM. Food and water were freely available. The animals were conditioned to the housing for 5 days before the start of the experiment and were treated at all times in a manner consistent with Department of Health, Education, and Welfare *Guidelines for the Care and Use of Laboratory Animals....* The animals were matched according to weight and a total of 30 were randomly selected for tumor implant, leaving 30 healthy animals as controls." (pp. 132-133)

8. **Data collection.** "The food was placed in conical dishes inside a metal cup to catch any spillage. The dishes were weighed each morning on a portable electric digital scale which was zeroed before each weighing.... The rats were weighed daily and at the end of the experiment the tumors were excised and weighed.... On day 27 of tumor growth, animals were lightly anesthetized with ether fumes and exsanguinated by cardiac puncture between 8 and 10 AM to control for any circadian variations in plasma hormone levels. The blood was allowed to coagulate and serum samples for 48 animals were frozen at $-20°$ C (12 specimens were inadvertently destroyed)." (p. 133)

9. **Results.** The extensive study results were presented in five figures and narrative of the article. "There was a significant main effect of tumor growth, $F_{(1,56)} = 26.6$, $p < .001$, diet, $F_{(1,56)} = 4.1$, $p = .05$, and days, $F_{(4,224)} = 29.6$, $p < .001$, on the grams of food eaten by the rats.... Due to the effect of tumor growth on food intake, the tumor-bearing animals were consuming less protein than healthy controls by day 15, $F_{(1,59)} = 16$, $p < .001$. On day 18, 3 days after the diet switch, protein intake was significantly different by tumor, $F_{(1,59)} = 377$ ($p < .001$) and by diet, $F_{(1,59)} = 176$, $p < .001$...body weight of tumor-bearing rats was significantly less than controls over the course of the experiment, $F_{(1,56)} = 20.5$, $p < .001$...there was a significant effect of tumor growth on mean serum insulin, $F_{(1,4)} = 4.7$, $p = .03$, but no effect of diet.... Similarly, serum IGF-1 was significantly lower in tumor-bearing rats than healthy controls, $F_{(1,47)} = 25.7$, $p < .001$, and was not affected by diet." (pp. 133-136)

10. **Discussion.** Findings and suggestions for further research. "Increasing the protein density of food from the standard 20% formulation to 40% resulted in a decline in total grams of food intake, and an increase in total grams protein intake of both control and tumor-bearing rats. The increased protein intake of tumor-bearing animals fed the 40% protein diet did not affect the nutrient status of these animals as indicated by body weight, or serum levels of total protein, insulin, or

IGF-1, nor did it affect tumor size in the tumor-bearing animals.... These data suggest that the lower serum levels of IGF-1 and insulin in hypophagic tumor-bearing animals are not the direct results of their reduced food, or in this case, protein intake.... Increasing the protein density of food resulted in a decrease in food intake in both healthy control and tumor-bearing animals." (p. 136)

"The regulation of food intake in humans is more complex than in animals which are maintained on standardized diets and feeding schedules. There is a need for studies to determine the effects of high calorie or high protein nutrition supplements on the total caloric and protein intake and, specifically, meal taking, of cancer patients. There is some evidence that use of nutritional supplements by patients with head and neck cancers results in a significant decline in food-derived calories and protein, though the caloric and protein density of the supplements produces a net increase in total calorie and protein intake.... However, there is little evidence that increase nutritional intake affects morbidity and mortality in weight-losing cancer patients.... Clearly, there is a need for further study of the metabolic impact of nutritional interventions, as well as the impact of calorie and/or protein dense nutritional supplements on meal taking and food appetite of cancer patients." (p. 137)

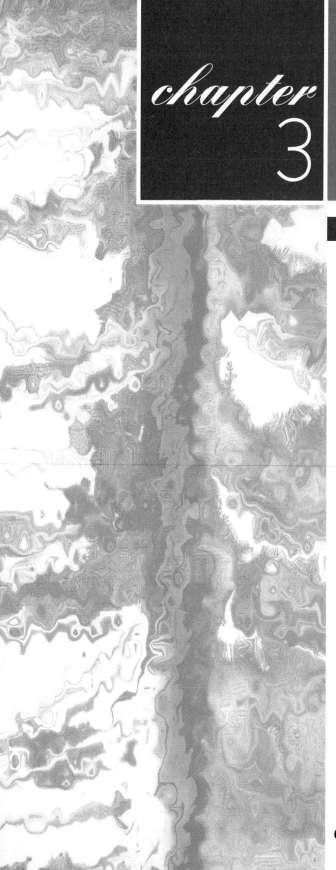

chapter 3

Research Problems, Purposes, and Hypotheses

Be sure to check out the free exercises on-line at
www.wbsaunders.com/MERLIN/Burns/
understanding

MERLIN

OUTLINE—cont'd

Hypotheses
    Types of Hypotheses
    Testable Hypothesis
Critiquing Research Objectives, Questions, and Hypotheses in Published Studies
Understanding Study Variables
    Types of Variables
        Independent and Dependent Variables
        Research Variables or Concepts
        Extraneous Variables
        Demographic Variables
    Conceptual and Operational Definitions of Variables
Critiquing Research Variables in Published Studies

OBJECTIVES

Completing this chapter should enable you to:
1. Define the concepts research topic, problem, and purpose.
2. Differentiate the research problem from the purpose.
3. Identify research topics, problems, and purposes in published quantitative, qualitative, and outcomes studies.
4. Examine the significance of research problems and purposes in published studies.
5. Critique the feasibility of a study problem and purpose by examining the researcher's expertise; money commitment; availability of subjects, facilities, and equipment; and the study's ethical considerations.
6. Examine the use of objectives, questions, and hypotheses in published studies.
7. Differentiate among the types of hypotheses (simple versus complex, nondirectional versus directional, associative versus causal, and statistical versus research).
8. Critique the quality of objectives, questions, and hypotheses presented in published studies.
9. Describe the different types of variables.
10. Differentiate between conceptual and operational definitions of variables.
11. Critique the conceptual and operational definitions of variables in published studies.
12. Use critical thinking in determining the significance and clarity of the problems, purposes, objectives, questions, hypotheses, and definitions of variables in published studies.

RELEVANT TERMS

Conceptual definition	Research purpose
Hypothesis	Research question
Associative hypothesis	Research topic
Causal hypothesis	Sample characteristics
Complex hypothesis	Variables
Directional hypothesis	Confounding variables
Nondirectional hypothesis	Demographic variables
Null (statistical) hypothesis	Dependent (response or outcome)
Research hypothesis	variable
Simple hypothesis	Environmental variables
Testable hypothesis	Extraneous variables
Operational definition	Independent (treatment or experimen-
Research objective	tal) variable
Research problem	Research variables or concepts

We are constantly asking questions to gain a better understanding of ourselves and the world around us. This human ability to wonder and ask creative questions is the first step in the research process. By asking questions, clinical nurses and nurse researchers are able to identify significant research topics and problems that will generate research findings that can ultimately be used to make changes in practice. A *research topic* is a concept or broad issue that is important to nursing, such as acute and chronic pain management, coping with illness, or health promotion. Each topic contains numerous potential research problems to guide quantitative, qualitative, and outcomes studies. For example, chronic pain management is a research topic that includes such potential problems as, What is chronic pain? and What is it like to live with chronic pain? Qualitative research might be used to investigate these problems or areas of concern in nursing. Quantitative research might be used to study such problems as, How can chronic pain be assessed accurately? and What are effective interventions for managing chronic pain? Outcomes research methodologies might be used to examine patient outcomes and the cost effectiveness of care provided in a chronic pain management clinic.

The problem or area of concern provides the basis for developing the research purpose. The purpose or goal of a study guides the development of the objectives, questions, or hypotheses. The objectives, questions, or hypotheses bridge the gap between the more abstractly stated problem and purpose and the detailed design for conducting the study. Objectives, questions, and hypotheses include the variables, the relationships among the variables, and often the population to be studied.

This chapter includes content that will assist in differentiating a problem from a purpose and critiquing the problems and purposes in published quantitative, qualitative, and outcomes studies. Objectives, questions, and hypotheses are also discussed, and the different types of study variables are introduced. The chapter concludes with critical-thinking exercises that guide the critique of the objectives, questions, hypotheses, and variables in published studies.

WHAT ARE RESEARCH PROBLEMS AND PURPOSES?

A *research problem* is an area of concern where there is a gap in the knowledge base needed for nursing practice. Research is required to generate essential knowledge to address the practice concern, with the ultimate goal of providing evidence-based nursing care (Brown, 1999; Fields, 2000). In a published study the research problem identifies an area of concern for a particular population and outlines the need for additional study. Not all published studies include a clearly expressed problem, but the problem can usually be identified in the first or second paragraph of the article. The research problem from Foster-Fitzpatrick, Ortiz, Sibilano, Marcantonio, and Braun's study of *The Effects of Crossed Leg on Blood Pressure Measurement* (1999, p. 105) is presented as an example.

"Blood pressure monitoring is one of the most commonly used techniques in the diagnosis and treatment of various health care problems. Accurate measurement of blood pressure is especially crucial in the assessment of hypertension. Consequently, all efforts should be made to eliminate errors in measuring blood pressure.

Numerous factors influence an individual's blood pressure measurement including medications, arm and body position, noise, extreme temperatures, constrictive clothing, faulty equipment, white-coat effect, attitude of the person taking the measurement, anxiety, improper cuff length or width, and talking.... Additionally, an overall diurnal variability in blood pressure has been observed. Blood pressure typically falls by approximately 15% during the night in people who are active during the day, although a lesser nocturnal decrease in blood pressure has been noted in some hypertensive subjects. During the early morning hours, some individuals exhibit an abrupt rise in blood pressure, which has been associated with cardiovascular complications (Kaplan, 1998).

Although not an acceptable practice, a single blood pressure measurement often is the basis for clinical decisions, such as adjustment of a person's antihypertensive drug dosage. Thus, it is crucial to eliminate all possible sources of error in measuring a person's blood pressure (Hill & Grim, 1991).

Some guidelines for accurately measuring blood pressure specify that the patient should keep feet flat on the floor. **However, research is lacking on the effect of crossing the leg at the knee during blood pressure measurement.**" (pp. 105-106)

In this example, the first paragraph clearly identifies the area of concern for a particular population, and paragraphs two through four provide concise background and significance for this concern. The concern is accurate blood pressure measurement, and the population is individuals having their blood pressures measured in a clinical setting. This is a significant problem since blood pressure measurement is used in the diagnosis and treatment of several health care problems and as a basis for clinical decisions related to adjustment of antihypertensive medications. The background provided by previous research indicates that there are numerous factors that influence accurate blood pressure measurement. The discussion of the problem concludes with a concise *problem statement* in **boldface** print in the example) that indicates the gap in the knowledge based needed for practice.

This example research problem includes concepts such as accurate measurement of blood pressure, factors influencing blood pressure measurement, and nursing intervention to promote accurate blood pressure measurement. A variety of nursing interventions could be implemented to determine their effects on blood pressure measurement. Thus each problem provides the basis for generating a variety of research purposes. In this study the knowledge gap regarding the effects of crossed legs on blood pressure measurement provides clear direction for the formulation of the research purpose.

The *research purpose* is a clear, concise statement of the specific aim or goal of a study. The goal of a study might be to identify, describe, or explain a situation or predict a solution to a problem. The purpose also includes the variables, the population, and often the setting for the study. A clearly stated research purpose can capture the essence of a study in a single sentence and is essential for directing the remaining steps of the research process (Creswell, 1994). In a published study the purpose statement is often presented after the problem or the literature review. In addition, the purpose is often reflected in the title of the study and is the first line of the study abstract. Foster-Fitzpatrick et al. (1999) identified the purpose of their study in the article title and abstract and then after the problem statement. The researchers clearly stated that the purpose of their study was "...to determine if blood pressure measurement is affected by the leg crossed at the knee as compared with feet flat on the floor" (p. 106).

The goal of this study was to examine the effects of two positions (legs crossed at knees and feet flat on the floor) on blood pressure measurement. This quasi-experimental study was conducted to determine the effects of two independent variables or treatments (legs crossed at knees and feet flat) on the dependent variable or outcome blood pressure measurement. The results indicated that systolic and diastolic blood pressure readings were significantly increased ($p < .0001$) with the crossed leg position. Thus, patients should be instructed to place their feet flat on the floor when their blood pressure is measured to eliminate a source of error (Foster-Fitzpatrick et al., 1999).

IDENTIFYING THE PROBLEM AND PURPOSE IN QUANTITATIVE, QUALITATIVE, AND OUTCOMES STUDIES

Quantitative, qualitative, and outcomes research approaches enable nurses to investigate a variety of research problems and purposes. Examples of research topics, problems, and purposes for different types of quantitative, qualitative, and outcomes studies are presented in this section.

Problems and Purposes in Types of Quantitative Studies

Example research topics, problems, and purposes for the different types of quantitative research (descriptive, correlational, quasi-experimental, and experimental) are presented in Table 3-1. If little is known about a topic, the researcher usually starts with a descriptive study and progresses to quasi-experimental and experimental studies. By examining the problems and purposes in Table 3-1, the differences and similarities among the types of quantitative research can be noted. Most published studies include a clearly expressed problem and purpose; however, the problem and purpose may need to be extracted from the introduction section of a research report.

The research purpose usually reflects the type of study that was conducted. The purpose of descriptive research is to describe concepts or variables, identify possible relationships, and describe differences among groups. Edel, Houston, Kennedy, and LaRocco (1998) conducted a comparative descriptive study that described the number and types of microbes found on artificial, polished, and natural nails, following a 5-minute surgical scrub. These authors found that artificial nails harbored a significantly higher number of bacteria than polished or natural nails, and that polished nails harbored a significantly higher number of bacteria than natural nails. These study findings are consistent with the conclusions of previous research. Thus nurses have empirical evidence that natural nails are safer in preventing the transmission of bacteria in clinical practice than are polished or artificial nails.

The purpose of correlational research is to examine the strength (low, moderate, or high) and type (positive or negative) of relationships among study variables. Bournaki (1997, p. 147) conducted a correlational study to examine the "relationships of children's age, gender, exposure to past painful experiences, temperament, fears, and child-rearing practices to the pain-related responses to venipuncture in school-age children" (see Table 3-1). The researcher found that age, past medical fears, and temperament were predictive of children's pain-related responses to venipuncture. These findings support the multidimensionality of children's pain responses and the need to assess and manage each child's pain in practice.

Quasi-experimental studies are conducted to determine the effect of a treatment or independent variable on designated dependent or outcome variables. Artinian, Washington, and Templin (2001) examined the effects of two independent variables (home telemonitoring [HT] and community-based monitoring [CBM]) on the dependent variable blood pressure control in a population of African American women (see

TABLE 3-1

QUANTITATIVE RESEARCH: TOPICS, PROBLEMS, AND PURPOSES

TYPE OF RESEARCH	RESEARCH TOPIC	RESEARCH PROBLEM AND PURPOSE
Descriptive Research	Aseptic technique (scrubbing for operating room), microbial flora, hygiene of fingernails	*Title of Study:* "Impact of a 5-minute scrub on the microbial flora found on artificial, polished, or natural fingernails of operating room personnel." (Edel, Houston, Kennedy, & LaRocco, 1998) *Problem:* "For many years, maintaining short and polish-free fingernails has been part of the Recommended Standards of Practice for scrubbing and gowning of operating room (OR) personnel.... However, in recent years as artificial nails have become more popular, some physicians, OR nurses, and other health care providers have challenged these guidelines, claiming that nails with frequent care provided by nail technicians are healthier than unmanicured natural nails.... A limited number of studies have been conducted to determine the relationship of artificial nails to bacterial colonization.... Only one study has examined bacterial colonization associated with polished nails." (Edel et al., 1998, pp. 54-55) *Purpose:* "The purpose of this study was to determine whether differences exist in the presence and type of microbes found on the nails and nail beds of OR personnel with natural, polished, or artificial nails before and after a 5-minute surgical scrub." (Edel et al., 1998, p. 55)
Correlational Research	Pain-related responses, venipuncture	*Title of Study:* "Correlates of pain-related responses to venipunctures in school-age children." (Bournaki, 1997) *Problem:* "Venipunctures are described as painful procedures by hospitalized children (Van Cleve, Johnson, & Pothier, 1996; Wong & Baker, 1988) and the most difficult to deal with by adolescent oncology survivors.... However, not all children respond similarly to venipunctures. Between 4% and 17% of school-age children rated their pain intensity to a venipuncture as severe... and 38% of children ages 3 to 10 had to be physically restrained during a venipuncture.... In a recent study by Van Cleve et al. (1996), hospitalized school-age children were found to rate venipuncture or intravenous cannulation as moderately painful. Factors that account for variability in children's responses to venipunctures have not been fully identified." (Bournaki, 1997, p. 147)

TABLE **3-1**		

QUANTITATIVE RESEARCH: TOPICS, PROBLEMS, AND PURPOSES—cont'd

TYPE OF RESEARCH	RESEARCH TOPIC	RESEARCH PROBLEM AND PURPOSE
		Purpose: "The purpose of this study, therefore, was to examine the relationship of a set of correlates, including age, gender, past painful experiences, temperament, general and medical fears, and child-rearing practices, on school-age children's subjective, behavioral, and heart rate responses to a venipuncture." (Bournaki, 1997, p. 147)
Quasi-Experimental Research	Blood pressure, treatment of hypertension, home tele-monitoring, community-based monitoring	*Title of the Study:* "Effects of home telemonitoring and community-based monitoring on blood pressure (BP) control in urban African Americans: A pilot study." (Artinian, Washington, & Templin, 2001)
		Problem: "One in four adults has hypertension (HTN), which highlights the prevalence of HTN as a cardiovascular risk factor (American Heart Association, 1999).... According to the World Health Organization (WHO) (WHO Expert Committee, 1996), HTN is the second most common reason for physician office visits worldwide. African Americans have a higher prevalence and greater severity of HTN than do other minorities and whites.... Although scientific evidence has established that there is an array of both non-pharmacologic and pharmacologic strategies that reduce BP, the rate of awareness, treatment, and control of HTN in the US population is declining, increasing danger for African Americans in particular (JNC-VI-Joint National Committee on Detection, Evaluation, and Treatment of High Blood Pressure, 1997). Inadequate BP monitoring is an important factor that affects BP control.... One way to improve HTN awareness and control is to facilitate access to care by realizing that the point of access need not be limited to a clinic, emergency department, or physician office. The need for tertiary alternative strategies to promote BP control is high." (Artinian et al., 2001, pp. 191-192)
		Purpose: Therefore, the purpose of this study was to determine the "effects of home telemonitoring and community-based monitoring on blood pressure control in urban African Americans." (Artinian et al., 2001, p. 191)

Continued

TABLE **3-1**		

QUANTITATIVE RESEARCH: TOPICS, PROBLEMS, AND PURPOSES—cont'd

TYPE OF RESEARCH	RESEARCH TOPIC	RESEARCH PROBLEM AND PURPOSE
Experimental Research	Sleep deprivation, wound healing	*Title of Study:* "Effects of 72 hours of sleep deprivation on wound healing in the rat." (Landis & Whitney, 1997) *Problem:* "Sleep is thought to be essential for recovery from injury, and lost or disturbed sleep is believed to hinder postinjury wound healing (tissue repair). Disrupted and lost sleep are common experiences in the immediate postoperative period ...and patients often express concern about losing sleep after surgery.... The consequences of lost sleep are of particular concern to nurses and other clinicians who provide or guide care for patients after acute surgical or accidental injury and are in a position to facilitate or educate patients about sleep. Questions regarding the possible effects of sleep loss on tissue repair and mechanisms by which sleep loss might negatively affect wound healing have been raised (Lee & Stotts, 1990), but no investigators have systematically evaluated the impact of sleep loss on tissue repair at cellular and subcellular levels." (Landis & Whitney, 1997, p. 259) *Purpose:* "The purpose of this study was to determine the effects of 72 hours of sleep loss on cellular markers of the proliferative and early collagen biosynthesis phases of wound healing." (Landis & Whitney, 1997, p. 261)

Table 3-1). At three months follow-up, women in both the HT and the CBM groups had significantly lower systolic and diastolic blood pressures than women in the comparison group. With additional study, these two interventions (HT and CBM) might provide an effective way for nurses to monitor minority patients' blood pressures to promote control of their hypertension.

Experimental studies are conducted in highly controlled settings, under highly controlled conditions to determine the effect of one or more independent variables on one or more dependent variables. Landis and Whitney (1997) conducted an experimental study of the effects of 72 hours of sleep deprivation on wound healing of rats in a laboratory setting. In this basic research, the investigators found that sleep deprivation does decrease wound healing, however, additional human research is needed before the findings will have implications for nursing practice.

Problems and Purposes in Types of Qualitative Studies

The problems formulated for qualitative research identify areas of concern that require investigation to gain new insights, expand understanding, or improve comprehension of the whole (Munhall, 2001). The purpose of a qualitative study indicates the focus of the study, which might be a concept such as pain, an event such as loss of a child, or a facet of a culture such as the healing practices of the American Indian. In addition, the purpose often identifies the qualitative approach used and the basic assumptions for this approach (Creswell, 1994). Examples of research topics, problems, and purposes for the types of qualitative research (phenomenological, grounded theory, ethnography, and historical) commonly conducted in nursing are presented in Table 3-2.

Phenomenological research is conducted to promote an understanding of human experiences from an individual researcher's perspective, such as working Americans' lived experience of being medically uninsured (Orne, Fishman, Manka, & Pagnozzi, 2000). Orne and colleagues (2000) identified four themes: (1) marginalized life, (2) up against rocks and hard places, (3) making choices—chancing it, and (4) getting by—more or less, that summarize the lived experience of being medically uninsured. This study provides insight to and promotes understanding of the urgent problem of the increasing number of working Americans without medical insurance.

In grounded theory research, the problem identifies the area of concern and the purpose indicates the focus of the theory to be developed from the research (Munhall, 2001). For example, Logan and Jenny (1997) investigated patients' work during mechanical ventilation and weaning to develop a theory of ventilator weaning. This theory could be used to facilitate the weaning of patients from ventilators in a variety of health care facilities.

In ethnographical research, the problem and purpose identify the culture and the specific attributes of the culture that are to be examined, described, analyzed, and interpreted (Germain, 2001). Kauffman (1995) described the haven provided by a senior center for elderly African-Americans in an inner city ghetto known for drug-related violence and crime. The study findings indicated that the elders' social interactions and mental health were improved by active participation in the center. The researcher encouraged policy makers and health care professionals to recognize the needs of inner city residents and to provide culturally competent health care to these individuals.

The problem and purpose in historical research focus on a specific individual, a characteristic of society, an event, or a situation in the past, as well as identify the time period in the past that was examined by the study (Fitzpatrick, 2001). For example, Krisman-Scott (2000) conducted a historical study of disclosure of terminal status from 1930 to 1990. The study conclusions were that disclosure of terminal status has slowly changed over time from concealment in the 1930s to more general acceptance of disclosure today. The groundwork for the change took place in the 1950s and 1960s and culminated in the 1970s. This change is based on the expanding view of individual rights, perceptions of death, and health care providers' responsibilities.

TABLE 3-2

QUALITATIVE RESEARCH: TOPICS, PROBLEMS, AND PURPOSES

TYPE OF RESEARCH	RESEARCH TOPIC	RESEARCH PROBLEM AND PURPOSE
Phenomenological Research	Phenomenon, medically uninsured, living on the edge, lived experience	*Title of the Study:* "Living on the edge: A phenomenological study of medically uninsured working Americans." (Orne, Fishman, Manka, & Pagnozzi, 2000) *Problem:* "The circumstance of being medically uninsured is a formidable barrier to millions of Americans in need of health care.... A 1997 national survey found that one in three adults had been without insurance for some period of time in the previous 2 years and that 57% of these respondents had been employed full-time...." (Kuttner, 1999) Although statistical evidence describing the problem of American workers who are without medical insurance mounts, little is known about how this phenomenon effects one's emotional, social, and physical well being. There is a paucity of research on their personal impact of this lived experience. Understanding this perspective, however, is imperative if health care providers, administrators, and policy-makers are to develop effective strategies to address the problems of this vulnerable population. This is particularly so for nurses, the caregivers who often have closer contact, over more extended periods of time, and in a wider variety of settings than other health care providers." (Orne et al., 2000, pp. 204-205) *Purpose:* "This study was designed to explore the experience of being medically uninsured from the perspective of American workers who have lived it. The purpose of this study was to describe and explicate what this experience means to the individual and the impact it has on daily life." (Orne et al., 2000, p. 205)
Grounded Theory Research	Mechanical ventilation, weaning, patient's experience	*Title of Study:* "Qualitative analysis of patients' work during mechanical ventilation and weaning." (Logan & Jenny, 1997) *Problem:* "Mechanical ventilation and weaning present significant challenges for clinicians. A substantial minority of patients who receive mechanical ventilation support have considerable weaning difficulties and account for a disproportionate amount of health care costs.... Predictors of weaning success have been studied extensively, primarily from physiologic and technologic perspectives. Less attention has been paid to

TABLE 3-2

QUALITATIVE RESEARCH: TOPICS, PROBLEMS, AND PURPOSES—cont'd

TYPE OF RESEARCH	RESEARCH TOPIC	RESEARCH PROBLEM AND PURPOSE
Grounded Theory Research (cont'd)		patients' subjective experience of mechanical ventilation and weaning, even though psychologic factors have been proposed as important determinants of outcomes in some patients, particularly for those requiring prolonged ventilator support." (Logan & Jenny, 1997, p. 140) *Purpose:* "The purpose of this study was to examine patients' subjective experiences of mechanical ventilation and weaning to validate and extend previous work. The study also contributes another perspective to an evolving theory of ventilator weaning." (Logan & Jenny, 1997, p. 141)
Ethnography Research	Inner city ghettos, survival, elders, drug activity	*Title of Study:* "Center as haven: Findings of an urban ethnography." (Kauffman, 1995) *Problem:* "In underserved, inner city ghettos known for drug-related violence and crime, active participation in community life is dangerous and even life-threatening. This is especially true for elders burdened with the infirmities of aging and lacking the means to provide for alternatives to social isolation. Few researchers have ventured into inner-city communities known for troublesome and dangerous public spaces.... Therefore, little is known about the social lives of people in these communities, in particular, vulnerable older people who are frequently victims of illegal drug activity." (Kauffman, 1995, p. 231) *Purpose:* "This urban ethnography was conducted over a period of three years in a predominantly African American inner-city ghetto. The main question to be answered was: How do elders survive in the midst of 'drug warfare' in an inner-city community known for its dangerous streets and public spaces?" (Kauffman, 1995, p. 231)
Historical Research	Disclosure, terminal status, death, dying, historical analysis	*Title of Study:* "An historical analysis of disclosure of terminal status." (Krisman-Scott, 2000) *Problem:* "In the last century the manner and place in which Americans experience death has changed. Sudden death has decreased and slow dying has increased.... Often, in response to both avoidance and denial, the dying pretend to be unaware. This cycle of pretense, instead of being helpful, robs a person of the opportunity to make appropriate end-of-life decisions and maintain power and control over what remains of life....

Continued

TABLE **3-2**		
QUALITATIVE RESEARCH: TOPICS, PROBLEMS, AND PURPOSES—cont'd		
TYPE OF RESEARCH	**RESEARCH TOPIC**	**RESEARCH PROBLEM AND PURPOSE**
Historical Research (cont'd)		Nurses, for a variety of reasons, have for the most part avoided telling people they are close to death, even though secrecy creates serious problems in caring for the dying.... The amount of information given to patients about illness, treatment, and prognosis has changed over time. Movement toward greater disclosure of health information to patients has occurred in the past 60 years." (Krisman-Scott, 2000, p. 47)
		Purpose: "The purpose of this study was to examine the concept of disclosure as it relates to terminal prognosis and trace its historical development and practice in the United States over the last 60 years.... An individual's ability to make appropriate end-of-life decisions, exert some control over the place and manner of death, and prepare self and significant others for this loss depends on knowing that life is drawing to a close." (Krisman-Scott, 2000, p. 47)

Problems and Purposes in Outcomes Research

Outcomes research is conducted to examine the end results of care. Table 3-3 includes the topics, problem, and purpose from an outcomes study by Rudy et al. (1995). This study was conducted to determine the outcomes for patients who are chronically critically ill in the special care unit (SCU) compared with the intensive care unit (ICU). Common outcomes of cost, patient satisfaction, length of stay, complications, and readmissions were examined to determine the impact of care in these two units on the patients and the health care system. The findings from this 4-year study demonstrated that nurse case-managers in an SCU setting can produce patient outcomes equal to or better than those obtained in the traditional ICU environment, for long-term critically ill patients. In addition, caring for patients in the SCU was more cost effective than caring for those in the ICU.

DETERMINING THE SIGNIFICANCE OF A STUDY PROBLEM AND PURPOSE

A research problem is significant in nursing when it has the potential to generate or refine relevant knowledge for practice. While critiquing the significance of the problem and purpose in a published study, you need to determine whether the knowl-

TABLE 3-3		

OUTCOMES RESEARCH: TOPICS, PROBLEMS, AND PURPOSES

TYPE OF RESEARCH	RESEARCH TOPIC	RESEARCH PROBLEM AND PURPOSE
Outcomes Research	Patient outcomes, special care unit, intensive care unit, chronically critically ill	*Title of Study:* "Patient outcomes for the chronically critically ill: Special care unit versus intensive care unit." (Rudy et al., 1995, p. 324) *Problem:* "The original purpose of intensive care units (ICUs) was to locate groups of patients together who had similar needs for specialized monitoring and care so that highly trained health care personnel would be available to meet these specialized needs. As the success of ICUs has grown and expanded, the assumption that a typical ICU patient will require only a short length of stay in the unit during the most acute phase of an illness has given way to the recognition that stays of more than one month are not uncommon.... These long-stay ICU patients represent a challenge to the current system, not only because of costs, but also because of concern for patient outcomes.... While ample evidence confirms that this subpopulation of ICU patients represents a drain on hospital resources, few studies have attempted to evaluate the effects of a care delivery system outside the ICU setting on patient outcomes, costs, and nurse outcomes." (Rudy et al., 1995, p. 324) *Purpose:* "The purpose of this study was to compare the effects of a low-technology environment of care and a nurse case management care delivery system (specific care unit, SCU) with the traditional high-technology environment (ICU) and primary nursing care delivery system on the patient outcomes of length of stay, mortality, readmission, complications, satisfaction, and cost." (Rudy et al., 1995, p. 324)

edge generated in the study (1) influences nursing practice, (2) builds on previous research, (3) promotes theory testing or development, and (4) addresses current concerns or priorities in nursing (Burns & Grove, 2001; Moody, Vera, Blanks, & Visscher, 1989).

Influences Nursing Practice

The practice of nursing needs to be based on empirical knowledge or knowledge that is generated through research. Thus studies that address clinical concerns and generate findings to improve nursing practice are considered significant. Several research problems and purposes have focused on the effects of nursing interventions or on ways to improve these interventions. For example, researchers have examined the effects of (1) pelvic muscle exercises on stress urinary incontinence (Johnson, 2001), (2) exercise training on chronic obstructive pulmonary disease (COPD) (Carrieri-Kohlman et al., 2001), and (3) warm and cold applications on the resolution of intravenous infiltrations (Hastings-Tolsma, Yucha, Tompkins, Robson, & Szeverenyi, 1993). These studies generated knowledge that has the potential to improve the care provided to patients and their families.

Builds on Previous Research

A significant study problem and purpose are based on previous research. In a research article, the introduction and literature review sections include relevant studies that provide a basis for a study. Often a summary of the current literature indicates what is known and not known in the area being studied. The gaps in the current knowledge base provide support for and document the significance of the study's purpose. For example, Foster-Fitzpatrick et al. (1999) provided documentation from a variety of sources that blood pressure (BP) measurement was influenced by numerous factors. However, what was not known was the effect of crossing the leg at the knee on the systolic and diastolic BP measurements of hypertensive patients. What was not known about the topic of BP measurement became the focus of the Foster-Fitzpatrick et al. (1999) study. The intent was to generate additional knowledge to improve the assessment of hypertensive patients' BP measurements in clinical settings.

Promotes Theory Testing or Development

Significant problems and purposes are supported by theory, and the study may focus on either testing or developing theory (Chinn & Kramer, 1998). For example, Jemmott and Jemmott (1991) tested the theory of reasoned action (Ajzen & Fishbein, 1980) in their study of condom use among black women. They tested the following proposition or relational statement from the theory: "A behavioral intention is seen as determined by the attitude toward the specific behavior and the subjective norm regarding that behavior" (p. 228). They then linked the proposition to their study by stating: "Thus, a woman's intention to use condoms is a function of her attitude—positive or negative—toward using condoms and her perception of what significant others [subjective norm] think she should do" (p. 229). Based on this theoretical proposition, Jemmott and Jemmott (1991) developed the following hypotheses:

"First, women who express more favorable attitudes toward condoms will report stronger intentions to use condoms than will women who express less favorable attitudes. Second, women who perceive subjective norms [significant others] more supportive of condom use will report stronger intentions to use condoms than will their counterparts who perceive subjective norms less supportive of condom use." (pp. 229-230)

By conducting this study, Jemmott and Jemmott (1991) tested the theory of reasoned action to determine its usefulness in describing people's attitudes and behavior about condom use. The study findings supported the hypotheses that attitudes and perceived subjective norms influence black women's use of condoms. Thus the proposition from the theory was supported.

Addresses Nursing Research Priorities

Since 1975, expert researchers, specialty groups, and funding agencies have identified a variety of nursing research priorities. Lindeman (1975) developed an initial list of research priorities for clinical practice that included nursing interventions focused on care of the elderly, pain management, and patient education. Nurses continue research in these areas today, with the goal of developing evidence-based nursing practice.

Many professional organizations have identified research priorities that are communicated through their web sites. For example, the American Association of Critical-Care Nurses (AACN) published its most current research priorities on its web site, at http://www.aacn.org/. These priorities include the following: (1) effective and appropriate use of technology to achieve optimal patient assessment, management, and outcomes; (2) creation of a healing, humane environment; (3) development of processes and systems that foster the optimal contribution of critical-care nurses; (4) effective approaches to symptom management; and (5) prevention and management of complications. This web site might be of assistance when determining the significance of studies conducted in the area of critical care.

The American Organization of Nurse Executives (AONE) established the following research priorities for the year 2000: (1) workforce, (2) patient care advocacy, and (3) technology. The workforce topic includes research focused on diversity, composition, professional growth, accountability, and recruitment and retention. Patient care advocacy includes research to address such areas as: relationships in the community, among health professionals, and in health care settings; efficient use of resources, new management methods, and techniques; and improvement in healthcare processes and outcomes across the continuum. In the area of technology, investigations need to examine the outcomes of technology adaptations, systems improvement and infrastructure changes to accommodate new technology, and leadership in managing technological change. AONE provides a discussion of their research priorities on their web site at: http://www.aone.org/practiceresearch/research_priorities.htm.

A major nursing research funding agency is the National Institute for Nursing Research (NINR). The NINR develops the National Nursing Research Agenda, which includes the following: identifying nursing research priorities, outlining a plan for implementing priority studies, and obtaining resources to support these priority projects. NINR has developed four goals to direct the institute's activities over 5 years (2000-2004). Goal 1 is to identify and support research opportunities that will achieve scientific distinction and produce significant contributions to health. The priority areas selected include the following: end of life and palliative care research, chronic illness experiences, quality of life and quality of care, health promotion and disease prevention research, symptom management of illness and treatment, telehealth interventions and monitoring, and cultural and ethnic considerations in health and illness. Goal 2 is to identify and support future areas of opportunity to advance research on high quality, cost-effective care and to contribute to the scientific base for nursing practice. The priorities related to this goal include research of the following: chronic illness and long-term care, health promotion and risk behaviors, cardiopulmonary health and critical care, neurofunction and sensory conditions, immune responses and oncology, and reproductive and infant health. Goal 3 is to communicate and disseminate research findings resulting from NINR-funded research, and Goal 4 is to enhance the development of nurse researchers though training and career development opportunities. Details about NINR mission, goals, and areas of funding are available on their web site at: http://www.nih.gov/ninr/.

Another federal agency that is funding health care research is the Agency for Healthcare Research and Quality (AHRQ), formerly the Agency for Health Care Policy and Research (AHCPR). The purpose of AHRQ is to enhance the quality, appropriateness, and effectiveness of health care services, as well as the access to such services, through the establishment of a broad base of scientific research and through the promotion of improvements in clinical practice and in the organization, financing, and delivery of health care services. Some of the current funding priorities are research on the effectiveness of children's mental health and substance abuse; cancer prevention, screening, and care; care at the end of life; and primary care practice. For a complete list of funding opportunities and grant announcements, see the AHRQ web site at http://www.ahcpr.gov.

Expert researchers, professional organizations, and federal agencies have identified research priorities to direct the future conduct of health care research. When critiquing a study, the focus should be on determining whether the problem and purpose are based on previous research, theory, and current research priorities. Whether the findings will have an impact on nursing practice should also be determined. These four elements discussed in this section document the significance of the study in developing and refining nursing knowledge.

EXAMINING THE FEASIBILITY OF A PROBLEM AND PURPOSE

When critiquing a study, the feasibility of the problem and the purpose of the study should be determined. The feasibility of a research problem and purpose is determined by examining the researchers' expertise; money commitment; availability of subjects, facilities, and equipment; and the study's ethical considerations (Kahn, 1994; Rogers, 1987). The feasibility of the Foster-Fitzpatrick et al. (1999) study of the effects of crossed legs on blood pressure measurement is critiqued and presented as an example.

Researcher Expertise

The research problem and purpose studied need to be within the area of expertise of the researchers. Research articles usually identify the education of the researchers and their current positions. This information indicates their research expertise and their area of clinical specialization.

The following questions might be used to assess the researchers' expertise in a research report:

1. **Were the researchers adequately prepared to conduct the study?** Nurses with a doctorate degree, who have a strong background in conducting research, often collaborate with master's-prepared nurses, who have strong clinical expertise, to conduct studies.
2. **Do the researchers have the clinical experience or expertise to conduct the study?**
3. **Do the researchers cite other studies they have conducted in this area?**
4. **Do the researchers acknowledge the assistance of others in the conduct of the study?**

Five nurses collaborated to study the effects of crossed legs on blood pressure measurement in 100 hypertensive male subjects (Foster-Fitzpatrick et al., 1999). The lead author, Foster-Fitzpatrick, was master's-prepared and a case manager in a major hospital. The second author, Ortiz, was a baccalaureate-prepared nurse, who was also a case manager in the same clinical agency. Sibilano was a doctorally prepared pulmonary clinical nurse specialist, Marcantonio was a doctorally prepared senior quality assurance analyst, and Braun was a doctorally prepared professor and nurse practitioner. These authors' credentials and positions indicate strong research and clinical expertise for conducting this study. This study demonstrates that nurses of all levels of educational preparation (bachelor to doctoral degree) can have an active role in the conduct of research.

Money Commitment

The problem and purpose studied are influenced by the amount of money available to the researcher. The cost of a research project can range from a few dollars for a student's small study to hundreds of thousands of dollars for complex projects. When critiquing a study, one of the points that should be analyzed is whether the researchers' financial resources were adequate to complete a quality study.

Sources of funding for a study are usually identified in the article. For example, the study might have been funded by a federal research grant or by a professional organization such as Sigma Theta Tau or the American Nurses Association. The researchers might have received financial assistance from companies that provided necessary equipment. Receiving funding for a study indicates that it was reviewed by peers, who chose to support the research financially. Foster-Fitzpatrick et al. (1999) did not indicate that their study was funded; however, this study could have been accomplished without external funding. The agencies where these individuals work probably provided support for data collection, entry, and analysis.

Availability of Subjects, Facilities, and Equipment

Researchers need to have adequate sample size, facilities, and equipment to implement their study. Most published studies indicate the sample size and setting(s) in the methods section of the research report.

The following questions might be used to assess the adequacy of the sample, setting, and equipment:
1. Was the sample size adequate to address the research purpose?
2. Was the facility appropriate and adequate for the research problem and purpose?
3. Was an adequate sample size obtained from the designated setting?
4. Did the study require a highly specialized laboratory, or was a natural setting appropriate?
5. Did the study require special equipment?
6. Was adequate equipment obtained to conduct the study?
7. Did the equipment function accurately during the study?

Most nursing studies are conducted in natural or partially controlled settings, such as a home, hospital unit, or clinic. Many of these facilities are easy to access, and the hospitals and clinics provide access to large numbers of patients. Foster-Fitzpatrick et al. (1999) obtained an adequate sample size of 100 hypertensive male patients from outpatient medical clinics of a Veterans Administration medical center.

Review the methods section of the research article to determine if adequate, accurate equipment was available. Nursing studies frequently require a limited amount of equipment, such as a tape or video recorder for interviews, or physiological instruments, such as an electrocardiogram (ECG) or thermometer. The Foster-Fitzpatrick et al. (1999) study required the following equipment: (1) A blood pressure (BP) monitor, IVAC Vital.Check® Vital Signs Measurement System, Model 4200 and (2) two cuff sizes, normal adult (24 × 42 cm) and large adult (33 × 56 cm). Before the beginning of the study, the BP monitor was calibrated for accuracy according to the IVAC Corporation Service Manual.

Ethical Considerations

The purpose selected for investigation must be ethical, which means that the subjects' rights and the rights of others in the setting are protected (Burns & Grove, 2001).

The following questions might be used to assess the ethical nature of a study:

1. Does the study purpose appear to infringe upon the rights of the subjects? There are usually some risks in every study, but the value of the knowledge generated should outweigh the risks.
2. Was it ethical to conduct this study based on the risks and benefits?
3. What is the benefit-risk ratio for the study? Chapter 6 includes the steps for determining the benefit-risk ratio of a study.

In the Foster-Fitzpatrick et al. (1999) study, the benefits of determining the effects of crossed legs on blood pressure measurement are significant in diagnosing and treating hypertension. The risks of the study are minimal and might include time, fatigue, and arm pressure caused by additional BP measurements. The subjects gave their verbal consent to participation in the study. Thus the researchers appeared to have protected the rights of the subjects and implemented a study where the benefits greatly outweigh the risks.

CRITIQUING PROBLEMS AND PURPOSES IN PUBLISHED STUDIES

The problem and purpose should be clearly and concisely expressed in a published study. In addition, the significance and feasibility of the problem and purpose should be examined.

The following questions might be helpful in critiquing the problem and purpose in a study.

1. Is the problem clearly and concisely expressed early in the study?
2. Is the problem sufficiently delimited in scope without being trivial?
3. Is the purpose clearly expressed?
4. Does the purpose narrow and clarify the focus or aim of the study?
5. Does the purpose identify the variables, population, and setting for the study?
6. Are the problem and purpose significant in generating nursing knowledge? Is the study based on previous research, theory, and current research priorities? Will the findings have an impact on nursing practice?
7. Was it feasible for the researchers to study the problem and purpose identified? Did the researchers have the expertise to conduct the study? Did they have adequate money, subjects, setting, and equipment to conduct the study? Was the purpose of the study ethical?

EXAMINING RESEARCH OBJECTIVES, QUESTIONS, AND HYPOTHESES IN RESEARCH REPORTS

Research objectives, questions, and hypotheses evolve from the problem, purpose, and study framework, and direct the remaining steps of the research process. In a published study the objectives, questions, or hypotheses are usually presented after the literature review section and right before the methods section. The content in this section is provided to assist in identifying and critiquing objectives, questions, and hypotheses in published studies.

Research Objectives

A *research objective* is a clear, concise, declarative statement that is expressed in the present tense. For clarity, an objective usually focuses on one or two variables and indicates whether they are to be identified or described. Sometimes the purpose of objectives is to identify relationships among variables or to determine differences between two groups regarding selected variables. Sometimes the purpose statement is divided into two or three objectives. A descriptive study by Brown (1997) demonstrates the logical flow from research problem and purpose to research objectives.

Research Problem

"In the United States, cardiovascular disorders cause more deaths among adults than all other diseases combined. Approximately one third of all deaths in the United States are caused by ischemic heart disease, and of these, one half result from an acute myocardial infarction (AMI).... Today, there is a new population at risk for the development of cardiovascular disease, the cocaine user.... The use of cocaine as a recreational drug by young adults has increased markedly since the early 1980s and has resulted in a significant increase in hospital emergency room admissions, mortality, and morbidity.... Traditionally, only case studies, animal studies, and small samples of patients with AMI attributed to cocaine use have been reported. **Little is known about chest pain syndromes after cocaine use, the patient's clinical symptomatology in the emergency department, or the risk factor profile of the cocaine user.**" (p. 136)

Research Purpose

"The purpose of this study was to examine the incidence of chest pain and cocaine use in 18-40 year olds who were seen in a public inner city emergency department." (p. 136)

Research Objectives

The objectives of this study were expressed in a detailed purpose statement indicating that the study was conducted "(1) to describe the incidence of cocaine use in 18-40 year old persons seen in a hospital emergency department with complaints of chest pain, and (2) to determine if there is a relationship among demographics, physiological, diagnostic, and patient history data associated with chest pain and cocaine use." (p. 136)

The cardiac problems that were identified by Brown (1997) as occurring with cocaine use are a significant health care concern that is increasing in prevalence in today's society. The purpose of Brown's (1997) study identifies the goal or aim of the research and includes the study variables (cocaine use and risk profile of the cocaine user), population (cocaine users with chest pain), and setting (emergency departments). The purpose of the first objective is to describe the incidence of cocaine use (variable) in 18- to 40-year-old individuals who complain of chest pain and are seen in hospital emergency departments. The second objective focuses on the examination of relationships among selected variables that comprise the risk-factor profile of a cocaine user (demographic, physiological, diagnostic, and patient history data) and the incidence of chest pain occurring with cocaine use. The problem statement (bold print in the example) provides a basis for the purpose, and the objectives evolve from the purpose and clearly indicate the focus of the study.

Research Questions

A *research question* is a concise interrogative statement that is worded in the present tense and includes one or more variables (or concepts). The foci of research questions are description of variable(s) or concept(s), examination of relationships among variables, and determination of differences between two or more groups regarding selected variable(s). Bostrom et al. (1996) conducted a descriptive correlational study to examine the nursing practices, costs, and outcomes of preventing the breakdown of skin. The problem, purpose, and research questions used to guide this study are logically developed and clearly expressed.

Research Problem

"Operating efficiently within the constraints of shrinking financial parameters is a major concern of nursing administrators. Nurses are challenged to determine not only which nursing interventions are effective but also the cost impact of the various interventions. One nursing intervention that holds great potential for possible refinement of protocol and resultant cost reduction is prevention and management of skin breakdown. The cost of treatments for maintaining skin

Continued

integrity ranges from $20 for a barrier dressing to several thousand dollars for a specialty bed.... A variety of intervention studies aimed at prevention of pressure sores have been conducted with patients identified at risk for altered skin integrity.... **Cost analyses related to the use of these various interventions have not been published."** (Bostrom et al., 1996, pp. 184-185)

Research Purpose

"The specific purpose of the investigation was to assess the relationships between the development of pressure ulcers during acute hospitalization and (a) skin breakdown risk and (b) types and costs of prevention strategies used by nurses." (p. 184)

Research Questions

The following questions were addressed in this study:
1. "What is the relationship between the Braden risk-factors scores for skin breakdown and actual skin breakdown in acute settings?
2. What is the relationship between the Braden risk-factors scores for skin breakdown and the strategies chosen for prevention of skin breakdown?
3. What is the relationship of both Braden risk-factors scores and strategies chosen for prevention of skin breakdown to actual skin breakdown?
4. What are the costs of skin breakdown prevention strategies?" (p. 185)

Skin breakdown is a significant health care problem that requires cost-effective nursing interventions to prevent. The research purpose clearly identifies the aim of the study: to examine the relationships between the development of pressure ulcers and skin breakdown risk and the types and costs of prevention strategies (variables) used on patients (population) during acute hospitalization (setting). The first, second, and third research questions focus on examining relationships (associations) among the study variables (Braden risk-factors scores for skin breakdown, incidence of skin breakdown, and prevention strategies). The fourth research question focuses on describing the costs of strategies to prevent skin breakdown. The research questions reflect the problem statement (in bold in the example) and purpose and clearly indicate the focus of the study. These questions were presented immediately before the methods section of the article and were used to direct the implementation of the study procedures and the analysis of study data.

Qualitative researchers sometimes identify research questions to focus their studies. The questions in qualitative studies identify the variable(s) or concept(s) that will be examined, and often clarify the focus of the study, which might be describing a lived experience, understanding a health practice in a specific culture, or clarifying the history of a nursing intervention. Orne et al. (2000) conducted a phenomenological study of medically-uninsured, working Americans. The problem and purpose of this study were presented earlier in Table 3-2. The researchers also state an objective (aim) and question to direct their study.

> "The aim was to heighten nurses' awareness, broaden understanding and answer the question: What is the lived experience of being employed but medically uninsured?" (Orne et al., 2000, p. 205)

The aim of this qualitative study was to increase awareness and understanding in nurses of the problem of employed, medically-uninsured Americans. The focus was also on describing the lived experience of being uninsured for these individuals. Describing the lived experience of individuals related to a particular phenomenon is the common focus of phenomenological research (Munhall, 2001).

Hypotheses

A *hypothesis* is a formal statement of the expected relationship(s) between two or more variables in a specified population. The hypothesis translates the research problem and purpose into a clear explanation or prediction of the expected results or outcomes of the study. A clearly stated hypothesis includes the variables to be manipulated or measured, identifies the population to be examined, and indicates the proposed outcomes for the study. Hypotheses also influence the study design, sampling technique, data collection and analysis methods, and interpretation of findings. In this section, types of hypotheses are described and a testable hypothesis is discussed.

Types of Hypotheses

Different types of relationships and numbers of variables are identified in hypotheses. A study might have one, three, five, or more hypotheses, depending on its complexity. The type of hypothesis developed is based on the purpose of the study. Hypotheses can be described using four categories: (1) associative versus causal, (2) simple versus complex, (3) nondirectional versus directional and (4) null versus research.

Associative versus causal hypotheses. The relationships identified in hypotheses are associative or causal. An *associative hypothesis* proposes relationships among variables that occur or exist together in the real world, and when one variable changes, the other changes (Reynolds, 1971). Associative hypotheses are usually expressed using the following formats:

1. Variable X is related to variables Y and Z in a specified population (predicts relationships among variables but does not indicate the types of relationships).
2. Variable X increases as variable Y increases in a specified population (predicts a positive relationship).
3. Variable X decreases as variable Y decreases in a specified population (predicts a positive relationship).
4. Variable X increases as variable Y decreases in a specified population (predicts a negative relationship).

Associative hypotheses identify relationships among variables in a study but do not indicate that one variable causes an effect on another variable. Lanza, Kayne, Pattison, Hicks, and Islam (1996) studied the relationship between behavioral cues and assaultive behavior and formulated the following problem, purpose, and associative hypotheses.

Research Problem

"Violence is now the Center for Disease Control's (CDC's) top priority (Rosenberg, 1993). Assault by patients on other patients and staff is reaching epidemic proportions both within hospital units and outpatient areas. The high rate of assault is a significant problem across types of institutions.... The assault rate increase in hospitals, reflecting the rising violence in society, has become a major public health problem.... **Better understanding of the problem of assaultive behavior will enable clinicians to make more accurate assessments and design more effective interventions to reduce assault incidence.**" (pp. 6-7)

Research Purpose

"The purpose of this study was to characterize patients who assaulted one or more times during the period of observation and to compare them to patients who had not assaulted. Factors compared were behavioral assessments and sociodemographic variables." (p. 8)

Hypotheses

"1. Patients who assault during the period of observation will differ from patients who do not in being more likely to have a history of violence and being more likely to have a history of alcohol abuse;
2. Patients who assault will exhibit more visibility cues (hostile verbalizations, increased motor activity, suspiciousness) than will nonassaultive patients;
3. Patients who assault and exhibit high-visibility cues (hostile verbalization, increased motor activity, suspiciousness) will score lower on the Withdrawal-Retardation Subscale...." (p. 10)

The problem indicates the area of concern, that is, violence in health care settings, and the need for further study to manage this problem (see problem statement in **boldface**). The purpose is based on the problem and clearly identifies the goal of the study. The purpose also identifies the study variables (assaults, behavioral assessment, and socio-demographic variables) and population (patients) and indicates the setting (hospital). Hypotheses 1 and 2 state positive associations, which means that as one variable increases, there is an increase in other variables. Hypothesis 1 predicts that an increase in assaults is associated with an increase in history of violence and alcohol abuse (positive [+] relationship).

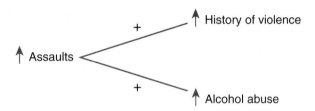

Hypothesis 2 predicts that an increase in assaults is related to an increase in visibility cues (positive [+] relationship).

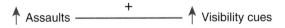

Hypothesis 3 predicts that patients who commit more assaults and demonstrate high-visibility cues have lower scores on the Withdrawal-retardation subscale (negative [−] or inverse relationship).

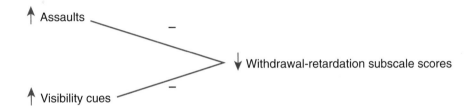

These hypotheses clearly identify the study variables and population and indicate the study outcomes. The results from the study only partially supported the hypotheses. Assaultive behavior was linked to a history of violence but not to alcohol dependence. Threatening language and increased motor activity were important signs of assault, but suspiciousness was not. There was no difference between the scores of the assaultive and nonassaultive patients on the Withdrawal-Retardation Subscale (Lanza et al., 1996).

A *causal hypothesis* proposes a cause-and-effect interaction between two or more variables, which are referred to as independent and dependent variables. The independent variable (treatment or experimental variable) is manipulated by the researcher to cause an effect on the dependent variable. The dependent variable (outcome or criterion variable) is measured to examine the effect created by the independent variable. A format for stating a causal hypothesis is the following: The subjects in the experimental group, who are exposed to the independent variable demonstrate greater change, as measured by the dependent variable, than do the subjects in the control group, who are not exposed to the independent variable.

Artinian et al. (2001, p. 191) studied the "effects of the home telemonitoring and community-based monitoring on blood pressure control in urban African Americans." The causal hypothesis on the following page was used to direct their study.

"Persons who participate in nurse-managed home telemonitoring (HT) plus usual care or who participate in nurse-managed community-based monitoring (CBM) plus usual care will have greater improvement in blood pressure (BP) from baseline to 3 months' follow-up than will persons who receive usual care only." (p. 191)

The independent variables are the two types of nurse-managed BP monitoring, HT and CBM, and the dependent variable is BP control. The population is clearly identified as African Americans with hypertension, who were recruited from a family community center in Detroit (setting). The findings from this study supported the hypothesis, indicating that the two monitoring interventions were effective in improving BP control in hypertensive African Americans. A causal arrow (➜) is used to show the relationship among these independent and dependent variables.

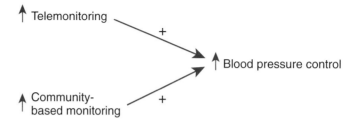

Simple versus complex hypotheses. A *simple hypothesis* states the relationship (associative or causal) between two variables. Moser and Dracup (2000) studied the impact of cardiopulmonary resuscitation (CPR) training on the perception of control felt by the spouses of patients recovering from cardiac disease. These researchers stated two simple hypotheses to direct their study.

Hypothesis 1: Higher levels of perceived control would be associated with less emotional distress in spouses of patients recovering from cardiac disease.

Hypothesis 2: CPR training would enhance the level of perceived control in spouses of patients recovering from cardiac disease.

Hypothesis 1 is associative and simple, and it states a negative or inverse relationship between two variables.

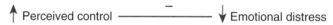

Hypothesis 2 is causal and simple and states that the independent variable (CPR) would cause an increase in the dependent variable (perceived control).

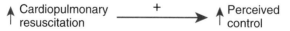

A *complex hypothesis* predicts the relationship (associative or causal) among three or more variables. Artinian et al. (2001) stated a complex, causal hypothesis that includes two independent variables and one dependent variable. The hypothesis and the variables are identified in Table 3-4. Moore and Dolansky (2001) conducted a quasi-experimental study "to test the effects of an early home recovery information intervention on physical functioning, psychological distress, and symptom frequency 1 month following coronary artery bypass graft surgery (CABG)" (p. 93). This complex, causal hypothesis is presented in Table 3-4, which identifies the number and types of variables studied.

A *nondirectional hypothesis* states that a relationship exists but does not predict the nature of the relationship. If the direction of the relationship being studied is not clear in clinical practice or in the theoretical or empirical literature, the researcher has no clear indication of the nature of the relationship. Under these circumstances, nondirectional hypotheses are developed, such as those developed by Jirovec and Kasno (1990) to direct their study.

"1. Elderly nursing home residents' self-appraisals of their self-care abilities are related to the basic conditioning factors of sex [gender], socio-cultural orientation, health, and family influences.

2. Elderly nursing home residents' self-appraisals of their self-care abilities are related to their perceptions of the nursing-home environment." (p. 304)

TABLE 3-4

COMPLEX, CAUSAL HYPOTHESES AND THEIR VARIABLES

HYPOTHESES	INDEPENDENT VARIABLES	DEPENDENT VARIABLES
"Persons who participate in nurse-managed home telemonitoring (HT) plus usual care or who participate in nurse-managed community-based monitoring (CBM) plus usual care will have greater improvement in blood pressure from baseline to 3 months' follow-up than will persons who receive usual care only." (Artinian, Washington, & Templin, 2001, p. 191)	Home telemonitoring Community-based monitoring	Blood pressure
"Both men and women who participated in the CHIP (Cardiac Home Information Program) intervention would have lower levels of psychological distress, higher levels of physical functioning, and fewer adverse symptoms than would women and men who did not participate in such a program." (Moore & Dolansky, 2001, p. 94)	Cardiac Home Information Program (CHIP)	Psychological distress Physical functioning Adverse symptoms

The first hypothesis is complex (five variables), associative, and nondirectional. The second hypothesis is simple (two variables), associative, and nondirectional. Both hypotheses state that a relationship exists but do not indicate the direction of the relationship. The hypotheses also clearly identify the study variables (self-appraisals of self-care abilities, basic conditioning factors, and perceptions of nursing-home environment), population (elderly), and setting (nursing home) and indicate the expected outcomes of the study.

A *directional hypothesis* states the nature (positive or negative) of the interaction between two or more variables. Directional hypotheses are developed from theoretical statements (propositions), findings of previous studies, and clinical experience. As the knowledge on which a study is based increases, the researcher is able to make a prediction about the direction of a relationship between the variables being studied. For example, Baker, Garvin, Kennedy, and Polivka (1993) developed a directional hypothesis to study the effect of environmental sound and communication on the heart rate (HR) and BP of patients in the coronary care unit. They developed their study hypothesis from previous research and theory, as indicated by the following quotation:

> "Overall, the findings of previous studies suggest that ambient and social stressors in coronary care are associated with cardiovascular (CV) changes in patients. However, it is not known if different CV effects occur with background sounds than with communication. Since stress is viewed as a person-environment relationship (Lazarus, Delongis, Folkman, & Gruen, 1985), the goal of this study was to examine factors in the natural environment that are associated with the stress response. The assumption was made that naturally occurring sounds, such as conversation and equipment, have personal meaning to subjects. The patient appraises the meaning through cognitive processes which in turn can produce autonomic CV arousal. Data suggest that persons with CV disease are more reactive to mental stress than persons without CV disease (Contrada & Krantz, 1988). It was *hypothesized* [emphasis added] that there would be an increase in patients' HR and BP during the high ambient stressors (environmental sounds) and social stressors (room and hall conversation) as compared to low ambient (background) sounds." (p. 416)

The use of terms such as *less, more, increase, decrease, greater, higher,* and *lower* in a hypothesis indicates the direction of the relationship. In Baker et al.'s (1993) complex, associative, directional hypothesis, environmental sounds and room and hall conversation are positively related to patient HR and BP. Thus as the environmental sounds and room and hall conversation increase, the patient's HR and BP increase.

A causal hypothesis predicts the effect of an independent variable on a dependent variable, specifying the direction of the relationship. The independent variable either increases or decreases each dependent variable. Thus all causal hypotheses are directional. Examine the causal hypotheses in Table 3-4 and note the effect of the independent variables on the dependent variables in these two studies.

Null versus research hypotheses. The *null hypothesis* (H_0), also referred to as a *statistical hypothesis,* is used for statistical testing and for interpreting statistical outcomes. Even if the null hypothesis is not stated, it is implied, because it is the converse of the research hypothesis (Kerlinger & Lee, 1999). Some researchers state the null hypothesis because it is more easily interpreted based on the results of statistical analyses. The null hypothesis is also used when the researcher believes there is no relationship between two variables and when there is inadequate theoretical or empirical information to state a research hypothesis.

A null hypothesis can be simple or complex and associative or causal. An example of a simple, associative, null hypothesis is the following: "There is no relationship between the number of experiences performing a developmental assessment skill and learning of the skill" (Koniak, 1985, p. 85). Fahs and Kinney (1991) developed the following causal, null hypothesis to direct their study: "There is no difference in the occurrence of bruise at injection site with low-dose heparin therapy when administered in three different subcutaneous sites [abdomen, thigh, and arm]" (p. 204). There was no statistically significant difference in bruising at 60 and 72 hours post-injection for the three sites. Thus this null hypothesis was supported and provides direction for giving heparin in clinical practice.

A *research hypothesis* is the alternative hypothesis (H_1 or H_A) to the null hypothesis and states that there is a relationship between two or more variables. All the hypotheses stated in previous sections of this chapter were research hypotheses. Research hypotheses can be simple or complex, nondirectional or directional, and associative or causal. Jadack, Hyde, and Keller (1995) formulated both research and null hypotheses to "examine gender differences in knowledge about HIV, the reported incidence of risky sexual behavior, and comfort with safer sexual practices among young adults" (p. 313). The hypotheses might be more clearly and concisely stated in the present tense versus the future tense. Each of the hypotheses is listed with a description indicating the type of hypothesis.

1. "There will be (is) no difference between men and women in knowledge about HIV transmission routes (sexual, needle sharing, casual)" (Jadack et al., 1995, p. 315). The type of hypothesis is null, associative, simple, and nondirectional, with two variables of gender and knowledge about HIV transmission routes.
2. "[T]here will be (is) no difference between men and women in knowledge about the effectiveness of measures to prevent sexual transmission of HI." (Jadack et al., 1995, p. 315). The type of hypothesis is null, simple, associative, and nondirectional, with two variables of gender and knowledge about effectiveness of measures to prevent sexual transmission of HIV.

Continued

3. "[M]en and women will differ with respect to reported frequency and type of behaviors that could lead to the transmission of HIV" (Jadack et al., 1995, p. 315). This hypothesis is research, associative, complex, and nondirectional. The variables are gender, frequency of behaviors, and types of behaviors. This hypothesis is nondirectional because there is no indication of how men and women will differ and associative because a relationship is stated with no indication of cause and effect.

4. "[M]en and women will differ with respect to reported level of comfort and safer sexual practices" (Jadack et al., 1995, p. 315). This hypothesis is research, complex, associative, and nondirectional. The variables are gender, level of comfort, and safer sexual practices. The hypothesis is nondirectional, with no indication of how men and women will differ, and associative because the relationship does not indicate cause and effect between variables.

Testable Hypothesis

A testable hypothesis is clearly stated, predicting a relationship between two or more variables. Hypotheses are clearer without the phrase, "There is no *significant* difference," because the level of significance is only a statistical technique applied to sample data. In addition, hypotheses should not identify methodological points, such as techniques of sampling, measurement, and data analysis (Kerlinger & Lee, 1999). Therefore such phrases as *"measured by,"* "in a *random sample* of," and *"using ANOVA"* (analysis of variance) are inappropriate since they limit the hypotheses to the measurement methods, sample, or analysis techniques identified for one study. In addition, hypotheses need to reflect the variables and population outlined in the research purpose and should be expressed in the present tense, not the future tense. Expressing the hypotheses in the present tense does not limit them to the study being conducted and enables them to be used in additional research.

The value of a hypothesis is ultimately derived from whether it is testable in the real world. A *testable hypothesis* is one that contains variables that are measurable or able to be manipulated. Thus the independent variable must be clearly defined, often by a protocol, so that it can be implemented precisely and consistently as a treatment in the study. The dependent variable must be precisely defined to indicate how it will be accurately measured.

A testable hypothesis also needs to predict a relationship that can be "supported" or "not supported" based on data collection and analysis. If the hypothesis states an associative relationship, correlational analyses are conducted on the data to determine the existence, type, and strength of the relationship between the variables studied. The hypothesis that states a causal link between the independent and dependent variables is evaluated using statistics that examine differences between the experimental and control groups, such as the *t*-test and ANOVA. It is the null hypothesis (stated or implied) that is tested to determine whether the independent variable produced a significant effect on the dependent variable.

CRITIQUING RESEARCH OBJECTIVES, QUESTIONS, AND HYPOTHESES IN PUBLISHED STUDIES

The research objectives, questions, and hypotheses need to be clearly focused and concisely expressed in studies. Both objectives and questions are used in qualitative studies and descriptive and correlational quantitative studies, but questions are more common. Some correlational studies focus on predicting relationships and might include hypotheses. Quasi-experimental and experimental studies need to be directed by hypotheses.

The following questions might be helpful during a critique of the objectives, questions, and hypotheses in a study.

1. Are the objectives, questions, or hypotheses formally stated in the study? If they were not stated, were they needed to direct the conduct of the study? If the study is quasi-experimental or experimental, hypotheses are needed to direct the study.
2. Are the objectives, questions, or hypotheses clearly focused and concisely expressed in the study? Do they clearly identify the variables and population to be studied?
3. Are the study objectives, questions, or hypotheses based on the purpose? They should not contain new concepts or variables that were not identified in the problem or purpose.
4. Are the variables and relationships among the variables identified in the objectives, questions, or hypotheses linked to the study framework?
5. Does each hypothesis predict a relationship between the variables?
6. Are the hypotheses associative or causal, simple or complex, directional or nondirectional, and research or null?
7. Are the hypotheses testable in this study? Thus are they clearly stated in the present tense, with measurable dependent variables and appropriate independent variables that can be consistently implemented during the study?

UNDERSTANDING STUDY VARIABLES

The research purpose and objectives, questions, and hypotheses include the variables or concepts to be examined in a study. *Variables* are qualities, properties, or characteristics of persons, things, or situations that change or vary. Variables are also concepts at different levels of abstraction that are concisely defined to promote their measurement or manipulation within a study (Chinn & Kramer, 1998). In this section, different types of variables are described, and conceptual and operational definitions of variables are discussed.

Types of Variables

Variables are classified into a variety of types to explain their use in research. Some variables are manipulated; others are controlled. Some variables are identified but not measured; others are measured with refined measurement devices. The types of variables presented in this section include independent, dependent, research, extraneous, and demographic.

Independent and Dependent Variables

The relationship between independent and dependent variables is the basis for formulating hypotheses for correlational, quasi-experimental, and experimental studies. An *independent variable* is a stimulus or activity that is manipulated or varied by the researcher to create an effect on the dependent variable. The independent variable is also called a *treatment* or *experimental variable*. A *dependent variable* is the response, behavior, or outcome that the researcher wants to predict or explain. Changes in the dependent variable are presumed to be caused by the independent variable.

The null hypothesis tested by Lim-Levy (1982) was the following: "Oxygen inhalation by nasal cannula of up to 6 LPM [liters per minute] does not affect oral temperature" (p. 150). The independent variable is oxygen inhalation by nasal cannula, and the oxygen was administered at three levels: 2, 4, and 6 LPM. The dependent variable was oral temperature measured by an electronic thermometer. This null hypothesis was supported in the study, indicating that oxygen inhalation by nasal cannula does not affect oral temperature. These findings provide clear direction for a nurse, while taking the temperature of a patient who is receiving oxygen nasally.

Research Variables or Concepts

Qualitative studies and some quantitative (descriptive and correlational) studies involve the investigation of research variables or concepts. *Research variables* or *concepts* are the qualities, properties, or characteristics identified in the research purpose and objectives or questions that are observed or measured in a study. Research variables or concepts are used when the intent of the study is to observe or measure variables as they exist in a natural setting without the implementation of a treatment. Thus no independent variables are manipulated, and no cause-and-effect relationships are examined. Logan and Jenny (1997) conducted a qualitative study to describe patients' recollections of their experiences during mechanical ventilation and weaning, and to extend an evolving nursing theory of weaning. The authors used grounded theory techniques to investigate the following concepts: (1) experiences with mechanical ventilation and (2) experiences during weaning.

Extraneous Variables

Extraneous variables exist in all studies and can affect the measurement of study variables and the relationships among these variables. Extraneous variables are of primary concern in quantitative studies because they can interfere with obtaining a clear understanding of the relational or causal dynamics within these studies. These variables are classified as recognized or unrecognized and controlled or uncontrolled. Some extraneous variables are not recognized until the study is in progress or is completed, but their presence influences the study outcome.

Researchers attempt to recognize and control as many extraneous variables as possible in quasi-experimental and experimental studies, and specific designs have been developed to control the influence of these variables. Lim-Levy (1982) controlled some of the extraneous variables in her study of the effect of oxygen inhalation by nasal cannula on oral temperature with specific sample exclusion criteria. The subjects who were mouth breathing or hyperventilating or who had an oral inflammatory process were excluded, because these characteristics might have influenced the oral temperature.

The extraneous variables that are not recognized until the study is in process, or are recognized before the study is initiated but cannot be controlled, are referred to as *confounding variables*. Sometimes extraneous variables can be measured during the study and controlled statistically during analysis. Analysis of covariance (ANCOVA) was used by Moore and Dolansky (2001) to control the effects of the extraneous variables of age, comorbidity, and presurgical cardiac functional status that might have influenced the outcomes from a Cardiac Home Information Program (CHIP), which was provided to patients who had coronary artery bypass graft (CABG) surgery. However, extraneous variables that cannot be controlled or measured are a design weakness and can hinder the interpretation of findings. As control in quasi-experimental and experimental studies decreases, the potential influence of confounding variables increases.

Environmental variables are a type of extraneous variable composing the setting in which the study is conducted. Examples of these variables include climate, family, health care system, and governmental organizations. If a researcher is studying humans in an uncontrolled or natural setting, it is impossible and undesirable to control all the extraneous variables. In qualitative and some quantitative (descriptive and correlational) studies, little or no attempt is made to control extraneous variables. The intent is to study subjects in their natural environment without controlling or altering that setting or situation. The environmental variables in quasi-experimental and experimental research can be controlled by using a laboratory setting or a specially constructed research unit in a hospital. Environmental control is an extremely important part of conducting an experimental study.

Demographic Variables

Demographic variables are characteristics or attributes of subjects that are collected to describe the sample. Some common demographic variables are age, education, gender, ethnic origin (race), marital status, income, job classification, and medical diagnosis(es). When a study is completed, the demographic data are analyzed to provide a picture of the sample and are called *sample characteristics*. A study's sample characteristics can be presented in table format or narrative. As discussed earlier in this chapter, Moore and Dolansky (2001) conducted a randomized trial of a home recovery intervention following CABG surgery in a sample of 180 patients. The demographic variables examined in this study included age, education, number of grafts, gender, length of stay, comorbidity, New York Heart Association (NYHA) classification, race, marital status, and employment status. Table 3-5 presents the demographic profile of the subjects in the study by Moore and Dolansky (2001); this profile is also referred to as the sample characteristics or demographics for the study.

> Sample characteristics can also be presented in narrative format in the research report. For example, in a grounded theory study of patients' work during mechanical ventilation and weaning, Logan and Jenny (1997) described their sample of 20 subjects as follows:
>
> "...11 were women and 9 were men. Their ages ranged from 19 to 83 years (mean 57.5 years). Twelve participants were married. Eleven patients had a variety of medical diagnoses, and 9 had had surgical procedures. Severity of illness as measured by the Acute Physiological and Chronic Health Evaluation (APACHE III) scale ranged from 5 to 44 (mean 20.8) at the time of admission. Patients receive mechanical ventilator support from 5 to 214 days (mean 31.5, median 14.5 days).... Length of time for weaning ranged from 1 to 45 days (mean 15.1, median 6.24 days)." (p. 141)

TABLE 3-5

SAMPLE DEMOGRAPHICS

	CONTROL (n = 90)	EXPERIMENTAL (n = 90)
Age (years)	63.2 ± 10.0	62.0 ± 10.8
Education (years)	13.5 ± 3.3	12.8 ± 3.0
Number of grafts	3.5 ± 1.0	3.3 ± 1.2
Length of stay	6.5 ± 2.8	6.0 ± 1.7
Comorbidity	1.2 ± 1.4	1.1 ± 1.2
	PERCENTAGE	**PERCENTAGE**
NYHA CLASS		
I	32.2	35.6
II	26.7	22.2
III	26.7	28.9
IV	14.4	13.3
MARITAL STATUS		
Married	62.2	71.1
RACE		
Caucasian	88.9	83.3
African American	11.1	14.4
Asian/Hispanic	0.0	2.3
EMPLOYMENT		
Employed	41.1	51.1

*NYHA, New York Heart Association.

From Moore, S. M., & Dolansky, M. A. (2001). Randomized trial of a home recovery intervention following coronary artery bypass surgery. *Research in Nursing & Health, 24*(2), 96.

Conceptual and Operational Definitions of Variables

A variable is operationalized in a study by the development of conceptual and operational definitions. A *conceptual definition* provides the theoretical meaning of a variable (Chinn & Kramer, 1998), and it is often derived from a theorist's definition of a related concept. In a published study, the framework includes concepts and their definitions, and the variables are selected to represent the concepts. Thus the variables are conceptually defined, indicating the link with the concepts in the framework. An *operational definition* is derived from a set of procedures or progressive acts that a researcher performs to receive sensory impressions (such as sound, visual, or tactile impressions) that indicate the existence or degree of existence of a variable (Reynolds, 1971). Operational definitions need to be independent of time and setting so that variables can be investigated at different times and in different settings using the same operational definitions. An operational definition is developed so that a variable can be measured or manipulated in a concrete situation, and the knowledge gained from studying the variable will increase the understanding of the theoretical concept that this variable represents.

Corff, Seideman, Venkataraman, Lutes, and Yates (1995) conducted a study to determine the "effectiveness of facilitated tucking, a nonpharmacologic nursing intervention, as a comfort measure in modulating preterm neonates' physiologic and behavioral responses to minor pain" (p. 143). The hypothesis for this prospective study was that "preterm neonates would have less variation in heart rate, oxygen saturation, and sleep state (shorter crying and sleep disruption time and less fluctuation in sleep states) in response to the painful stimulus of a heelstick with facilitated tucking than without" (Corff et al., 1995, p. 144). The variables from this study are identified and defined conceptually and operationally in the next section.

Independent Variable—Facilitated Tucking

CONCEPTUAL DEFINITION. A nonpharmacological comfort measure that involves the motoric containment of an infant's arms and legs.

OPERATIONAL DEFINITION. The infant's arms and legs are contained in "a flexed, midline position close to the infant's trunk with the infant in a side-lying or supine position" (p. 144) (Fig. 3-1).

Dependent Variables—Heart Rate and Oxygen Saturation

CONCEPTUAL DEFINITION. Physiological cardiovascular responses that are influenced by painful stimuli.

OPERATIONAL DEFINITION. Heart rate and oxygen saturation per pulse oximetry "were recorded visually and were graphed using a System VI Air Shields Infant Monitor With Data Logger" (p. 145).

Dependent Variable—Sleep State

CONCEPTUAL DEFINITION. Behavioral responses of crying, sleep disruption time, and fluctuation in sleep state that are influenced by painful stimuli.

Continued

OPERATIONAL DEFINITION. "Sleep states were recorded by one of two observers who reached 90% reliability in reading sleep states, as defined in the Neonatal Individualized Developmental Care and Assessment Program. Sleep states are defined as state 1 = deep sleep; state 2 = light sleep; state 3 = drowsiness; state 4 = awake, alert; state 5 = aroused, fussy; and state 6 = crying.... Sleep states were recorded during a 12-minute baseline period, the heelstick period, and a 15-minute post-stick period for both control and experimental trials." (p. 145)

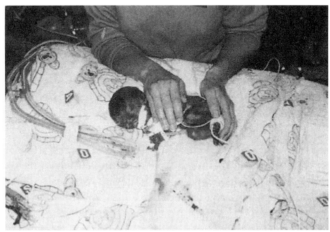

Fig. 3-1 Facilitated tucking of a premature infant. *(From Corff, K. E., Seideman, R., Venkataraman, P. S., Lutes, L., & Yates, B. [1995]. Facilitated tucking: A nonpharmacologic comfort measure for pain in preterm neonates.* Journal of Obstetric, Gynecologic and Neonatal Nursing, 24[2], 144. Reprinted with permission.)

The variables in quasi-experimental and experimental research are narrow and specific in focus and can be quantified (converted to numbers) or manipulated using specified steps that are often developed into a protocol. In addition, the variables are objectively defined to decrease researcher bias, as indicated in the previous example. The research variables or concepts in descriptive and correlational quantitative studies and sometimes qualitative studies are usually more abstract and broadly defined. In many qualitative studies, the focus of the study is to define the concept(s) being studied. For example, Orne et al. (2000) conducted their study "with the goal of constructing a vivid depiction of the lived experience of being employed but medically uninsured" (p. 205). The conceptual definition for being employed but medically uninsured was identified in the analysis section of the research report in a table format.

Research Concept—Being Employed but Medically Uninsured

CONCEPTUAL DEFINITION. Table 3-6 illustrates the definition.

OPERATIONAL DEFINITION. The concept of being employed but medically uninsured was investigated with face-to-face interviews using an unstructured format.

Thus the focus of Orne et al.'s (2000) study was to define and describe the concept of being employed but medically uninsured. The findings from this study could become the basis for additional research to expand our understanding and ability to manage the problem of the medically uninsured.

TABLE 3-6

THEMATIC ANALYSIS

THEME CLUSTERS	THEMES
A Marginalized Life	Vulnerable on All Fronts
	Limits, Loss and Hard Times
Up Against Rocks and Hard Places	The Paradox of Middle Ground
	Entangled in Power and Politics
Making Choices—Chancing It	Setting Priorities—Weighting the Odds
	Living with Compromise
	A Game of Russian Roulette
Getting By—More or Less	Lucky So Far
	Resilience
	Resigned to Adversity
	The Emotional Price Tag

Orne, R. M., Fishman, S. J., Manka, M., Pagnozzi, M. E. (2000). Living on the edge: A phenomenological study of medically uninsured working Americans. *Research in Nursing & Health, 23*(3), Table 1, p. 207.

CRITIQUING RESEARCH VARIABLES IN PUBLISHED STUDIES

Variables need to be identified clearly and defined conceptually and operationally in a published study.

The following questions might be helpful during a critique of the variables in a study.

1. Are the independent, dependent, or research variables or concepts identified?
2. Are the variables that are manipulated or measured in the study consistent with the variables identified in the purpose or the objectives, questions, or hypotheses?
3. Are the variables reflective of the concepts identified in the study framework?
4. Are the variables clearly defined conceptually and operationally based on theory and previous research?
5. Is the conceptual definition of the variable consistent with the operational definition?
6. Were the essential demographic variables examined and summarized?
7. Were the extraneous variables identified and controlled as necessary in the study?
8. Are there uncontrolled extraneous variables that may have influenced the findings? Is the potential impact of these variables on the findings discussed?

SUMMARY

This chapter provides an introduction to the research problem and purpose and the objectives, questions, and hypotheses that are used to direct studies. The problem is an area of concern where there is a gap in the knowledge base needed for nursing practice. The research purpose is a concise, clear statement of the specific goal or aim of the study. The goal of a study might be to identify, describe, explain, or predict a solution to a situation in clinical practice.

The problem and purpose of a study need to have professional significance and potential or actual significance for society. When critiquing the significance of the problem and purpose in a published study, you need to determine if the knowledge generated by the study influences nursing practice, builds on previous research, promotes theory development, and/or addresses current concerns or priorities in nursing. The feasibility of studying an identified problem and purpose is also examined in a research critique. Study feasibility is evaluated by examining the researchers' expertise; money commitments; availability of subjects, facilities, and equipment; and the study's ethical considerations. Guidelines are provided to direct the critique of problems and purposes in quantitative, qualitative, and outcomes research reports.

Research objectives, questions, or hypotheses are formulated to bridge the gap between the more abstractly stated research problem and purpose and the detailed design and data analysis. Research objectives are clear, concise, declarative statements that are expressed in the present tense. Research questions are concise, interrogative statements that are worded in the present tense and include one or more variables. Objectives and questions focus on description of variables, examination of rela-

tionships among variables, and determination of differences between two or more groups regarding selected variables.

A hypothesis is the formal statement of the expected relationship(s) between two or more variables in a specified population. The hypothesis translates the research problem and purpose into a clear explanation or prediction of the expected results or outcomes of the study. Hypotheses can be described using four categories: (1) associative versus causal, (2) simple versus complex, (3) nondirectional versus directional, and (4) null versus research. Testable hypotheses contain variables that are measurable or manipulable, and these hypotheses are evaluated using statistical analyses. Guidelines are provided for use in critiquing objectives, questions, and hypotheses in published studies.

The research purpose and objectives, questions, or hypotheses identify the variables to be examined in a study. Variables are qualities, properties, or characteristics of persons, things, or situations that change or vary. The types of variables discussed in this chapter include independent, dependent, research, extraneous, environmental, and demographic. An independent variable is a stimulus or activity that is manipulated or varied by the researcher to create an effect on the dependent variable. A dependent variable is the response, behavior, or outcome that the researcher wants to predict or explain. Research variables or concepts are the qualities, properties, or characteristics that are observed or measured in a study. Research variables are often examined in descriptive and correlational quantitative studies, and research concepts or variables might be examined in qualitative studies. Extraneous variables exist in all studies and can affect the measurement of study variables and the relationships among these variables. Environmental variables are a type of extraneous variable that make up the setting in which the study is conducted. Demographic variables are characteristics or attributes of the subjects that are collected and analyzed to describe the study sample.

A variable is operationalized in a study by developing conceptual and operational definitions. A conceptual definition provides the theoretical meaning of a variable and is derived from a theorist's definition of a related concept. The conceptual definition provides a basis for formulating an operational definition. An operational definition is derived from a set of procedures or progressive acts that a re-searcher performs to receive sensory impressions that indicate the existence or degree of existence of a variable. Operational definitions indicate how a treatment or independent variable will be implemented and how the dependent variable will be measured. Operational definitions need to be independent of time and setting so that variables can be investigated at different times and in different settings using the same definitions. The chapter concludes with guidelines to direct the critique of study variables in research reports.

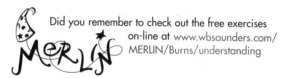

Did you remember to check out the free exercises on-line at www.wbsaunders.com/ MERLIN/Burns/understanding

REFERENCES

Ajzen, I., & Fishbein, M. (1980). *Understanding attitudes and predicting social behavior.* Englewood Cliffs, NJ: Prentice-Hall.

American Heart Association. (1999). *1999 heart and stroke statistical update.* Dallas: American Heart Association.

Artinian, N. T., Washington, O. G., & Templin, T. N. (2001). Effects of home telemonitoring and community-based monitoring on blood pressure control in urban African Americans: A pilot study. *Heart & Lung: The Journal of Critical Care, 30*(3), 191-199.

Baker, C. F., Garvin, B. J., Kennedy, C. W., & Polivka, B. J. (1993). The effect of environmental sound and communication on CCU patients' heart rate and blood pressure. *Research in Nursing & Health, 16*(6), 415-421.

Bostrom, J., Mechanic, J., Lazar, N., Michelson, S., Grant, L., & Nomura, L. (1996). Preventing skin breakdown: Nursing practices, costs, and outcomes. *Applied Nursing Research, 9*(4), 184-188.

Bournaki, M. C. (1997). Correlates of pain-related responses to venipunctures in school-age children. *Nursing Research, 46*(3), 147-154.

Brown, S. C. (1997). Chest pain and cocaine use in 18 to 40 year-old persons: A retrospective study. *Applied Nursing Research, 10*(3), 136-142.

Brown, S. J. (1999). *Knowledge for health care practice: A guide to using research evidence.* Philadelphia: Saunders.

Burns, N., & Grove, S. K. (2001). *The practice of nursing research: Conduct, critique, and utilization* (4th ed.). Philadelphia: Saunders.

Carrieri-Kohlman, V., Gormley, J. M., Eiser, S., Demir-Deviren, S., Nguyen, H., Paul, S. M., et al. (2001). Dyspnea and the affective response during exercise training in obstructive pulmonary disease. *Nursing Research, 50*(3), 136-146.

Chinn, P. L., & Kramer, M. K. (1998). *Theory and nursing: Integrated knowledge development.* St. Louis: Mosby.

Contrada, R. J., & Krantz, D. S. (1988). Stress, reactivity, and type A behavior: Current status and future directions. *Annals of Behavioral Medicine, 10*(2), 64-70.

Corff, K. E., Seideman, R., Venkataraman, P. S., Lutes, L., & Yates, B. (1995). Facilitated tucking: A nonpharmacologic comfort measure for pain in preterm neonates. *Journal of Obstetric, Gynecologic, & Neonatal Nursing, 24*(2), 143-147.

Creswell, J. W. (1994). *Research design: Qualitative and quantitative approaches.* Thousand Oaks, CA: Sage.

Edel, E., Houston, S., Kennedy, V., & LaRocco, M. (1998). Impact of a 5-minute scrub on the microbial flora found on artificial, polished, or natural fingernails of operating room personnel. *Nursing Research, 47*(1), 54-59.

Fahs, P. S. S., & Kinney, M. R. (1991). The abdomen, thigh, and arm as sites for subcutaneous sodium heparin injections. *Nursing Research, 40*(4), 204-207.

Fields, S. D. (2000). Clinical practice guidelines: Finding and appraising useful, relevant recommendations for geriatric care. *Geriatrics, 55*(1), 59-64.

Fitzpatrick, M. L. (2001). Historical research: The method. In P. L. Munhall, (Ed.), *Nursing research: A qualitative perspective* (pp. 403-415). Boston, MA: National League for Nursing Press.

Foster-Fitzpatrick, L., Ortiz, A., Sibilano, H., Marcantonio, R., & Braun, L. T. (1999). The effects of crossed leg on blood pressure measurement. *Nursing Research, 48*(2), 105-108.

Germain, C. P. (2001). Ethnography: The method. In P. L. Munhall, (Ed.), *Nursing Research: A qualitative perspective* (pp. 277-306). Boston, MA: National League for Nursing Press.

Hastings-Tolsma, M. T., Yucha, C. B., Tompkins, J., Robson, L., & Szeverenyi, N. (1993). Effect of warm and cold applications on the resolution of IV infiltrations. *Research in Nursing & Health, 16*(3), 171-178.

Hill, M. N., & Grim, C. M. (1991). How to take a precise blood pressure. *American Journal of Nursing, 91*(2), 38-42.

Jadack, R. A., Hyde, J. S., & Keller, M. L. (1995). Gender and knowledge about HIV, risky sexual behaviors, and safer sex practices. *Research in Nursing & Health, 18*(4), 313-324.

Jemmott, L. S., & Jemmott, J. B., III. (1991). Applying the theory of reasoned action to AIDS risk behavior: Condom use among black women. *Nursing Research, 40*(4), 228-234.

Jirovec, M. M., & Kasno, J. (1990). Self-care agency as a function of patient-environmental factors among nursing home residents. *Research in Nursing & Health, 13*(5), 303-309.

Johnson, V. Y. (2001). Effects of a submaximal exercise protocol to recondition the pelvic floor musculature. *Nursing Research, 50*(1), 33-41.

JNC-IV-National Committee on Detection, Evaluation, and Treatment of High Blood Pressure. (1997). *The sixth report of the Joint National Committee on prevention, detection, evaluation, and treatment of high blood pressure.* NIH Publication No. 98-4080. Bethesda, MD: National Institutes of Health.

Kahn, C. R. (1994). Picking a research problem: The critical decision. *The New England Journal of Medicine, 330*(21), 1530-1533.

Kaplan, N. M. (1998). *Clinical hypertension.* Baltimore: Williams & Wilkins.

Kauffman, K. S. (1995). Center as haven: Findings of an urban ethnography. *Nursing Research, 44*(4), 231-236.

Kerlinger, F. N., & Lee, H. B. (1999). *Foundations of behavioral research* (4th ed.). New York: Harcourt Brace.

Krisman-Scott, M. A. (2000). An historical analysis of disclosure of terminal status. *Journal of Nursing Scholarship, 32*(1), 47-52.

Koniak, D. (1985). Autotutorial and lecture-demonstration instruction: A comparative analysis of the effects upon students' learning of a developmental assessment skill. *Western Journal of Nursing Research, 7*(1), 80-100.

Kuttner, R. (1999). The American health care system—Health insurance coverage. *The New England Journal of Medicine, 340*(3), 163-168.

Landis, C. A., & Whitney, J. D. (1997). Effects of 72 hours of sleep deprivation on wound healing in the rat. *Research in Nursing & Health, 20*(3), 259-267.

Lanza, M. L., Kayne, H. L., Pattison, I., Hicks, C., & Islam, S. (1996). The relationship of behavioral cues to assaultive behaviors. *Clinical Nursing Research, 5*(1), 6-27.

Lazarus, R. S., Delongis, A., Folkman, S., & Gruen, R. (1985). Stress and adaptational outcomes: The problem of confounded measures. *American Psychologist, 40*(7), 770-779.

Lee, K. A., & Stotts, N. A. (1990). Support of the growth hormone-somatomedin system to facilitate healing. *Heart & Lung, 19*(2), 157-164.

Lim-Levy, F. (1982). The effect of oxygen inhalation on oral temperature. *Nursing Research, 31*(3), 150-152.

Lindeman, C. A. (1975). Delphi survey of priorities in clinical nursing research. *Nursing Research, 24*(6), 434-441.

Logan, J., & Jenny, J. (1997). Qualitative analysis of patients' work during mechanical ventilation and weaning. *Heart & Lung, 26*(2), 140-147.

Moody, L., Vera, H., Blanks, C., & Visscher, M. (1989). Developing questions of substance for nursing science. *Western Journal of Nursing Research, 11*(4), 393-404.

Moore, S. M., & Dolansky, M. A. (2001). Randomized trial of a home recovery intervention following coronary artery bypass surgery. *Research in Nursing & Health, 24*(2), 93-104.

Moser, D. K., & Dracup, K. (2000). Impact of cardiopulmonary resuscitation training on perceived control in spouses of recovering cardiac patients. *Research in Nursing & Health, 23*(4), 270-278.

Munhall, P. L. (2001). *Nursing research: A qualitative perspective.* Boston, MA: National League for Nursing Press.

Orne, R. M., Fishman, S. J., Manka, M., & Pagnozzi, M. E. (2000). Living on the edge: A phenomenological study of medically uninsured working Americans. *Research in Nursing & Health, 23*(3), 204-212.

Reynolds, P. D. (1971). *A primer in theory construction.* Indianapolis: Bobbs-Merrill.

Rogers, B. (1987). Research corner: Is the research project feasible? *American Association of Occupational Health Nurses Journal, 35*(7), 327-328.

Rosenberg, M. (November 15, 1993). *Understanding violence—A public health perspective.* Paper presented at the American Academy for Nursing Conference, Violence: Nursing Debates the Issues. Washington, DC.

Rudy, E. B., Daly, B. J., Douglas, S., Montenegro, H. D., Song, R., & Dyer, M. A. (1995). Patient outcomes for the chronically critically ill: Special care unit versus intensive care unit. *Nursing Research, 44*(6), 324-330.

Van Cleve, L., Johnson, L., & Pothier, P. (1996). Pain responses of hospitalized infants and children to venipuncture and intravenous cannulation. *Journal of Pediatric Nursing, 11*(3), 161-168.

WHO Expert Committee. (1996). *Hypertension control.* Geneva: World Health Organization.

Wong, D. L., & Baker, C. M. (1988). Pain in children: Comparison of assessment scales. *Pediatric Nursing, 14*(1), 9-17.

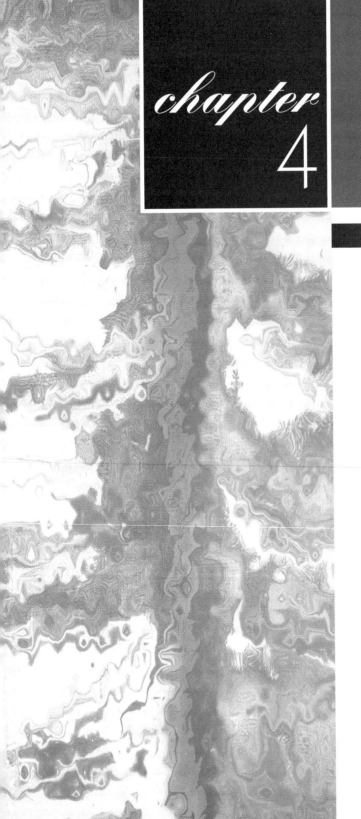

chapter 4

Review of Literature

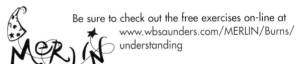

Be sure to check out the free exercises on-line at
www.wbsaunders.com/MERLIN/Burns/
understanding

OUTLINE—cont'd

Clarifying Evidence for Best Practices through Literature Reviews
   Integrated Literature Reviews—State of the Science
   Meta-Analyses
Writing a Review of Literature

OBJECTIVES

Completing this chapter should enable you to:
1. Describe the sources and content of a literature review in a research report.
2. Differentiate between theoretical and empirical sources.
3. Discuss the purposes for reviewing the literature in quantitative and qualitative studies.
4. Critique the literature review section of a published study.
5. Discuss the process for identifying and locating research sources.
6. Conduct a computerized search of the literature.
7. Use the Internet to search for relevant electronic publications.
8. Use a variety of sources in developing a literature review.
9. Summarize the research literature in an area of interest to promote the use of evidence-based knowledge in nursing practice.

RELEVANT TERMS

Academic library
Benchmarking
Bibliographical database
Citation
Clustered
Complex search
Dissertation
Electronic journal
Empirical literature
Evidence for best practices
Full-text databases
Integrative review of research
Interlibrary loan department
Keywords
Landmark studies
Library sources

Linking
Meta-analyses
Monographs
Paraphrasing
Periodicals
Primary source
Public library
Relevant studies
Review of literature
Search field
Secondary source
Special library
Surfing the Web
Synthesis of sources
Theoretical literature
Thesis

The amount of research information available continues to escalate, with the production of approximately 6000 new scientific articles a day. At this rate, scientific knowledge will double about every 5 years (Naisbitt & Aburdene, 1990). The number of nursing journals has increased by more than 575% since 1961, and a multitude of these research reports are available on the Internet. Thus the literature review process is much more enlightening today than in the past, and computerized databases have greatly facilitated the process of searching the literature. The result of a literature review is a summary of current theoretical and scientific knowledge about a particular problem, and this summary includes a synthesis of what is known and not known about the problem. A *review of literature* may be conducted to summarize the research-based knowledge for practice or to guide the development of a study to increase the evidence needed to guide practice. This chapter provides essential information to assist you in critiquing the literature review sections of quantitative and qualitative studies, reviewing the literature, and synthesizing research findings to guide practice. A literature review on the prediction and prevention of pressure ulcers is presented as an example of research knowledge that is ready for use in practice.

UNDERSTANDING THE LITERATURE REVIEW IN PUBLISHED STUDIES

In published studies researchers present literature reviews to provide the reader with a background for the problem studied. The review of literature section will include a description of the current knowledge of a practice problem, the gaps in this knowledge base, and the contribution of the present study to the development of knowledge in this area. The scope of a literature review should be broad enough to allow the reader to become familiar with the research problem and narrow enough to include predominantly relevant sources. *Relevant sources* means that the literature being reviewed has a direct bearing on the problem studied. To increase your understanding of the literature reviews presented in published studies, the following areas are addressed: (1) the sources included in a literature review and (2) the purposes of the literature review in quantitative and qualitative studies.

SOURCES INCLUDED IN A LITERATURE REVIEW

Two main types of sources are cited in the review of literature for research: theoretical and empirical. The word *empirical* is defined as knowledge derived from research. Other types of published information, such as descriptions of clinical situations, educational literature, and position papers, are examined by the researcher in the process of reviewing the literature but are rarely cited in a research publication because of their subjectivity (Pinch, 1995). *Citation* is when the author quotes a source, uses it as an example, or brings it forward as support for a position taken. Theoretical and empirical sources can be primary or secondary in origin, but usually only primary sources are cited in a literature review. This section describes the theoretical and empirical literature cited in published studies and clarifies the differences between primary and secondary sources in literature reviews.

Theoretical and Empirical Literature

Theoretical literature includes concept analyses, models, theories, and conceptual frameworks that support a selected research problem and purpose. Theoretical sources can be found in periodicals and monographs. *Periodicals,* such as journals, are published over time, and are numbered sequentially for the years published. *Monographs,* such as books, booklets of conference proceedings, or pamphlets, are usually written once and may be updated with a new edition. Periodicals and monographs are available in a variety of media, such as print, on-line, or CD-ROM. In a published study, theoretical and conceptual sources are described and summarized to reflect the current understanding of the research problem and to provide a basis for the study framework.

Empirical literature includes published studies, usually in journals or books, and unpublished studies, such as master's theses and doctoral dissertations. A *thesis* is a research project completed by a master's student as part of the requirements for a master's degree. A *dissertation* is an extensive, usually original research project that is completed as the final requirement for a doctoral degree. The empirical literature reviewed depends on the study problem and the type of research conducted. Research problems that have been frequently studied or are currently being investigated have more extensive empirical literature than new or unique problems. Descriptive studies are usually conducted in new areas of research, so the number of studies available for review is limited compared to those for a quasi-experimental or experimental study.

Primary and Secondary Sources

The published literature includes primary and secondary sources. A *primary source* is written by the person who originated or is responsible for generating the ideas published. In empirical publications, a primary source is written by the person(s) who conducted the research. A primary theoretical source is written by the theorist who developed the theory or conceptual content. A *secondary source* summarizes or quotes content from primary sources. Thus authors of secondary sources paraphrase the works of researchers and theorists. The problem with secondary sources is that the author has interpreted the works of someone else, and this interpretation is influenced by that author's perception and bias. Sometimes errors and misinterpretations have been spread by authors using secondary sources rather than primary sources. Predominantly, primary sources are cited in research reports. Secondary sources are used only if primary sources cannot be located or if the secondary source provides creative ideas or a unique organization of information not found in a primary source.

PURPOSE OF THE LITERATURE REVIEW IN QUANTITATIVE RESEARCH

The review of literature in quantitative research is conducted to direct the development and implementation of a study. The major literature review is conducted at the beginning of the research process, and a limited review is conducted during the generation of the research report to identify new studies. The purpose of the literature review is similar for the different types of quantitative studies (descriptive, correlational, quasi-experimental, and experimental). Relevant sources are cited throughout a quantitative research report in the introduction, methods, results, and discussion sections. In the introduction section, the background and significance of the research problem are summarized from relevant sources. The review of literature section includes both theoretical and empirical sources that document the current knowledge of the problem studied. The framework section is developed from the theoretical literature and sometimes from empirical literature, depending on the focus of the study. The methods section of the research report describes the design, sample, measurement methods, treatment, and data collection process that are based on previous research. In the results section, the analysis of the data is conducted with knowledge of the results of previous studies. The discussion section of the research report provides conclusions that are a synthesis of the findings from previous research and those from the present study.

PURPOSE OF THE LITERATURE REVIEW IN QUALITATIVE RESEARCH

In qualitative research the purpose and timing of the literature review vary based on the type of study to be conducted (Table 4-1). Phenomenologists believe the literature should be reviewed after data collection and analysis so that the information in the

TABLE 4-1	
PURPOSES OF THE LITERATURE REVIEW IN QUALITATIVE RESEARCH	
TYPE OF QUALITATIVE RESEARCH	**PURPOSE OF THE LITERATURE REVIEW**
Phenomenological research	Compare and combine findings from the study with the literature to determine current knowledge of a phenomenon
Grounded theory research	Use the literature to explain, support, and extend the theory generated in the study
Ethnographical research	Review the literature to provide a background for conducting the study, as in quantitative research
Historical research	Literature is reviewed to develop research questions and is a source of data in the study

literature will not influence the researcher's openness (Munhall, 2001). For if a researcher decided to describe the phenomenon of dying, the review of li would include Kübler-Ross's (1969) five stages of grieving. Knowing the de these stages could influence the way the researcher views the phenomenon data collection and analysis. However, after data analysis, the information fro literature is compared with findings from the present study to determine simila and differences. Then the findings are combined to reflect the current knowledg the phenomenon.

In grounded theory research, a minimal review of relevant studies is done at the beginning of the research process. This review is only a means of making the researcher aware of what studies have been conducted, but the information from these studies is not used to direct data collection or theory development for the current study. The literature is primarily used by the researcher to explain, support, and extend the theory generated in the study (Munhall, 2001).

The review of literature in ethnographic research is similar to that in quantitative research. The literature is reviewed early in the research process to provide a general understanding of the variables to be examined in a selected culture. The literature is usually theoretical because few studies have typically been conducted in the area of interest. From these sources a framework is developed for examining complex human situations in the selected culture (Munhall, 2001). The literature review also provides a background for conducting the study and interpreting the findings.

In historical research an initial literature review is conducted to select a research topic and to develop research questions. Then the investigator develops an inventory of sources, locates these sources, and examines them; thus the literature is a major source of data in historical research. Since historical research requires an extensive review of literature that is sometimes difficult to locate, the researcher can spend months and even years locating and examining sources. The information gained from the literature is analyzed and organized into a report to explain how an identified phenomenon has evolved over a particular time period (Munhall, 2001).

CRITIQUING THE LITERATURE REVIEW IN A PUBLISHED STUDY

The literature review section of a research report needs to be identified and critiqued for quality. The review of literature might be a clearly identified section in the report or part of the introduction. A quality literature review logically builds a case for the study being reported. Thus reading the literature review should provide a basic understanding of the study problem and evidence that the study conducted was appropriate based on the current knowledge of this problem. This section provides guidelines for critiquing the literature review in a published study and an example literature review critique.

GUIDELINES FOR CONDUCTING A CRITIQUE OF THE LITERATURE REVIEW

Critiquing the literature review of a published study involves examining the quality of the content and sources presented. The content of the literature review includes what is known and not known about the study problem and identifies the focus of the present study. Thus the review needs to provide a basis for the study purpose and is often organized according to the variables in the purpose. The sources cited need to be relevant and current for the problem and purpose of the study. To determine if sources cited in a research report are relevant, the sources or abstracts of the sources must be located and reviewed. This is very time consuming and is usually not done when critiquing an article. However, you can review the reference list and determine the focus of the sources, the number of empirical and theoretical sources cited, and where and when the sources were published.

The literature review should include current sources (5 to 10 years before publication of the report). Sources cited should be comprehensive as well as current, and that depends on whether the problem studied has existed for years or is relatively new. Some problems have been studied for decades, and the literature review often includes landmark studies that were conducted years ago. *Landmark studies* are significant research projects that generate knowledge that influences a discipline and sometimes society. These studies are frequently replicated or are the basis for the generation of additional studies. For example, Williams (1972) studied factors that contribute to skin breakdown, and these findings provided the basis for numerous studies on the prevention and treatment of pressure ulcers. Many of these studies have been summarized to provide guidelines for the prediction and prevention of pressure ulcers in clinical practice (Barczak, Barnett, Childs, & Bosley, 1997; Bergstrom et al., 1994; Cullum, Deeks, Sheldon, Song, & Fletcher, 2001; Harrison, Wells, Fisher, & Prince, 1996; National Pressure Ulcer Advisory Panel, 1989; Panel for the Prediction and Prevention of Pressure Ulcers in Adults, 1992; Whittemore, 1998).

 Critiquing the literature review section of a published study is often difficult for students because they are less familiar with the topic than are the authors of the article. In addition, the literature review sections frequently are too concise to present the current knowledge on selected topics because the review is often reduced to comply with space limitations for publication (Downs, 1999a,b). Asking the following questions might help in assessing the quality of a literature review in a study.

1. Are primary sources cited in the review?
2. Are the references current?
3. Are relevant studies identified and described?
4. Are relevant theories identified and described?
5. Are relevant landmark studies described?
6. Are relevant studies critiqued?

7. **Are the sources paraphrased to promote the flow of the content presented?**
8. **Is the current knowledge about the research problem described?**
9. **Does the literature review identify the gap in the knowledge base that provides a basis for the study conducted?**
10. **Is the literature review clearly organized, logically developed, and concisely written?**

Example Critique of a Study's Literature Review

The review of literature section from Vyhlidal, Moxness, Bosak, Van Meter, and Bergstrom's (1997) study of the effects of selected mattress surfaces on the incidence of pressure ulcers is presented as an example. "The purpose of the study was to compare the incidence of pressure ulcers in 40 newly admitted at-risk (Braden Scale score <18) skilled nursing–facility residents, randomly assigned to Iris 3000 (Bio Clinic of Sunrise Medical Corp, Ontario, CA) foam mattress overlays ($n = 20$) or a MAXIFLOAT (BG Industries, Northridge, CA) foam mattress replacements ($n = 20$)" (p. 111). The literature review is presented on pages 112–113 of the research article, and the references are on page 120.

Background or Literature Review

"Landis (1930) found that the average arteriolar capillary pressure among healthy subjects was 32 mm Hg. Based largely on the Landis findings, practitioners and developers of support surfaces contend that unrelieved pressure greater than 32 mm Hg creates tissue ischemia which can lead to pressure ulcer development (Hedrick-Thompson, Halloran, Strader, & McSweeney, 1993; Jester & Weaver, 1990; Krouskop, Williams, Krebs, Herszkowicz, & Garber, 1985; Panel for the Prediction and Prevention of Pressure Ulcers in Adults, 1992). Furthermore, high pressures of short duration and low pressures of long duration are known to be capable of producing pressure ulcers (Husain, 1953; Kosiak, 1959). Manufacturers of support surfaces use the 32 mm Hg capillary closing pressure as a benchmark to evaluate product pressure reduction capabilities. Support surfaces that reduce pressure between skin overlying bony prominences and support surfaces (interface pressure) below 32 mm Hg should hypothetically reduce the risk of pressure ulcer development.

Product studies have examined interface pressure using healthy subjects rather than subjects at risk for developing ulcers (Hedrick-Thompson et al., 1993; Jester & Weaver, 1990). The Jester and Weaver study compared families of products [using a sample of] low risk or normal volunteers lying on the support surfaces for unknown periods of time. MAXIFLOAT replacement foam mattresses had lower interface pressure readings among four product groups (overlays, air mattresses, foam mattresses, and other mattresses), but these pressures were not

Continued

as low as air-fluidized or low air-loss specialty beds. A study of 4-in. convoluted foam mattress overlays reported the overlays to have significantly lower pressure readings than the standard bed (Krouskop et al., 1985). Hedrick-Thompson et al. (1993) also found 4-in. foam overlays to have lower pressure readings than the standard bed but higher pressures than air mattress overlays and air-loss beds.

A more informative way of evaluating product efficacy is to examine a patient-centered outcome, whether or not patients develop pressure ulcers. However, few investigators have evaluated product efficacy in terms of this outcome. No studies could be found testing the efficacy of the MAXIFLOAT or Iris 3000 foam support surfaces. A few studies were found on other brands of 4-in. foam overlays. Subjects in these studies were usually hospitalized or skilled nursing facility residents. One study reported no statistical difference in skin outcome between 4-in. foam overlays and alternating air pressure mattresses (Whitney, Fellows, & Larson, 1984). In contrast, Stoneberg, Pitcock, and Myton (1986) noted a higher number and greater severity of pressure ulcers with 4-in. foam overlays than with alternating pressure pads. Kemp et al. (1993) found [that] solid 4-in. foam overlays produced statistically fewer ulcers than the convoluted foam overlays when taking into account Braden Scale mobility subscale scores.

Research involving MAXIFLOAT foam mattresses is limited to explaining interface pressures. No research specifically examined the Iris 3000 foam overlay, but conflicting findings on pressure reduction and pressure ulcer incidence were reported with other 4-in. foam overlay products. This study compares these two foam products based on pressure ulcer incidence in an at-risk population. Results will provide clinicians with meaningful data to aid in the selection of a cost-effective beneficial product." (Vyhlidal et al., 1997, pp. 112–113)

The literature review, though brief, includes quality content and relevant sources that provide a basis for the conduct of this study. The review of literature is well organized and focuses on the study variables (pressure ulcer, Iris 3000 foam mattress overlays, and MAXIFLOAT foam mattress replacements). The first two paragraphs describe what is known about the research problem, and the third paragraph focuses on what is not known or the gap in the knowledge base needed for practice. The last paragraph briefly summarizes the major points of the literature review and addresses the importance of the current study in contributing to the development of knowledge for practice.

The researchers cited quality, relevant primary sources from excellent medical and nursing research journals, such as the *Journal of the American Medical Association, Journal of ET Nursing, Ostomy/Wound Management, Research in Nursing & Health, Archives of Physical Medicine and Rehabilitation, Journal of Rehabilitation Research and Development, Heart,* and *Journal of Gerontological Nursing.* The clinical practice guideline for the prediction and prevention of pressure ulcers is an excellent source that was developed by health professionals (physicians and nurses), politicians, and consumers who are experts in the field of pressure ulcer prevention, assessment, and treatment (Panel for the Prediction and Prevention of Pressure Ulcers in Adults, 1992). The sources are current and comprehensive, ranging from 1930 to 1995. The research by Landis (1930) is a landmark study that documented the pressure at which pressure ulcers develop. Most of the sources were published in the late 1980s and 1990s.

The study by Vyhlidal and colleagues (1997) did produce useful findings for practice. They found that the MAXIFLOAT foam mattress replacements were significantly more effective in preventing pressure ulcers than the Iris 3000 foam mattress overlay, even when the subjects on the MAXIFLOAT were heavier and used the mattress more days than the subjects on the Iris 3000. "MAXIFLOAT proved to be more effective in preventing pressure ulcers in an at-risk skilled-care population and was cost-effective" (p. 111). This knowledge is valuable in making decisions about the bed surfaces for elderly patients at risk for pressure ulcers.

PERFORMING A LITERATURE REVIEW

A background in reading research reports and critiquing the literature review sections of published studies should provide assistance during a review of the literature in an area of interest. This section focuses on reviewing relevant literature to generate a picture of what is known and not known about a problem and to determine whether the knowledge is ready for use in practice. For example, maybe you have noted that many hospitalized patients are elderly, and far too many of them develop pressure ulcers during their hospital stay. Reviewing the research literature might provide possible solutions for this practice problem. The steps for reviewing the literature include the following: (1) using the library, (2) identifying relevant research sources, and (3) locating these sources.

USING THE LIBRARY

This section provides you with information about libraries and some tips on using them. There are three major categories of libraries: public, academic, and special (Strauch, Linton, & Cohen, 1989). The *public library* serves the needs of the community in which it is located and usually contains few research reports. The *academic library* is located within an institution of higher learning. It contains numerous research reports in journals and books and provides access to many other sources online. Most academic libraries have an *interlibrary loan department,* which can be useful when you cannot find a particular research report. This department can frequently locate and obtain books, booklets, conference proceedings, and articles from other libraries within 1 or 2 weeks.

The *special library* contains a collection of materials on a specific topic or specialty area, such as nursing or medicine. Large hospitals, health care centers, and health research centers have special libraries that contain sources relevant to health care providers and researchers. For example, the most comprehensive collection of national and international nursing literature is available at the Center for Nursing Scholarship in Indianapolis, Indiana. Specialty libraries, such as those in hospitals, often have a librarian who will assist nurses in conducting a literature search.

The process of using a library and searching the literature has changed dramatically as the use of computers has increased. Today, good libraries provide access to large numbers of electronic databases that supply a broad scope of the available literature nationally and internationally. Thus library users are able to identify relevant sources quickly and also to print full-text versions of many of these sources immediately. Photocopies can be made from journals held by the library, and photocopies of articles not otherwise available can often be obtained through Interlibrary Loan arrangements between your library and other libraries across the country. It may not even be necessary to go to a library to use the services you need. Authorized users can access many library services at any time and location by using the Internet. Library consultations, database searching, Interlibrary loan services, full-text article downloads, and more, are often available to faculty and student researchers, even those who live far from the university. The Internet can provide a link to the university library, through direct modem connections and through e-mail. Computers are also available for users within the library. However, each library's computerized resources differ. Written documentation will usually provide step by step explanations of how to use electronic resources. When you use library services for the first time, you might ask the library personnel for an orientation to their services or search for orientation material available electronically. Library personnel in the reference department are familiar with the library's collections and operations and can provide assistance in using the computers to access electronic resources, as well as indexes, abstracts, and reference materials in the library. Common *library sources* for research reports include journals, books, conference proceedings, master's theses, and doctoral dissertations (Strauch et al., 1989).

IDENTIFYING RELEVANT RESEARCH SOURCES

Once a problem in clinical practice is identified, the literature can be searched for studies related to this problem. Before you begin searching the literature, you should consider exactly what information you are seeking. A written plan of the search strategy can save considerable time. The plan should include selecting databases to search, selecting keywords, locating relevant literature, and storing the references using reference management software. Several electronic searches, not just one, may be required to obtain the studies needed.

Selecting Databases to Search

A *bibliographical database* is a compilation of citations. A *citation* provides the information necessary to locate a reference. For example, the author's name, year of publication, title, journal name, volume number, issue number, and page numbers are all needed to find a journal article. A database may consist of citations relevant to a specific discipline or may be a broad collection of citations from a variety of disciplines. The most relevant nursing database is CINAHL, accessible at http://www.cinahl.com, which contains citations of nursing literature published after 1955. Another database commonly used by nurse researchers is MEDLINE, the on-line version of *Index Medicus*. The National Library of Medicine provides free access to MEDLINE through PubMed available at http://www.ncbi.nih.gov/entrez/query.fcgi. For a variety of reasons, including the cost of receipt and storage and convenience to library users, many libraries are discontinuing subscriptions to paper versions of journals and, instead, subscribing to services that provide access to electronic versions. Libraries subscribe to vendors who, for a fee, provide software, such as Silver Platter, OVID, and PaperChase, which can be used to access multiple bibliographical databases. *Full-text databases* of journal articles are now available for some journals. This means that you can conduct a computer search on a topic, get a list of citations, identify the citations that seem useful, and select the "full-text" option to read the text online, print it, or save it as a computer file. What a time saver! CINAHL now provides access to the full text of some articles.

Selecting Keywords

Keywords are the major concepts or variables of a research problem or topic. These terms will be your keywords to begin a search. In most databases, phrases can be used as well as single terms. As relevant studies are identified, they can be reviewed for other terms to be used as keywords. Alternative terms (synonyms) for concepts or variables might also be used as keywords. Most databases have a thesaurus that can be used to identify keyword search terms. The thesaurus can be accessed by logging on to the database. Truncating words may allow you to locate more citations related to that term. For example, authors might have used *intervene, intervenes, intervened, intervening, intervention,* or *intervenor*. To capture all of these terms, a truncated term, such as *interven, interven*,* or *interven$* (the form depends on the rule of the search engine you are using), can be used in a search. Irregular plurals, such as woman and women, should also be considered as search terms. If an author is frequently cited, a search using the author's name can be performed. In this case, the term should be identified as an author term, not a keyword term.

Each search term that is used should be listed in a written search plan. As new terms are discovered, they should be added to the list. For each search, the following should be recorded: (1) the name of the database that is used, (2) the date the search is performed, (3) the exact search strategy that is used, (4) the number of articles that are found, and (5) the percentage of relevant articles that are found. You can even develop a table to record this information from multiple search strategies (Table 4-2). The results of each search should be saved on your computer's hard drive, a floppy disk, or a zip disk for later reference. The filename of the saved search results should be written in the search record.

TABLE 4-2

WRITTEN SEARCH RECORD

DATABASE SEARCHED	DATE OF SEARCH	SEARCH STRATEGY	NUMBER OF ARTICLES FOUND	PERCENTAGE OF ARTICLES RELEVANT
CINAHL				
MEDLINE				
Academic Search Premier				
Cochrane Library				

Using Reference Management Software

Reference management software can make tracking the references that have been obtained through searches considerably easier. This type of software can be used to conduct searches and to store the information on all search fields for each reference obtained in a search, including the abstract. Once this is done, all of the needed citation information and the abstract are readily available electronically when the literature review is written. As each article is read, comments about it can be inserted into the reference file.

Reference management software has been developed to interface directly with the most commonly used word processing software to organize the reference information using whatever citation style you stipulate. Citations can be inserted directly into a paper with just a keystroke or two. The two most commonly used software packages, along with the Web sites with information about them, are as follows:

ProCite: http://www.isiresearchsoft.com/pc/PChome.asp

EndNote: http://www.endnote.com/

A trial version of either software package can be downloaded from the Web site and used to write one or two papers. In this way, you can judge each program's effectiveness in helping track and cite references and decide whether to purchase it.

Locating Relevant Literature

Within each database, a search is initiated by performing a separate search of each keyword that has been identified. Search engines are unforgiving of misspellings, so spelling should be carefully watched. Most databases allow you to indicate quickly where in the database records you wish to search for the term—in the article titles, journal names, keywords, formal subject headings, or full texts of the articles. Citations are usually listed with the most recent ones first.

Most databases provide abstracts of the articles in which the term is cited, allowing you to get some sense of their content, so you may judge whether the term is useful in relation to your selected topic. If an important reference is found, it should be saved to a file.

At this time, not all of the listed citations should be examined. Instead, the number of citations (or "hits") that were found in the search should be noted. In some cases, the number of hits may be far too large to examine all of them. For example, in April 2002, a search of an on-line database using the keyword "coping" yielded 5039 hits. The keyword "social support" yielded 9191 hits.

After a search has been completed, the results should be saved as a file, the number of citations should be recorded, and the next keyword should be searched. When you have completed this activity, you should have some sense of the extent of available literature in your area of interest. At this point, you should also have enough information to plan more complex searches.

Performing Complex Searches

A *complex search* combines two or more concepts or synonyms in one search. Selection of the concepts or synonyms to combine may be based on the results of previous searches. The method of performing more complex searches varies with the bibliographical database, so when a particular database is used for the first time, it is best to look for instructions and consider consulting a librarian.

In some bibliographical databases, the word *and* is used to combine terms. In some databases, the word *AND* must be in uppercase. Sometimes quotation marks must be placed around the concepts—for example, "coping" and "social support." In others, just typing *coping* and *social support* will find the references needed. While using CINAHL and OVID software, you can perform searches for individual terms and then initiate a complex search by selecting the "Combine" option at the top of the screen. A new screen appears, listing the previous searches you have performed. You may select two or more of the previous searches to combine. For example, you might wish to combine the concepts "coping" *AND* "social support." In April 2002, selecting the "Combine AND" option in CINAHL for the "coping" search and the "social support" search yielded 1064 hits.

Searches for some topics may reveal that many hits are not useful because the selected search term also includes another term that is of no interest. For example, you may want to examine studies of coping but not those discussing coping in relation to support. To eliminate references with the term *support*, use as your search phrase "coping" NOT "support."

A number of other complex operations can be used to search databases, but the search methods described here will get you started. Instructions about how to use search options should be available in the database you are using. Some databases provide an advanced search option in which separate boxes are available for inclusion of multiple terms. For example, you might wish to include an author's last name, one or more key terms, and a journal title in a single search.

Limiting the Search

Several strategies may be used to limit a search if, after performing complex searches, there are still too many hits. The limits that can be imposed vary with the database. In CINAHL, for example, a search may be limited to English language articles. You can also limit the years of a search. For example, a search might be limited to articles published in the last 10 years. Searches can be limited to find only papers that are research, are reviews, are published in consumer health journals, include abstracts, or are available in full text.

When the combined search for "coping" and "social support," described in the last section, was limited to research papers in English, there were 641 hits. In CINAHL, a search can be limited by clicking on the icon above the search history labeled "Limit." The icon figure is a bull's-eye with a red arrow. Limiting the search to research papers in English published between 1997 and 2002 yielded 260 hits. A search limited to research papers in English with full text available yielded 32 hits. A search for only full-text articles severely limits the relevant sources currently available using CINAHL; however, CINAHL is adding an increasing number of full-text articles and this search approach should be viable in the near future.

Based on the titles, the hits that seem most relevant to a topic can be selected by clicking the box to the left of the reference in the list of citations (OVID software). Then the citations that have been selected can be either printed or saved to a file. Saving the citation to a file and then printing it with a word processing program takes considerably less paper than trying to print directly from the database. The full-text option can be selected for hits with full text available. These papers can be either printed or saved to files for printing later or reading later on the computer screen.

Selecting Search Fields

Search fields indicate the various pieces of information provided about an article by the bibliographical database. The fields vary with the bibliographical database. In CINAHL, selecting the Search Fields option at the top of the search page allows you to choose the search fields that you would like to be listed for the references you select. The following list explains the search fields available in CINAHL:

Accession number. The number that is assigned to the citation when it was entered into the CINAHL database.

Special fields contained. List of the special fields available for a particular citation. Special fields include abstracts and cited references.

Authors. Names of the authors, last name first, then initials of first names. Author names are in blue and underlined. The underlining indicates that clicking on the name will result in a search listing all of the citations in the database in which that individual is an author. This option allows you to identify other publications by authors who are central to building the body of knowledge of the topic you have selected to study.

Institution. The institution(s) at which the author(s) was affiliated at the time the article was published. This information might be useful if you wished to contact the author.

Title. Title of the article.

Source. Journal title, volume number, issue number, page numbers, year, month, and number of references.

Abbreviated source. Abbreviated version of the journal title, volume number, issue number, page numbers, year, month, and number of references.

Document delivery. The National Library of Medicine (NLM) serial identifier number. This number is useful if you plan to request delivery of the document by fax, e-mail, or postal delivery. In many cases, there is a rather large fee for this service.

Journal subset. The categories to which the journal has been assigned. For example, the journal may be classified as a core nursing journal, a nursing journal, a peer-reviewed journal, or a U.S. journal.

Special interest category. The categories of specialization to which the journal has been assigned. For example, the journal may be classified in the category of "Onco-logic Care."

CINAHL subject headings. The key words from the CINAHL thesaurus, which have been assigned to the article. Examination of these subject headings across the references obtained in a search can suggest additional keywords to be added to the keyword list.

Instrumentation. A list of measurement instruments used in the study.

Abstract. An abstract of the study.

ISSN. The International Standard Serial Number, an identifier number for the journal.

Publication type. The type of article. For example, journal article, research journal article, dissertation. Also indicates the presence of tables, graphs, and charts.

Language. The language in which the article is written. In many cases, articles that are not in English have English abstracts.

Entry month. The month in which the citation was included in CINAHL.

Cited references. List of full references for all citations included in the paper. These references can be valuable because they allow you to cross-check the completeness of your computer searches.

A cross-check is performed by comparing the database's cited references list with the list of citations obtained from your searches. This is very easy to do if reference-managing software is used. In many cases you will find "treasures" that would have been missed if you had relied only on the computer search. Some of the references, which may not be journals or books listed in the databases that have been searched, may provide clues to other databases that might offer additional useful sources. These references suggest new keywords for another computer search in the databases you have been using.

Linking

Linking moves you from one Web site to another Web site. In citation databases such as CINAHL, linking allows you to go from the underlined word <u>full text</u> directly to a full-text electronic version of an article. This is possible because a link has been established between the database and an archive of full-text journal articles. In the coming years, nursing databases will provide links from one electronic article to another and eventually to electronic books. This type of linking will allow the user to click on a citation in the text or the reference list of an electronic article and be connected directly with the full text of the referenced article. The time required to locate and obtain the majority of literature on a selected topic will be greatly reduced. Currently, there are multiple archives of full-text nursing journal articles, but the various archives are not interconnected. Efforts are underway to develop linking capabilities across databases (Barber, 2001).

Searching Electronic Journals

A number of new nursing journals have been developed that are published only in electronic form and are referred to as *electronic journals.* Because of the high costs of publishing and distributing a printed journal, a publishing company risks losing money unless there is a very large market for the journal. Most of the electronic journals are targeted to specialty audiences that are relatively small. These journals may have more current information on a topic than can be found in traditional journals, because articles submitted by authors are reviewed and published in electronic journals within 3 to 4 months. For articles submitted to printed journals, the time from submission to publication is 1 to 2 years (Fitzpatrick, 2001).

Many electronic journals have been established at universities by faculty members interested in a particular specialty area. In some cases, subscribing to the online journal may be the only way to gain access to the articles. Some electronic journals are listed in available bibliographic databases, and full-text articles from the electronic journal can be accessed through the database. However, many electronic journals are not yet in the bibliographic databases or may not be in the database you are using. Ingenta (http://www.ingenta.com/) is a commercial Web site that allows the search of thousands of on-line journals from many disciplines.

Relevant articles from an electronic journal can be obtained by first locating the journal on the Internet and then scanning the titles of the published articles. Many libraries have contracts with the vendors that enable their affiliated users to have off-campus access to some of these journals and databases. Some contracts require that nonaffiliated users may use the resources only within the library. Still other contracts require that all use of the resources must occur in the library or other specified buildings or terminals. A list of the current electronic nursing journals is available at the following Web addresses:

http://www.nursefriendly.com/nursing/linksections/nursingjournals.html

http://www.healthweb.org (select "nursing" from list)

http://www.thornbury-nre.co.uk/index.asp (under search, select "Journals [Home Pages]". Under category, select countries desired. Home pages of nursing journals around the world are provided.)

Many libraries provide lists of the electronic journals available to their affiliated users that can be examined. If you are affiliated with the library, you may be able to obtain articles quite easily.

Searching the World Wide Web

It is unlikely that studies relevant to a topic can be found by searching the Web; however, you may find other relevant information. One advantage of information obtained from the Web is that it is likely to be more current than material found in books. One disadvantage is that the information is uneven in terms of accuracy. There is no screening process for information placed on the Web. Thus a considerable amount of misinformation can be found, as well as some "gems" that might not be found elsewhere. It is important to check the source of any information obtained on the Web so that its validity can be judged.

A wide range of search engines are available for conducting Web searches. Search engines vary in the following ways: (1) the approach used to search the Web, (2) the extent of the Web that is covered (most do not cover the entire Web so you may need to use more than one engine), (3) the frequency with which the search engine updates the Web sites that are indexed, and (4) the ease with which they are used. New search engines appear on the scene almost daily, so identifying the "best" search engine in this text is not particularly useful. Many university libraries provide a list of good search engines.

When a promising site is found, its location can be stored in the Web browser (called "Bookmarks" in Netscape and "Favorites" in Internet Explorer). Remember, however, that if a Web site will be used as a reference in a bibliography, the date it was viewed and the address (URL, Uniform Research Locator) it had at that time are required for proper citation.

Storing a Web site's address on a browser simplifies return visits to check information on the Web site. Additionally, many Web sites are frequently updated and can be regularly checked for new information. Sometimes clicking on a link (underlined or highlighted name) on one Web site will reveal other Web sites with helpful information. Following these links, referred to as *surfing the Web*, is an important part of a Web search. Information overload is one problem that may be encountered while surfing the Web; you may find too much information and need to be selective about what you retrieve.

Although both Internet Explorer and Netscape store a history of the Web sites you have visited as you move from one to another, it is wise to store their locations in the browser to avoid having to retrace the steps back through the links. Also, Web sites are often changed or deleted, so it is wise to save a particularly useful Web page as a file. Text, graphics, or both may be saved from the Web. If space on your hard drive is a problem, a "zip" (file compression) program can be used to store the file in a smaller form.

Metasearchers offer relatively new approaches to searching the Web. These programs perform a search by using multiple search engines, enabling a single search to cover more of the Web. As of the writing of this chapter, our favorite metasearcher is Dogpile, which can be found at http://www.dogpile.com. Dogpile uses an innovative strategy for searching that increases the number of hits on a topic.

Systematically Recording References

The bibliographical information on a source should be recorded in a systematic manner, according to the format that will be used in the reference list. Many journals and academic institutions use the format developed by the American Psychological Association (APA) (2001). The reference lists in this text are presented in a modified APA format. Computerized lists of sources usually contain complete citations for references and should be filed for future use. You can also easily search a computerized database with a computer and obtain complete reference citations.

Sources that will be cited in a paper or recorded in a reference list should be cross-checked two or three times to prevent errors. Damrosch and Damrosch (1996) have identified some of the common errors that authors make when applying the APA format, and they provide guidelines for how to avoid them. The sources cited in the reference list should follow the correct format for print and on-line full-text versions.

Print Version

Plawecki, H. M. (1996). Improving a manuscript's chances for acceptance. *Journal of Holistic Nursing, 14*, 3–5.

On-Line Full-Text Version

Plawecki, H. M. (1996). Improving a manuscript's chances for acceptance. *Journal of Holistic Nursing, 14*, 3–5. Available: OVID File: Periodical Abstracts Research II Item: 02993150.

CLARIFYING EVIDENCE FOR BEST PRACTICES THROUGH LITERATURE REVIEWS

The process of reviewing the literature in preparation for conducting a study involves careful critique of the methodology and an examination of the existing literature. Findings from each research report are clarified by the reviewer and then paraphrased. *Paraphrasing* involves expressing an author's findings clearly and concisely in your own words. A new study is then designed to improve the methodology and to strengthen the evidence for practice. In recent years, it has become increasingly urgent that the literature also be reviewed to define the state of the science in a given area of practice through integrated literature reviews and meta-analyses.

Integrated Literature Reviews—State of the Science

An *integrative review of research* is conducted to identify, analyze, and synthesize the results from independent studies to determine the current knowledge (what is known and not known) in a particular area (Ganong, 1987; Hearn, Feuer, Higginson, & Sheldon, 1999; Jadad, Moher, & Klassen, 1998; Smith & Stullenbarger, 1991). A group of nurses on a nursing unit might find a need for an integrated review regarding a particular patient care problem. If a review cannot be found in the literature, it might be necessary to perform one specific to the needs of the unit. The results could guide the development of a protocol for the procedure or be used in developing a critical pathway. The studies are selected for inclusion based on their quality and their relationship to a selected practice problem. Thus initially, the studies should be read and critiqued. Then the studies that are of the highest quality should be selected, and their purposes, methods, results, and findings should be compared. It might help to develop a table that includes essential information from each study so that comparisons can be made (Table 4-3) (Martin, 1997). It might also help to identify the findings that are common among the different studies and to compare and contrast

TABLE 4-3

SYNTHESIZING STUDIES TO GENERATE A REVIEW OF LITERATURE

AUTHOR AND YEAR	PURPOSE	SAMPLE	MEASUREMENT	TREATMENT	RESULTS	FINDINGS
Allman (1991)						
Bergstrom, Braden, Laguzza, & Holman (1987)						
Berlowitz & Wilking (1989)						
Braden & Bergstrom (1987)						
Harrison, Wells, Fisher, & Prince (1996)						
Norton (1989)						
Norton, McLaren, & Exton-Smith (1975)						
Okamoto, Lamers, & Shurtleff (1983)						

the outcomes of these studies. Table 4-4 was developed as an example, using the studies conducted on the prediction and prevention of pressure ulcers in adults. Then the focus should be on integrating the findings from all of the studies. The type of reasoning used during the integration of findings is synthesis. *Synthesis of sources* involves compiling the findings from all of the selected studies, and analyzing and interpreting the clustered findings. Finally the meanings obtained from all sources are combined, or *clustered,* to specify the current state of research-based knowledge for a particular area of clinical practice. A number of integrated reviews of research have been written on pressure ulcer prevention.*

Expert researchers and clinicians have developed publications that summarize nursing knowledge on a variety of topics. In 1983 the first volume of the *Annual Review of Nursing Research* was published. The integrative reviews of research included in these annual publications cover relevant topics about nursing practice, nursing care delivery, nursing education, and the nursing profession. Integrative reviews have also been published in a variety of clinical and research journals. The Sigma Theta Tau *Online Journal of Nursing Synthesis* publishes only integrated reviews. The international Cochrane Collaboration (http://www.cochrane.org) and the Agency for Health Care Research and Quality (http://www.ahrq.gov/) commission systematic reviews on critical areas of health care. The journal *Evidence-Based Nursing* also participates in identifying clinical research for practice (Sermeus & Vanhaecht, 2000).

*Anthony, 1996; Armstrong & Bortz, 2001; Carlson & King, 1990; Cooper, 1987; Draper & Denis, 1996; Hedrick-Thompson, 1992; Land, 1995; Panel for the Prediction and Prevention of Pressure Ulcers in Adults, 1992; Rutledge, Donaldson, & Pravikoff, 2000; Witko & Whittemore, 1998.

TABLE 4-4

COMPARISON AND CONTRAST STUDY FINDINGS ON THE PREDICTION AND PREVENTION OF PRESSURE ULCERS

AUTHOR AND YEAR	FINDING 1	FINDING 2	FINDING 3
Allman (1991)			
Bergstrom, Braden, Laguzza, & Holman (1987)			
Berlowitz & Wilking (1989)			
Braden & Bergstrom (1987)			
Harrison, Wells, Fisher, & Prince (1996)			
Norton (1989)			
Norton, McLaren, & Exton-Smith (1975)			
Okamoto, Lamers, & Shurtleff (1983)			

Meta-Analyses

Meta-analyses go beyond the integrated review by performing statistical analyses using summative findings from multiple published studies. Using these strategies, it is possible to provide a global estimate of such things as the mean number of days of hospitalization following a particular procedure, or the reduction in the number of hours a patient spends in a coronary care unit as a result of a particular nursing intervention. The results from meta-analyses are sometimes referred to as *benchmarking* (Rudy, Lucke, Whitman, & Davidson, 2001). Meta-analyses are discussed in greater detail in Chapter 13.

WRITING A REVIEW OF LITERATURE

A literature review should document the current knowledge of a selected topic and indicate the findings that are ready for use in practice. Often a detailed outline is developed to guide the writing of a literature review. The review of literature begins with an introduction, includes a presentation of relevant studies, and concludes with a summary of current knowledge (Burns & Grove, 2001). The headings and essential content of a literature review are briefly described as follows:

1. ***Introduction.*** The introduction indicates the focus or purpose of the review; describes the organization of sources; and indicates the basis for ordering the sources—for example, from least to most important or from least to most current. This section should be brief and interesting enough to capture the attention of the reader. The introduction may be rewritten several times based on the development of other sections of the literature review.

2. ***Empirical literature.*** Empirical literature includes quality studies that are relevant for a selected utilization project. For each study, the purpose, sample size, design, and specific findings should be presented, with a scholarly but brief critique of the study's strengths and weaknesses. This critique should be clear and concise and include only the most relevant studies. The content from these sources is best paraphrased or summarized in your own words. If a direct quotation is used, it should be kept short to promote the flow of ideas. Long quotations are often unnecessary and interfere with the reader's train of thought.

   Ethical issues must be considered in presenting research sources (Gunter, 1981). The content from studies must be presented honestly and not distorted to support a selected utilization project. The weaknesses of a study need to be addressed, but it is not necessary to be highly critical of a researcher's work. The criticism should be focused on the content, be related in some way to the proposed project, and be stated as possible or plausible explanations, so that it is neutral and scholarly rather than negative and blaming. Additionally, the researchers' works that are cited in the literature review should be accurately documented.

3. ***Summary.*** The summary includes a concise presentation of the research knowledge about a selected topic, including what is known and not known. The Panel for the Prediction and Prevention of Pressure Ulcers in Adults (1992) has summarized the research literature related to the prevention of pressure ulcers in adults. The following quotation presents key information from their summary of risk assessment tools and risk factors.

Risk Assessment Tools and Risk Factors

GOAL: "Identify at risk individuals needing prevention and the specific factors placing them at risk.

Bed- and chair-bound individuals or those with impaired ability to reposition should be assessed for additional factors that increase risk for developing pressure ulcers. These factors include immobility, incontinence, nutritional factors such as inadequate dietary intake and impaired nutritional status, and altered level of consciousness. Individuals should be assessed on admission to acute care and rehabilitation hospitals, nursing homes, home care programs, and other health care facilities. A systematic risk assessment can be accomplished by using a validated risk assessment tool such as the Braden Scale or Norton Scale. Pressure ulcer risk should be reassessed at periodic intervals. All assessments of risk should be documented.

RATIONALE: To prevent pressure ulcers, individuals at risk must be identified so that risk factors can be reduced through intervention. The primary risk factors for pressure ulcers are immobility and limited activity levels (Allman, compiled, 1991; Berlowitz & Wilking, 1989; Norton, McLaren, & Exton-Smith, 1975; Okamoto, Lamers, & Shurtleff, 1983). Therefore, persons with impaired ability to reposition themselves or those whose activity is limited to bed or any chair should be assessed for their risk of developing a pressure ulcer. To determine the magnitude of risk, the degree to which mobility and activity levels are limited can be quantified. Both the Norton Scale (Norton et al., 1975) and the Braden Scale (Bergstrom, Braden, Laguzza, & Holman, 1987; Braden & Bergstrom, 1987) assess these factors.

Other risk factors for pressure ulcer development include incontinence, impaired nutritional status, and altered level of consciousness. Incontinence is assessed by the Moisture subscale of the Braden Scale (Braden & Bergstrom, 1987) and the Incontinence component of the Norton Scale....Nutritional factors are considered indirectly in the General Condition component of the Norton Scale (Norton, 1989) and the Nutritional Status subscale of the Braden Scale.... Altered level of consciousness is assessed by the Norton Scale's Mental Condition subscale and the Braden Scale's Sensory Perception subscale.

Numerous risk assessment tools exist; however, only the Braden Scale and the Norton Scale (original and modified) have been tested extensively. The Braden Scale has been evaluated in diverse sites that include medical-surgical units, intensive care units, and nursing homes. The Norton Scale has been tested with elderly subjects in hospital settings.

The reported sensitivity and specificity of these risk assessment tools have varied greatly. This variability probably reflects differences in study settings, populations, and outcome measures.... The degree to which preventative interventions have been implemented in response to the findings of the risk assessments in these studies may have also contributed to the variability in their reported performance....

Despite the limitations of the Norton and Braden scales, their use ensures systematic evaluation of individual risk factors. No information is currently available to suggest that adaptations of these risk assessment tools or the assessment of any single risk factor or a combination of risk factors predict risk as well as the overall scores obtained by the tools.

The condition of an individual admitted to a health care facility is not static; consequently, pressure ulcer risk requires routine reexamination. The frequency with which such reevaluations need to be done is unknown. However, if an individual becomes bed- or chair-bound or develops difficulty with repositioning, pressure ulcer risk needs to be assessed. Accurate and complete documentation of all risk assessments ensures continuity of care and may be used as a foundation for the skin care plan." (Panel for the Prediction and Prevention of Pressure Ulcers in Adults, 1992, pp. 13–15)

Once the research literature has been read and summarized, a decision should be made about whether there is adequate knowledge to make a change in clinical practice. For example, what changes would you make in your practice after reading the summary of research literature on risk assessment tools and risk factors for prevention of pressure ulcers? Research has shown that the Braden (Braden & Bergstrom, 1987) and Norton scales (Norton, 1989) are effective in assessing patients at risk for developing pressure ulcers. In addition, both scales have been effective in assessing pressure ulcer risk in the elderly. Both scales might be submitted to your agency so that the administration and staff might select one for use in practice. The next step involves developing a plan to change practice based on research. The process for using research findings in practice is the focus of Chapter 13.

SUMMARY

The review of literature in a research report is a summary of current knowledge about a particular practice problem and includes what is known and not known about this problem. The literature is reviewed to summarize knowledge for use in practice or to provide a basis for conducting a study. To increase your understanding of the literature reviews presented in published studies, the following areas are addressed: (1) the sources included in a literature review and (2) the purposes of the literature review in quantitative and qualitative studies. A literature review often includes theoretical literature (concept analyses, maps or models, and theories) and empirical literature (studies) that support the research problem and purpose studied. Usually primary sources are cited, but not secondary sources. The purpose of the literature review in quantitative research is to direct the development and implementation of the study and is the same for the different types of studies (descriptive, correlational, quasi-experimental, and experimental). In qualitative research, the purpose and timing of the literature review vary based on the type of study to be conducted. The purposes for conducting literature reviews for phenomenological, grounded theory, ethnographic, and historical research are addressed.

This chapter also provides guidelines for critiquing the literature review section in a published study. Questions are identified to help with determining the quality of a study's literature review. The literature review from Vyhlidal et al. (1997) on the effects of mattress surfaces on the incidence of pressure ulcers is presented as an example, and a critique of this literature review is provided.

The process of searching the literature has changed dramatically as the use of computers has increased. Through the use of electronic databases, a large volume of references can be located quickly. Before beginning a search of the literature, a written plan of your search strategy should be developed. The bibliographical databases you plan to search should be selected. Keywords for conducting your search should be selected. Keywords are the major concepts or variables that must be included in a search. A search should be initiated by performing a separate search of each keyword that has been identified. Then the results of two or more searches should be combined to limit the number of references to a reasonable number. Reference management software should be used to track the references obtained through the searches.

The final step in the literature review process is summarizing relevant studies to determine the current body of knowledge. Summarizing research literature involves selecting the relevant studies, synthesizing the study findings, and writing the review. A comprehensive, scholarly synthesis of the literature is evident in published integrative reviews of research. These reviews are conducted to identify, analyze, and synthesize the results from independent studies to determine the current knowledge in a particular area. The literature review usually begins with an introduction, includes empirical sources, and concludes with a summary of current knowledge. A brief summary of the research literature related to prevention of pressure ulcers in adults is presented as an example.

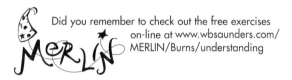

Did you remember to check out the free exercises on-line at www.wbsaunders.com/ MERLIN/Burns/understanding

REFERENCES

Allman, R. M. (1991). *Pressure ulcers among bedridden hospitalized elderly.* Division of Gerontology/Geriatrics, University of Alabama at Birmingham. Unpublished data compiled.

American Psychological Association. (2001). *Publication manual of the American Psychological Association* (5th ed.). Washington, DC: Author.

Anthony, D. (1996). The treatment of decubitus ulcers: A century of misinformation in the textbooks. *Journal of Advanced Nursing, 24*(2), 309–316.

Armstrong, D., & Bortz, P. (2001). An integrative review of pressure relief in surgical patients. *AORN Journal, 73*(3), 645, 647–648.

Barber, D. (April, 2001). A guide to electronic journal archives. *Online Journal of Issues in Nursing, 5*(11), Manuscript 7. Retrieved February 19, 2002 from http://www.nursingworld.org/ojin/topic11_7.htm

Barczak, C. A., Barnett, R. I., Childs, E. J., & Bosley, L. M. (1997). Fourth national prevalence pressure ulcer prevalence survey. *Advances in Wound Care, 10*(4), 18–26.

Bergstrom, N. et al. (1994). *Treatment of pressure ulcers.* Clinical Practice Guideline, Number 15. AHCPR Publication No. 95-0652. Rockville, MD: Agency for Health Care Policy and Research, Public Health Service, U. S. Department of Health and Human Services.

Bergstrom, N., Braden, B. J., Laguzza, A., & Holman, V. (1987). The Braden Scale for predicting pressure sore risk. *Nursing Research, 36*(4), 205–210.

Berlowitz, D. R., & Wilking, S. V. (1989). Risk factors for pressure sores. A comparison of cross-sectional and cohort-derived data. *Journal of the American Geriatrics Society, 37*(11), 1043–1050.

Braden, B., & Bergstrom, N. (1987). A conceptual schema for the study of the etiology of pressure sores. *Rehabilitation Nursing, 12*(1), 8–12.

Burns, N., & Grove, S. K. (2001). *The practice of nursing research: Conduct, critique, and utilization* (4th ed.). Philadelphia: Saunders.

Carlson, C. E., & King, R. B. (1990). Prevention of pressure sores. In J. J. Fitzpatrick, R. L. Taunton, & J. O. Benoliel (Eds.), *Annual review of nursing research* (Vol. 8, pp. 35–56). New York: Springer.

Cooper, D. M. (1987). Pressure ulcers: Unpublished research 1976–1986: Process to outcome. *Nursing Clinics of North America, 22*(2), 475–492.

Cullum, N., Deeks, J., Sheldon, T. A., Song, F., Fletcher, A. W. (2001). Beds, mattresses and cushions for pressure sore prevention and treatment. *The Cochrane Library (Oxford), 2*(20), 1–20.

Damrosch, S., & Damrosch, G. D. (1996). Methodology corner. Avoiding common mistakes in APA style: The briefest of guidelines. *Nursing Research, 45*(6), 331–333.

Downs, F. S. (1999a). How much is enough? *Applied Nursing Research, 12*(3), 164–165.

Downs, F. S. (1999b). How to cozy up to a research report. *Applied Nursing Research, 12*(4), 215–216.

Draper, S., & Denis, N. (1996). Preventing heel pressure ulcers: A review of studies evaluating body support surfaces and heel devices. *Orthoscope, 2*(3): 5–6.

Fitzpatrick, J. J. (2001). Scholarly publishing: Current issues of cost and quality, fueled by the rapid expansion of electronic publishing. *Applied Nursing Research, 14*(1), 1–2.

Ganong, L. H. (1987). Integrative reviews of nursing research. *Research in Nursing & Health, 10*(1), 1–11.

Gunter, L. (1981). Literature review. In S. D. Krampitz & N. Pavlovich (Eds.), *Readings for nursing research* (pp. 11–16), St. Louis: Mosby.

Harrison, M. B., Wells, G., Fisher, A., & Prince, M. (1996). Practice guidelines for the prediction and prevention of pressure ulcers: Evaluating the evidence. *Applied Nursing Research, 9*(1), 9–17.

Hearn, J., Feuer, D., Higginson, I. J., & Sheldon, T. (1999). Issues in research: Systematic reviews. *Palliative Medicine, 13*(1), 75–80.

Hedrick-Thompson, J. K. (1992). A review of pressure reduction device studies. *Journal of Vascular Nursing, 10*(4), 3–5.

Hedrick-Thompson, J., Halloran, T., Strader, T., & McSweeney, M. (1993). Pressure-reduction products: Making appropriate choices. *Journal of ET Nursing, 20*(6), 239–244.

Husain, T. (1953). An experimental study of some pressure effects on tissues with reference to the bed-sore problem. *Journal of Pathology and Bacteriology, 66*, 347–358.

Jadad, A. R., Moher, D., & Klassen, T. P. (1998). Guides for reading and interpreting systematic reviews. *Archives of Pediatrics & Adolescent Medicine, 152*(8), 812–817.

Jester, J., & Weaver, V. (1990). A report of clinical investigation of various tissue support surfaces used for the prevention, early intervention, and management of pressure ulcers. *Ostomy/Wound Management, 26*, 39–45.

Kemp, M. et al. (1993). The role of support surfaces and patient attributes in preventing pressure ulcers in elderly patients. *Research in Nursing & Health, 16*(2), 89–96.

Kosiak, M. (1959). Etiology and pathology of decubitus ulcers. *Archives of Physical Medicine and Rehabilitation, 42*, 19–29.

Krouskop, T., Williams, R., Krebs, M., Herszkowicz, I., & Garber, S. (1985). Effectiveness of mattress overlays in reducing interface pressures during recumbency. *Journal of Rehabilitation Research and Development, 22*(3), 7–10.

Kübler-Ross, E. (1969). *On death and dying.* New York: Macmillan.

Land, L. (1995). A review of pressure damage prevention strategies. *Journal of Advanced Nursing, 22*(2), 329–337.

Landis, E. (1930). Micro-injection studies of capillary blood pressure in human skin. *Heart, 15*, 209–278.

Martin, P. A. (1997). Ask an expert: Writing a useful literature review for a quantitative research project. *Applied Nursing Research, 10*(3), 159–162.

Munhall, P. L. (2001). *Nursing research: A qualitative perspective* (3rd ed.). Sudbury, MA: Jones & Bartlett.

Naisbitt, J., & Aburdene, P. (1990). *Megatrends 2000: Ten new directions for the 1990's.* New York: Morrow.

National Pressure Ulcer Advisory Panel (1989). *Pressure Ulcers: Incidence, economics, risk assessment. Consensus development conference statement.* West Dundee, IL: S-N Publications.

Norton, D. (1989). Calculating the risk: Reflections on the Norton Scale. *Decubitus, 2*(3), 24–31.

Norton, D., McLaren, R., & Exton-Smith, A. N. (1975). *An investigation of geriatric nursing problems in hospital.* London: Churchill Livingstone.

Okamoto, G. A., Lamers, J. V., & Shurtleff, D. B. (1983). Skin breakdown in patients with myelomeningocele. *Archives of Physical Medicine Rehabilitation, 64*(1), 20–23.

Panel for the Prediction and Prevention of Pressure Ulcers in Adults. (1992). *Pressure ulcers in adults: Prediction and prevention.* Clinical practice guidelines. AHCPR Publication No. 92–0047. Rockville, MD: Agency for Health Care Policy and Research, Public Health Service, U.S. Department of Health and Human Services.

Pinch, W. J. (1995). Synthesis: Implementing a complex process. *Nurse Educator, 20*(1), 34–40.

Rudy, E. B., Lucke, J. F., Whitman, G. R., & Davidson, L. J. (2001). Benchmarking patient outcomes. *Journal of Nursing Scholarship, 33*(2), 185–189.

Rutledge, D. N., Donaldson, N. E., & Pravikoff, D. S. (2000). Protection of skin integrity: Progress in pressure ulcer prevention since the AHCPR 1992 guideline. *Online Journal of Clinical Innovations, 3*(5), 1–67.

Sermeus, W., & Vanhaecht, K. (2000). WISECARE to support evidence in practice, *Applied Nursing Research, 13*(3), 159–161.

Smith, M. C., & Stullenbarger, E. (1991). A prototype for integrative review and meta-analysis of nursing research. *Journal of Advanced Nursing, 16*(11), 1272–1283.

Stoneberg, C., Pitcock, N., & Myton, C. (1986). Pressure sores in the homebound: One solution. *American Journal of Nursing, 86*(4), 426–428.

Strauch, K., Linton, R., & Cohen, C. (1989). *Library research guide to nursing: Illustrated search strategy and sources.* Ann Arbor, MI: Pierian Press.

Vyhlidal, S. K., Moxness, D., Bosak, K. S., Van Meter, F. G., & Bergstrom, N. (1997). Mattress replacement or foam overlay? Prospective study on the incidence of pressure ulcers. *Applied Nursing Research, 10*(3), 111–120.

Whitney, J., Fellows, B., & Larson, E. (1984). Do mattresses make a difference? *Journal of Gerontological Nursing, 10*(10), 20–25.

Whittemore, R. (1998). Pressure-reduction support surfaces: A review of the literature. *Journal of Wound, Ostomy, and Continence Nursing, 25*(1), 6–24.

Williams, A. (1972). A study of factors contributing to skin breakdown. *Nursing Research, 21*(3), 238–243.

Witko, A. (1998). A review of the literature on pressure-reduction support surfaces: Something is missing. Pressure-reduction support surfaces: A review of the literature. *Journal of Wound, Ostomy, and Continence Nursing, 25*(4), 177.

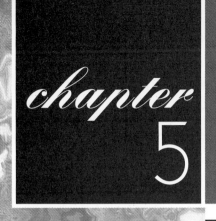

chapter 5

Understanding Theory and Research Frameworks

OBJECTIVES

Completing this chapter should enable you to:
1. Explain the purpose of study frameworks.
2. Identify the elements of a study framework (concept, relational statement, conceptual model, theory, and conceptual map).
3. Ascertain the framework of a published study and illustrate it using a conceptual map.

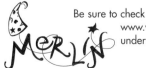

Be sure to check out the free exercises on-line at
www.wbsaunders.com/MERLIN/Burns/
understanding

135

OBJECTIVES—cont'd

4. Discuss the relationship of concepts and variables in research.
5. Explain the relationship between theory and research.
6. Critique a study framework.

RELEVANT TERMS

Abstract
Concept
Conceptual definition
Conceptual map
Conceptual model
Constructs
Existence statement
Framework
Implicit framework

Phenomenon (Phenomena)
Philosophical stance
Philosophies
Propositions
Relational statement
Statements
Theory
Variable

When an idea for a study first emerges, the researcher has a "theory" about what the study outcomes will be and why. That theory might not be formally stated or even written, but it is, nonetheless, a theory. If a researcher was telling you about her or his study ideas, you might ask why she or he planned to use a particular variable, or why she or he expected particular study outcomes. The explanation you received would be an expression of a theory about the study since the ideas that lead a researcher to develop a particular study have their roots in theory. Sometimes the researcher has read about the theory and may have used the theoretical ideas in clinical practice. Other studies the researcher read may have tested that theory. In other cases, the theoretical ideas may have not been previously put into writing. As a researcher develops a plan for conducting a study, the theory on which the study is based is expressed as the study framework. The framework spells out the logic that the researcher used in planning the study. When the study is carried out, the researcher can then answer the question Was my theory correct? Thus a study tests the accuracy of theoretical ideas. In explaining the study findings, the researcher will interpret those findings in relation to the theory.

An important part of critiquing the quality of a study is to identify and evaluate the framework. Understanding the theory on which a study is based also will help you determine whether it is appropriate to apply the study findings to your practice. To assist you, this chapter discusses what theories are and how they are tested, how a framework is developed, which strategies can be used to identify the framework in a published study, and how frameworks should be critiqued.

WHAT IS A THEORY?

We use theories to organize what we know about a phenomenon. Formally, a *theory* is defined as an integrated set of defined concepts and statements that present a view of a phenomenon and can be used to describe, explain, predict, and/or control that phenomenon. In Chapter 1 we indicated that the purpose of research can be either theory generation or theory testing. Most quantitative research is designed for theory testing. Theories are tested through research to determine the correctness of their descriptions, explanations, predictions, and strategies to control outcomes. Theories may be generated through qualitative research. These theories are developed as the outcome of a qualitative study rather than as a guide to the development of a study, which occurs in quantitative research.

Theories Guide Nursing Practice

Theories have been developed in nursing to explain phenomena important to clinical practice. For example, we have a theory of uncertainty in illness (Mischel, 1988), a theory of health promotion behavior (Pender, Murdaugh & Parsons, 2001), and a theory of mother-infant attachment (Walker, 1992). Sometimes we use theories developed in other disciplines, such as psychology or biology, and apply them to nursing situations. Although we use these theories to guide our practice, in many cases we have not tested them to determine whether the nursing actions proposed by the theory actually have the effects claimed.

In their theory of mother-infant bonding, Klaus and Kennell (1976), proposed that bonding between a mother and her newborn child occurred within hours or days of birth. They proposed that if skin-to-skin physical contact between mother and child did not occur during this short time frame, bonding would not occur, and the relationship between mother and child would be permanently impaired. Nurses leaped on this idea and focused intensely on ensuring that early physical contact occurred between mother and newborn. However, research testing this theoretical notion demonstrated that it was not true (Walker, 1992). Mother and newborn, although kept apart because of illness or other circumstances, were able to bond. This example supports the contention that theories should not be applied to clinical practice without first testing the ideas through research. In this case a theory of attachment, based on long-term studies of mothers and infants, emerged. These studies found that development of an attachment between mother and child was indeed critical but that the process occurred over a period of months rather than days. These findings, expressed as the theory of attachment, guide nurses in their care of mothers and their children.

Theories are Abstract

Theories are *abstract* rather than concrete. Abstract means that the theory is the expression of an idea apart from any specific instance. An abstract idea focuses on more general things. Concrete ideas are concerned with realities or actual instances; they are particular rather than general. For example, the word *anxiety* represents an abstract idea; a family member pacing in an intensive care waiting room is a particular instance of reality and thus is concrete. The abstract ideas in theories can be tested through research to verify that they hold true in a concrete reality. The abstract idea of the mother bonding with her newborn infant within a few hours or days did not hold true in a concrete reality. In some cases, theories are generated as a result of research. The specific instances discovered during the study are used by the researcher to develop more abstract (or general) ideas about the phenomenon of interest. Selye's (1976) theory of stress was developed through specific instances demonstrated in multiple studies. Since Selye was a physician, he used case studies as specific instances of the phenomenon he was describing. The specific instances discovered during a qualitative study are often used to generate theory. Critical thinking is required to generate theory, to test theory, or to relate concrete realities to abstract ideas.

CONCEPTUAL MODELS

Conceptual models are similar to theories and are sometimes referred to as theories. However, conceptual models are even more abstract than theories. A *conceptual model* broadly explains phenomena of interest, expresses assumptions, and reflects a philosophical stance. A *phenomenon* (the plural form is *phenomena*) is an occurrence or a circumstance that is observed, something that impresses the observer as extraordinary, or a thing that appears to and is constructed by the mind. Caring is a phenomenon. Assumptions are statements that are taken for granted or considered true, even though they have not been scientifically tested. For example, we might assume that people who are poor feel poor. *Philosophies* are rational intellectual explorations of truths, principles of being, knowledge, or conduct. A *philosophical stance* is a specific philosophical view held by a person or group of individuals. For example, a philosophical stance might hold that there is no single reality, that reality is different for each individual. Although conceptual models vary in their level of abstraction and in the breadth of phenomena they explain, they all provide an overall picture of the phenomena they explain. Conceptual models are not generally considered testable through research. However, theories derived from a conceptual model can be tested.

Most disciplines have several conceptual models, each with a distinctive vocabulary. A number of conceptual models have been developed in nursing. For example, Roy and Andrews' (1998) model describes adaptation as the primary phenomenon of interest to nursing. Her model identifies the elements she considers essential to adaptation and describes how the elements interact to produce adaptation. Orem (2001) considers self-care to be the phenomenon that is central to nursing. Her model explains how nurses facilitate the self-care of clients. Rogers and colleagues (1994) sees human beings as the central phenomenon of interest to nursing, and her model is designed to explain the nature of human beings. A conceptual model may use the same or similar terms as other models but define them in different ways. For example, Roy, Orem, and Rogers may all use the term *health* but define it in different ways.

FRAMEWORK

A *framework* is a brief explanation of a theory or those portions of a theory to be tested in a study. Every study has a framework. This is true whether the study is physiological or psychosocial. A clearly expressed framework is one indication of a well-developed study. Perhaps the researcher expects one variable to cause the other. In a well-thought-out study, the researcher would explain abstractly in the framework why one variable is expected to cause the other. The idea would be expressed concretely as a hypothesis to be tested through the study methodology.

Unfortunately, in some studies, the ideas that compose the framework remain nebulous and vaguely expressed. Although the researcher believes that the variables being studied are related in some fashion, this notion is expressed only in concrete terms. The researcher may make little attempt to explain why the variables are thought to be related. However, the rudiment of a framework is the expectation (perhaps not directly expressed) that there may be an important link(s) among the study variables. Sometimes, rudimentary ideas for the framework are expressed in the introduction or literature review, in which linkages among variables found in previous studies are discussed, but then the researcher stops without fully developing the ideas as a framework. These are referred to as *implicit frameworks.* In most cases, a careful reader can extract an implicit framework from the text. Unfortunately, many nursing studies have implicit frameworks.

As the body of knowledge related to a phenomenon increases, the development of a framework to express the knowledge becomes easier. Therefore frameworks for quasi-experimental and experimental studies, which usually have a background of descriptive and correlational studies, should be more easily and fully developed than frameworks for descriptive studies. Descriptive studies often examine multiple factors to understand a phenomenon not previously well studied. Theoretical work related to the phenomenon may be tentative or nonexistent. Therefore the framework may not be as well developed.

In some studies the framework is derived from a well-tested theory that has been used as the framework for many studies. Most theories used as nursing research frameworks are from other fields and are based on theoretical works from psychology (e.g., the theory of stress and coping; Lazarus & Folkman, 1984), physiology (e.g., the theory of biological rhythms; Luce, 1970), and sociology (e.g., the theory of internal versus external control; Rotter, 1966). In other studies the framework is developed from newly proposed theory. Newly proposed theories in nursing often emerge from questions related to identified nursing problems or from the clinical insight that a relationship exists between or among elements important to desired nursing outcomes. These situations tend to be concrete, and they require that the researcher, using critical reasoning, express these concrete ideas in abstract language. New theories may also be developed from conceptual models or from elements of existing theories not previously related.

ELEMENTS OF THEORY

The first step in understanding theories is to become familiar with the elements related to theoretical ideas and their application. These elements include the concept, relational statement, and conceptual map.

Concept

A *concept* is a term that abstractly describes and names an object or phenomenon, thus providing it with a separate identity or meaning. For example, the term *anxiety* is a concept. The concept is the basic element of a theory. A published study should include identification and definition of all of the concepts important to the framework. Two terms closely related to concept are *construct* and *variable*. In conceptual models, concepts have very general meanings and are sometimes referred to as *constructs*. A construct associated with the concept of anxiety might be "emotional responses." At a more concrete level, terms are referred to as variables and are narrow in their definition. A *variable* is more specific than a concept. The word *variable* implies that the term is defined so that it is measurable and suggests that numerical values of the term are able to vary (vari-able) from one instance to another. A variable related to anxiety might be "palmar sweating," because a specific method exists for assigning numerical values to varying amounts of palmar sweat. The linkages among constructs, concepts, and variables are illustrated in the following figure.

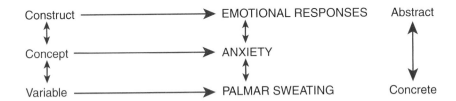

Defining Concepts

Defining concepts allows consistency in the way the term is used. A *conceptual definition* differs from the dictionary definition of a word. A conceptual definition is more comprehensive than a denotative (or dictionary) definition and includes associated meanings the word may have. A conceptual definition is referred to as connotative. Connotations of a term bring memories, moods, or images subtly or indirectly to mind (*The American Heritage Dictionary*, 2000). For example, a conceptual definition of fireplace might include the senses of hospitality and warm comfort that are often associated with fireplaces, whereas the dictionary definition is narrower and more specific: "An open recess for holding a fire at the base of a chimney." (*The American Heritage Dictionary*, 2000). Many terms commonly used in nursing language have not been clearly defined. The use of these terms in theory or research requires thoughtful exploration of the connotative meanings that the terms have within nursing and a clear statement of their meaning within the particular theory or study.

> The importance of going beyond the denotative dictionary definition of a concept is illustrated in a study designed to explore the meaning of the concept "caring" (Morse, Solberg, Neander, Bottorff, & Johnson, 1990) that was funded by the National Center for Nursing Research. The questions posed by these researchers illustrate the critical thought that must precede the development of a conceptual definition. Although the concept of caring is central to nursing, efforts to define it have been difficult. For example, the terms *caring, care,* and *nursing care* have different meanings. Caring may be an action such as "taking care of" or a concern such as "caring about." Caring may be viewed from the perspective of the nurse or the patient. The authors identified five categories of caring: (1) caring as a human trait, (2) caring as a moral imperative (ethically, one is obligated to provide it), (3) caring as an affect (feeling), (4) caring as an interpersonal relationship, and (5) caring as a therapeutic intervention. Caring has an effect on the subjective experience of the patient and the physical response of the patient.
>
> There are a number of questions about caring that need to be answered: (1) "Is caring a constant and uniform characteristic, or may caring be present in various degrees within individuals?" (2) "Is caring an emotional state that can be depleted?" (3) "Can caring be nontherapeutic?" "Can a nurse care too much?" (4) "Can cure occur without caring?" "Can a nurse provide safe practice without caring?" (5) "What difference does caring make to the patient?" (Morse et al., 1990, pp. 9–11). The authors' conclusion was that a clear conceptual definition of caring did not exist. The work of these authors generated considerable effort by others to develop further the conceptual definition of caring.

A related concept, "direct caregiving," has been carefully examined and defined by Swanson, Jensen, Specht, Johnson, and Maas (1997) to be "provision by a family care provider of appropriate personal and health care for a family member or significant other" (pp. 68–69). Caregiving addresses the care recipient's emotional, social, and physical needs. In order for direct caregiving to occur, the caregiver must have "a sense of responsibility, filial obligation, adequate financial resources, good health, and family and marital support. Social skills, spiritual support, the history of the relationship between caregiver and care recipient, and role acceptance have also been identified as important antecedents to direct caregiving." (p. 69)

Because of the significance of conceptual definitions, it is important that you identify the researcher's conceptual definitions of terms when you critique a study. Each variable in the study should be associated with a concept, a conceptual definition, and a method of measurement. The links among the conceptual definitions, the variables in the study, and the related measurement methods should be determined. (These linkages are discussed in Chapter 3.)

 To critique a framework, your critical thinking skills should be used to seek answers to the following questions about the concepts, conceptual definitions, variables, and measurement methods.

1. **What are the concepts in the framework?**
2. **How are the concepts defined?**
3. **Are the conceptual definitions clear and adequate?**
4. **What are the variables in the study?**
5. **Is each study variable associated with a concept and its definition?**
6. **What measurement methods are used in the study?**
7. **Is each measurement method consistent with its associated concept and conceptual definition?**

Critiquing a framework requires that you go beyond the framework itself to examine its linkages to other components of the study. To answer the previous questions, the concepts and conceptual definitions must first be extracted from the written text in the introduction, the literature review, or the discussion of the framework. Then the adequacy of the definitions and the linkages of concepts to variables and their measurement must be judged.

Example: How to Extract Concepts and Conceptual Definitions from a Published Study

The following framework was extracted from a study by Schmelzer, Case, Chappell, and Wright (2000) entitled "Colonic Cleansing, Fluid Absorption, and Discomfort Following Tap Water and Soapsuds Enemas." The study was published in *Applied Nursing Research*. Concepts have been circled and conceptual definitions have been underlined to show you how to identify and mark them in published studies. In physiologic studies, some concepts may not be defined because their meanings are commonly held within the discipline. These are referred to as primitive concepts.

"The ideal enema solution would effectively cleanse the colon with minimal side effects. The following sections describe the colonic cleansing mechanism and the dangers of excessive fluid absorption, rectal mucosal damage, and discomfort."

Colonic Cleansing

Enemas cleanse the colon by stimulating propulsion and secretion. Three major factors influence an enema's ability to stimulate defecation: enema volume, the presence of chemical irritants, and the osmolarity or tonicity of the solution (Wood, 1994). The instillation of a large fluid volume into the intestinal lumen stimulates propulsion; chemical irritants stimulate both propulsion and secretion to rapidly empty the colon (Chang, Sitrin, & Black, 1996). Hypertonic solutions such as sodium phosphate enemas stimulate defecation by drawing fluid from the body into the lumen of the colon through osmosis and by directly irritating rectal mucosa. To promote fluid absorption from the colon, hypotonic solutions are thought to slow propulsion (Chang et al., 1996; Woods, 1994). Because tap water, a hypotonic solution, does not irritate colonic mucosa (Niv, 1990), its effect must be the result of volume alone. Soapsuds solutions are also hypotonic, but both a large volume and chemical irritation stimulate defecation.

Few studies have addressed optimal enema volume and individual tolerance. Nursing texts recommend volumes ranging from 0.5 to 1 liter (Craven & Hirnle, 1996; Sorensen & Luckmann, 1986), but up to 2 liters have been given (Hageman & Goei, 1993). Because the adult rectal capacity is about 400 ml (Doughty & Jackson, 1993), larger volumes (500 to 2000 ml) would reach the sigmoid colon and beyond resulting in stretching of bowel lumen.

Fluid Absorption

Fluid absorption is one of the colon's major functions. Of the approximately 9 L of fluid that enter the colon daily, about 8.8 L is absorbed by the epithelial cells lining the lumen of the colon (Chang et al., 1996). Osmosis promotes absorption when luminal contents are hypotonic to plasma. Tap water enemas were used to rehydrate patients before intravenous access was available (Harmer & Henderson, 1944), but repeated tap water enemas can cause hyponatremia and fluid overload (Chertow & Brady, 1994).

The amount of fluid absorbed from stools is related to the length of time it is in contact with the colon's epithelial cells (Chang et al., 1996). After the enema is instilled, nurses report telling patients to resist defecating as long as possible (Schmelzer & Wright, 1996), and nursing textbooks suggest that longer retention produces better results (Craven & Hirnle, 1996; Sorensen & Luckmann, 1986). This practice, however, would seem to promote greater water absorption, decrease the available volume to stimulate defecation, and increase the risk of fluid overload.

Mucosal Irritation

When endocrine cells and sensory neurons detect chemical changes from foreign antigens, toxins or chemicals, they initiate a secretory response to dilute the irritant and powerful propulsive forces to eject it from the body (Wood, 1994). This response may be useful if the irritation is mild enough to stimulate defeca-

Continued

Margin annotations (left, top to bottom):
concept — concept — conceptual definition of enema — concept — concept — conceptual definition of hypertonic — concept — conceptual definition of fluid absorption — concept

Margin annotations (right, top to bottom):
concept — concept — concept — conceptual definition of osmolarity — conceptual definition of defecation — concept — concept — conceptual definition of hypotonic — concept — concept — conceptual definition of chemical irritate — concept

Margin annotations (bottom):
conceptual definition of secretory response — conceptual definition of stimulates propulsion

tion without damaging the mucosal cells; however, excessive irritation can damage mucosal cells and the resulting inflammation could dramatically increase secretion and propulsion (Chang et al., 1996).

Although tap water is not an irritation (Niv, 1990), soapsuds enemas have been associated with severe mucosal irritation and colitis (Kim, Cho, & Levinsohn, 1980; Orchard & Lawson, 1986; Toffler & Barry, 1972). Despite these reports, soapsuds enemas are still frequently used to treat constipation (Schmelzer & Wright, 1993; 1996).

"Extraneous Variables

The size of the enema returns can be influenced by certain factors including age, gender, and the time since the last bowel movement...."

Statements

Statements express claims that are important to the theory. An *existence statement* declares that a given concept exists or that a given relationship between concepts occurs. For example, an existence statement might claim that a condition referred to as *stress* exists and that there is a relationship between the concept of stress and the concept of health. A *relational statement* clarifies the type of relationship that exists between or among concepts. For example, one relational statement might propose that high levels of stress are related to declining levels of health. Another relational statement might propose that exercise is related to weight. It is the statements of a theory that are tested through research, not the theory itself. Testing a theory involves determining the truth of each relational statement in the theory. However, a single study might test only one relational statement. As more studies examine a single relational statement, increasing evidence of the truth or falsity of that statement is confirmed. Many studies are required to validate all the statements in a theory.

In theories, *propositions* (relational statements) can be expressed at various levels of abstraction. The statements found in conceptual models (general propositions) are at a high level of abstraction. Statements found in theories (specific propositions) are at a moderate level of abstraction. Hypotheses are at a low level of abstraction and are specific. As statements are expressed in a less abstract way, they become more narrow in scope (Fawcett & Downs, 1992), as shown in the following.

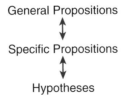

Statements at varying levels of abstraction that express relationships between or among the same conceptual ideas can be arranged in hierarchical form, from general to specific. This should allow the reader to see the logical links among the various levels of abstraction.

Roy and Roberts (1981) developed statement sets related to Roy's nursing model that could be used in frameworks for research, as shown in the following excerpts.

General Proposition

"The magnitude of the internal and external stimuli will positively influence the magnitude of the physiological response of an intact system."

Specific Proposition

"The amount of mobility in the form of exercising positively influences the level of muscle integrity."

Hypothesis

"If the nurse helps the patient maintain muscle tone through proper exercising, the patient will experience fewer problems associated with immobility" (Roy & Roberts, 1981, p. 90).

In critiquing a published study, critical reasoning should be used to identify the statements expressed as propositions and hypotheses. The following questions may help you identify and critique these statements:

1. **What statements are expressed within the publication?**
2. **Are all of the study concepts included within the statements?**
3. **Are the statements expressed as both propositions and hypotheses (or research questions)?**
4. **Are one or more statements being tested by the study design?**

Extracting Statements from a Published Study

In some studies, the statements are implied rather than clearly stated, and sometimes they are located within the introduction or literature review rather than within a clearly expressed framework. If the statements are implied and not clearly stated, critical reasoning should be used to extract them from the text and express them as statements. To begin, the introduction, the background and significance, the literature review, and the framework should be searched for sentences that seem to express relationships between concepts included in the study. The next step is to write down a single sentence that seems to be a relational statement and express it graphically. For example, the statement "exercise is related to weight" could be expressed as:

Exercise ⟷ Weight

The next statement can be identified as a relational statement and should be written down and expressed graphically. This step should be continued until all of the statements related to the selected concepts have been graphically expressed. If the linkages among the graphic statements you have developed are examined, the theoretical ideas embedded in the text should gradually become clearer.

The extraction of statements from text in a published study is illustrated with Schmelzer and colleagues' (2000) study. It should be noted that all of the concepts previously identified are included in these statements. General propositions are underlined, specific propositions are underlined with a wavy line, and hypotheses are underlined with a double rule. If you were marking text in an article, a variety of colored highlighters could be used to differentiate these various types of statements. Notes could also be written in the margins.

Background

"The ideal enema solution would effectively cleanse the colon with minimal side effects. The following sections describe the colonic cleansing mechanism and the dangers of excessive fluid absorption, rectal mucosal damage, and discomfort.

Colonic Cleansing

General proposition — Enemas cleanse the colon by stimulating propulsion and secretion. Three major factors influence an enema's ability to stimulate defecation: enema volume, the presence of chemical irritants, and the osmolarity or tonicity of the solution (Wood, 1994). — Specific proposition

The instillation of a large fluid volume into the intestinal lumen stimulates propulsion; chemical irritants stimulate both propulsion and secretion to rapidly empty the colon (Chang, Sitrin, & Black, 1996). — Specific proposition

Hypertonic solutions, such as sodium phosphate enemas, stimulate defecation by drawing fluid from the body into the lumen of the colon through osmosis and by directly irritating rectal mucosa. — Specific proposition

To promote fluid absorption from the colon, hypotonic solutions are thought to slow propulsion (Chang et al., 1996; Woods, 1994). — Specific propositio

Because tap water, a hypotonic solution, does not irritate colonic mucosa (Niv, 1990), its effect must be the result of volume alone. — Specific proposition

Soapsuds solutions are also hypotonic, but both a large volume and chemical irritation stimulate defecation.

Few studies have addressed optimal enema volume and individual tolerance. Nursing texts recommend volumes ranging from 0.5 to 1.0 liter (Craven & Hirnle, 1996; Sorensen & Luckmann, 1986), but up to 2 liters have been given (Hageman & Goei, 1993). Because the adult rectal capacity is about 400 ml (Doughty & Jackson, 1993), larger volumes (500 to 2000 ml) would reach the sigmoid colon and beyond.

Fluid Absorption

Fluid absorption is one of the colon's major functions. Of the approximately 9 liters of fluid that enter the colon daily, about 8.8 liters is absorbed by the epithelial cells lining the lumen of the colon (Chang et al., 1996). Osmosis promotes absorption when luminal contents are hypotonic to plasma. — General proposition

Tap water enemas

were used to rehydrate patients before intravenous access was available (Harmer & Henderson, 1944), but repeated tap water enemas can cause hyponatremia and fluid overload (Chertow & Brady, 1994).

The amount of fluid absorbed from stools is related to the length of time it is in contact with the colon's epithelial cells (Chang et al., 1996). After the enema is instilled, nurses report telling patients to resist defecating as long as possible (Schmelzer & Wright, 1996), and nursing textbooks suggest that longer retention produces better results (Craven & Hirnle, 1996; Sorensen & Luckmann, 1986). This practice, however, would seem to promote greater water absorption, decrease the available volume to stimulate defecation, and increase the risk of fluid overload.

    Specific proposition

Mucosal Irritation

When endocrine cells and sensory neurons detect chemical changes from foreign antigens, toxins or chemicals, they initiate a secretory response to dilute the irritant and powerful propulsive forces to eject it from the body (Wood, 1994). This response may be useful if the irritation is mild enough to stimulate defecation without damaging the mucosal cells; however, excessive irritation can damage mucosal cells and the resulting inflammation could dramatically increase secretion and propulsion (Chang et al., 1996).

    Specific proposition

Although tap water is not an irritation (Niv, 1990), soapsuds enemas have been associated with severe mucosal irritation and colitis (Kim, Cho, & Levinsohn, 1980; Orchard & Lawson, 1986; Toffler & Barry, 1972). Despite these reports, soapsuds enemas are still frequently used to treat constipation (Schmelzer & Wright, 1993; 1996).

"Extraneous Variables

The size of the enema returns can be influenced by certain factors including age, gender, and the time since the last bowel movement…. Renal function, serum albumin, and overall hydration status influence an individual's response to a large fluid load. Serum blood urea nitrogen (BUN) and creatinine reflect renal function, and hematocrit and sodium levels provide information about hydration status."

    Specific proposition

Conceptual Map

One strategy for expressing a theory is a *conceptual map* that graphically shows the interrelationships of the concepts and statements (Artinian, 1982; Fawcett & Downs, 1992; Moody, 1989; Newman, 1979; Silva, 1981). A conceptual map is developed to explain which concepts contribute to or partially cause an outcome. The map should be supported by references from the literature. A conceptual map summarizes and integrates what is known about a phenomenon more succinctly and clearly than does a literary explanation and allows one to grasp the wholeness of a phenomenon.

A conceptual map includes all of the major concepts in a theory or framework. These concepts are linked by arrows expressing the proposed linkages between concepts. Each linkage shown by an arrow is a graphic illustration of a relational state-

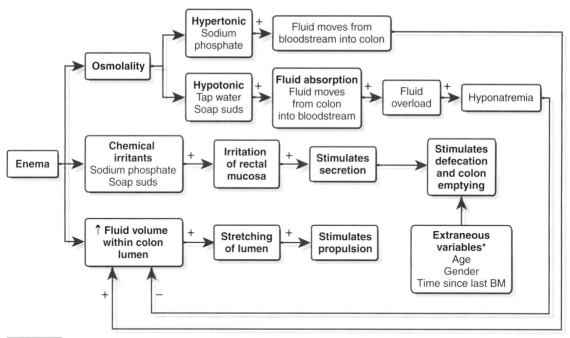

Fig. 5-1   Conceptual map constructed from statements extracted from study. *(Data from Schmelzer, M., Case, P., Chappell, S. M., & Wright, K. B. [2000]. Colonic cleansing, fluid absorption, and discomfort following tap water and soapsuds enemas.* Applied Nursing Research, 13*[2], 83-91.)*

BM, Bowel movement.
*Effect might be explained by variations in colon muscle tone.

ment (proposition) of the theory. Mapping is useful in identifying gaps in the logic of the theory and reveals inconsistencies, incompleteness, and errors (Artinian, 1982). Schmelzer, and colleagues (2000) did not provide a conceptual map with their framework. The statements extracted from their published study were used to construct the map in Fig. 5-1.

In critiquing a conceptual map, critical reasoning should be used to seek answers to the following questions:
1. Is the framework expressed as a conceptual map?
2. Are all of the concepts in the study included on the map?
3. Does the author provide conceptual definitions of each concept on the map?
4. Does the author provide statements for each linkage between concepts shown on the map?
5. Does the author provide references from the literature to support the linkages between concepts shown on the map?
6. Is it clear which linkages on the map are being tested by the published study? If no conceptual map is provided, a map that represents the study's framework should be developed and described.

FRAMEWORKS FOR PHYSIOLOGICAL STUDIES

Until recently, physiological studies tended to lack a clearly defined framework. Some physiological researchers discounted the importance of the theoretical dimension of research. This was due, in part, to the emphasis in nursing on psychosocial theories. In addition, some researchers tended to discount biological knowledge. The theoretical basis for physiological studies is derived from physics, physiology, and pathophysiology and may not be considered theory by some researchers. The knowledge in these areas is well tested through research, and theoretical relationships are often referred to as laws and principles. The theoretical relationships may be considered facts rather than theories. However, propositions can be developed and tested using these laws and principles and then applied to nursing problems. Developing a framework to clearly express the logic on which the study is based is helpful both to the researcher and to those reading the published study. The critique of a physiological framework is no different than that of other frameworks. However, concepts and conceptual definitions in physiological frameworks may be less abstract than concepts and conceptual definitions in many psychosocial studies. Concepts in physiological studies might be such terms as cardiac output, dyspnea, wound healing, blood pressure, tissue hypoxia, metabolism, and functional status.

Timmerman and Stevenson (1996) developed a physiological framework for a study of the relationship between severity of binge eating and body fat in women who do not purge after a binge. The following is their description of their framework.

"The conceptual framework for this study was the set point theory of energy regulation in which body fat is regulated within specific parameters or a set point. In defense of the body's set point, variations in food intake are counteracted by adjustments in the level of energy expended. The body responds to increased consumption by increasing the energy expended and to decreased consumption by reducing the energy expended (Keesey, 1986). This theory explains why weight gains and losses cannot be predicted solely on changes in caloric intake. Obesity occurs when body fat is regulated at an elevated set point. Although further research is needed on how the set point becomes elevated, consumption of long-term, high fat diets is one factor identified as potentially increasing the set point (Hill, Dorton, Sykes, & Digirolamo, 1989).

According to the set point theory, the body would defend its set point against intermittent binge episodes by increasing energy expenditure. However, when severity of binge eating increases (larger amounts ingested and binges more frequent), the body's set point would be elevated. A long history of habitual binge eating may contribute to [the] degree of obesity by progressively elevating the set point. Thus, individuals with different levels of binge eating severity should, hypothetically, have different amounts of body fat." (p. 390)

The purpose of this study was to clarify the relationship between binge eating severity and degree of body fat by using more precise measurements of binge eating severity (caloric intake) and body fat (underwater weight) than [those]

Continued

used in previous studies. In addition, length of binge eating history was measured as a separate variable to determine its role in the accumulation of body fat. Other factors identified from the literature (total caloric intake, age, parity, weight cycling, activity level, genetic predisposition to obesity, and age of obesity onset) also were measured in order to examine their influence on degree of body fat in the nonpurge binge eating population.

"The research questions were: (a) What is the relationship between binge eating severity and body fat (percent of body fat and BMI [body mass index]) in nonpurge binge eating women? and (b) What are the best predictors for body fat (percent of body fat and BMI) among nonpurge binge eating women?" (p. 391)

FRAMEWORKS INCLUDING CONCEPTUAL NURSING MODELS

Relatively few nursing studies have frameworks that include a conceptual nursing model. Moody and colleagues (1988), who examined nursing practice research from 1977 to 1986, found an increase in studies using a nursing model as a framework from 8% in the first half of the decade under study to 13% in the second half. The most frequently used models were those of Orem, Rogers, and Roy. Silva (1986), who studied the extent to which five nursing models (those of Johnson, Roy, Orem, Rogers, and Newman) had been used as frameworks for nursing research, found 62 studies published between 1952 and 1985 that used one of these models as a framework. However, only nine of these studies met Silva's specified criteria as an actual test of nursing theory. Only in these nine studies did the study design extract and test statements from the nursing theory.

Building a body of knowledge related to a particular conceptual model requires an organized program of research. This program of research is referred to as a "research tradition." A group of scholars dedicated to conducting research related to the model develop theories compatible with the model, including propositions for testing. An organized plan for testing these propositions is agreed upon. Researchers conducting studies consistent with a particular research tradition often maintain a network of communication regarding their work. In some cases annual conferences focused on the model are held to share research findings, explore theoretical ideas, and maintain network contacts. Conceptual models of nursing do not have well established research traditions (Fawcett, 1989). However, research traditions are being developed for some nursing models.

One example of a nursing model with an emerging research tradition is Orem's (2001) model of self-care. This model focuses on the domain of nursing practice and on what nurses actually do when they practice nursing. Orem proposes that individuals generally know how to take care of themselves (self-care). If they are dependent in some way (e.g., by being very young, aged, or handicapped), family members usually take on this responsibility (dependent care). If individuals are ill or have some pathology (e.g., diabetes or a colostomy), they or their family members often acquire special skills to provide that care (therapeutic self-care). An individual's capacity to provide self-care is referred to as "self-care agency." A self-care

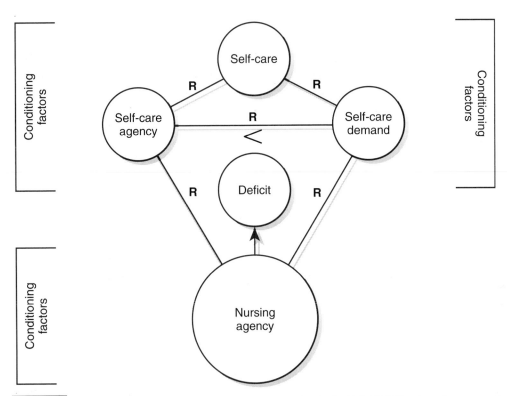

Fig. 5-2 A conceptual framework for nursing. *(From Orem, D. E. [1995].* Nursing: Concepts of practice *[5th ed.]. St. Louis: Mosby. Used with permission.).*

R, Relationship; <, deficit relationship, current or projected.

deficit occurs when self-care demand exceeds self-care agency. These ideas are expressed graphically in Fig. 5-2.

Nursing care is provided only when there is a deficit in the self-care or dependent care that the individual and the family provides (self-care deficit). In this case the nurse (or nurses) develops a nursing system to provide the needed care. This system involves prescribing, designing, and providing the needed care. The goal of nursing care is to facilitate resumption of self-care by the person, their family, or both. There are three types of nursing systems: wholly compensatory, partly compensatory, and supportive-educative. Selection of one of these systems is based on the capacity of the person to perform self-care.

The notion of self-care as an important construct for nursing has drawn nurse researchers to Orem's work. Multiple studies have been performed examining self-care in a variety of nursing situations. Instruments, consistent with Orem's model, have been developed to measure some of her concepts. Orem developed three theories related to her model: the "Theory of Self-Care Deficits," the "Theory of Self-Care," and the "Theory of Nursing Systems" (also referred to as the "General Theory of Nursing"). However, few propositions emerging from Orem's theories have been tested.

For a number of years, Dodd and colleagues have been conducting studies based on Orem's model.* Many of these studies have been funded through the National Institutes of Health (NIH). This is an important example of the carefully planned programs of research that are necessary to validate the usefulness of a nursing theory in guiding nursing practice.

In 1996, Dodd et al. conducted a study funded by the National Cancer Institute to test the effectiveness of a nurse-initiated systematic oral hygiene teaching program to prevent chemotherapy-induced oral mucositis in patients. In previous studies Dodd and colleagues (1986-1990; 1988-1992), had found that nursing management of mucositis in patients receiving chemotherapy for cancer was "in disarray." Because most patients are receiving chemotherapy as outpatients, it is not possible to monitor closely the condition of a patient's mouth.

"Many patients were told that they might experience oral problems because of their chemotherapy, but they were not instructed in any type of preventive mouth care. Therefore, most patients who experienced mouth problems initially tried to self-manage using a trial-and-error approach. When patients sought assistance from their physicians or nurses, they were offered a variety of remedies with instructions to `swish and spit.' Many patients indicated that this approach was not only ineffective, it actually increased their discomfort and mouth problems (Dodd et al., 1996, p. 922).

Basing her claims on Orem's theory of self-care agency, Dodd proposed that a nurse-initiated systematic oral hygiene teaching program, (PRO-SELF: Mouth Aware [PSMA] Program) that is offered before the development of mucositis, would enhance the patient's self-care agency and result in a decrease in the incidence and severity of mucositis (Fig. 5-3). The Oral Assessment Guide (Eilers, Berger, & Peterson, 1988) was used to guide clinician ratings of chemotherapy-related changes in the oral mucosa. The study developed to validate this proposition also tested the effectiveness of two mouthwashes used in the mouth-care protocol: chlorhexidine and a placebo control (sterile water). The findings of the study validated Orem's concept of self-care agency. "The PSMA program provided patients with the knowledge and skills needed to perform the systematic oral hygiene protocol. Evidence exists that the patients used the PSMA program as instructed.... Data from this study suggest that the use of a systematic oral hygiene program prescribed in the PSMA program may have reduced the incidence of chemotherapy-induced mucositis from an *a priori* estimate of 44% to less than 26%." (p. 926)

---

*Dibble, Padilla, Dodd, & Miaskowski, 1998; Dodd, 1982a,b, 1983a,b, 1984a,b,c, 1987a,b, 1988a,b, 1991, 1996; 1997; 1999; 2000; Dodd & Dibble, 1993; Dodd, Dibble, Miaskowski, et al., 2001; Dodd, Dibble, & Thomas, 1992a,b; Dodd, Janson, et al., 2001; Dodd, Lindsey, et al., 1986–1990; Dodd, Larson et al., 1996; Dodd et al., 1986–1990; Dodd, Lindsay, Stetz, et al., 1988-1992; Dodd, Lovejoy, et al., 1992; Dodd, Miaskowski, et al., 2000; Dodd & Mood, 1981; Dodd, Miaskowski, & Paul, 2001; Dodd, Thomas, & Dibble, 1991; Dodd, West, et al., 2000; Facione & Dodd, 1995; Facione, Dodd, Holzemer, & Meleis, 1997; Larson, Dodd, & Aksamit, 1998; Larson et al., 1998; Lovely, Miaskowski, & Dodd, 1999; Mandrell, Ruccione, Dodd, et al., 2000; Messias, Yeager, Dibble, & Dodd, 1997; Musci & Dodd, 1990; Piper, Dibble, Dodd, Weiss, Slaughter, & Paul, 1998.

No significant difference was found in the effectiveness of the two mouth-washes used in the study. Thus Dodd and colleagues recommend the use of water in implementing the PSMA program. This study was selected for the 1996 Oncology Nursing Society (ONS)/Schering Corporation Excellence in Cancer Nursing Research Award.

Mouth Care

Each day you MUST:
1. **Look** at your whole mouth, including your lips and tongue *every morning* before brushing, flossing, and rinsing. **Check** for problems listed below.
2. **Brush** your teeth for 90 seconds *twice a day*—after breakfast and before bedtime.
3. **Floss** your teeth at least *once a day.*
4. **Rinse** your mouth with one capful of the medicated mouthwash for 30 seconds *twice a day*—after breakfast and before bedtime. Swish thoroughly and spit out.
5. **Do NOT eat or drink ANYTHING, including WATER, FOR 30 MINUTES** after using the medicated mouthwash.
6. **Avoid** smoking, alcoholic beverages, and spicy foods.

Mouth Problems to Check for Daily
*If you have any of the following **problems,*** you must call your nurse AS SOON AS POSSIBLE.
1. **Sores** in your mouth
2. **White spots** in your mouth
3. **Pain** in your mouth
4. **Difficulty** eating or drinking
5. Unusual amount of **bleeding**
   Nurse's name _____
   Phone number _____

*Specific instructions for denture wearer were provided.

Fig. 5-3   PRO-SELF Mouth Aware Prevention Program for Non-Denture Wearers. *(From Dodd et al. [1996]. Randomized clinical trial of chlorhexidine versus placebo for prevention of oral mucositis in patients receiving chemotherapy. Oncology Nursing Forum, 23[6], 921. Used with permission.)*

Critiquing a framework that includes both a conceptual model and a theory is more complex than critiquing a framework based only on a theory. Constructs and their definitions, and concepts and their definitions should be identified. Both general and specific propositions need to be identified and linked to the hypotheses or research questions. Including a conceptual model as well as a theory in a framework is a relatively new idea in nursing. Therefore few published studies have frameworks that include a conceptual model, a theory, and a conceptual map illustrating the linkage between the model and the theory. The map for such a framework must include both the conceptual model and a testable theory. Fig. 5-4 shows an example of a map including both. Tulman and Fawcett (1990) developed this map to illustrate a framework designed to study functional status after diagnosis of breast cancer. The map is based on Roy's Model of Adaptation (Roy, 1984).

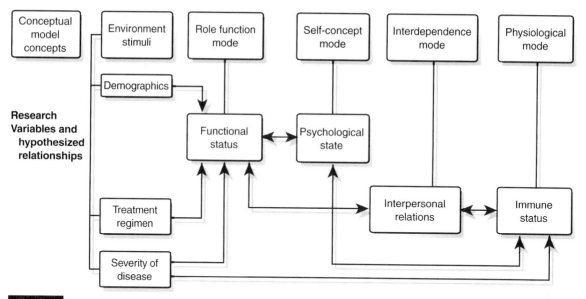

Fig. 5-4 Conceptual map includes a conceptual nursing model (Roy) and a tentative theory: framework for studying functional status after diagnosis of breast cancer. *(From Tulman, L., & Fawcett, J. [1990]. A framework for studying functional status after diagnosis of breast cancer. Cancer Nursing, 13[2], 98. Used with permission.)*

Critiquing a Framework

A framework must be critiqued within the context of the overall study. Therefore critical reasoning should be used to critique the logical structure of the framework itself, and to address the following questions:

1. **Did the framework guide the methodology of the study? To determine this, the following criteria should be used:**
   a. **The concepts are linked with variables that are measured.**
   b. **The concepts are represented by variables in hypotheses, research questions, or objectives.**
   c. **The study hypotheses, research questions, or objectives emerge from propositions in the framework.**
   d. **The hypotheses, research questions, or objectives are tested statistically.**
2. **Were the study findings related to the framework? Examine the discussion of findings. Look for comments connecting the findings to specific elements of the framework. The author may discuss the adequacy of the variables and measurements as reflections of the concepts. Comments discussing the implications of the findings in terms of the truth or falsity of framework propositions should be identified. The author may make evaluative statements about the overall framework or suggest modifications based on study findings.**

3. Are the findings for each hypothesis, question, or objective consistent with those proposed by the framework? The truth or falsity of the framework propositions should be judged on the basis of the study findings.
4. What do the findings tell you about the usefulness of the framework for clinical practice and future studies?
5. If the findings are not consistent with the framework, was the methodology adequate to test the hypothesis, research question, or objective? This question will need to be answered individually for each hypothesis, research question, or objective. You may need to become familiar with the content of Chapters 7 (research designs), 8 (sampling), 9 (measurement), and 10 (statistical analysis) to answer this question adequately.
6. Are the findings consistent with those of other studies using the same framework (or testing the same propositions)? Your ability to answer this question depends on whether the author provided information in the published study about other studies that have tested the same propositions.

SUMMARY

Research is based on theory. We use theories to organize what we know about a phenomenon. A theory is defined as an integrated set of defined concepts and statements that present a view of a phenomenon and can be used to do one or more of the following: describe, explain, predict, or control that phenomenon. Theories are abstract rather than concrete. Abstract means that the theory is the expression of an idea apart from any specific instance. Concrete ideas are concerned with realities or actual instances. Conceptual models are similar to theories and are sometimes referred to as theories. Conceptual models are even more abstract than theories. A conceptual model broadly explains phenomena of interest, expresses assumptions, and reflects a philosophical stance. A framework is a brief explanation of a theory or those portions of a theory to be tested in a study. Every study has a framework, although some frameworks are poorly expressed. The framework must identify and define the concepts and the relational statements being tested. Because frameworks are important in the conduct of research, essential elements of a study critique are the identification and evaluation of the framework. To critique a framework, the structure of theories and the logic on which they are based should be understood.

The first step in understanding theories is to become familiar with the terms related to theoretical ideas and their application. These terms include concept, relational statement, and conceptual map. A concept abstractly describes and names an object or a phenomenon, thus providing it with a separate identity or meaning. Defining a concept allows consistency in the way the term is used. A statement expresses a claim that is important to the theory. Existence statements declare that a given concept exists or that a given relationship occurs. Relational statements clarify the type of relationship that exists between or among concepts. Statements can be expressed at various levels of abstraction. The statements found in conceptual models (general propositions) are expressed at a high level of abstraction. Statements found in theories (specific propositions) are expressed at a moderate level of abstraction. Hypotheses are expressed at a low level of abstraction and are specific. One strategy for expressing a theory is a conceptual map that diagrammatically shows the interrelationships of the concepts and statements. A conceptual map includes all of the major concepts in the theory. These concepts are linked together by arrows that indicate the proposed linkages between concepts. Testing a theory involves determining the truth of each relational statement in the theory. Critiquing a framework requires the identification and evaluation of the concepts, their definitions, and the statements linking the concepts. Questions are provided throughout the chapter to assist you in this process. Examples of critiques of pub-

lished studies are included to illustrate the critique process.

Relatively few nursing studies have frameworks that include a conceptual nursing model. An organized program of research is important for building a body of knowledge related to the phenomena explained by a particular conceptual model. This program of research is referred to as a research tradition. One example of a nursing model with an emerging research tradition is Orem's model of self-care. An example of a framework that includes Roy's model is presented to illustrate the development of a framework with both a model and a theory.

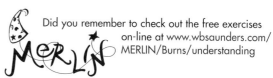

Did you remember to check out the free exercises on-line at www.wbsaunders.com/ MERLIN/Burns/understanding

REFERENCES

The American Heritage Dictionary of the English Language, (2000) (4th ed.) Boston: Houghton Mifflin.

Artinian, B. (1982). Conceptual mapping. Development of the strategy. *Western Journal of Nursing Research, 4*(4), 379–393.

Chang, E., Sitrin, M., & Black, D. (1996). *Gastrointestinal, hepatobiliary, and nutritional physiology.* Philadelphia: Lippincott-Raven.

Chertow, G. M., & Brady, H. R. (1994). Hyponatremia from tap-water enema [Letter] *Lancet, 344*(8924), 748.

Craven, R., & Hirnle, C. (1996). *Fundamentals of nursing— Human health and function.* (2nd ed., pp. 1249–1253). Philadelphia: Lippincott.

Dibble, S. L., Padilla, G. V., Dodd, M. J., & Miaskowski, C. (1998). Gender differences in the dimensions of quality of life. *Oncology Nursing Forum, 25*(3), 577–583.

Dodd, M. J. (1982a). Chemotherapy knowledge in patients with cancer: Assessment and informational interventions. *Oncology Nursing Forum, 9*(3), 39–44.

Dodd, M. J. (1982b). Assessing patient self-care for side effects of cancer chemotherapy—Part I. *Cancer Nursing, 5*(6), 447–451.

Dodd, M. J. (1983a). Assessing patient self-care for side effects of cancer chemotherapy—Part II. *Cancer Nursing, 5*(6), 63–67.

Dodd, M. J. (1983b). Self-care for side effects of cancer chemotherapy: An assessment of nursing interventions. *Cancer Nursing, 6*(1), 63–67.

Dodd, M. J. (1984a). Patterns of self-care in cancer patients receiving radiation therapy. *Oncology Nursing Forum, 10*(3), 23–27.

Dodd, M. J. (1984b). Self-care for patients with breast cancer to prevent side effects of chemotherapy: A concern for public health nursing. *Public Health Nursing, 1*(4), 202–209.

Dodd, M. (1984c). Measuring informational intervention for chemotherapy knowledge and self-care behavior. *Research in Nursing & Health, 7*(1), 43–50.

Dodd, M. J. (1987a). *Managing side effects of chemotherapy and radiation therapy: A guide for patients and nurses.* Norwich, CT: Appleton & Lange.

Dodd, M. J. (1987b). Efficacy of proactive information on self-care in radiation therapy patients. *Heart & Lung, 16*(5), 538–544.

Dodd, M. J. (1988a). Efficacy of proactive information on self-care in chemotherapy patients. *Patient Education and Counseling, 11*(3), 215–225.

Dodd, M. J. (1988b). Patterns of self-care in patients with breast cancer. *Western Journal of Nursing Research, 10*(1), 7–14.

Dodd, M. J. (1991). *Managing the side effects of chemotherapy and radiation: A guide for patients and their families* (2nd ed.). Englewood Cliffs, NJ: Prentice Hall.

Dodd, M. J. (1996). *Managing the side effects of chemotherapy and radiation therapy: A guide for patients and their families* (3rd ed.). San Francisco: University of California, School of Nursing Press.

Dodd, M. J. (1997). Self Care: Ready or not! *Oncology Nursing Forum, 24*(6), 983-990.

Dodd, M. J. (1999). Self-care: Not as simple as we hoped…. 32nd Annual Communicating Nursing Research Conference/13th Annual WIN Assembly, "Nursing Research: For the Health of Our Nation," held April 22-24, 1999, at the Bahia Hotel, San Diego. *Communicating Nursing Research, 32,* 43–56.

Dodd, M. J. (2000). Improving pain management: An ongoing journal. Introduction: Portrait of a scientist…Christine Miaskowski. *Oncology Nursing Forum, 27*(6), 935–937.

Dodd, M. J., & Dibble, S. L. (1993). Predictors of self-care: A test of Orem's model. *Oncology Nursing Forum, 20*(6), 895–901.

Dodd, M. J. et al. (2001). A comparison of the affective state and quality of life of chemotherapy patients who do and do not develop chemotherapy-induced oral mucositis. *Journal of Pain & Symptom Management, 21*(6), 498–505.

Dodd, M. J., Dibble, S. L., & Thomas, M. L. (1992a). Outpatient chemotherapy: Patients' and family members' concerns and coping strategies. *Journal of Public Health Nursing, 9*(1), 37–44.

Dodd, M. J., Dibble, S. L., & Thomas, M. L. (1992b). Self-care for patients experiencing cancer chemotherapy side effects: A concern for home care nurses. *Home Healthcare Nurse, 9*(1), 21–26.

Dodd, M. et al. (2001). Advancing the science of symptom management. *Journal of Advanced Nursing, 33*(5), 668–676.

Dodd, M. J. et al. (1996). Randomized clinical trial of chlorhexidine versus placebo for prevention of oral mucositis in patients receiving chemotherapy. *Oncology Nursing Forum, 23*(6), 921–927.

Dodd, M. J. et al. (1986–1990). *Coping and self-care of cancer families: Nurse prospectus* (Final report). Funded by the National Institutes of Health, R01 CA 1440.

Dodd, M. J. et al. (1988–1992). *Self-care interventions to decrease chemotherapy morbidity* (Final Report). Funded by the National Institutes of Health and the National Cancer Institute, R01 CA 48312.

Dodd, M. J. et al. (1992). *Self-care intervention to decrease chemotherapy morbidity.* Invited paper presented at the Seventeenth Annual Congress of the Oncology Nursing Society, San Diego, CA.

Dodd, M. J., Miaskowski, C., & Paul, S. M. (2001). Symptom clusters and their effect on the functional status of patients with cancer. *Oncology Nursing Forum, 28*(3), 465–470.

Dodd, M. J.et al. (2000). Factors influencing oral mucositis in patients receiving chemotherapy. *Cancer Practice: A Multidisciplinary Journal of Cancer Care, 8*(6), 291–297.

Dodd, M. J., & Mood, D. W. (1981). Chemotherapy: Helping patients to know the drugs they are receiving and their possible side effects. *Cancer Nursing, 4*(4), 311–318.

Dodd, M. J., Thomas, M. L., & Dibble, S. L. (1991). Self-care for patients experiencing cancer chemotherapy side effects: A concern for home care nurses. *Home Healthcare Nurse, 9*(6), 21–26.

Dodd, M., West, C., Tripathy, D., Miaskowski, C., Paul, S., & Koo, P. (2000). A RCT of the effectiveness of the PRO-SELF Pain Control Program…. 33rd Annual Communicating Nursing Research Conference/14th Annual WIN Assembly, "Building on a Legacy of Excellence in Nursing Research," held April 13–15, 2000 at the Adam's Mark Hotel, Denver, Colorado. *Communicating Nursing Research, 33*:242, 2000.

Doughty, D. B., & Jackson, D. B. (1993). *Gastrointestinal disorders.* St. Louis: Mosby.

Eilers, J., Berger, A. M., & Peterson, M. C. (1988). Development, testing, and application of the oral assessment guide. *Oncology Nursing Forum, 15*(3), 325–330.

Facione, N., & Dodd, M. J. (1995). Women's narratives of help seeking for breast cancer. *Cancer Practice, 3*(4), 219–225.

Facione, N. C., Dodd, M. H., Holzemer, W., & Meleis, A. I. (1997). Helpseeking for self-discovered breast symptoms: Implications for early detection. *Cancer Practice: A Multidisciplinary Journal of Cancer Care, 5*(4), 220–227.

Fawcett, H., & Downs, F. (1992). *The relationship of theory and research* (2nd ed.). Norwalk, CT: Appleton-Century-Crofts.

Fawcett, J. (1989). *Analysis and evaluation of conceptual models of nursing* (2nd ed.). Philadelphia: Davis.

Hageman, M., & Goei, R. (1993). Cleansing enema prior to double-contrast barium enema examination: Is it necessary? *Radiology, 187*(1), 109–112.

Harmer, B., & Henderson, V. (1944). *Textbook of the principles and practice of nursing* (p. 663). New York: Macmillan.

Hill, J., Dorton, J., Sykes, M., & Digirolamo, M. (1989). Reversal of dietary obesity is influenced by its duration and severity. *International Journal of Obesity, 13*(5), 711–722.

Keesey, R. (1986). A set point theory of obesity. In K. Brownell & J. Foreyt (Eds.). *Handbook of eating disorders* (pp. 63-87). New York: Basic Books.

Kim, S. K., Cho, C., & Levinsohn, E. M. (1980). Caustic colitis due to detergent enema. *American Journal of Roentgenology, 134*(2), 397–398.

Klaus, M. H., & Kennell, J. H. (1976). *Maternal-infant bonding: The impact of early separation or loss on family development.* St. Louis: Mosby.

Larson P. J., Dodd M. J., & Aksamit I. (1998). A symptom-management program for patients undergoing cancer treatment: The Pro-Self Program. *Journal of Cancer Education, 13*(4), 248–252.

Larson, P. J. et al. (1998). The PRO-SELF Mouth Aware program: An effective approach for reducing chemotherapy-induced mucositis. *Cancer Nursing, 21*(4), 263–268.

Lazarus, R., & Folkman, S. (1984). *Stress, appraisal, and coping.* New York: Springer.

Lovely, M. P., Miaskowski, C., & Dodd, M. (1999). Relationship between fatigue and quality of life in patients with glioblastoma multiformae. *Oncology Nursing Forum, 26*(5), 921–925.

Luce, G. (1970). *Biological rhythms in psychiatry and medicine.* Washington, DC: U.S. Public Health Service.

Mandrell, B. N. et al. (2000). Consensus statements: Applying the concept of self-care to pediatric oncology patients. *Seminars in Oncology Nursing, 16*(4), 315–316.

Messias, D. K. H., Yeager, K. A., Dibble, S. L., & Dodd, M. J. (1997). Patients' perspectives of fatigue while undergoing chemotherapy. *Oncology Nursing Forum, 24*(1), 43–48.

Mischel, M. H. (1988). Uncertainty in illness. Image: *Journal of Nursing Scholarship, 20*(4), 225–232.

Moody, L. E. (1989). Building a conceptual map to guide research. *Florida Nursing Review, 4*(1), 1–5.

Moody, L. E., Wilson, M. E., Smyth, K., Schwartz, R., Tittle, M., & Van Cott, M. L. (1988). Analysis of a decade of nursing practice research: 1977–1986. *Nursing Research, 37*(6), 374–379.

Morse, J. M., Solberg, S. M., Neander, W. L., Bottorff, J. L., & Johnson, J. L. (1990). Concepts of caring and caring as a concept. *Advances in Nursing Science, 13*(1), 1–14.

Musci, I., & Dodd, M. (1990). Predicting self-care with patients and family members' affective states and family function. *Oncology Nursing Forum, 17*(3), 394–400.

Newman, M. A. (1979). *Theory development in nursing.* Philadelphia: Davis.

Niv, Y. (1990). Enema preparation for proctosigmoidoscopy does not cause mucosal changes (Letter to the editor). *Southern Medical Journal, 79*(11), 1459–1460.

Orchard, J., & Lawson, R. (1986). Severe colitis induced by soap enemas. *Southern Medical Journal, 79*(11), 1459–1460.

Orem, D. E. (1995). *Nursing: Concepts of practice* (5th ed.). St. Louis: Mosby.

Orem, D. E. (2001). *Nursing: Concepts of practice* (6th ed.). St. Louis: Mosby.

Pender, N. J., Murdaugh, C. L., & Parsons, M. A. (2001). *Health promotion in nursing practice* (4th edition). Upper Saddle River, NJ: Prentice Hall.

Piper, B. F., Dibble, S. L., Dodd, M. J., Weiss, M. C., Slaughter, R. E., & Paul, S. M. (1998). The revised Piper Fatigue Scale: psychometric evaluation in women with breast cancer. *Oncology Nursing Forum, 25*(4), 677–684.

Rogers, M. E., Malinski, V. M., & Barrett, E. A. M. (1994). *Martha E. Rogers: Her life and her work.* Philadelphia: Davis.

Rotter, J. (1966). Generalized expectancies for internal versus external control of reinforcement. *Psychological Monographs, 80*(1), 1–28.

Roy, C. (1984). *Introduction to nursing: An adaptation model* (2nd ed.). Englewood Cliffs, NJ: Prentice-Hall.

Roy, C., & Andrews, H. A. (1998). *Roy adaptation model.* Norwalk, CT: Appleton & Lange.

Roy, C., & Roberts, S. L. (1981). *Theory construction in nursing: An adaptation model.* Englewood Cliffs, NJ: Prentice-Hall.

Schmelzer, M., Case, P., Chappell, S. M., & Wright, K. B. (2000). Colonic cleansing, fluid absorption, and discomfort following tap water and soapsuds enemas. *Applied Nursing Research, 13*(2), 83–91.

Schmelzer, M., & Wright, K. (1993). Say nope to soap, *American Journal of Nursing, 93*(3), 21.

Schmelzer, M., & Wright, K. (1996). Enema administration techniques used by experienced registered nurses. *Gastroenterology Nursing, 19*(5), 171–175.

Selye, H. (1976). *The stress of life.* New York: McGraw-Hill.

Silva, M. C. (1981). Selection of a theoretical framework. In S. D. Krampitz & N. Pavlovich (Eds.). *Readings for nursing research* (pp. 17–28). St. Louis: Mosby.

Silva, M. C. (1986). Research testing nursing theory: State of the art. *Advances in Nursing Science, 9*(1), 1–11.

Sorensen, K., & Luckmann, J. (1986). *Basic nursing: A physiologic approach* (2nd ed., pp. 839–842). Philadelphia: Saunders.

Swanson, E. A., Jensen, D. P., Specht, J., Johnson, M. L., & Maas, M. (1997). Caregiving: Concept analysis and outcomes. *Scholarly Inquiry for Nursing Practice: An International Journal, 11*(1), 65–79.

Timmerman, G. M., & Stevenson, J. S. (1996). The relationship between binge eating severity and body fat in nonpurge binge eating women. *Research in Nursing & Health, 19*(5), 389–398.

Toffler, R. B., & Barry, J. M. (1972). Colonic mucosal slough following detergent enemas. *American Journal of Gastroenterology, 58*(6), 638–640.

Tulman, L., & Fawcett, J. (1990). A framework for studying functional status after diagnosis of breast cancer. *Cancer Nursing, 13*(2), 95–99.

Walker, L. O. (1992). *Parent-infant nursing science: Paradigms, phenomena, methods.* Philadelphia: Davis.

Wood, J. (1994). Physiology of the enteric nervous system. In L. R. Johnson, (Ed.), *Physiology of the gastrointestinal tract* (3rd ed., pp. 423-482). New York: Raven Press.

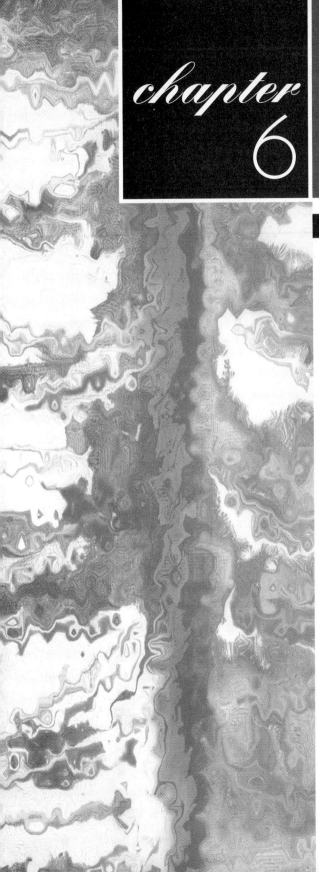

chapter 6

Examining Ethics in Nursing Research

Be sure to check out the free exercises on-line at
www.wbsaunders.com/MERLIN/Burns/
understanding

MeRLiN

OUTLINE—cont'd

OBJECTIVES

Completing this chapter should enable you to:
1. Identify the historical events influencing the development of ethical codes and regulations for research.
2. Describe three ethical principles that are important in conducting research on human subjects.
3. Discuss the human rights that require protection in research.
4. Describe the informed consent process.
5. Evaluate the consent process in a research project.
6. Describe the functions of institutional review boards in research.
7. Examine the benefit-risk ratio of studies conducted in clinical agencies.
8. Describe the types of scientific misconduct that are occurring in the conduct, reporting, and publication of research today.
9. Discuss the use of animals in research.
10. Critique the ethical information provided in a published study.

RELEVANT TERMS

Anonymity
Autonomous agents
Benefit-risk ratio
Breach of confidentiality
Coercion
Confidentiality
Consent form
Covert data collection
Deception

Diminished autonomy
Discomfort and harm
Ethical principles
    Principle of beneficence
    Principle of justice
    Principle of respect for person(s)
Fabrication
Falsification
Human rights

What is unethical research? Are unethical studies that violate subjects' rights or involve scientific misconduct conducted today? One would like to believe that unethical studies, such as the Nazi experiments of World War II, are a thing of the past. However, this is not the case, since more recent studies in nursing and other disciplines include evidence of scientific misconduct with the violation of subjects' rights and the publication of inaccurate scientific information (Njie & Thomas, 2001; Rankin & Esteves, 1997).

Misconduct can occur during the conduct, reporting, and publication of studies. *Scientific misconduct* in research includes such fraudulent practices as fabrication, falsification, or forging of data; dishonest manipulation of the design or methods with protocol violations; misrepresentation of findings; and plagiarism (Rankin & Esteves, 1997). Scientific misconduct is a major problem, and over half of the top 50 research institutions in the United States have been investigated for fraud. Thus the ethical aspects of published studies and of research conducted in clinical agencies should be critiqued. Most published studies include ethical information about subject selection and the data collection process in the methods section of the report. An institutional review board (IRB) should review studies conducted in clinical agencies to determine whether the studies are ethical.

To provide a background for examining ethical aspects of studies, this chapter describes the ethical codes and regulations that currently guide the conduct of biomedical and behavioral research. The following elements of ethical research are detailed: (1) protecting subjects' rights, (2) balancing the benefits and risks in a study, (3) obtaining informed consent, and (4) obtaining institutional approval for research. The role of nurses as patient advocates when research is conducted in their agencies is also discussed. Two timely ethical issues, scientific misconduct and the use of animals in research, are discussed. The chapter concludes with critique guidelines to assist you in determining whether a study is ethical or unethical.

HISTORICAL EVENTS INFLUENCING THE DEVELOPMENT OF ETHICAL CODES AND REGULATIONS

Since the 1940s four experimental projects have been highly publicized for their unethical treatment of human subjects: the Nazi medical experiments, the Tuskegee Syphilis Study, the Willowbrook Study, and the Jewish Chronic Disease Hospital

Study (Berger, 1990; Levine, 1986). Although these were biomedical studies and the primary investigators were physicians, the evidence suggests that nurses understood the nature of the research, identified potential research subjects, delivered treatments to the subjects, and served as data collectors. These unethical studies demonstrate the importance of ethical conduct for nurses while they are reviewing, participating in, or conducting nursing or biomedical research (Carico & Harrison, 1990; Njie & Thomas, 2001). These four studies also influenced the formulation of ethical codes and regulations that currently direct the conduct of research.

Nazi Medical Experiments

From 1933 to 1945 the Third Reich in Europe performed atrocious unethical medical activities. The programs of the Nazi regime included sterilization, euthanasia, and medical experimentation for the purpose of producing a population of racially pure Germans who were destined to rule the world. The medical experiments were conducted on prisoners of war and persons considered to be racially valueless, such as Jews, who were confined in concentration camps. The experiments involved exposing subjects to high altitudes, freezing temperatures, malaria, poisons, spotted fever (typhus), untested drugs, and surgeries, usually without any form of anesthesia. Extensive examination of the records from some of these studies indicated that they were poorly conceived and conducted. Thus little if any useful scientific knowledge was generated by this research (Berger, 1990; Steinfels & Levine, 1976).

The Nazi experiments violated numerous rights of the research subjects. The selection of subjects for these studies was racially based and unfair, and the subjects had no choice; they were prisoners who were forced to participate. As a result of these experiments, subjects were frequently killed, or they sustained permanent physical, mental, and social damage (Levine, 1986).

Nuremberg Code

Those involved in the Nazi experiments were brought to trial before the Nuremberg Tribunals, and their unethical research received international attention. The mistreatment of human subjects in these studies led to the development of the Nuremberg Code in 1949 (Table 6-1). This code includes guidelines that should help you evaluate the consent process, the protection of subjects from harm, and the balance of benefits and risks in a study (Nuremberg Code, 1986).

Declaration of Helsinki

The Nuremberg Code provided the basis for the development of the Declaration of Helsinki, which was adopted in 1964 and revised in 1975, 1983, 1989, 1996, and 2000 by the World Medical Association (Levine, 1986). A major focus of the initial document was the differentiation of therapeutic research from nontherapeutic research. *Therapeutic research* provides patients with an opportunity to receive an experimental treatment that might have beneficial results. *Nontherapeutic research* is conducted

TABLE 6-1

NUREMBERG CODE

1. The voluntary consent of the human subject is absolutely essential....
2. The experiment should be such as to yield fruitful results for the good of society, unprocurable by other methods or means of study, and not random and unnecessary in nature.
3. The experiment should be so designed and based on the results of animal experimentation and a knowledge of the natural history of the disease or other problem under study that the anticipated results will justify the performance of the experiment.
4. The experiment should be so conducted as to avoid all unnecessary physical and mental suffering and injury.
5. No experiment should be conducted where there is an *a priori* reason to believe that death or disabling injury will occur, except, perhaps, in those experiments where the experimental physicians also serve as subjects.
6. The degree of risk to be taken should never exceed that determined by the humanitarian importance of the problem to be solved by the experiment.
7. Proper preparations should be made and adequate facilities provided to protect the experimental subject against even remote possibilities of injury, disability, or death.
8. The experiment should be conducted only by scientifically qualified persons. The highest degree of skill and care should be required through all stages of the experiment of those who conduct or engage in the experiment.
9. During the course of the experiment the human subject should be at liberty to bring the experiment to an end if he has reached the physical or mental state where continuation of the experiment seems to him to be impossible.
10. During the course of the experiment the scientist in charge must be prepared to terminate the experiment at any stage, if he has probable cause to believe, in the exercise of the good faith, superior skill and careful judgment required of him that a continuation of the experiment is likely to result in injury, disability, or death to the experimental subject....

From Nuremberg Code (1949). In R. J. Levine (Ed.). *Ethics and regulations of clinical research* (2nd ed., pp. 425–426). Baltimore-Munich: Urban & Schwarzenberg.

to generate knowledge for a discipline; the results of the study might benefit future patients but will probably not benefit those acting as research subjects. The Declaration of Helsinki includes the following ethical principles: (1) the investigator should protect the life, health, privacy, and dignity of human subjects; (2) the investigator should exercise greater care to protect subjects from harm in nontherapeutic research; and (3) the investigator should only conduct research where the importance of the objective outweighs the inherent risks and burdens to the subjects. The ethical principles of the Declaration of Helsinki can be reviewed on-line at http://www.wma.net/e/policy/17-c_e.html. Most institutions conducting clinical research adopted the Nuremberg Code and Declaration of Helsinki; however, episodes of scientific misconduct continued to occur in biomedical and behavioral research (Levine, 1986).

Tuskegee Syphilis Study

In 1932 the U.S. Public Health Service initiated a study of syphilis in African-American men in the small rural town of Tuskegee, Alabama (Levine, 1986; Rothman, 1982). The study, which continued for 40 years, was conducted to determine the natural course of syphilis in African-American men. Many of the subjects who consented to participate in the study were not informed about the purpose and procedures of the research. Some were unaware that they were subjects in a study. By 1936 it was apparent that the men with syphilis had developed more complications than the men in the control group. Ten years later the death rate among those with syphilis was twice as high as it was for the control group. The subjects were examined periodically but were not treated for syphilis, even when penicillin was determined to be an effective treatment for the disease in the 1940s. Information about an effective treatment for syphilis was withheld from the subjects, and deliberate steps were taken to deprive them of treatment (Brandt, 1978).

Published reports of the Tuskegee Syphilis Study started appearing in 1936, and additional papers were published every 4 to 6 years. No effort was made to stop the study; in fact, in 1969 the Centers for Disease Control and Prevention (then called the Center for Disease Control) decided that the study should continue. In 1972, an account of the study in the *Washington Star* sparked public outrage; only then did the Department of Health, Education, and Welfare stop the study. The study was investigated and found to be ethically unjustified (Brandt, 1978).

Willowbrook Study

From the mid-1950s to the early 1970s, Dr. Saul Krugman conducted research on hepatitis at Willowbrook, an institution for the mentally retarded in Staten Island, New York (Rothman, 1982). The subjects were children who were deliberately infected with the hepatitis virus. During the 20-year study, Willowbrook closed its doors to new inmates because of overcrowded conditions. However, the research ward continued to admit new inmates, and parents had to give permission for their child to be in the study to gain admission to the institution (Levine, 1986).

From the late 1950s to the early 1970s, Krugman's research team published several articles describing the study protocol and findings. In 1966, Beecher cited the Willowbrook Study in the *New England Journal of Medicine* as an example of unethical research. The investigators defended injecting the children with the virus because they believed most of the children would acquire the infection upon admission to the institution. They also stressed the benefits the subjects received, which were a cleaner environment, better supervision, and a higher nurse-patient ratio on the research ward (Rothman, 1982). Despite the controversy, this unethical study continued until the early 1970s.

Jewish Chronic Disease Hospital Study

Another highly publicized unethical study was conducted at the Jewish Chronic Disease Hospital in New York in the 1960s. The purpose of this study was to determine patients' rejection responses to live cancer cells. Twenty-two patients were injected with a suspension containing live cancer cells that had been generated from human cancer tissue (Levine, 1986). Because these patients were not informed that they were taking part in research or that the injections they received were live cancer cells, their rights were not protected. In addition, the study was never presented for review to the research committee of the Jewish Chronic Disease Hospital, and the physicians caring for the patients were unaware that the study was being conducted. The physician directing the research was an employee of the Sloan-Kettering Institute for Cancer Research, and there was no indication that this institution had conducted a review of the research project (Hershey & Miller, 1976). This unethical study was conducted without the informed consent of the subjects and without institutional review and had the potential to injure, disable, or cause the death of the human subjects.

Department of Health, Education, and Welfare 1973 Regulations for the Protection of Human Research Subjects

The continued conduct of harmful, unethical research from the 1960s to the 1970s made additional controls necessary. In 1973, the Department of Health, Education, and Welfare (DHEW) published its first set of regulations for the protection of human research subjects. These regulations also provided protection for persons having limited capacity to consent, such as people who are ill, mentally impaired, or dying (Levine, 1986). According to the DHEW regulations, all research involving human subjects had to undergo full institutional review, which increased the protection of human subjects. However, reviewing all studies without regard for the degree of risk involved greatly increased the time for study approval and reduced the number of studies conducted.

National Commission for the Protection of Human Subjects of Biomedical and Behavioral Research

Because the issue of protecting human subjects in research was not resolved by the DHEW regulations, the National Commission for the Protection of Human Subjects of Biomedical and Behavioral Research (1978) was formed. This commission was established by the National Research Act (Public Law 93-348), which was passed in 1974. The commission identified three *ethical principles* that are relevant to the conduct of research involving human subjects: respect for persons, beneficence, and justice. The *principle of respect for persons* indicates that persons should be treated as autonomous agents with the right to self-determination and the freedom to participate or not participate in research. Those persons with diminished autonomy, such as children, people who are terminally or mentally ill, and prisoners, are entitled to additional protection. The *principle of beneficence* encourages the researcher to do good and "above all, do no harm." The *principle of justice* states that human subjects should be treated fairly in terms of the benefits and the risks of research. Before it was dissolved in 1978, the commission developed ethical research guidelines based on these three principles and made recommendations to the Department of Health and Human Services (DHHS) in the *Belmont Report.* Information on the *Belmont Report* and the three ethical principles, respect of persons, beneficence, and justice, can be obtained on-line at http://ohrp.osophs.dhhs.gov/humansubjects/guidance/, and then selecting belmont.htm from the list of options.

Current Federal Regulations for the Protection of Human Subjects

In response to the recommendations of The National Commission for the Protection of Human Subjects of Biomedical and Behavioral Research, the DHHS developed a set of federal regulations (Code of Federal Regulations Title 45, Part 46 Protection of Human Subjects) (DHHS, 1991). These regulations include the following: (1) general requirements for informed consent and documentation of informed consent; (2) criteria for the membership, functions, and operations of an IRB for review of research; and (3) directives for dealing with and reporting of scientific misconduct (DHHS, 1981, 1983, 1989, 1991). These DHHS regulations remain the established guidelines for evaluating the ethical aspects of research today. The federal regulations can be accessed on-line at http://ohrp.osophs.dhhs.gov/humansubjects/guidance/45cfr46.htm. The Office for Human Research Protection (OHRP) is responsible for interpreting and overseeing the implementation of these regulations regarding the protection of human subjects. Extensive information about the operations and functions of OHRP can be found at their web site, http://ohrp.osophs.dhhs.gov/.

PROTECTING HUMAN RIGHTS

What are human rights? How are these rights protected during research? *Human rights* are claims and demands that have been justified in the eyes of an individual or by the consensus of a group of individuals. Nurses who critique published studies, review research for conduct in their agencies, or assist with data collection for a study have an ethical responsibility to determine whether the rights of the research subjects are protected. The human rights that require protection in research include the rights to the following: (1) self-determination, (2) privacy, (3) anonymity and confidentiality, (4) fair treatment, and (5) protection from discomfort and harm (American Nurses Association, 2001; American Psychological Association, 1982; Silva, 1995).

Right to Self-Determination

The right to self-determination is based on the ethical principle of respect for persons, and it indicates that humans are capable of controlling their own destiny. Thus humans should be treated as *autonomous agents,* who have the freedom to conduct their lives as they choose without external controls. Subjects are treated as autonomous agents in a study if the researcher: (1) informed them about the study,

(2) allowed them to choose whether to participate, and (3) allowed them to withdraw from the study at any time without penalty (Levine, 1986). Flynn (1997) studied the health practices of homeless women and documented that her subjects were treated as autonomous agents.

> "The study was approved by the university's Institutional Review Board for the protection of human subjects. To ensure protection of human rights, all prospective participants were informed, both verbally and in writing, of the maintenance of confidentiality, their right to refuse to participate, and [that] the refusal to participate would in no way affect their status or services received at the shelter." (p. 74)

Violation of the Right to Self-Determination

A subject's right to self-determination can be violated through the use of coercion, covert data collection, and deception. *Coercion* occurs when one person intentionally presents an overt threat of harm or an excessive reward to another to obtain compliance. Some subjects are coerced to participate in research because they fear harm or discomfort if they do not participate. For example, some patients feel that their medical and nursing care will be negatively affected if they do not agree to be research subjects. Other subjects are coerced to participate in studies because they believe that they cannot refuse the excessive rewards offered, such as large sums of money, special privileges, or jobs (Rudy, Estok, Kerr, & Menzel, 1994).

With *covert data collection*, subjects are unaware that research data are being collected (Reynolds, 1979). For example, in the Jewish Chronic Disease Hospital Study, most of the patients and their physicians were unaware of the study. The subjects were informed that they were receiving an injection of cells, but the word "cancer" was omitted (Beecher, 1966).

The use of *deception* (the actual misinforming of subjects for research purposes) (Kelman, 1967) can also violate a subject's right to self-determination. A classic example of deception is the Milgram (1963) study, in which the subjects thought they were administering electric shocks to another person, but the person was really a professional actor who pretended to feel the shocks. If deception is used in a study, the research report should indicate how the subjects were deceived and that the subjects were informed of the actual research activities and the findings at the end of the study.

Persons with Diminished Autonomy

Some persons have *diminished autonomy*, which means that they are vulnerable and less advantaged because of legal or mental incompetence, terminal illness, or confinement to an institution (DHHS, 1991; Levine, 1986). These persons require additional protection of their right to self-determination because of their decreased ability or inability to give informed consent. In addition, these persons are vulnerable to coercion and deception. The research report should include justification for the use of subjects with diminished autonomy, and the need for justification increases as the subject's risk and vulnerability increase.

Legally and mentally incompetent subjects. Children (minors), mentally impaired patients, and unconscious patients are legally and mentally incompetent to give informed consent. These individuals often lack the ability to comprehend information about a study and to make decisions about participating in or withdrawing from the study. These persons have a range of vulnerability from minimal to absolute. The use of persons with diminished autonomy as research subjects is more acceptable if the following are true: (1) the research is therapeutic, that is, the subjects might benefit from the experimental process; (2) the researcher is willing to use both vulnerable and nonvulnerable individuals as subjects; (3) the risk is minimized in the study, and (4) the consent process is strictly followed to ensure the rights of the prospective subjects (Levine, 1986; Watson, 1982).

Children. The laws defining the minor status of a child are statutory and vary from state to state. Often a child's competence to give consent is operationalized by age, with incompetence being irrefutable up to age 7 (Broome & Stieglitz, 1992; Thompson, 1987). However, by age 7 children can think in terms of concrete operations and can provide meaningful assent to participation as research subjects (Thompson, 1987). With advancing age and maturity the child should play a stronger role in the consent process.

The DHHS regulations require "soliciting the assent of the children (when capable) and the permission of their parents or guardians. Assent means a child's affirmative agreement to participate in research…. Permission means the agreement of parent(s) or guardian to the participation of their child or ward in research" (DHHS, 1991, Section 46.402; http://ohrp.osophs.dhhs.gov/humansubjects/guidance/45cfr46.htm). The decision about using children as research subjects is also influenced by the therapeutic nature of the research and the risks versus benefits. Thompson (1987) developed a guide for obtaining informed consent based on the child's level of competence, the therapeutic nature of the research, and the risks versus benefits (Table 6-2).

There is an increased need for ethical research using children as subjects. Researchers are being urged to conduct clinical trials with children to determine the effectiveness of selected pharmacological and nonpharmacological treatments for various age groups (Rosato, 2000). Tigges (2001) studied affiliation preferences and condom use in Hispanic and non-Hispanic white adolescents. The methods section of the article documented the consent of the parents and the assent of the adolescents to participate in the study.

> "Students in two public high schools in a city of 60,000 in northern New Mexico participated in this study. The schools were chosen because of their willingness to participate in the study about sexual behavior. A total of 457 students anonymously completed structured questionnaires…. Two weeks before ques-

> tionnaire administration, letters were mailed to the parents of all 12th-grade students. Parents were instructed to return the form if they did not want their child to participate in the study. Students could also decline participation at the time of questionnaire administration. Nonparticipation occurred because of parental refusals (n = 6, 1%), student refusals (n = 8, 1%), and student absence on the days of survey administration (n = 135, 22%)." (p. 233)

Adults. Certain adults, because of mental illness, cognitive impairment, or a comatose state, are incompetent and incapable of giving informed consent. Persons are said to be incompetent if, in the judgment of a qualified clinician, they have those attributes that ordinarily provide the grounds for designating incompetence (Levine, 1986). Incompetence can be temporary (e.g., inebriation), permanent (e.g., advanced senile dementia), or subjective or transitory (e.g., behavior or symptoms of psychosis). If an individual is judged incompetent and incapable of giving consent, the researcher must seek approval from the prospective subject and his or her legally authorized representative. A legally authorized representative is an individual or another body authorized under applicable law to consent on behalf of a prospective subject to the subject's participation in the research procedure(s) (DHHS, 1991, Sec-

TABLE 6-2

GUIDE TO OBTAINING INFORMED CONSENT, BASED ON THE RELATIONSHIP BETWEEN A CHILD'S LEVEL OF COMPETENCE, THE THERAPEUTIC NATURE OF THE RESEARCH, AND RISK VERSUS BENEFITS

	NONTHERAPEUTIC		THERAPEUTIC	
	MMR-LB	MR-LB	MR-HB	MMR-HB
CHILD, INCOMPETENT (GENERALLY 0-7 YR)				
Parents' consent	Necessary	Necessary	Sufficient*	Sufficient
Child's assent	Optional[†]	Optional[†]	Optional	Optional
CHILD, RELATIVELY COMPETENT (7 YR AND OLDER)				
Parents' consent	Necessary	Necessary	Sufficient[‡]	Recommended
Child's assent	Necessary	Necessary	Sufficient[§]	Sufficient

MMR, More than minimal risk; *MR*, minimal risk; *LB*, low benefit; *HB*, high benefit.

*A parent's refusal can be superceded by the principle that a parent has no power to forbid the saving of a child's life.

[†]Children making a "deliberate objection" would be precluded from participation by most researchers.

[‡]In cases not involving the privacy rights of a "mature minor."

[§]In cases involving the privacy rights of a "mature minor."

tion 46.102). However, individuals can be judged incompetent and still assent to participate in certain minimal risk research, if they are able to understand what they are being asked to do (Levine, 1986).

To and Chan (2000) conducted a study to examine the effectiveness of a progressive muscle relaxation program in reducing the aggressive behaviors of mentally handicapped patients. Since these patients were incompetent to give informed consent, the researchers followed a detailed process for obtaining their assent and their parents or guardians' permission for participation in the study. The following example provides direction for critiquing a study conducted with subjects with diminished autonomy.

> ### "Consent for Study
>
> Before the study, informed consent that described the purpose of the study, potential risk/benefits, right to confidentiality, and right to withdrawal, were distributed and explained to all subjects and their parents/guardians. Because of the subjects' limited cognitive abilities, it was believed that comprehension of the informed consent might pose some difficulty. Therefore, special care and effort were taken to ensure the subjects' understanding of the information in the document. For example, the researchers played a tape about the muscle relaxation training and asked the subjects whether they wanted to learn the exercises. Moreover, all subjects were told that the training would help them to decrease their aggressive behaviors. They were told that the training would enable them to learn new behavior that could be useful when they were unhappy. After a detailed explanation, all subjects showed an understanding of the study. Written consent was gained from the subjects (assent) and subjects' parents/guardians (permission)." (p. 41)

Terminally ill subjects. Participating in research could have increased risks and minimal or no benefits for terminally ill subjects. In addition, the dying subject's condition could affect the study results and lead the researcher to misinterpret the results (Watson, 1982). For example, cancer patients have become an over-studied population. It is not unusual for the majority of blood work, bone marrow scans, lumbar punctures, and biopsies to be conducted in cancer patients for purposes of research to fulfill protocol requirements (Strauman & Cotanch, 1988). These biomedical research treatments can easily compromise the care of these individuals, which poses ethical dilemmas for clinical nurses. More nurses will be responsible for ensuring adherence to ethical standards in research as they participate in institutional review of research and serve as patient advocates in the clinical setting (Davis, 1989; Njie & Thomas, 2001).

McCorkle, Robinson, Nuamah, Lev, and Benoliel (1998) studied the "effects of home nursing care for patients during terminal illness on the bereaved's psychological distress" (p. 2). The investigators were cautious in obtaining permission from the patients and their spouses to participate in the study. The patients were contacted first by their physician or the physician's designee to determine if the patient was willing to participate. Only those patients who agreed to be contacted were then called by the investigators and asked to participate in the study. Only 100 of the 127 patients contacted agreed to participate. The spouses of these patients were also asked to participate; only 91 completed the study because some chose to withdraw after the death of their spouse. It is important to study terminally ill patients so that essential knowledge for their care may be generated, but the rights of these individuals should be closely guarded during the conduct of a study.

Subjects confined to institutions. Prisoners are individuals who are confined to institutions and are designated as having diminished autonomy by federal law (DHHS, 1991, Subpart C, Section 46.301-46.306). Prison inmates might feel coerced to participate in research because they fear harm or desire the benefits of early release, special treatment, or monetary gain (Levine, 1986).

Hospitalized patients are a vulnerable population but are not designated as having diminished autonomy by law. However, patients are vulnerable because they are ill and are confined in settings that are controlled by health care personnel. Some hospitalized patients feel obligated to be research subjects because they want to assist a particular nurse or physician with his or her research. Others feel coerced to participate because they fear that their care will be adversely affected if they refuse. Thus researchers should be cautious about protecting the rights of patients in health care agencies who participate in research.

In critiquing studies, nursing students should evaluate the subjects' capacity for self-determination and assess whether the rights of subjects with diminished autonomy were protected. The following questions may be used as a guide during the critique of a study.

1. Were the subjects informed about the research project?
2. Did the subjects voluntarily give their consent to be in the study?
3. Did the subjects have the freedom to withdraw from the study?
4. Did the subjects have diminished autonomy because of legal or mental incompetence, terminal illness, or confinement to an institution? If they did, were special precautions taken in obtaining consent from these subjects and their parents or guardians?

Right to Privacy

Privacy is the freedom an individual has to determine the time, extent, and general circumstances under which private information will be shared with or withheld from others. Private information includes a person's attitudes, beliefs, behaviors, opinions, and records. The research subject's privacy is protected if the subject is informed, consents to participate in a study, and voluntarily shares private information with a researcher (Levine, 1986).

Invasion of Privacy

An *invasion of privacy* occurs when private information is shared without an individual's knowledge or against his or her will. The invasion of subjects' right to privacy brought about the Privacy Act of 1974. As a result of this act, individuals have the right to provide or prevent access of others to their records (Levine, 1986). A research report will often indicate that the subjects' privacy was protected and might include the details of how this was accomplished.

Right to Anonymity and Confidentiality

Based on the right to privacy, the research subject has the right to anonymity and the right to assume that the data collected will be kept confidential. Complete *anonymity* exists when the subject's identity cannot be linked, even by the researcher, with his or her individual responses (American Nurses Association, 2001). For example, Mullins (1996) promised her subjects anonymity when she studied nurse caring behaviors desired by patients with acquired immunodeficiency syndrome (AIDS) or human immunodeficiency virus (HIV).

> "A letter explaining the study, the CBA (Caring Behavior Assessment) tool, a letter to participants, and the demographic sheet were sent to administrators of health care agencies…. After access to agency clients was obtained, potential subjects who met the sampling criteria were asked if they would like to participate in the study. Those potential subjects who expressed interest in the study were given a packet containing the CBA tool, a letter describing the study, and a demographic sheet…. By completing the CBA tool and the demographic sheet, the subject agreed to participate in the study. Subjects did not indicate their names or addresses on the tools or demographic sheets, thus allowing participants to be anonymous. Tools and demographic sheets were not coded in any way to link them with agencies or subjects." (p. 20)

In most studies, researchers know the identity of their subjects, and they promise them that their identity will be kept anonymous from others and that the research data will be kept confidential. *Confidentiality* is the researcher's management of private information shared by a subject. The researcher must refrain from sharing that information without the authorization of the subject. Confidentiality is grounded in the following premises: "(1) Individuals can share personal information to the extent they wish and are entitled to have secrets; (2) one can choose with whom to share personal information; (3) those accepting information in confidence have an obligation to maintain confidentiality; and (4) professionals, such as researchers, have a duty to maintain confidentiality that goes beyond ordinary loyalty." (Levine, 1986, p. 164)

A *breach of confidentiality* can occur when a researcher, by accident or direct action, allows an unauthorized person to gain access to the raw data of a study. Confidentiality can also be breached in reporting or publishing a study if a subject's identity is accidentally revealed, violating the subject's right to anonymity (Ramos, 1989). Breach of confidentiality is of special concern in qualitative studies that have few subjects and involve the reporting of long quotes made by the subjects. These long quotes might reveal the identity of a subject to others, resulting in a breach of confidentiality (Sandelowski, 1994). Breaches of confidentiality that can be especially harmful to subjects include those regarding religious preferences; sexual practices; income; racial prejudices; drug use; child abuse; and personal attributes such as intelligence, honesty, and courage.

The research report should be examined for evidence that subject confidentiality was maintained during data collection and analysis. In addition, the research findings should be reported so that a subject or group of subjects cannot be identified by their responses. Brudenell (2000) conducted a "qualitative study that explored women's concurrent experiences of alcohol/drug recovery while parenting their infant" (p. 82). The participants in this study were from a vulnerable population with "a history of polydrug use, such as methamphetamine and alcohol..." (p. 83). Brudenell (2000) detailed how she protected her subjects' right to privacy and self-determination in the procedure section of the article.

"Procedure

Approval for the study was granted by the Institutional Review Board from Oregon Health Sciences University and from cooperating agencies in the location for the research, a metropolitan area in the western United States. The researcher obtained a signed informed consent agreement from each participant after the study was explained. The consent form included a clause concerning the mandatory reporting of suspected child abuse and neglect by the nurse researcher. The researcher reexplained the study and verified continuing consent at subsequent interviews. Confidentiality and anonymity of participants were carefully protected. For example, all tapes, transcripts, and notes were coded without participants' names and kept in a locked compartment." (p. 83)

In this study, data were analyzed as a group for the sample of 11 subjects, and the results were presented so that individual subjects could not be identified by their responses.

In critiquing a published study, you might examine whether the subjects' right to anonymity and confidentiality was protected by addressing the following questions:

1. Were the subjects' identities kept anonymous?
2. Were the subjects ensured confidentiality or anonymity by the researchers?
3. Were the research data kept confidential?
4. Were the data analyzed and the findings presented in a way to ensure the anonymity of the subjects in the research report?

Right to Fair Treatment

The right to fair treatment is based on the ethical principle of justice. According to this principle, people should be treated fairly and should receive what they are due or owed. The research report should indicate that the selection of subjects and their treatment during the study were fair.

Fair Selection and Treatment of Subjects

In the past, injustice in subject selection resulted from social, cultural, racial, and sexual biases in society. For many years research was conducted on categories of individuals who were thought to be especially suitable as research subjects, such as poor people, charity patients, prisoners, slaves, peasants, dying persons, and others who were considered undesirable (Reynolds, 1979). Researchers often treated these subjects carelessly and had little regard for the harm and discomfort they experienced. The Nazi medical experiments, the Tuskegee Syphilis Study, the Willowbrook Study, and the Jewish Chronic Disease Hospital Study all exemplify unfair subject selection.

Another concern with subject selection is that some researchers select subjects because they like them and want them to receive the specific benefits of a study. Other researchers have been swayed by power or money to make certain patients subjects so these patients can receive potentially beneficial treatments. Random selection of subjects can eliminate some of the researcher's biases that might influence subject selection.

Researchers and subjects should have a specific agreement regarding the researcher's role and the subject's participation in a study (American Psychological Association, 1982). While conducting the study, the researcher should treat the subjects fairly and respect that agreement. For example, the activities or procedures that the subject is to perform should not be changed without the subject's consent. The benefits promised to the subjects should be provided. In addition, subjects who participate in studies should receive equal benefits regardless of age, race, or socioeconomic level.

The research report should indicate that the selection and treatment of the subjects were fair. Subjects should have been selected for reasons directly related to the problem being studied and not for their easy availability, compromised position, manipulability, or friendship with the researcher (National Commission for the Protection of Human Subjects of Biomedical and Behavioral Research, 1978). In addition, the procedures section of the research report should indicate fair and equal treatment of the subjects during data collection. Introduced earlier in this chapter, the Mullins (1996) study of nursing care behaviors desired by patients with AIDS or HIV demonstrates fair selection and treatment of subjects.

"…The sample for this study included persons with a diagnosis of AIDS/HIV who agreed to participate in the study and met specific criteria for the sample's subjects…. Criteria for this study were as follows. Subjects in the sample were at least 18 years of age and had the diagnosis of either AIDS or HIV-seropositive status. Subjects had to be alert and could not be confused to be able to give reliable responses…. Patients who were initially diagnosed as having AIDS or as HIV-seropositive during the present hospitalization or clinic visit were not included in the sample. This criterion was included to allow the patient newly diagnosed with AIDS/HIV time to begin to accept the reality of being diagnosed with a fatal disease." (pp. 19-20)

Mullins (1996) demonstrated fair selection of subjects by allowing any potential subject the option of participating or not in the study. Patients who were cognitively impaired or newly diagnosed with AIDS or HIV were excluded. This procedure indicates that the researcher was attempting to protect the individuals with diminished autonomy by not including them in the study. The subjects were treated the same way throughout the study and were only asked to complete a demographic sheet and a study scale.

Right to Protection from Discomfort and Harm

The right to protection from discomfort and harm from a study is based on the ethical principle of beneficence, which states that one should do good and, above all, do no harm. According to this principle, members of society should take an active role in preventing discomfort and harm and promoting good in the world around them. In research, *discomfort and harm* can be physical, emotional, social, economic, or any combination of these four (Weider, 2000). Reynolds (1972) identified five categories of studies based on levels of discomfort and harm: no anticipated effects, temporary discomfort, unusual levels of temporary discomfort, risk of permanent damage, and certainty of permanent damage.

No Anticipated Effects

In some studies no positive or negative effects are expected for the subjects. For example, studies that involve reviewing patients' records, students' files, pathology reports, or other documents have no anticipated effects on the research subjects. In this type of study, the researcher does not interact directly with the subjects; however, there is still a potential risk of invading a subject's privacy.

Temporary Discomfort

Studies that cause temporary discomfort are described as minimal risk studies, in which the discomfort is similar to what the subject would encounter in his or her daily life and is temporary, ending with the termination of the experiment (DHHS, 1991). Many nursing studies require the completion of questionnaires or participation in interviews, which usually involve minimal risk or are a mere inconvenience for the subjects. The physical discomfort might include fatigue, headache, or muscle tension. The emotional and social risks might include anxiety or embarrassment associated with answering certain questions. The economic risks might include the time commitment for the study or travel costs to the study site.

Most clinical nursing studies examining the effect of a treatment involve minimal risk. For example, a study might involve examining the effects of exercise on the blood glucose levels of diabetic subjects. For the study the subjects would be asked to test their blood glucose level one extra time per day. Discomfort occurs when the blood is drawn, and there is a potential risk of physical changes that might occur with exercise. The subjects might also feel anxiety and fear associated with the additional blood testing, and the testing could be an added expense. The diabetic subjects in this study would encounter similar discomforts in their daily lives, and the discomfort would cease with the termination of the study.

Unusual Levels of Temporary Discomfort

In studies that involve unusual levels of temporary discomfort, subjects frequently have discomfort both during the study and after it has been completed. For example, subjects might have prolonged muscle weakness, joint pain, and dizziness after participating in a study that required them to be confined to bed for 10 days to determine the effects of immobility. Studies that require subjects to experience failure, extreme fear, or threats to their identity or to act in unnatural ways involve unusual levels of temporary discomfort. In some qualitative studies, subjects are asked questions that open old wounds or involve reliving traumatic events (Ford & Reuter, 1990). For example, asking subjects to describe their rape experience could precipitate feelings of extreme anger, fear, sadness, or any combination of these emotions. In such studies, investigators should indicate in their research report that they were vigilant in assessing the subjects' discomfort and referred them as necessary for appropriate professional intervention.

Risk of Permanent Damage

In some studies, subjects might sustain permanent damage; this is more common in biomedical research than in nursing research. For example, medical studies of new drugs and surgical procedures have the potential to cause subjects permanent physical damage. Some topics investigated by nurses have the potential to permanently damage subjects emotionally and socially. Studies examining sensitive information, such as sexual behavior, child abuse, AIDS or HIV status, or drug use, can be very risky for subjects. These studies have the potential to cause permanent damage to a subject's personality or reputation. There are also potential economic risks, such as those resulting from a decrease in job performance or loss of employment.

Certainty of Permanent Damage

In some research, such as the Nazi medical experiments and the Tuskegee Syphilis Study, the subjects experienced permanent damage. Conducting research that will permanently damage subjects is highly questionable, regardless of the benefits that will be gained. Frequently the benefits gained from such a study are not experienced by the research subjects but by others in society. Studies causing permanent damage to subjects violate the fifth principle of the Nuremberg Code (see Table 6-1) (Levine, 1986).

In critiquing a published study, the level of discomfort and harm experienced by the subjects should be determined.

1. What was the level of risk of the study: no anticipated effects, temporary discomfort, unusual levels of temporary discomfort, risk of permanent damage, or certainty of permanent damage?
2. Was this level of risk reasonable for the study based on the potential benefit of the knowledge generated?
3. Should the study have been revised or cancelled because the risk level was too great? If revision is suggested, how might the study have been revised?

UNDERSTANDING INFORMED CONSENT

What is informed consent? How is informed consent obtained from research subjects? Informing is the transmission of essential ideas and content from the investigator to the prospective subject. Consent is the prospective subject's agreement to participate in a study as a subject. Every prospective subject, to the degree that he or she is capable, should have the opportunity to choose whether to participate in research (Brent, 1990; Cassidy & Odd, 1986). *Informed consent* includes four elements: (1) disclosure of essential study information to the subject, (2) comprehension of this information by the subject, (3) competence of the subject to give consent, and (4) voluntary consent of the subject to participate in the study.

Essential Information for Consent

Informed consent requires the researcher to disclose specific information to all prospective subjects. The following information is identified as essential for obtaining informed consent from research subjects (DHHS, 1991; Levine, 1986).

1. *Introduction of research activities.* The initial information presented to prospective subjects clearly indicates that a study is to be conducted and that the individuals are being asked to participate as subjects.
2. *Statement of the research purpose.* The researcher states the immediate purpose of the research and any long-range goals related to the study.
3. *Selection of research subjects.* The researcher explains to prospective subjects why they were selected as possible subjects.
4. *Explanation of procedures.* Prospective subjects receive a complete description of the procedures to be followed and identification of any procedures that are experimental in the study (DHHS, 1991, Section 46.116a).
5. *Description of risks and discomforts.* Prospective subjects are informed of any reasonably foreseeable risks or discomforts (physical, emotional, social, and economic) that might result from the study (DHHS, 1991, Section 46.116a).
6. *Description of benefits.* The investigator describes any benefits to the subjects or to other people or future patients that may reasonably be expected from the

research (DHHS, 1991, Section 46.116a), including any financial advantages or other rewards for participating in the study.

7. *Disclosure of alternatives.* The investigator discloses the appropriate alternative procedures or courses of treatment, if any, that might be advantageous to the subjects (DHHS, 1991, Section 46.116a). For example, the researchers of the Tuskegee Syphilis Study should have informed the subjects with syphilis that penicillin was an effective treatment for the disease.

8. *Assurance of anonymity and confidentiality.* Prospective subjects should know the extent to which their responses and records will be kept confidential. Subjects are promised that their identity will remain anonymous in reports and publications of the study.

9. *Offer to answer questions.* The researcher offers to answer any questions the prospective subjects may have.

10. *Noncoercive disclaimer.* Subjects are asked to sign a noncoercive disclaimer, which is a statement that participation is voluntary and that refusal to participate will involve no penalty or loss of benefits to which the subject is otherwise entitled (DHHS, 1991, Section 46.116a).

11. *Option to withdraw.* Subjects are informed that they may discontinue participation (withdraw from a study) at any time without penalty or loss of benefits (DHHS, 1991, Section 46.116a).

12. *Consent to incomplete disclosure.* In some studies, subjects are not completely informed of the study purpose because that knowledge would alter their actions. However, prospective subjects must be told when certain information is being withheld deliberately.

A consent form is a written document that includes the elements of informed consent required by the DHHS Regulations (1991, Section 46.116). In addition, a consent form might include other information required by the institution where the study is to be conducted or by the agency funding the study. An example of a consent form is presented in Fig. 6-1; descriptors indicate the essential consent information.

Comprehension of Consent Information

Informed consent implies not only that the researcher has imparted information to the subjects, but also that the prospective subjects have comprehended that information. The researcher should take the time to teach the subjects about the study. The amount of information to be taught depends on the subjects' knowledge of research and the specific research topic. The benefits and risks of a study should be discussed in detail, with examples that the potential subject can understand. Patient advocates in a clinical agency should assess whether patients involved in research understand the purpose and the potential risks and benefits of their participation in a study.

Competence to Give Consent

Autonomous individuals, who are capable of understanding the benefits and risks of a proposed study, are competent to give consent. Persons with diminished autono-

Consent Form

Study Title: The Needs of Family Members of Critically Ill Adults
Investigator: Linda L. Norris, R.N.

Ms. Norris is a registered nurse studying the emotional and social needs of family members of patients in the Intensive Care Units **(research purpose)**. Although the study will not benefit you directly, it will provide information that might enable nurses to identify family members' needs and to assist family members with those needs **(potential benefits)**.

The study and its procedures have been approved by the appropriate people and review boards at The University of Texas at Arlington and X hospital **(IRB approval)**. The study procedures involve no foreseeable risks or harm to you or your family **(potential risks)**. The procedures include: (1) responding to a questionnaire about the needs of family members of critically ill patients and (2) completing a demographic data sheet **(explanation of procedure)**. Participation in this study will take approximately 20 minutes **(time commitment)**. You are free to ask any questions about the study or about being a subject and you may call Ms. Norris at (999) 999-9999 (work) or (111) 111-1111 (home) if you have further questions **(offer to answer questions)**.

Your participation in this study is voluntary; you are under no obligation to participate **(voluntary consent)**. You have the right to withdraw at any time and the care of your family member and your relationship with the health care team will not be affected **(option to withdraw)**.

The study data will be coded so it will not be linked to your name. Your identity will not be revealed while the study is being conducted or when the study is reported or published. All study data will be collected by Ms. Norris, stored in a secure place, and not shared with any other person without your permission **(assurance of anonymity and confidentiality)**.

I have read this consent form and voluntarily consent to participate in this study.

_____   *(if appropriate)*
                                     _____
Subject's signature   Date   Legal representative   Date

                                     _____
                                     Relationship to subject

I have explained this study to the above subject and have sought his/her understanding for informed consent.

_____
Investigator's signature   Date

Fig. 6-1 Sample consent form.

my because of legal or mental incompetence, terminal illness, or confinement to an institution are frequently not legally competent to consent to participate in research (see the section "Right to Self-Determination" earlier in this chapter). Frequently, the researcher determines the competence of the subject (Douglas & Larson, 1986). In the research report the investigator will often indicate the competence of the subjects and the process that was used for obtaining informed consent.

Voluntary Consent

Voluntary consent means the prospective subject has decided to take part in a study of his or her own volition without coercion or any undue influence (Douglas & Larson, 1986). Voluntary consent is obtained after the prospective subject has been given the essential information about the study and has shown comprehension of this information.

A research report will often discuss the consent process and identify some of the essential consent information that was provided to the potential subjects. All research reports should have some mention of the consent process for that study, but the depth of the discussion will vary based on the research purpose and the types of subjects included in the study. Wilson, Pittman, and Wold (2000) conducted a qualitative study of school-aged migrant children's perceptions of their own health. They detailed the consent process for parents and children in the procedure section of their article.

> **"Procedure**
>
> An explanation of the study was given, and permission to approach parents and children attending a summer-school program for children of migrant farm workers in south Georgia was granted by school officials. [Written] Informed consent was granted by a parent, and verbal assent was obtained from each child participating. We met with the teachers of grades 3 through 8 and arranged a convenient time to talk with students. An explanation of the study was given to the children, and those children who had parental permission and wanted to join a group went with us to the designated room. Before beginning each focus-group session, we developed a rapport with the children by allowing each child to say something into the tape recorder. When their voices were played back, some children seemed surprised at hearing their voices. Some laughed, and others were intrigued at hearing their friends' voices. Each child was asked if he or she still wanted to participate in the group and his or her 'yes' on the tape was the assent to participate. None of the children's names were recorded on the tape, to assure confidentiality, and all results were reported as group data." (p. 140)

Wilson and colleagues (2000) provided the parents and children detailed information about the study to promote their comprehension regarding participation. Rapport was developed with the children and they were able to play with the tape recorder to promote their comfort in participating in the study. During data collection, the children were given opportunities to withdraw from the study if they desired. Consent was documented for both parents and children; signed consent form for the parents and tape-recorded assent for the children. Consent and participation seemed to be voluntary for both parents and children.

A critique of a research report requires examining the ethics of the consent process. The following questions might be used to direct a critique.

1. Was the information that was essential for consent provided?
2. Were the subjects capable of comprehending the information?
3. Did the researcher take any action to ensure that the subjects comprehended the consent information?
4. Were the subjects competent to give consent?
5. If the subjects were not competent to give consent, who acted as their legally authorized representatives?
6. Did it seem that the subjects participated voluntarily in the study?

UNDERSTANDING INSTITUTIONAL REVIEW

In an *institutional review,* a committee of peers (institutional review board or IRB) examines studies for ethical concerns. You might be part of an IRB that examines studies in your agency. Thus you should know the activities of an IRB and the guidelines used in determining the ethical acceptability of a study. The membership, functions, and guidelines for IRBs are available on-line at http://ohrp.osophs.dhhs.gov/humansubjects/guidance/45cfr46.htm.

The functions of an IRB involve reviewing research to determine whether: (1) the rights and welfare of the subjects were protected, (2) the methods used to secure informed consent were appropriate, and (3) the potential benefits of the study were greater than the risks (Martin, 1996). The DHHS regulations (1991) identify three levels of review: exempt from review, expedited review, and complete review. The IRB chairperson, the committee, or both determine the level of the review required for each study.

Studies are usually *exempt from review* if they involve no apparent risks for the research subjects. Research qualifying for exemption from review by the DHHS (1991, Section 46.101b) is described in Table 6-3. Nursing studies that have no foreseeable risks or are a mere inconvenience for subjects are usually identified as exempt from review by the chairperson of the IRB. Studies with risks that are considered minimal are expedited in the review process. *Minimal risk* means that the risks of harm anticipated in the proposed research are no greater, in probability and magnitude, than those ordinarily encountered in daily life or during the performance of routine physical or psychological examinations or tests (DHHS, 1991, Section 46.102i). Under *expedited review* procedures, the review may be carried out by the IRB chairperson or by one or more experienced IRB reviewers designated by the chairperson. Table 6-4 describes research that qualifies for expedited review.

TABLE 6-3

RESEARCH QUALIFYING FOR EXEMPTION FROM IRB REVIEW

Unless otherwise required by department or agency heads, research activities in which the only involvement of human subjects will be in one or more of the following categories are exempt from review.

1. Research conducted in established or commonly accepted educational settings, involving normal educational practices, such as:
   (i) research on regular and special education instructional strategies, or
   (ii) research on the effectiveness of or the comparison among instructional techniques, curricula, or classroom management methods.
2. Research involving the use of educational tests (cognitive, diagnostic, aptitude, achievement), survey procedures, interview procedures or observation of public behavior, unless:
   (i) information obtained is recorded in such a manner that human subjects can be identified, directly or through identifiers linked to the subjects; and
   (ii) any disclosure of the human subjects' responses outside the research could reasonably place the subjects at risk of criminal or civil liability or be damaging to the subjects' financial standing, employability, or reputation.
3. Research involving the use of educational tests (cognitive, diagnostic, aptitude, achievement), survey procedures, interview procedures, or observation of public behavior that is not exempt under paragraph (b) (2) of this section, if:
   (i) the human subjects are elected or appointed public officials or candidates for public office; or
   (ii) federal statute(s) require(s) without exception that the confidentiality of the personally identifiable information will be maintained throughout the research and thereafter.
4. Research involving the collection or study of existing data, documents, records, pathological specimens, or diagnostic specimens, if these sources are publicly available or if the information is recorded by the investigator in such a manner that subjects cannot be identified, directly or through identifiers linked to the subjects.
5. Research and demonstration projects, which are conducted by or subject to the approval of Department or Agency heads, and which are designed to study, evaluate, or otherwise examine:
   (i) public benefit or service programs;
   (ii) procedures for obtaining benefits or services under those programs;
   (iii) possible changes in or alternatives to those programs or procedures; or
   (iv) possible changes in methods or levels of payment for benefits or services under those programs.
6. Taste and food quality evaluation and consumer acceptance studies:
   (i) if wholesome foods without additives are consumed, or
   (ii) if a good is consumed that contains a food ingredient at or below the level and for a use found to be safe, or agricultural chemical or environmental contaminant at or below the level found to be safe, by the Food and Drug Administration or approved by the Environmental Protection Agency or the Food Safety and Inspection Service of the U.S. Department of Agriculture.

Excerpted from the *Federal Register* of June 18, 1991 (DHHS, 1991, Section 46.101b).

TABLE 6-4

RESEARCH QUALIFYING FOR EXPEDITED IRB REVIEW

Expedited review (by committee chairpersons or designated members) for the following research involving no more than minimal risk is authorized:

1. Collection of hair and nail clippings, in a nondisfiguring manner; deciduous teeth and permanent teeth if patient care indicates a need for extraction.
2. Collection of excreta and external secretions including sweat, uncannulated saliva, placenta removed at delivery, and amniotic fluid at the time of rupture of the membrane prior to or during labor.
3. Recording of data from subjects 18 years of age or older using noninvasive procedures routinely employed in clinical practice. This includes the use of physical sensors that are applied either to the surface of the body or at a distance and do not involve input of matter or significant amounts of energy into the subject or an invasion of the subject's privacy. It also includes such procedures as weighing, testing sensory acuity, electrocardiography, electroencephalography, thermography, detection of naturally occurring radioactivity, diagnostic echography and electroretinography. It does not include exposure to electromagnetic radiation outside the visible range (for example, x-rays, microwaves).
4. Collection of blood samples by venipuncture, in amounts not exceeding 450 ml in an 8-week period and no more than two times per week, from subjects 18 years of age or older and who are in good health and not pregnant.
5. Collection of both supragingival and subgingival dental plaque and calculus, provided the procedure is not more invasive than routine prophylactic scaling of the teeth and the process is accomplished in accordance with accepted prophylactic techniques.
6. Voice recordings made for research purposes such as investigations of speech defects.
7. Moderate exercise by healthy volunteers.
8. The study of existing data, documents, records, pathological specimens, or diagnostic specimens.
9. Research on individual or group behavior or characteristics of individual, such as studies of perception, cognition, game theory, or test development, where the investigator does not manipulate subjects' behavior and research will not involve stress to subjects.
10. Research on drugs or devices for which an investigational new drug exemption or an investigational devise exemption is not required.

Excerpted from the *Federal Register* of June 18, 1991 (DHHS, 1991, Section 46.101). Additional regulations that apply to research involving fetuses, pregnant women, human in vitro fertilization, and prisoners are available in the *Federal Register,* 1991, part 46.

Studies that have greater than minimal risks must receive a *complete review* by an IRB. To obtain IRB approval, researchers should ensure the following:

1. Risks to subjects are minimized.
2. Risks to subjects are reasonable in relation to anticipated benefits.
3. Selection of subjects is equitable.
4. Informed consent is sought from each prospective subject or the subject's legally authorized representative.
5. Informed consent is appropriately documented.
6. The research plan makes adequate provision for monitoring data collection for subjects' safety.
7. Adequate provisions are made to protect the privacy of subjects and maintain the confidentiality of data. (DHHS, 1991, Section 46.111a)

In a research report, the investigator will usually indicate that the study was approved by the appropriate IRB(s). Brudenell (2000), who studied a woman parenting her infant during her alcohol recovery, clearly indicated that she had obtained IRB approval for her study from the university and the clinical agencies serving as settings for the study.

> "Approval for the study was granted by the Institutional Review Board from Oregon Health Sciences University and from cooperating agencies in the location of the research, a metropolitan area in the western United States." (p. 83)

EXAMINING THE BENEFIT-RISK RATIO OF A STUDY

Nurses who serve on an IRB for their agencies, act as a patient advocate when research is conducted in their agencies, or are asked to collect data for a study should examine the balance of benefits and risks in studies. To determine this balance, or *benefit-risk ratio*, the benefits and risks of the sampling method, consent process, procedures, and potential outcomes of the study should be assessed (Fig. 6-2). Informed consent should be obtained from subjects, and selection and treatment of subjects during the study must be fair. An important outcome of research is the development and refinement of knowledge. The type of knowledge that might be obtained from the study and who will be influenced by the knowledge should be assessed.

The type of research conducted (therapeutic or nontherapeutic) affects the potential benefits for the subjects. In therapeutic research, subjects might benefit from the study procedures in areas such as skin care, range of motion, touch, and other nursing interventions. The benefits might include improved physical condition, which could facilitate emotional and social benefits. Some researchers have noted that participation in descriptive research has encouraged subjects to process and disclose thoughts regarding life-altering events, and that these actions have been beneficial to the subjects' health and well-being (Carpenter, 1998). Nontherapeutic nursing research does not benefit subjects directly, but it is important because it generates and refines nursing knowledge for future patients, the nursing profession, and society (King, 2000). All research subjects benefit by having an increased understanding of the research process and knowing the findings from a particular study.

Examining the benefit-risk ratio also involves assessing the type, degree, and number of risks that subjects might encounter while participating in a study. The risks involved depend on the purpose of the study and the procedures used to conduct the study. Risks can be physical, emotional, social, and economic, and can range from the level of no anticipated risk or mere inconvenience to the level of certain risk of permanent damage (see the "Right to Protection from Discomfort and Harm" section earlier in this chapter) (Levine, 1986; Reynolds, 1972). If the risks outweigh the benefits, the study is probably unethical and should not be conducted. If the benefits outweigh the risks, the study is probably ethical and has the potential to add to nursing's knowledge base (Fig. 6-2).

Let us examine the benefit-risk ratio for a study that focused on the effects of an exercise and diet program on the subjects' serum lipid values and cardiovascular (CV) risk level. The serum lipid levels examined were serum cholesterol, low-density lipoprotein (LDL) and high-density lipoprotein (HDL). The subjects voluntarily agreed to participate in the study and signed a consent form. All subjects were treated fairly during subject selection and data collection. The potential benefits to the participants included (1) increased knowledge about exercise and diet, (2) increased knowledge about serum lipid values and CV risk level at the start of the program and 1 year later, (3) improved levels of serum lipids, (4) lowered CV risk level, and

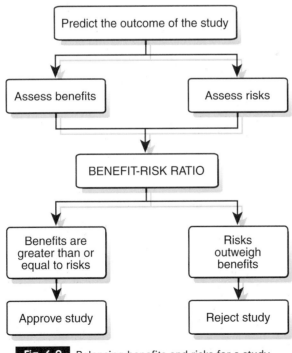

Fig. 6-2 Balancing benefits and risks for a study.

(5) improved exercise and diet habits. The risks included the discomfort of having blood drawn twice and the time spent participating in the study (Bruce, 1991; Bruce & Grove, 1994). These discomforts were temporary; they ended with the termination of the study. In addition, the discomforts did not exceed what the subjects would experience in their daily lives. The amount of time that the subjects spent participating in the study was minimized through efficient organization and precise scheduling of research activities.

In examining the benefit-risk ratio, we note that the benefits appear to be greater in number and importance than the risks; the risks are temporary and can be minimized by the researcher. The researcher received approvals from the university and clinical agency IRBs, and obtained informed consent from each subject. The informed consent process involved the following: (1) providing each subject with essential information about the study, both orally and in writing; (2) giving each subject the choice of whether to participate in the study; and (3) having each subject read and sign a consent form. Thus this study was ethical, and provided benefits both to the subjects and their families and to the development of nursing knowledge regarding the effects of exercise and diet on serum lipid levels and CV risk level.

If you were a member of the IRB that reviewed this study, you and the other committee members would probably recommend approving the study for implementation in your agency. Because the risks of the study are minimal, the review process would probably be expedited. If you were a patient advocate, you would examine the risks and benefits, determine whether the study had received IRB approval, and examine the appropriateness of the informed consent process. Because the study meets ethical guidelines, you would probably encourage patients to be subjects in this study so that they might receive the identified benefits. You would also probably be willing to identify potential subjects or collect data for the researcher.

Critiquing the Ethics of a Study

The ethical aspects of a study include having the research project approved by the IRB for the setting and obtaining informed consent from the subjects. This information should be included in published studies. The following questions could be used to critique the ethical aspects of a study.

1. Was the study approved by the appropriate IRB?
2. Was informed consent obtained from the subjects?
3. If the subjects were legally or mentally incompetent, terminally ill, or confined to an institution, were special precautions taken in obtaining their consent? Did the incompetent subjects assent to participate in the study? Did their legally authorized representative give permission for them to participate in the study?
4. Were the rights of the subjects protected during sampling, data collection, and data analysis?
5. Was the privacy of the subjects protected during the study and in the research report?
6. Was the benefit-risk ratio of the study acceptable? Did the benefits outweigh the risks?

UNDERSTANDING SCIENTIFIC MISCONDUCT

The goal of research is to generate sound scientific knowledge, which is possible only through the honest conduct, reporting, and publication of quality research. However, during the last 20 years an increasing number of fraudulent studies have been published in prestigious scientific journals. In the late 1980s scientific misconduct was deemed a serious problem that was investigated by the DHHS (1989). In 1989 two new federal agencies were organized for reporting and investigating scientific misconduct. The Office of Scientific Integrity Review (OSIR) was established to manage scientific misconduct by grant recipients. The Office of Scientific Integrity (OSI) supervises the implementation of the rules and regulations related to scientific misconduct and manages any investigations (DHHS, 1989; Hawley & Jeffers, 1992). The investigations by the OSIR and OSI revealed a variety of fraudulent behaviors. In some situations the fraudulent studies were never conducted, and the researchers fabricated the data and study results. In other cases, the findings were consciously distorted. Some of the common types of dishonest or fraudulent research are identified and described in Table 6-5.

An example of scientific misconduct was evident in the publications of Dr. Robert Slutsky, a heart specialist at the University of California, San Diego, School of Medicine. He resigned in 1986 when confronted with inconsistencies in his research publications. His publications contained "statistical anomalies that raised the question of data fabrication" (Friedman, 1990, p. 1416). In 6 years, Slutsky published 161 articles,

---

TABLE 6-5

DISHONESTY IN RESEARCH

TYPE	DESCRIPTION
Fabrication, falsification, or forging	Deliberate invention of nonexistent information
Manipulation of design or methods	Intentional planning of the study design or data collection methods so that the results will be biased toward the research hypothesis
Selective retaining or manipulation of data	Choosing only data that are consistent with the research hypothesis and discarding the rest
Plagiarism	Intentional representation of the work or ideas of others as one's own, or rewording one's own work to produce a new paper based on the same data; abuse of confidentiality of information from others
Irresponsible collaboration	Failure to participate appropriately in an investigative team or fulfill responsibilities as a co-author

From Larson, E. (1989). Maintaining quality in clinical research and evaluation: When corrective action is necessary. Reprinted from the *Journal of Nursing Quality Assurance, 3*(4), 30. Used with permission of Aspen Publishers, Inc., © 1989.

and at one time he was completing an article every 10 days. Eighteen of the articles were found to be fraudulent and have retraction notations, and 60 articles were questionable (Friedman, 1990).

Dr. Stephen Breuning, a psychologist at the University of Pittsburgh, engaged in deceptive and misleading practices in reporting his research on retarded children. He used his fraudulent research to obtain more than $300,000 in federal grants. In 1988 he was criminally charged with research fraud. He pleaded guilty, was fined $20,000, and faced up to 10 years in prison (Chop & Silva, 1991).

In 1996 a review and revision of the existing scientific misconduct policy was initiated to (1) develop a research misconduct policy that would be uniform across the agencies of the federal government, (2) establish a policy that would address behavior that had the potential to affect the integrity of the research record, and (3) develop a procedure that would safeguard the handling of allegations of research misconduct. In this policy, *"research misconduct* is defined as fabrication, falsification, or plagiarism in proposing, performing, or reviewing research, or in reporting research results. *Fabrication* is making up results and recording or reporting them. *Falsification* is manipulating research materials, equipment, or processes, or changing or omitting data or results such that the research is not accurately represented in the research record. *Plagiarism* is the appropriation of another person's ideas, processes, results, or words without giving appropriate credit, including those obtained through confidential review of others' research proposals and manuscripts. Research misconduct does not include honest error or honest differences of option" (DHHS ORI, 2001; on-line at http://ori.dhhs.gov/).

An act of research misconduct requires a significant departure from the acceptable practice of the scientific community for maintaining the integrity of the research record. The act must be committed intentionally, and the allegation must be proven by a preponderance of evidence. The DHHS (2001) policy also addresses the responsibilities that federal agencies and research institutions have in maintaining the integrity of the research process. Guidelines are provided to assist agencies and research institutions in developing fair and timely procedures for responding to allegations of research misconduct. The administrative actions taken in a situation depend on the seriousness of the misconduct. The available actions include, "but are not limited to, letters of reprimand; the imposition of special certification or assurance requirements to ensure compliance with applicable regulations or terms of an award; suspension or termination of an active award; or suspension and debarment" (DHHS, 2001).

The publication of fraudulent research is a major concern in medicine and a growing concern in nursing. The decrease in funds available for research and the increase in emphasis on research publications could lead to an increase in the incidence in fraudulent publications (Njie & Thomas. 2001). A survey by Rankin and Esteves (1997) suggested that the following acts of scientific misconduct had occurred in many institutions: plagiarism, deception in data collection, misrepresentation of findings, violation of protocol, violations of missing data, falsification of bibliographies, and improper representation of authorship. All nursing professionals should clearly understand the difference between ethical and unethical research practice and promote ethical behavior in research. Scientific misconduct must be identified and reported to maintain the quality of nursing research (Burns & Grove, 2001).

EXAMINING THE USE OF ANIMALS IN RESEARCH

The use of animals as research subjects is a controversial issue of growing concern to nurse researchers (Burns & Grove, 2001). A small but increasing number of nurse scientists are conducting physiological studies that require the use of animals. Many scientists, especially physicians, believe the current animal rights movement could threaten the future of health research. These groups are active in antiresearch campaigns and are backed by massive resources, with a treasury that was estimated at $50 million in 1988 (Pardes, West, & Pincus, 1991). Some of the animal rights groups are trying to raise the consciousness of researchers and society to ensure that animals are used wisely in the conduct of research and are treated humanely.

Two important questions should be addressed: (1) Should animals be used as subjects in research? (2) If animals are used in research, what mechanisms ensure that they are treated humanely? The type of research project influences the selection of subjects. Animals are just one of a variety of subjects used in research; others include human beings, plants, and computer data sets. If possible, most researchers use nonanimal subjects because they are generally less expensive. If the studies are low risk, which most nursing studies are, human beings are frequently used as subjects. However, some studies require the use of animals to answer the research question. Approximately 17 to 22 million animals are used in research each year, and 90% of them are rodents. The combined percentage of dogs and cats used in research is only 1% to 2% (Goodwin & Morrison, 2000).

Since animals are deemed valuable subjects for selected research projects, what mechanisms ensure that animals are treated humanely? At least five separate types of regulations exist to protect research animals from mistreatment. The federal government, state governments, independent accreditation organizations, professional societies, and individual institutions work to ensure that research animals are used only when necessary and only under humane conditions. At the federal level, animal research is conducted according to the guidelines of the Public Health Service (PHS) Policy on Humane Care and Use of Laboratory Animals, which was adopted in 1986 and reprinted essentially unchanged in 1996 (National Institutes of Health, Office for Protection from Research Risks [NIH OPRR], 1996). The PHS Policy on Humane Care and Use of Laboratory Animals defines *animal* as any live, vertebrate animal that is used or intended to be used in research, research training, experimentation, or biological testing or for a related purpose. Any institution proposing research involving animals must have a written Animal Welfare Assurance statement acceptable to the PHS that documents compliance with the PHS policy. All assurances are evaluated by the NIH's OPRR to determine the adequacy of the institution's proposed program for the care and use of animals in PHS conducted or supported activities (NIH OPRR, 1996).

Compliance with the PHS Policy has promoted the humane care and treatment of animals in research. In addition, over 700 institutions conducting health-related research have sought accreditation by the American Association for Accreditation of Laboratory Animal Care (AAALAC), which was developed to ensure the humane treatment of animals in research (Goodwin & Morrison, 2000). In conducting research, the subjects should be carefully selected; and if animals are used as subjects, they should be humanely treated.

SUMMARY

We would like to believe that unethical research, such as the Nazi experiments of World War II, is a thing of the past. However, this is not the case; more recently published studies include evidence that subjects' rights were violated. Thus the ethical aspects of published studies and of research conducted in agencies must be critiqued. Historical events, ethical codes, and regulations are presented in this chapter as guidelines for determining whether a study was conducted ethically.

Since the 1940s, four experimental projects have been highly publicized for their unethical treatment of human subjects: (1) the Nazi medical experiments, (2) the Tuskegee Syphilis Study, (3) the Willowbrook Study, and (4) the Jewish Chronic Disease Hospital Study. The unethical aspects of each are discussed. In response to these studies, a number of codes and regulations have been implemented. Two historical documents (the Nuremberg Code and the Declaration of Helsinki) have had a strong impact on the conduct of research. More recently, the DHHS (1981, 1983, 1991) passed regulations to promote ethical conduct in research, including: (1) general requirements for informed consent and (2) guidelines for IRB review of research.

Conducting research ethically requires protection of the human rights of subjects. The rights that require protection in research include the following: (1) self-determination, (2) privacy, (3) anonymity and confidentiality, (4) fair treatment, and (5) protection from discomfort and harm. Nurses can help protect the rights of research subjects by: (1) understanding the informed consent process, (2) being involved in the institutional review of research in their agencies, and (3) examining the benefits and risks of studies conducted in their agencies.

Informed consent involves the following: (1) transmission of essential study information to the potential subject, (2) comprehension of that information by the potential subject, (3) competence of the potential subject to give consent, and (4) voluntary consent by the potential subject to participate in the study. In an institutional review, a committee of peers (an IRB) examines a study for ethical concerns. The IRB conducts three levels of review: exempt, expedited, and complete. The chapter includes guidelines for obtaining informed consent and institutional review of research studies.

To balance the benefits and risks of a study, the type, degree, and number of risks are examined, and the potential benefits are identified. If possible the risks should be minimized and the benefits maximized to achieve the best possible benefit-risk ratio. Patient advocates should determine that the research conducted on patients in their care is ethical. The chapter provides questions that might be asked during a critique of the ethical aspects of a research report.

The chapter concludes with two current ethical issues: scientific misconduct in research and animal use in studies. Serious ethical problems of the last two decades are the conduct, reporting, and publication of fraudulent research. Researchers have fabricated data and research results for publication, distorted or incorrectly reported research findings, and mismanaged the implementation of study protocols. Researchers in all disciplines should be aware of the potential for scientific misconduct and act responsibly to protect the integrity of scientific knowledge. Another ethical concern in research is the use of animals in studies. Some of the animal rights groups are threatening the future of health-care research with their antiresearch campaigns. Over the years, animal research has provided knowledge that is essential for conducting human research. Currently animals are used infrequently in research, but if a study requires animals, they should be treated humanely.

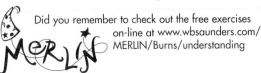

Did you remember to check out the free exercises on-line at www.wbsaunders.com/ MERLIN/Burns/understanding

REFERENCES

American Nurses Association. (2001). *Code of ethics for nurses with interpretive statements.* Washington, DC: American Nurses Association. Draft on-line http://ana.org/ethics/code9.htm.

American Psychological Association. (1982). *Ethical principles in the conduct of research with human participants.* Washington, DC: American Psychological Association.

Beecher, H. K. (1966). Ethics and clinical research. *New England Journal of Medicine, 274*(24), 1354-1360.

Berger, R. L. (1990). Nazi science: The Dachau hypothermia experiments. *New England Journal of Medicine, 322*(20), 1435-1440.

Brandt, A. M. (1978). Racism and research: The case of the Tuskegee syphilis study. *Hastings Center Report, 8*(6), 21-29.

Brent, N. J. (1990). Legal issues in research: Informed consent. *Journal of Neuroscience Nursing, 22*(3), 189-191.

Broome, M. E., & Stieglitz, K. A. (1992). The consent process and children. *Research in Nursing & Health, 15*(2), 147-152.

Bruce, S. L. (1991). *The effect of a coronary artery risk evaluation program on the serum lipid values of a selected military population.* Unpublished master's thesis, University of Texas at Arlington.

Bruce, S. L., & Grove, S. K. (1994). The effect of a coronary artery risk evaluation program on serum lipid values and cardiovascular risk levels. *Applied Nursing Research, 7*(2), 67-74.

Brudenell, I. (2000). Parenting an infant during alcohol recovery. *Journal of Pediatric Nursing, 15*(2), 82-88.

Burns, N., & Grove, S. K. (2001). *The practice of nursing research: Conduct, critique, and utilization* (4th ed.). Philadelphia: Saunders.

Carico, J. M., & Harrison, E. R. (1990). Ethical considerations for nurses in biomedical research. *Journal of Neuroscience Nursing, 22*(3), 160-163.

Carpenter, J. S. (1998). Methodology corner: Informing participants about the benefits of descriptive research. *Nursing Research, 47*(1), 63-64.

Cassidy, V. R., & Odd, L. F. (1986). Legal and ethical aspects of informed consent: A nursing research perspective. *Journal of Professional Nursing, 2*(6), 343-349.

Chop, R. M., & Silva, M. C. (1991). Scientific fraud: Definitions, policies, and implications for nursing research. *Journal of Professional Nursing, 7*(3), 166-171.

Davis, A. J. (1989). Informed consent process in research protocols: Dilemmas for clinical nurses. *Western Journal of Nursing Research, 11*(4), 448-457.

Department of Health and Human Services (DHHS) (January 26, 1981). Final regulations amending basic HHS policy for the protection of human research subjects. *Code of Federal Regulations,* Title 45 Public Welfare, Part 46.

Department of Health and Human Services (DHHS) (March 8, 1983). Protection of human subjects. *Code of Federal Regulations,* Title 45 Public Welfare, Part 46.

Department of Health and Human Services (DHHS) (1989). Final rule: Responsibilities of awardee and applicant institutions for dealing with and reporting possible misconduct in science. *Federal Register, 54,* 32446-32451.

Department of Health and Human Services (DHHS) (June 18, 1991). Protection of human subjects. *Code of Federal Regulations,* Title 45 Public Welfare, Part 46.

Department of Health and Human Services (DHHS), Office of Research Integrity (ORI) (2001). *Introduction to the ORI* [On-line]. Available at: http://ori.dhhs.gov/. Accessed 2001.

Douglas, S., & Larson, E. (1986). There's more to informed consent than information. *Focus on Critical Care, 13*(2), 43-47.

Flynn, L. (1997). The health practices of homeless women: A causal model. *Nursing Research, 46*(2), 72-77.

Ford, J. S., & Reuter, L. I. (1990). Ethical dilemmas associated with small samples. *Journal of Advanced Nursing, 15*(2), 187-191.

Friedman, P. J. (1990). Correcting the literature following fraudulent publication. *Journal of the American Medical Association, 263*(10), 1416-1419.

Goodwin, F. K., & Morrison, A. R. (2000). Science and self-doubt. *Reason, 32*(5), 22-28.

Hawley, D. J., & Jeffers, J. M. (1992). Scientific misconduct as a dilemma for nursing. *Image: Journal of Nursing Scholarship, 24*(1), 51-55.

Hershey, N., & Miller, R. D. (1976). *Human experimentation and the law.* Germantown, MD: Aspen.

Kelman, H. C. (1967). Human use of human subjects: The problem of deception in social psychological experiments. *Psychological Bulletin, 67*(1), 1-11.

King, N. M. (2000). Defining and describing benefit appropriately in clinical trials. *Journal of Law, Medicine & Ethics, 28*(2000), 332-343.

Larson, E. (1989). Maintaining quality in clinical research and evaluation: When corrective action is necessary. *Journal of Nursing Quality Assurance, 3*(4), 30.

Levine, R. J. (1986). *Ethics and regulation of clinical research* (2nd ed.). Baltimore and Munich: Urban & Schwarzenberg.

Martin, P. A. (1996). Member responsibilities on a nursing research committee. *Applied Nursing Research, 9*(3), 154-157.

McCorkle, R., Robinson, L., Nuamah, I., Lev, E., & Benoliel, J. Q. (1998). The effects of home nursing care for patients during terminal illness on the bereaved's psychological distress. *Nursing Research, 47*(1), 2-10.

Milgram, S. (1963). Behavioral study of obedience. *Journal of Abnormal and Social Psychology, 67*(4), 371-378.

Mullins, I. L. (1996). Nurse caring behaviors for persons with acquired immunodeficiency syndrome/human immunodeficiency virus. *Applied Nursing Research, 9*(1), 18-23.

National Commission for the Protection of Human Subjects of Biomedical and Behavioral Research (1978). *Belmont report: Ethical principles and guidelines for research involving human subjects.* DHEW Publication No. (05) 78-0012. Washington, DC: U.S. Government Printing Office.

National Institutes of Health, Office for Protection from Research Risks (NIH OPRR) (1996). *Public health service policy on humane care and use of laboratory animals* [Online]. Available: http://grants1.nih.gov/grants/olaw/references/phspol.htm (3/5/2002).

Njie, V. P. S., & Thomas, A. C. (2001). Quality issues in clinical research and the implications on health policy (QICRHP). *Journal of Professional Nursing, 17*(5), 233-242.

Nuremberg Code (1986). In R. J. Levine (Ed.), *Ethics and regulation of clinical research* (2nd ed., pp. 425-426). Baltimore and Munich: Urban & Schwarzenberg.

Pardes, H., West, A., & Pincus, H. A. (1991). Physicians and the animal-rights movement. *New England Journal of Medicine, 324*(23), 1640-1643.

Ramos, M. C. (1989). Some ethical implications of qualitative research. *Research in Nursing & Health, 12*(1), 57-63.

Rankin, M., & Esteves, M. D. (1997). Perceptions of scientific misconduct in nursing. *Nursing Research, 46*(5), 270-275.

Reynolds, P. D. (1972). On the protection of human subjects and social science. *International Social Science Journal, 24*(4), 693-719.

Reynolds, P. D. (1979). *Ethical dilemmas and social science research.* San Francisco: Jossey-Bass.

Rosato, J. (2000). The ethics of clinical trials: A child's view. *Journal of Law, Medicine & Ethics, 28*(2000), 362-378.

Rothman, D. J. (1982). Were Tuskegee and Willowbrook studies in nature? *Hastings Center Report, 12*(2), 5-7.

Rudy, E. B., Estok, P. J., Kerr, M. E., & Menzel, L. (1994). Research incentives: Money versus gifts. *Nursing Research, 43*(4), 253-255.

Sandelowski, M. (1994). Focus on qualitative methods: The use of quotes in qualitative research. *Research in Nursing & Health, 17*(6), 479-482.

Silva, M. (1995). *Ethical guidelines in the conduct, dissemination, & implementation of nursing research.* Washington, DC: American Nurses Association.

Steinfels, P., & Levine, C. (1976). Biomedical ethics and the shadow of Nazism. *Hastings Center Report, 6*(4), 1-20.

Strauman, J. J., & Cotanch, P. H. (1988). Oncology nurse research issues: Over studied populations. *Oncology Nursing Forum, 15*(5), 665-667.

Thompson, P. J. (1987). Protection of the rights of children as subjects for research. *Journal of Pediatric Nursing, 2*(6), 392-399.

Tigges, B. B. (2001). Affiliative preferences, self-change, and adolescent condom use. *Journal of Nursing Scholarship, 33*(3), 231-237.

To, M. Y. F., & Chan, S. (2000). Evaluating the effectiveness of progressive muscle relaxation in reducing the aggressive behaviors of mentally handicapped patients. *Archives of Psychiatric Nursing, 14*(1), 39-46.

Watson, A. B. (1982). Informed consent of special subjects. *Nursing Research, 31*(1), 43-47.

Weider, C. (2000). The ethical analysis of risk. *Journal of Law, Medicine & Ethics, 28*(2000), 344-361.

Wilson, A. H., Pittman, K., & Wold, J. L. (2000). Listening to the quiet voices of Hispanic migrant children about health. *Journal of Pediatric Nursing, 15*(3), 137-147.

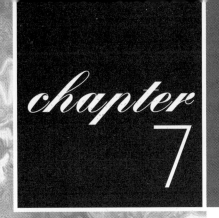

chapter 7

Clarifying Research Designs

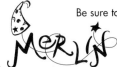

Be sure to check out the free exercises on-line at
www.wbsaunders.com/MERLIN/Burns/
understanding

OUTLINE—cont'd

Mapping the Design
Outcomes Research
Role of Replication Studies in Evidence-Based Practice

OBJECTIVES

Completing this chapter should enable you to:
 1. Identify the purpose of the research design.
 2. Explain the relationships among the study framework; research objectives, questions, or hypotheses; and the study design.
 3. Discuss the following concepts relevant to design: causality, multicausality, probability, bias, control, manipulation, and validity.
 4. Describe the role of validity in conducting research.
 5. Compare and contrast the four types of validity: statistical conclusion, internal, construct, and external.
 6. Describe the threats to the four types of design validity.
 7. Describe the elements of a good design: controlling the environment, controlling equivalence of subjects and groups, controlling the treatment, controlling measurement, and controlling extraneous variables.
 8. Identify the designs of published studies.
 9. Critique the quality of designs of quantitative nursing studies.
 10. Select studies sufficiently well designed to provide evidence on which practice can be based.
 11. Identify types of designs used in nursing research: descriptive, correlational, quasi-experimental, and experimental.
 12. Model designs of published studies.

RELEVANT TERMS

Approximate replication
Bias
Case study design
Causality
Comparative descriptive design
Concurrent replication
Construct validity
Control
Correlational design
Descriptive correlational design
Descriptive design
Design validity
Exact replication
Experimental design
External validity

Heterogeneous
Homogeneous
Internal validity
Intervention
Manipulation
Multicausality
Outcomes research
Predictive correlational design
Probability
Quasi-experimental design
Replication studies
Research design
Statistical conclusion validity
Systematic extension replication

A *research design* is a blueprint for conducting a study that maximizes control over factors that could interfere with the validity of the findings. Just as the blueprint for a house must be individualized to the specific house being built, so must the design be made specific to a study. The control provided by the design increases the probability that the study results will be accurate reflections of reality. Skill in identifying the study design and in evaluating the threats to validity resulting from design flaws is an important part of critiquing studies. Validity has become increasingly important in nursing research because studies must be well designed to contribute to evidence-based practice. The proportion of nursing studies designed to provide evidence that nursing interventions are effective in achieving desired outcomes must increase.

Many published studies do not identify the design used in the study. Determining the design may require putting together bits of information from various parts of the research report. Clues to the design can be found in the purpose; framework; research objectives, questions, or hypotheses; and variables. Elements that must be identified to determine the study design include the presence or absence of a treatment, number of groups in the sample, number and timing of measurements to be performed, sampling methods, time frame for data collection, planned comparisons between variables or groups, and strategies used to control extraneous variables.

After the design is identified, its adequacy to accomplish the study purpose should be critiqued. In addition to being important for class assignments, the skill of critiquing studies is becoming an important component of nursing practice. Evidence-based practice includes an expectation that practitioners will know the current research relevant to their practice. However, only those studies that are sufficiently well designed should be chosen to guide a practice. To provide the information necessary to identify and critique designs of published studies, this chapter includes the concepts important to design, identifies some designs commonly used in nursing studies, and describes the elements of a good design. The chapter also includes content related to defining experimental interventions, mapping designs, and identifying outcome studies and replication studies.

CONCEPTS IMPORTANT TO DESIGN

Many terms used in discussing research design have special meanings within this context. Understanding the meanings of these concepts is critical to understanding the purpose of a specific design. Some of the major concepts used in research design are causality, multicausality, probability, bias, control, manipulation, and validity.

Causality

According to *causality* theory, things have causes, and causes lead to effects. The original criteria for causation required that a variable "cause" an identified "effect" each time the cause occurred. It was also assumed that each effect had a single cause. Although these assumptions may be true in the basic sciences, such as chemistry or physics, they are unlikely to be true in the health sciences or social sciences. The term causality is currently defined with greater flexibility.

You may be able to determine whether the purpose of a study is to examine causality by perusing the purpose statement and the propositions within the framework. For example, the purpose of a causal study might be to examine the effect of a specific preoperative education program on length of hospital stay. The proposition might state that preoperative teaching results in a decreased hospitalization period. Preoperative teaching is not the only factor affecting length of hospital stay. Other important factors include the diagnosis, type of surgery, patient's age, initial physical condition of the patient, and complications that occurred after surgery. However, from the perspective of causality, it is important to design the study so that the effect of a single cause (preoperative education program) can be examined apart from the other factors that affect length of hospital stay. The researcher using a causal perspective would design the study to include only a specific type of surgery, select only subjects who were initially in good physical condition and were within a narrow age range, and exclude patients who had complications after surgery. Multiple studies would be performed to examine the effects of different types of surgery, subjects in different physical conditions, or complications on length of hospital stay. Experimental or quasi-experimental designs are commonly used to examine causality. The independent variable in a study is expected to be the cause, and the dependent variable is expected to reflect the effect of the independent variable. Statistical analyses are likely to be bivariate—that is, examining differences between two groups on a single dependent variable using statistical procedures such as the *t*-test.

Multicausality

Multicausality, the recognition that a number of interrelating variables can be involved in causing a particular effect, is a more recent idea related to causality. Very few phenomena in nursing can be clearly pinned down to a single cause and a single effect. Because of the complexity of causal relationships, a theory is unlikely to identify every concept involved in causing a particular phenomenon. However, the greater the proportion of causal factors that can be identified and examined in a single study, the clearer the understanding will be of the overall phenomenon. This greater understanding is expected to increase the ability to predict and control the effect. Thus in examining the effect of preoperative teaching on length of hospital stay, researchers using the perspective of multicausality would design the study to include a broad range of diagnoses, patient ages, patient conditions, and complications after surgery. Studies developed from a multicausal perspective will include more variables than those using a strict causal orientation. Hypotheses are likely to be complex and to include more than two variables. Statistical analysis procedures would be used to examine the combined effects of multiple independent variables on a single dependent variable.

Probability

Probability addresses relative rather than absolute causality. From the perspective of probability, a cause may not produce a specific effect each time that particular cause occurs. Using a probability orientation, the researcher would design the study to examine the probability that a given effect would occur under a defined set of circumstances or to examine the variations in a given effect that occurred based on the set of circumstances. The circumstances might be variations in multiple variables. For example, while examining the effect of multiple variables on length of hospitalization, the researcher might examine the probability of a given length of hospital stay under a variety of specific sets of circumstances. One specific set of circumstances might be that the patient had 15 minutes of preoperative teaching, underwent a specific type of surgery, was a certain age, had a particular level of health before surgery, and experienced a specific complication. The probability of a given length of hospital stay could be expected to vary as the set of circumstances varied. When examining probability, the researcher finds that hypotheses are complex, with multiple variables. Advanced statistical procedures would be used and might include regression analyses.

Bias

The term *bias* means a slant or deviation from the true or expected. Bias in a study distorts the findings from what the results would have been without the bias. Because studies are conducted to determine the real and the true, researchers place great value on identifying and removing sources of bias in their study or controlling their effects on the study findings. Designs are developed to reduce the possibility and effects of bias. Any component of a study that deviates or causes a deviation from a true measurement of the study variables leads to distorted findings. Many factors related to research can be biased; these include the researcher, the components of the environment in which the study is conducted, the individual subjects, the sample, the groups formed, the measurement tools, the data collection process, the data, and the statistics.

For example, some of the subjects for the study might have been taken from a unit of the hospital in which the patients were participating in another study involving high-quality nursing care; or one nurse, selecting patients for the study, might have assigned the patients who were most interested in the study to the experimental group. Each of these situations introduces a bias to the study.

An important focus in critiquing a study is to identify possible sources of bias. This requires careful examination of the researcher's report of the study methods, including strategies for obtaining subjects and performing measurements. However, not all biases can be identified from the published report of a study. The article may not provide sufficient detail about the methods to detect all of the biases.

Control

One method of reducing bias is to increase the amount of control in the design. *Control* means having the power to direct or manipulate factors to achieve a desired outcome. For example, in a study of preoperative teaching, subjects might be randomly selected and then randomly assigned to the experimental or control group. The researcher might control the duration of preoperative teaching sessions, the content taught, the method of teaching, and the identity of the teacher. The time that the teaching occurred in relation to surgery could be controlled, as well as the environment in which it occurred. Measurement of the length of hospital stay might be controlled by ensuring that the number of days or hours was calculated exactly the same way for each subject. Limiting the characteristics of subjects, such as diagnosis, age, type of surgery, and incidence of complications, is a form of control. Control is particularly important in experimental and quasi-experimental studies. The greater the researcher's control over the study situation, the more credible (or valid) the study findings. The purpose of research designs is to maximize control factors in the study situation.

 In critiquing a study, you should identify the elements that were controlled and those that could have been controlled to improve the study design. The feasibility of controlling particular elements of the study should be considered. In addition, you should consider the effect of not controlling certain elements on the validity of the study findings.

Manipulation

Manipulation is a form of control used most commonly in experimental or quasi-experimental research. Controlling the treatment or intervention is the most commonly used manipulation. In a study of the effects of preoperative teaching, the situation might be manipulated so that one group of subjects received preoperative teaching and another did not. In a study on oral care, the frequency of care might be manipulated.

When experimental designs are used to explore causal relationships in nursing research, the nurse must be free to manipulate the variables under study. If the freedom to manipulate a variable (e.g., the type, amount, or frequency of pain control measures) is under someone else's control (e.g., the physician or the staff nurses), a bias is introduced into the study. Thus the treatment each subject receives would differ. The researcher would be, so to speak, comparing apples and oranges. In descriptive and correlational studies, little or no effort is made to manipulate factors in the situation. Instead, the purpose is to examine the situation as it exists. Thus there is a greater possibility of biases influencing findings in these studies.

 In critiquing a study, you need to determine which elements of the design were manipulated and how they were manipulated. You need to judge the adequacy of the manipulation and identify elements that should have been manipulated to improve the validity of the findings.

Design Validity

Design validity is the determination of whether the study provides a convincing test of the framework propositions. Critical analysis of research involves being able to think through any threats to validity and make judgments about how seriously these threats affect the integrity of the findings. Validity provides a major basis for deciding which findings are useful for patient care.

Cook and Campbell (1979) described four types of design validity: statistical conclusion validity, internal validity, construct validity, and external validity. Each of these types should be evaluated as a component of critiquing the study design. The following paragraphs discuss briefly each type of design validity. For a more detailed discussion of the threats to design validity, see Burns and Grove (2001).

Statistical conclusion validity is concerned with whether the conclusions about relationships or differences drawn from statistical analyses are an accurate reflection of the real world. False conclusions can be reached when interpreting the results of statistical analyses. For example, a Type I error occurs when a researcher incorrectly concludes that a relationship or difference exists between variables or groups when in reality it does not. A Type II error occurs when a researcher concludes that no significant relationship or difference exists between variables or between groups when in reality it does. Researchers often examine the possibility of a Type II error by performing a power analysis of studies in which no significant difference or relationship was found.

A critique of a study should identify conclusions that may be false. In nursing studies, there is a greater risk of a Type II than a Type I error. Therefore, in critiquing a study in which the findings indicate no statistically significant differences, the validity of those findings should be questioned. The study should be examined for evidence that the researcher performed power analyses when no significant difference or relationship was found.

Internal validity is the extent to which the effects detected in the study are a true reflection of reality rather than the result of the effects of extraneous variables. Although internal validity should be a concern in all studies, it is addressed more frequently in relation to studies examining causality than in other studies. In studies examining causality, one needs to question whether the effect found in the study may have been caused by a third, often unmeasured, variable (an extraneous variable) rather than by the treatment. The possibility of an alternative explanation of cause is sometimes referred to as a "rival hypothesis." Any study can contain threats to internal validity, and these validity threats can lead to a false-positive or false-negative conclusion.

In critiquing a study, the following question should be considered: "Is there another reasonable (valid) explanation (rival hypothesis) for the finding other than that proposed by the researcher?"

Construct validity examines the fit between the conceptual definitions and operational definitions of variables. Concepts are defined within the framework (conceptual definitions). The conceptual definitions are used to develop the operational definitions of the variables. Operational definitions (methods of measurement) should reflect the concept. The threats to construct validity are related to the development and selection of measurement techniques.

In critiquing a study, the links between concepts, conceptual definitions, and methods of measurement for threats to construct validity should be examined carefully.

External validity is the extent to which study findings can be generalized beyond the sample used in the study. The most serious threat would lead to the findings being meaningful only for the group being studied. To some extent the significance of a study is dependent on the range of patients and situations to which the findings can be generalized. Sometimes the factors influencing external validity are subtle and may not be reported in research papers. Generalization is usually narrower for a single study than for multiple replications of a study using different samples (perhaps from different populations) in different settings.

In critiquing a study, you should identify the populations to which the findings can be generalized.

DESIGN FOR NURSING STUDIES

A variety of study designs are used in nursing research; the four types most commonly used are descriptive, correlational, quasi-experimental, and experimental. Descriptive and correlational studies examine variables in natural environments and do not include treatments imposed by the researcher. Quasi-experimental and experimental studies are designed to examine cause and effect. These studies are conducted to examine differences in dependent variables that are thought to be caused by independent variables (treatments). The following discussion briefly describes the four types of designs and provides specific examples of each. For more detail on specific designs, see Burns and Grove (2001).

The algorithm shown in Fig. 7-1 may be used to determine the type of study design used in a published study. The algorithm includes a series of "yes" or "no" responses to specific questions about the design. The algorithm starts with the question "Is there a treatment?" The answer leads to the next question, with the four types of design being identified in the algorithm. Then a second algorithm provided for each type of design can be used to identify the specific design used in the study.

Descriptive Design

The descriptive study is designed to gain more information about characteristics within a particular field of study. Its purpose is to provide a picture of a situation as it naturally happens. A descriptive design may be used to develop theories, identify problems with current practice, justify current practice, make judgments, or deter-

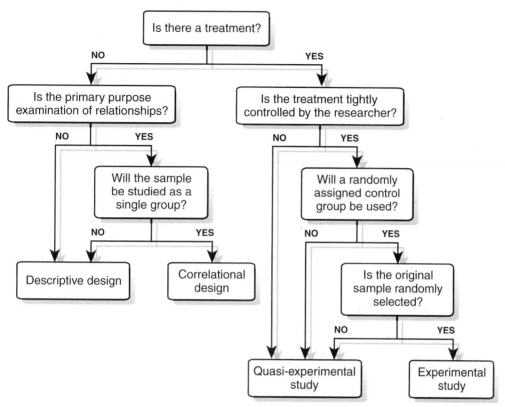

Fig. 7-1   Algorithm for determining type of study design.

mine what others in similar situations are doing (Waltz & Bausell, 1981). No manipulation of variables is involved in a descriptive design. Dependent and independent variables are not used because no attempt is made to establish causality. In many aspects of nursing there is a need for a clearer picture of the phenomenon before causality can be examined. Protection against bias is achieved through: (1) conceptual and operational definitions of variables, (2) sample selection and size, (3) valid and reliable instruments, and (4) data collection procedures that partially control the environment. Descriptive designs vary in level of complexity. Some contain only two variables; others may include multiple variables.

Typical Descriptive Design

The most commonly used design in the category of descriptive studies is presented in Fig. 7-2. The design is used to examine characteristics of a single sample. The *descriptive design* includes identifying a phenomenon of interest, identifying the variables within the phenomenon, developing conceptual and operational definitions of the variables, and describing the variables. The description of the variables leads to an interpretation of the theoretical meaning of the findings and the development of hypotheses.

CLARIFICATION ──▶ MEASUREMENT ──▶ DESCRIPTION ──▶ INTERPRETATION

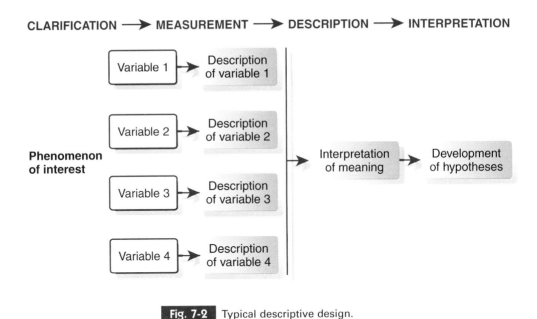

Fig. 7-2 Typical descriptive design.

An example of a descriptive design is Mimnaugh, Winegar, Mabrey, and Davis' (1999) study of sensations experienced during removal of selected tubes. Three masters-prepared nurses and one doctorally prepared nurse conducted this study. The following describes the design of the study.

"The major purpose of this study was to determine the types and intensity of sensations that patients experience when chest tubes (CTs) and Jackson-Pratt (JP) abdominal tubes are removed. A convenience sample of 62 hospitalized subjects, 31 with CTs and 31 with JP tubes, participated. Each subject was interviewed after tube removal. Sensations were identified, and intensity of sensation was marked on a 100-mm Visual Analogue Scale." (p. 78)

"The following research questions were addressed:
1. What sensations do patients experience when abdominal JP tubes are removed?
2. What sensations do patients experience when CTs are removed?
3. What is the intensity of the sensations patients experience when abdominal and chest tubes are removed?
4. What factors affect the perception and intensity of sensations that are experienced?
5. What types of information are patients commonly given before tube removal?
6. What types of information do patients indicate that they would like to receive before removal of abdominal or chest tubes?" (p. 79)

Findings

"Similar sensations were reported by both groups. Intensity of sensation was consistently higher in the JP group. The most frequently reported sensations were pain (77%) on JP tube removal and pulling (90%) upon CT removal" (p. 78).

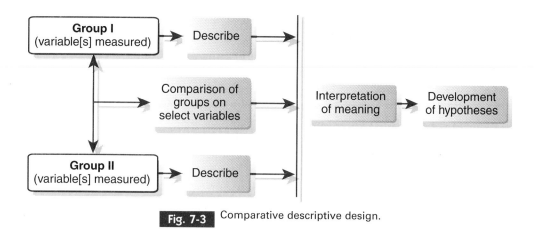

Fig. 7-3 Comparative descriptive design.

Comparative Descriptive Design

The *comparative descriptive design* (Fig. 7-3) is used to describe variables and to examine differences in variables in two or more groups that occur naturally in a setting. Descriptive and inferential analyses may be used to examine differences between or among groups. The results obtained from these analyses are frequently not generalized to a population. An example of this design is Sheahan's (2000) study comparing the documentation of health risks and the extent of health promotion counseling of two types of providers, nurse practitioners and physicians, working in a health department. This study was conducted by a doctorally prepared nurse practitioner. The following are excerpts from the study:

"The objectives of this two-group comparative study were to (a) compare medical record documentation of selected health risk factors and health promotion counseling by nurse practitioners and physicians and, (b) examine patient demographic factors and diagnoses associated with health risk identification and health promotion counseling. For 3 months, emergency service medical records (N = 305) of patients, aged 18 or older, who sought care in a level three, tertiary care center during the 3-11 shift, were selected by stratified random sampling.... The sample was stratified by providers and included 151 records by NPs and 154 records by physicians.... Records were reviewed for documentation of identification and counseling for the following health risk factors: an elevated blood pressure 140/90 or above, tobacco and alcohol use, presence of dental caries, and appropriate weight or evidence of descriptive terms or diagnoses of obesity or overweight." (pp. 246-247)

Continued

Conclusions

"Many opportunities for identification of health risks and follow-up counseling, as recommended in *Healthy People 2000* (U.S. Department of Health and Human Services, 1991) and by the U.S. Preventive Services Task Force (1996) were not documented. To meet the new goals of *Healthy People 2010* [U.S. Department of Health and Human Services, 2000], health care providers in all settings should identify health risk factors and document health promotion counseling during every patient encounter." (p. 245)

Case Study Design

The *case study design* involves an intensive exploration of a single unit of study, such as a person, very small number of subjects, family, group, community, or institution. Although the number of subjects tends to be small, the number of variables in a case study is usually large. In fact it is important to examine all variables that might have an impact on the situation being studied.

Case studies were commonly used in nursing 30 years ago but appear in the literature less frequently today. Well-designed case studies are a good source of descriptive information and can be used as evidence to support or invalidate theories. Information from a variety of sources can be collected on each concept of interest using different data collection methods. This strategy can greatly expand the understanding of the phenomenon under study. Case studies are also useful for demonstrating the effectiveness of a therapeutic technique. In fact the reporting of a case study can be the vehicle by which the technique is introduced to other practitioners. The case study design also has potential for revealing important findings that can generate new hypotheses for testing. Thus the case study can lead to the design of large sample studies to examine factors identified by the case study.

The case study design depends on the circumstances of the case but usually includes an element of time. The subject's history and previous behavior patterns are usually explored in detail. As the case study proceeds, the researcher may become aware of components important to the focus of the study that were not originally included in the study. Both quantitative and qualitative elements are likely to be incorporated into the case study design.

An example of a case study design is presented in Lillard and McFann's (1990) book, *A Marital Crisis: For Better or Worse.* The following is an excerpt from that book:

"A patient/family case history was selected for study based on the complexity of the marital relationship, an apparently unpredictable crisis occurring during a home visit by Hospice of Marin staff, and involvement of a maximum number of team members including nurses, chaplain, and counselor. Although there were adult children in the family constellation, the marital couple's relationship was pivotal and of major concern to the IDT [interdisciplinary team]. Consequently the study report focuses on the couple, presenting selected, relevant assessments and interventions that occurred during the course of hospice care. Names and demographics are changed in the report to assure family confidentiality." (p. 98)

The algorithm shown in Fig. 7-4 can be used to determine the type of descriptive design used in a published study.

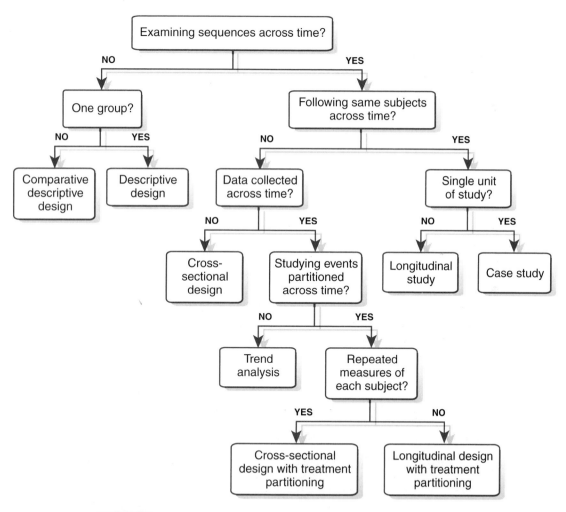

Fig. 7-4   Algorithm for determining type of descriptive design.

Excerpts of Descriptive Design Study to be Critiqued

Lennie, Christman, and Jadack (2001) conducted a study of "educational needs and altered eating habits following a total laryngectomy." The following describes the purpose, methods, and sample characteristics for that study. Two doctorally prepared nurses and a masters-prepared nurse conducted the study.

Method

Study design. Descriptive

Purpose. "The purpose of this study was to describe the eating-related experiences and informational needs of people with a total laryngectomy" (p. 668).

"Research Questions

1. What was the effect of total laryngectomy on eating patterns, enjoyment of eating, and food choice?
2. Which healthcare professionals provided information regarding alterations in eating and nutrition following total laryngectomy?
3. How satisfied were participants with the information received from health-care providers regarding alterations in eating and nutrition following total laryngectomy?
4. What were the characteristics of information that produced low and high satisfaction ratings from participants?
5. What information did participants feel should have greater emphasis during patient teaching about alterations in eating and nutrition following total laryngectomy?" (p. 668)

Sample. "Thirty-four people with laryngectomies were recruited from the online WebWhispers laryngectomy support group. WebWhispers (http://www.Webwhispers.org) is a national Internet support group for people who have undergone a laryngectomy. The site lists 183 people with a laryngectomy and caregivers as members…. All members with a total laryngectomy were e-mailed an invitation to participate and a description of the study. Interested individuals received a consent form and the survey in the mail. All surveys received were assigned numbers to ensure confidentiality. Actual names were not associated with the surveys. After data collection was complete, participants received a follow-up letter thanking them for their participation and encouraging them to contact the researchers if they had any questions. (p. 669)

"Thirty-four people returned completed questionnaires—an 83% return rate of those who expressed interest in participating in the study. Eighty-five percent of the participants were male, with a mean age of 62 years (range 47-76) and an average of five years since laryngectomy (range 0.25-16 years)." (p. 669)

Measures

"Background and demographic information: Background data included gender, marital status, age, race, education, and work history. Questions regarding living arrangement, children, and average household income were included. Participants were asked to indicate the date of surgery, type of surgery performed, length of hospital stay, presurgical diagnosis, and whether they received radiation treatment." (p. 669)

"Food, Eating Experiences, and Diet Questionnaire. The investigators designed the Food, Eating Experiences, and Diet (FEED) Questionnaire to describe experiences related to food and eating postlaryngectomy and to determine respondents' perceptions of the instructions and counseling they received from healthcare providers regarding nutrition and potential eating difficulties as a result of laryngectomy and related treatments. The instrument was pilot tested on five people with a total laryngectomy. Feedback regarding clarity and content was used to make modifications to the instrument prior to the study. The instrument consisted of five sections. The first three sections focused on potential changes related to different aspects of eating. The fourth section measured perceptions of hunger and appetite. The fifth section was designed to obtain perceptions of information received from healthcare providers regarding potential changes in eating following laryngectomy.... Space was provided in each section for participants to make comments or write explanations of their answers. Thus, both quantitative and qualitative data were collected in each section of the instrument." (p. 669)

"Key Points

1. The incidence of long-term alterations in eating and nutrition following total laryngectomy may be higher than many clinicians perceive.

2. Healthcare providers have not adequately prepared the large number of patients undergoing total laryngectomy for the alterations in eating that occur following this surgery.

3. Healthcare professionals working at large referral centers may find it particularly important to routinely verify that patients have received adequate teaching with respect to alterations in eating and nutrition following laryngectomy.

4. The most helpful intervention may be referral to a support group, as the task of solving eating-related problems following total laryngectomy can be made easier by consultation with others who have experienced similar problems." (p. 667)

Critique Comments

This interesting study used a descriptive design and a convenience sample. It addresses an issue of concern related to functional status of persons with laryngectomies after initial recovery. The framework of the study, which must be extracted from the literature review section of the article, is based on the pathophysiologic changes caused by the surgical procedure. Characteristic of descriptive studies, the design has few control factors other than the requirement of having experienced a total laryngectomy. The questionnaire used in the study has no documented validity other than the pilot test. However, the authors wanted an instrument to gather specific data that may not have been available in existing instruments. The study might have been strengthened if an instrument with documented validity had been available. The questionnaire was mailed to homes so the researchers had no assurance that the subject completed the questionnaire. Other family members might have completed it, introducing threats to validity. The authors do not report a power analysis

Continued

evaluating the adequacy of the sample size. The population was sufficiently educated and had the financial means to own a computer linked to the Internet. It's possible that those less fortunate patients might have even more difficulties than those found in this study.

Correlational Design

The purpose of a *correlational design* is to examine relationships between or among two or more variables in a single group. This examination can occur at several levels. The researcher can seek to describe a relationship (descriptive correlational), predict relationships among variables (predictive correlational), or simultaneously test all the relationships proposed by a theory (model testing design). In correlational designs, a large variance in the variable scores is necessary to determine the existence of a relationship. Thus the sample should reflect the full range of scores possible on the variables being measured. Some subjects should have very high scores, others very low scores, and the rest should be distributed throughout the possible range of scores. Because of the need for wide variation on scores, correlational studies generally require large sample sizes. Subjects are not divided into groups because group differences are not examined.

Descriptive Correlational Design

The purpose of a *descriptive correlational design* is to describe variables and examine relationships among these variables. Using this design will facilitate the identification of many interrelationships in a situation (Fig. 7-5). The study may examine variables in a situation that has already occurred or is currently occurring. No attempt is made to control or manipulate the situation. As with descriptive studies, variables must be clearly identified and defined.

An example of a descriptive correlational design is Rew, Taylor-Seehafer, Thomas, and Yockey's (2001) study titled "Correlates of Resilience in Homeless Adolescents." A doctorally prepared nurse and a doctorally prepared psychologist conducted this study.

MEASUREMENT

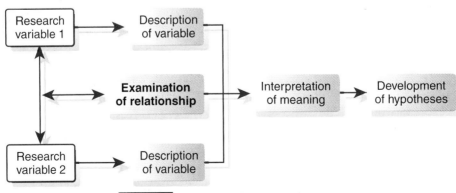

Fig. 7-5   Descriptive correlational design.

"Purposes. To (a) describe reasons adolescents give for their homelessness, (b) explore relationships among resilience and selected risk and protective factors, (c) identify differences in risk and protective factors by gender and sexual orientation, and (d) determine best predictors of resilience." (p. 33)

Design. "A descriptive and exploratory correlational design was used to collect and analyze data from a convenience sample of 59 homeless adolescents who sought health and social services from a community street-outreach project in central Texas in 1998." (p. 33)

Methods. "A paper and pencil survey consisting of valid measures (Resilience Scale, UCLA-Revised Loneliness Scale, Beck Hopelessness Scale, Social Connectedness Scale, and Death-Related Attitude Schedule) was administered in a street-outreach setting.

Findings. Nearly half the sample (47%) reported a history of sexual abuse and 36% self-identified as gay, lesbian, or bisexual in orientation. Over half (51%) were thrown out of their homes by their parents, 37% left home because their parents disapproved of their alcohol or drug use, and nearly one-third left home because parents sexually abused them. Lack of resilience was significantly related to hopelessness, loneliness, life-threatening behaviors, and connectedness, but not to gender or sexual orientation. Hopelessness and connectedness explained 50% of the variance in resilience.

Conclusions. Participants who perceived themselves as resilient, although disconnected from other people, were less lonely, less hopeless, and engaged in fewer life-threatening behaviors than were those who perceived themselves as not being resilient. They survived by adapting to street life and by becoming overly self-reliant. Findings may be useful in planning interventions to promote health and well-being in this vulnerable population." (p. 33)

Predictive Correlational Design

The purpose of a *predictive correlational design* is to predict the value of one variable based on values obtained for another variable(s). Prediction is one approach to examining causal relationships between variables. Because causal phenomena are being examined, the terms *dependent* and *independent* are used to describe the variables. One variable is classified as the dependent variable and all other variables as independent variables. The aim of a predictive design (Fig. 7-6) is to predict the level of the dependent variable from the independent variables. The independent variables that are most effective in prediction are highly correlated with the dependent vari-

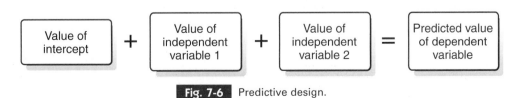

Fig. 7-6 Predictive design.

able but not highly correlated with other independent variables used in the study. Predictive correlational designs require the development of a theory-based mathematical hypothesis proposing variables expected to effectively predict the dependent variable. The hypothesis is then tested using regression analysis.

Dormire and Yarandi (2001) conducted a predictive correlational study of "Predictors of Risk for Adolescent Childbearing" (pp. 81-86). A doctorally prepared nurse and a doctorally prepared statistician conducted this study.

Purpose. The purpose of this study was to "develop a predictive model that identifies young women at risk for adolescent motherhood" (p. 81).

Variables. Variables in this study were self-esteem, perceptions of childbearing, race, social status, and relationships with family members and friends.

Sample. "A stratified sample of 357 adolescents was drawn from public health units and public schools in six randomly selected counties in North Central Florida" (p. 81).

Instruments. "Four research instruments in addition to a demographic instrument were used to obtain data: 1) Hollingshead Four Factor Index of Social Status (Hollingshead, 1975), 2) Parental Bonding Instrument (Parker, Tupling & Brown, 1979), 3) Rosenberg Self-Esteem Scale (Rosenberg, 1965), and 4) Parenting Perceptions Instrument (PPI) (Dormire, 1992)." (p. 83)

Procedure. "Those girls who consented to participate in the study first completed a demographic questionnaire that included the questions appropriate for calculation of social status. The demographic questionnaire included data regarding variables that are part of the social context (i.e., number of friends pregnant, years of education, and mother's age at first pregnancy), because other researchers have identified these factors as related to adolescent childbearing. While these factors were not the major focus of the research, they were conceptually a fit and provided additional social context data." (p. 83) Following this the three scales were administered.

Analysis. A stepwise logistic regression was used to investigate the combined effects of these variables for identification of risk for adolescent motherhood." (p. 81)

Findings. "In this [sic] data, the greatest likelihood of childbearing (97.66%) is represented by an [sic] 14-year-old African American adolescent who did not know her dad, lived in an unskilled laborer household, felt positively about being a mother at her current age, knew three friends who were pregnant, and had two friends who were mothers. The power of this combination of variables is evident in comparing probability for a 14-year-old with all of the same variable levels; her probability of motherhood is 80.6%. This comparison indicates that, although age is an important variable in adolescent motherhood, the social factors of the model presented in this research are critical to identifying those adolescents at greatest risk." (p. 84)

"Conversely, calculation of the probabilities for adolescents with differing social status characteristics finds reduction of motherhood probability. An

18-year-old adolescent who is White, lives in a home with a parent in a professional occupation, knows her father, does not want to be a mother at her current age, and has no friends either pregnant or parenting has only a 12.5% probability of motherhood. The 14-year-old with these same characteristics has a 1.4% probability." (p. 84)

Implications. "With instruments that are readily available to practitioners, nurses can evaluate these variables and determine the risk of adolescent motherhood to individuals. Several of the variables significant to risk assessment can be obtained through interview alone.... Subsequent nursing interventions can be directed toward prevention to those at greatest risk. Nurses in any clinical setting can refer adolescents identified to be at risk for early pregnancy to prevention programs available in their communities." (p. 86)

Model Testing Design

Some studies are designed specifically to test the accuracy of a hypothesized causal model. The design requires that all variables relevant to the model be measured. A large, heterogeneous sample is required. All the "paths" expressing relationships between concepts are identified, and a conceptual map is developed (Fig. 7-7). The analysis determines whether the data are consistent with the model.

Berger and Walker (2001) used a model testing design to "test an explanatory model of variables influencing fatigue in women during the first three cycles of adjuvant breast cancer chemotherapy and to determine the extent to which model variables explain fatigue at treatments and predict fatigue at cycle midpoints" (p. 42). The model being tested is shown in Fig. 7-8. Two doctorally prepared authors conducted this study.

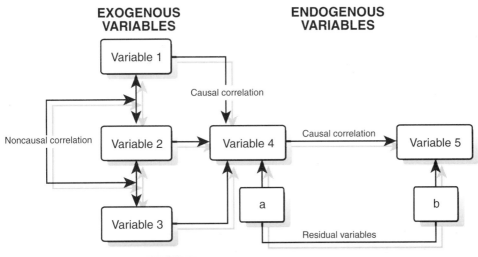

Fig. 7-7 Model testing design.

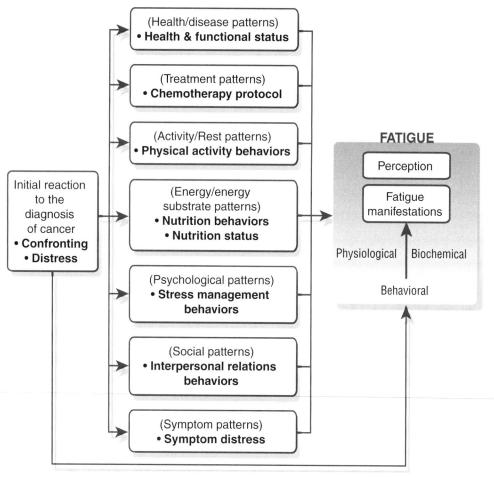

Fig. 7-8 Model testing design.

Sample. "The sample included 60 women who received chemotherapy after surgery for Stage I or II breast cancer" (p. 42).

Instruments. "Fatigue was measured by the Piper Fatigue Scale Predictor variables and measures were health and functional status (Medical Outcomes Study Short Form General Health Survey-36), chemotherapy protocol, health-promoting lifestyle behaviors (Health Promoting Lifestyle Profile II), nutritional status (hematocrit [Hct] and body mass index [BMI], symptom distress [Symptom Distress Scale], and initial reaction to the diagnosis of cancer [Reaction to the Diagnosis of Cancer Questionnaire])." (p. 42)

Findings. "The proposed model of factors influencing fatigue in women receiving breast cancer chemotherapy was partially supported.... The final

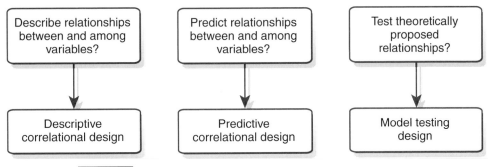

Fig. 7-9 Algorithm for determining type of correlational design.

models support the belief that fatigue is influenced by a variety of physiologic, psychological, and social factors. None of the conceptualized influencing factors were eliminated from both models; however, not all variables selected to represent these factors were retained, and the strength of the paths differed at treatment times and cycle midpoints." (p. 49)

To determine the type of correlational design used in a published study, use the algorithm shown in Fig. 7-9. For more detail on specific correlational designs referred to in this algorithm, see Burns and Grove (2001).

Critique of Example Correlational Design

In critiquing a correlational design, a large, representative sample is expected with a wide range of values on the measured variables. Berger and Walker's (2001) sample of 60 subjects was determined by power analysis to be adequate for the multiple regression analysis they performed. To allow for an anticipated 15% attrition, 72 subjects were recruited. "Seventy-seven eligible women were identified, 5 declined to participate, and 12 withdrew before completing the study, leaving a sample of 60" (p. 45). The time required to complete the instruments affects the willingness of individuals to participate. The small number who declined to participate is remarkable. Subjects were followed in the study for 10 to 12 weeks. Given the time and medical condition of subjects, the mortality rate is small. The instruments used in the study are valid and reliable and have been used in multiple studies. In a correlational study it is critical that a full range of scores for each of the variables is included in the correlational analyses. The authors report the range and distribution of scores on the measures taken in the study, allowing a critique of the adequacy of distribution. Examination of the distribution reveals a wide distribution of scores that should have been adequate for the analyses. The path analyses performed were appropriate to address the study purpose. Interpretation of the analysis results was performed with careful application to the theory being tested.

TESTING CAUSALITY

Designs developed to test causality emerged in the early 1900s, because of a need in agriculture to test the effectiveness of new methods for improving crop production (Fisher, 1935). The purpose of the experimental design is to provide the best method possible to obtain a true representation of cause and effect in the situation under study. This means providing the greatest amount of control possible to examine causality with the least error possible. To examine cause, the researcher must eliminate all factors influencing the dependent variable other than the cause (independent variable) being studied. The effects of some factors are eliminated by controlling them (e.g., sampling criteria). The study is designed to prevent other elements from intruding into the observation of the specific cause and effect that the researcher wishes to examine.

We consider the three essential elements of experimental research to be: (1) random assignment of subjects to groups; (2) researcher-controlled manipulation of the independent variable; and (3) researcher control of the experimental situation and setting, including a control or comparison group. There is disagreement about whether random sampling is essential for labeling a study as experimental. Randomization, in which nonrandomly obtained subjects are randomly assigned to groups, is considered by some to be an acceptable substitute for random samples. Control of variance is considered by all to be essential in experimental designs. Sample criteria are explicit, the independent variable is provided in a precisely defined way, the dependent variables are carefully operationalized, and the environment in which the study is conducted is rigidly controlled to prevent the interference of unstudied factors from modifying the dynamics of the process being studied.

In nursing and medical research, as well as in research in other disciplines, such as education and social work, achieving the control considered essential to an experimental design is difficult, and in some cases impossible. Much of the science used to guide clinical practice in nursing and medicine is derived from clinical trials, which are critically reviewed and considered to have the best designs possible. Clinical trials use randomization but do not have random samples. They have a convenience sample with the subjects randomly assigned to groups. Thus there is a reduced probability of equivalence between the experimental group and the comparison group and an increased risk that the sample is not representative of the target population.

Quasi-Experimental Design

Quasi-experimental designs facilitate the search for knowledge and examination of causality in situations in which complete control is not possible. These designs were developed to control as many threats to validity as possible in a situation in which some of the components of true experimental design are lacking. A nonequivalent comparison group, one in which the control group is not selected by random means, is commonly used in quasi-experimental studies. Some groups are more nonequivalent than others. In most quasi-experimental studies, experimental and comparison subjects are selected from the same pool of potential subjects. But in some quasi-experimental designs, comparison and treatment groups evolve naturally. For example, groups might include subjects who choose a treatment as the experimental group and subjects who chose not to receive a treatment as the comparison group. These groups cannot be considered equivalent because the individuals in the control group usually differ in important ways from those in the treatment group.

Quasi-experimental study designs vary widely. The most frequently used design in social science research is the untreated control group design with pretest and posttest (Fig. 7-10). With this design, the researcher has an experimental group who receives the experimental treatment (or intervention) and a comparison group who receives no treatment (or, in some cases, the usual treatment [care] provided in the circumstances under study). Another commonly used design is the posttest-only design with a comparison group (Fig. 7-11). This design is used in situations in which a pretest is not possible. For example, if the researcher is examining differences in the amount of pain that a subject feels during a painful procedure, and a nursing intervention is used to reduce pain for subjects in the experimental group, it might not be possible (or meaningful) to pretest the amount of pain before the procedure. This design has a number of threats to validity because of the lack of a pretest and thus is sometimes referred to as a "preexperimental design." The algorithm shown in Fig. 7-12 can be used to determine the type of quasi-experimental study design used in a published study. Burns and Grove (2001) contains more details about specific designs identified in this algorithm.

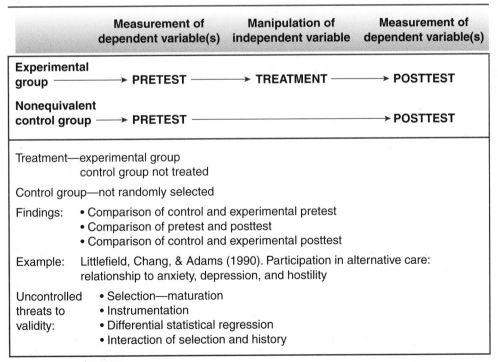

	Measurement of dependent variable(s)	Manipulation of independent variable	Measurement of dependent variable(s)
Experimental group ⟶	**PRETEST** ⟶	**TREATMENT** ⟶	**POSTTEST**
Nonequivalent control group ⟶	**PRETEST** ⟶		**POSTTEST**

Treatment—experimental group
          control group not treated

Control group—not randomly selected

Findings: • Comparison of control and experimental pretest
            • Comparison of pretest and posttest
            • Comparison of control and experimental posttest

Example: Littlefield, Chang, & Adams (1990). Participation in alternative care: relationship to anxiety, depression, and hostility

Uncontrolled   • Selection—maturation
threats to   • Instrumentation
validity: • Differential statistical regression
                • Interaction of selection and history

Fig. 7-10 Untreated comparison group design with pretest and posttest.

	Manipulation of independent variable	Measurement of dependent variable(s)
Experimental group	→TREATMENT	→ POSTTEST
Nonequivalent control group		→ POSTTEST

Treatment—often ex post facto
      may not be well defined

Experimental group—those who receive the treatment and the posttest

Pretest—inferred—norms of measures of dependent variable(s) of population from which pretreatment experimental group taken

Control group—not randomly selected—tend to be those who naturally in the situation do not receive the treatment

Findings: • Comparison of posttest scores of experimental and control groups
              • Comparison of posttest scores with norms

Example: Monahan (1991). Potential outcomes of clinical experience

Uncontrolled threats to validity: • No link between treatment and change
              • No pretest
              • Selection

Fig. 7-11 Posttest-only design with a comparison group.

Critique of Example Quasi-Experimental Design

Earl, Jackson, and Rickman (2001) conducted a quasi-experimental study to examine the effects of having ready access to an alcohol-based gel on rates of compliance with hand antisepsis guidelines. This study was published in *American Journal of Nursing (AJN)* accessible to a large number of practicing nurses. This study was conducted by an author with a master's degree in public health, another author was an RN with a PhD degree, and a physician.

AJN overview. "Hand antisepsis is arguably the single most effective means of preventing and controlling nosocomial infection. Yet it's often neglected, although nosocomial infections threaten the lives of approximately two million patients in the United States annually. Among the reasons health care workers give for non-compliance are the inconvenience and time involved in traditional soap-and-water handwashing and the drying effect this method has on skin.

These three researchers sought to discover whether making hand antisepsis a quicker and more convenient process would increase compliance. This 1999 observational study, which took place on two hospital intensive care units, established a baseline rate of soap-and-water handwashing compliance then offered health care workers an alternative: hand degerming using a rinse-free, alcohol-

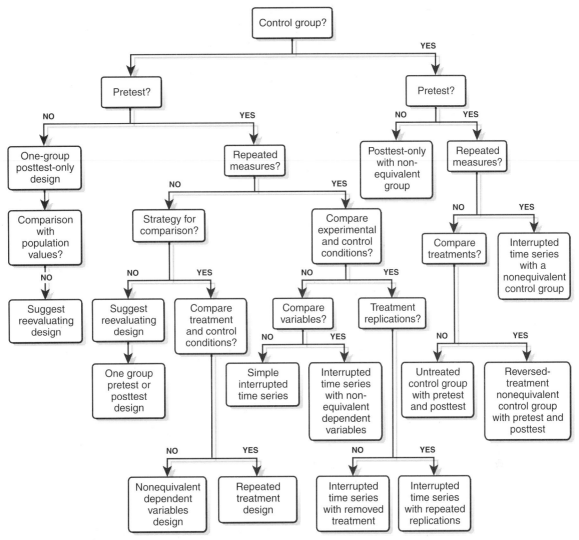

Fig. 7-12 Algorithm for determining type of quasi-experimental design.

based gel. Such gels are relatively inexpensive, and dispensers are easy to install and use. Seventy-three gel dispensers were installed inside and outside patient rooms, and compliance was evaluated over short- and long-term periods. The ready availability of the gel resulted in a sustained increase in hand antisepsis rates among health care workers. These findings support the use of these products as a viable method of increasing rates of hand antisepsis compliance." (p. 26)

Methods. "Between January and May 1999, we conducted a three-phase observational study on two intensive care units—the 20-bed surgical intensive care unit

Continued

(SICU) and the 13-bed medical intensive care unit (MICU)—at the University of California, San Diego, Medical Center. Phase I determined the baseline rates of soap-and-water handwashing. Seventy-three dispensers containing an alcohol-based gel were then installed both inside and outside patient rooms. Phase II evaluated their impact on rates of hand degerming two to six weeks post-installation, and Phase III measured compliance 10 to 14 weeks postinstallation.

The five observers, all public health graduate students, followed the guidelines for handwashing and hand antisepsis of the Association for Professionals in Infection Control and Epidemiology (APIC). They recorded episodes of patient contact that required hand antisepsis and noted whether this actually occurred. For each episode there was a maximum of two instances of compliance: before and after patient contact. Although the APIC guideline also mandates hand cleansing when shifting between unclean and clean sites during care of a single patient, the observers did not have the expertise to evaluate when this was necessary, and we did not record such instances.

Observation sessions were scheduled at varied times throughout the day and night in order to obtain an accurate picture of compliance on all shifts. Health care workers were classified as ancillary personnel (such as radiation technicians and physical therapists), nursing personnel (registered and licensed vocation nurses as well as nursing assistants), or physicians. Unit managers were informed of the study's purpose, but unit staff was not. When approached by staff members, observers said that they were conducting an infection control study for the medical center's Epidemiology Unit.

Results. In a total of 402 hours of observation during the three phases, 3015 opportunities for hand degerming were recorded and 1481 episodes were observed." (p. 28)

"The availability of alcohol-based gel in conveniently placed, wall-mounted dispensers produced a sustained, long-term increase in hand antisepsis rates on both units and at all levels of employment. Hand antisepsis increased 32.8% during phase II, two to six weeks after gel dispensers were installed, and the rate continued to increase (8.4%) at 10 to 14 weeks after installation. This result is consistent with those reported by Pittet and colleagues, whose three-year study found that the increase in compliance was sustained over the long term." (p. 31)

Experimental Designs

A variety of *experimental designs*, some relatively simple and others very complex, have been developed for a variety of studies focused on examining causality. In some cases, researchers may combine characteristics of more than one design to meet the needs of their study. Names of designs vary from one text to another. When reading and critiquing a published study, you determine the author's name for the design (some authors do not name the design used) and read the description of the design to determine the type of design used in the study. The algorithm shown in Fig. 7-13

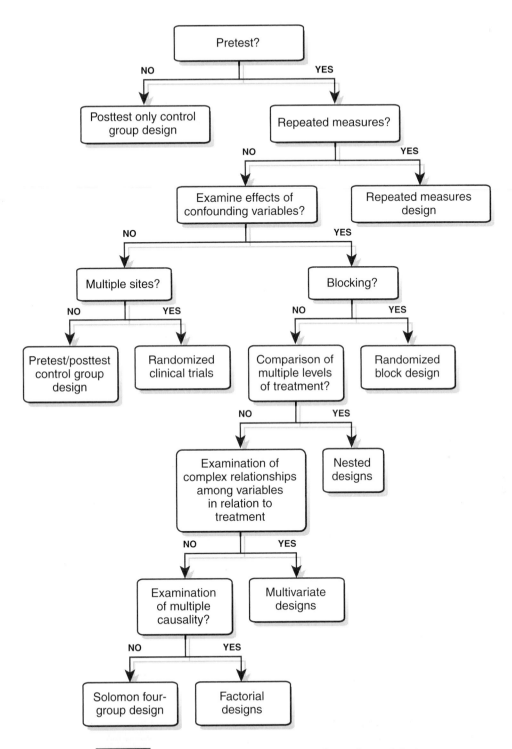

Fig. 7-13 Algorithm for determining type of experimental design.

can be used to determine the type of experimental study design used in a published study. Burns and Grove (2001) contains more details about specific designs referred to in Fig. 7-13.

Pretest-Posttest Design

The most common experimental design used in nursing studies is the pretest-posttest design. This design is similar to that shown in Fig. 7-10, except that the experimental study is more tightly controlled. Multiple groups (both experimental and control) can be used to great advantage in this design. For example, one control group can receive no treatment, whereas another control group receives a placebo treatment. Each one of multiple experimental groups can receive a variation of the treatment, such as a different frequency, intensity, or length of nursing care measures. These additions greatly increase the generalizability of study findings.

Factorial Design

The factorial design is a complex, multivariate experimental design. In a factorial design, two or more characteristics, treatments, or events are independently varied within a single study. This design is a logical approach to examining multicausality. The simplest arrangement is one in which two treatments or factors are involved, and within each factor, two levels are manipulated (e.g., the presence or absence of the treatment). This is referred to as a "2 × 2 factorial design." This design is illustrated in Fig. 7-14, using the two independent variables of relaxation and distraction as means of pain relief.

A 2 × 2 factorial design produces a study with four cells. Each cell must contain an equivalent number of subjects. Cells B and C allow examination of each separate intervention. Cell D subjects receive no treatment and serve as a control group. Cell A allows examination of interaction between the two independent variables. The design can be used to control for confounding variables. The confounding variable is included as an independent variable, and interactions between it and the other independent variable are examined (Spector, 1981).

	Level of distraction	
Level of relaxation	Distraction	No Distraction
Relaxation	A	B
No relaxation	C	D

Fig. 7-14 Example of factorial design.

Randomized Clinical Trial

The randomized clinical trial has been used in medicine since 1945. However, until recently it has not been used in nursing. The clinical trial uses large numbers of subjects to test the effects of a treatment and compare the results with those of a control group that has not received the treatment (or that has received a traditional treatment). Subjects are drawn from a reference population, using clearly defined criteria, and are then randomly assigned to treatment or control groups. Baseline states should be comparable in all groups included in the study. The treatment should be equal and consistently applied, and outcomes need to be measured consistently. Care should be taken to ensure that randomization procedures are rigidly adhered to in a study.

Because of the need to have large samples and to be able to generalize to a variety of clinical settings and patients, the study may be carried out simultaneously in multiple geographic locations coordinated by the primary researcher. Use of this design has the potential to greatly improve the scientific base for nursing practice (Fetter et al., 1989; Tyzenhouse, 1981).

Critique of Example Experimental Design

A study by Olsen et al. (2001) titled "The Effect of Aloe Vera Gel/Mild Soap versus Mild Soap Alone in Preventing Skin Reactions in Patients Undergoing Radiation Therapy" will be used as an example of an experimental study. Four of the researchers conducting this study have both an RN and a BSN. One author has a master's degree in public health, and one is a physician with a doctorate in science.

Purpose and objectives. "To determine whether the use of mild soap and aloe vera gel versus mild soap alone would decrease the incidence of skin reactions in patients undergoing radiation therapy" (p. 543).

Hypothesis. "The use of aloe vera gel/soap would decrease the incidence of skin changes (e.g., skin texture, erythema, itch, tanning) and lengthen the amount of time before radiation-induced dermatitis developed" (p. 544).

Design. Prospective, randomized, blinded, clinical trial.

Setting. Radiation therapy outpatient clinic in a cancer center affiliated with a major teaching medical facility.

Sample. "The mean age of the participants was 56 years. The group consisted of Caucasians (74%) and African Americans (26%). The ethnic mix was non-Hispanic (65%) and Hispanic (35%)" (p. 544).

Methods. "Prophylactic skin care began on the first day of radiation therapy. Patients cleansed the area with mild, unscented soap. Patients randomized into the experimental arm of the trial were instructed to liberally apply aloe vera gel to the area at various intervals throughout the day." (p. 544)

Study variables. "Age, sex, race, ethnicity, and skin type (light, medium, dark), prior or existing skin conditions, chemotherapy administration, and tumor sites. Dose at which the first skin change was noted was used as a grouping category in analysis. Skin change variables included itching, skin texture, tanning, erythema, and time to skin change." (p. 544)

Continued

Treatment. "Patients were directed to gently cleanse the irradiated area with mild, unscented soap that was provided. [The experimental group received soap and aloe vera gel, while the control group received only soap.] They were cautioned to protect the skin in the irradiated area from trauma; not to use band-aids or tape; to pat the cleansed area dry with a soft, clean towel or cloth; to avoid prolonged exposure to direct sunlight; and to wear loose-fitting clothing that would not rub the area. The average number of applications was six to eight times per day. Patients were further instructed that the gel should be rinsed off gently before their treatment each day so that no gel would be present on the skin prior to receiving radiotherapy. No other gels or creams were to be applied by either group." (p. 544)

At low cumulative dose levels < 2,700 cGy, no difference existed in the effect of adding aloe. When the cumulative dose was high (> 2,700 cGy), the median time was five weeks prior to any skin changes in the aloe/soap arm versus three weeks in the soap only arm. When the cumulative dose increases over time, there seems to be a protective effect of adding aloe to the soap regimen.

Implications for nursing practice. "Skin products used to treat radiation dermatitis vary among institutions. Nurses should be aware that some patients may be predisposed to skin problems. Nurses must be aware of newly developed products and research regarding these products so that effective treatment can be instituted." (p. 543)

"Key Points

1. Almost all patients undergoing external beam radiation therapy are expected to develop acute skin reactions.
2. Skin products currently in use are those that clinicians routinely have used in the past based on anecdotal data.
3. More controlled studies of radiotherapy and skin reactions area needed." (p. 543)

Critique

The study's purpose and the clinical problems encountered are clearly described in their article. The hypothesis is clearly stated and testable. The results of this study have potential practical clinical consequences: reducing skin damage due to radiation treatment for cancer. Ropka's (1996) questions for the critique of experimental studies will be used to examine Olsen and colleague's (2001) study.

Primary question 1. Was the assignment of patients to treatments randomized? Olsen and colleague's (2001) study used a strong design to answer questions of cause and effect—a prospective, randomized, controlled clinical trial. Subjects were randomly assigned to groups and the independent variable—the presence of aloe vera in the skin care regimen, was implemented the first day of radiation therapy. The study also included a control group that received soap but not aloe vera gel. Thus the first key criterion of random assignment was met. However, the extent to which subjects followed the regimen is not reported.

Primary question 2. Were all 73 patients who entered the trial properly accounted for and attributed at its conclusion? Were all measurements taken on all subjects and reported at the end? Primary question 2 can be answered by addressing four additional questions.

1. Were all subjects followed up for the entire study period? Olson and colleagues report that "data from 70 patients were available for analysis. One patient did not receive insurance authorization to receive radiotherapy at our institution. Another patient did not begin planned radiation because her medical oncologist made the decision to delay radiation until chemotherapy administration was completed. The third patient refused radiation therapy" (p. 544). Results related to ascertainment of the primary outcome variable, skin change, are reported for all 70 subjects who remained in the study.

2. Were patients analyzed in the groups to which they were randomized? Yes. All tables of data list 32 subjects in the experimental group and 38 subjects in the control group, for a total of 70 subjects.

3. Did subjects in one group experience different or more severe side effects, toxicities, or complications than subjects in the other group, making one skin treatment preferable to the other? No side effects were reported.

4. Was tolerance of, and thus adherence to, therapy greater with one treatment than the other, indicating that use of one would better improve skin condition?" The extent of adherence to the regimen was not reported.

The following secondary questions should be asked to evaluate design validity.

1. Were patients, health-care workers, and study personnel "blind" to the treatment? The study was blind, but not double-blind. Patients in the experimental group received a gel not received by the control group. Thus it is likely that the patients knew they were in the experimental group. Skin scoring was performed weekly using the Acute Radiation Morbidity Scoring Criteria. The authors report "in an effort to eliminate bias, clinicians were blinded to the treatment arm." (p. 544) Patients may have been instructed not to inform the clinician of their position in the study but this is not stated. It is possible that patients in the control group, knowing they were not in the experimental group, might not have adhered to the regimen as carefully as those in the experimental group. However, there was no difference between the groups in subjects who received lower levels of radiation. And differences in the two groups among those who received higher levels of radiation were in the expected direction.

2. Were the groups similar at the start of the trial? Based on clinical experience or prior research, investigators provided information regarding patient characteristics that they believed were potentially related to the primary outcome. Characteristics reported as similar at the start of the trial included skin type, tumor site, gender, race, and ethnicity. Characteristics with some differences between groups included age and cumulative dose of radiation.

3. Aside from the experimental interventions, were the groups treated equally? Clinically relevant aspects of interventions performed in all groups are com-

Continued

parable, excluding the type of soap or gel received. Methods used to measure the dependent variable (skin change) were also similar in all groups, including use of a standard measure of skin change.

Will the Results Assist Nurses in Caring for Patients?

As Ropka (1996, p. 68) points out in evaluating an earlier study, "one can decide whether to apply a study's results when caring for a patient only if the study's validity has been established. To gain a clear understanding of this study, readers of the article must understand the difference between random selection and random assignment of subjects to treatment groups. Subjects in this study presumably constitute a convenience sample of patients who met the eligibility criteria of the study and were available in the established setting at that time. Therefore these subjects were not randomly selected. Because of the potential sampling bias, generalization of findings to other patients…should be limited."

DEFINING EXPERIMENTAL INTERVENTIONS

In quasi-experimental and experimental studies, an *intervention* is developed that is expected to result in differences in posttest measures of the treatment and control or comparison groups. This intervention may be physiologic, psychosocial, educational, or a combination of these. The details of the intervention should have been carefully planned and a rationale given for providing the intervention in a particular way. The researcher should describe the intervention in detail in the published study. Labels for interventions, such as "preoperative teaching," limit the reader's ability to understand the exact nature of the intervention. We may be easily led astray since each of us has our own expectations of what should occur during preoperative teaching. Nursing is currently developing classifications of nursing interventions. These classifications should be useful to the researcher in clarifying the intervention provided (Egan, Snyder, & Burns, 1992). The intervention should maximize the differences between the groups. Thus it should be the best intervention that can be provided under the circumstances of the study, an intervention that should make a difference in the experimental group.

Although control and comparison groups traditionally received no intervention, this circumstance is not possible in many nursing studies. For example, it would be unethical not to provide preoperative teaching to a patient. In addition, in many studies it is possible that just spending time with a patient or having a patient participate in activities that he or she considers beneficial may itself cause an effect. Therefore the study often includes a control or comparison group intervention. This intervention is usually the treatment the patient would receive if a study were not being conducted. The researcher should describe in detail the intervention the control or comparison group receives so that the study can be adequately critiqued. Because the quality of this usual treatment is likely to vary considerably among subjects, variance in the control or comparison group is likely to be high, and the risk of a Type II error is greater than when the control or comparison group receives no treatment.

Johnson, Fieler, Wlasowicz, Mitchell, and Jones (1997) studied the effects of nursing care guided by self-regulation theory on coping with radiation therapy. They describe their nursing intervention as follows:

"The control-group patients received the routine nursing care that was usual practice at the institution. The aspect of care relevant to the study was patient information. The only specific standards for patient teaching were that it had to take place and be documented. What was taught, when it was taught, and amount of detail included varied among nurses. In general, nurses would 'catch' a patient during the first week of treatment, and they would meet for 10 to 15 minutes in any space that was available. The nurses would provide a brief overview of the procedures involved in RT [radiation therapy] and inform the patients about possible side effects. Some of the nurses would talk about self-care management of the side effects, and others would tell the patient 'Let me know when you have [the side effect], and I will give you more information.' Patient teaching sheets that contained general information about RT and self-care activities for specific side effects were available. Nurses usually gave the sheets to patients during the first week of treatment.

The theory-based nursing care consisted of interventions delivered at four points in time: (a) before the simulation (treatment planning) procedure, (b) the first week of treatment, (c) the last week of treatment, and (d) one month post-treatment. Nurses made 30-minute appointments with patients to deliver the interventions. At the beginning of each appointment, nurses told patients the topics that would be covered and that the information would help them to handle the experience of receiving RT because they would know what to expect. At the end of each intervention session, patients were told the time of the next appointment and the topics that would be covered.... The expected experiences were described by the nurses in concrete, objective terms without reference to subjective features such as severity and amount of distress that might be experienced." (p. 1043)

In critiquing the interventions in a study, you might be asked the following questions:
1. Was the experimental intervention described in detail?
2. Was justification from the literature provided for development of the experimental intervention?
3. Was the experimental intervention the best that could be provided given current knowledge?
4. Was a protocol developed to ensure consistent or reliable implementation of the treatment with each subject throughout the study?
5. Did the study report indicate who implemented the treatment? If more than one person implemented the treatment, were they trained to ensure consistency in the delivery of the treatment?
6. Was any control group intervention described?

MAPPING THE DESIGN

In quasi-experimental and experimental studies, the design can be mapped to clarify the points at which measurements are taken and treatments are provided for various groups in the study. Generally, the symbol "O" is used for an observation or a measurement. Several measurements or observations may be indicated by this symbol. The symbol "T" is used for a treatment. For example, in a study with two groups, experimental and control, who received a pretest and posttest (pretest-posttest control group design), the design could be mapped as follows.

	Pretest		Posttest
Experimental group	O	T	O
Control group	O		O

This design map could be used for a quasi-experimental or an experimental study. In the quasi-experimental study, the control group would be called the "comparison" (or "nonequivalent") group." Experimental design subjects are randomly selected and then randomly assigned to groups. If the study included several posttests at monthly intervals, the design could be mapped as follows:

| | Pretest | | POSTTEST | | | |
			1 mo	2 mo	3 mo	4 mo
Experimental group	O_1	T	O_2	O_3	O_4	O_5
Control group	O_1		O_2	O_3	O_4	O_5

Variations in the design map could be expressed for more than two groups, by adding more rows, for repeated treatments, by placing the "T" at each place the treatment is administered, or for multiple treatments. Multiple treatments could be labeled T_1, T_2, T_3, and so on.

OUTCOMES RESEARCH

Outcomes research is a relatively new approach to research design that focuses on the end results of patient care. Those who promote outcomes research demand that providers justify the selection of patient care interventions and systems of care based on evidence of improvements in patients' lives and increases in cost effectiveness. The strategies used in outcomes research are, to some degree, a departure from the accepted design strategies referred to as the "scientific method." Design methods for outcomes research have emerged from epidemiology, evaluation methods, and economic theory. Outcome studies provide rich opportunities to build a stronger scientific underpinning for nursing practice. Using the design strategies of outcomes research, nursing can document the impact of care provided by nurses. Some dimensions of nursing that lend themselves to outcome studies are decision-making processes, case management, outcomes of nurse practitioner care, and community health care. Hospitals are a major target of outcomes research, and yet the patient outcomes are attributed either to the hospital as a whole or to physicians. Nursing practice in the hospital setting is invisible as a force influencing patient outcomes (Clark & Lang, 1992; Kelly, Huber, Johnson, McCloskey, & Maas, 1994).

Research designs and methodologies for outcomes studies are still emerging. The preferred methods of obtaining samples are different in outcomes studies; random sampling is not considered desirable and is seldom used. *Heterogeneous* (subjects with a wide variety of characteristics) rather than *homogeneous* (subjects with similar characteristics) samples are obtained. Rather than using sampling criteria that restrict subjects who are included in the study to decrease possible biases, outcomes researchers seek large, heterogeneous samples that reflect as much as possible all patients who would be receiving care in the real world. Samples are expected to include, for example, patients with various comorbidities and patients with varying levels of health status. Burns and Grove (2001) contains additional information on outcomes studies.

ROLE OF REPLICATION STUDIES IN EVIDENCE-BASED PRACTICE

Replication studies involve reproducing or repeating a study to determine whether similar findings will be obtained (Taunton, 1989). Replication is essential for knowledge development since it: (1) establishes the credibility of the findings, (2) extends the generalizability of the findings over a range of instances and contexts, (3) provides support for theory development, and (4) decreases the acceptance of erroneous results (Beck, 1994). Thus replication studies are essential to generate knowledge that can be used in practice.

Four different types of replication studies have been conducted to generate scientific knowledge for nursing: (1) exact, (2) approximate, (3) concurrent, and (4) systematic extension (Beck, 1994; Haller & Reynolds, 1986). An *exact,* or identical, *replication* involves duplicating the initial researcher's study to confirm the original findings. All conditions of the original study must be maintained; thus "there must be the same observer, the same subjects, the same procedure, the same measures, the same locale, and the same time" (Haller & Reynolds, 1986, p. 250). Exact replications might be thought of as ideal to confirm original study findings but are frequently not attainable. An *approximate,* or operational, *replication* involves repeating the original study under similar conditions, following the original methods as closely as possible (Beck, 1994; Haller & Reynolds, 1986). The intent is to determine whether the findings from the original study hold up despite minor changes in the research conditions. If the findings generated through replication are consistent with the original study findings, these findings are more credible and have the potential to be used in practice.

A *concurrent,* or internal, *replication* involves the collection of data for the original study and their replication simultaneously to provide a check of the reliability of the original study (Beck, 1994). The confirmation, through replication, of the original study findings is part of the original study's design. For example, a research team might collect data simultaneously at two different hospitals and compare and contrast the findings. Consistency in the findings increases the credibility and generalizability of the findings. A *systematic extension,* or constructive, *replication* is done under distinctly new conditions. The researchers conducting the replication do not follow the design or methods of the original researchers; rather, "the second investigative team begins with a similar problem statement but formulates new means to verify the first investigator's findings" (Haller & Reynolds, 1986, p. 250). The aim of this type of replication is to extend the findings of the original study and test the limits of generalizability.

Beck (1994) conducted a computerized and manual review of the nursing literature from 1983 through 1992 and found only 49 replication studies. Possibly, the number of replication studies is limited because replication is viewed by some as less scholarly or less important than original research. However, the lack of replication studies severely limits the development of a scientific knowledge base for nursing (Beck, 1994; Martin, 1995). Thus, replication of studies is an important priority for nursing because it will greatly influence the generation of nursing knowledge that can be synthesized for use in practice (Burns & Grove, 2001).

SUMMARY

A research design is a blueprint for conducting a study that maximizes control over factors that could interfere with the validity of the findings. Elements central to the study design include the presence or absence of a treatment, number of groups in the sample, number and timing of measurements to be performed, method of sampling, time frame for data collection, planned comparisons, and control of extraneous variables.

Selecting a design requires an understanding of certain concepts: causality, multicausality, probability, bias, control, manipulation, and validity. In causality, there is an assumption that situations have causes and that causes lead to effects. Multicausality is the recognition that a number of interrelating variables can be involved in causing a particular effect. Probability deals with the likelihood that a specific effect will occur following a particular cause. Bias is of great concern in research because of the potential effect on the meaning of the study findings. Any component of the study that deviates or causes a deviation from the true measurement of variables leads to distorted findings. Manipulation is moving around or controlling the movement, such as manipulating the independent variable. If the freedom to manipulate a variable is under someone else's control, a bias is introduced into the study. Control means having the power to direct or manipulate factors to achieve a desired outcome. The greater the control the researcher has over the study situation, the more credible the study findings will be.

Validity is a measure of the truth or accuracy of a claim. When conducting a study, the researcher is confronted with major decisions regarding four types of validity: statistical conclusion validity, internal validity, construct validity, and external validity. Statistical conclusion validity refers to whether the conclusions about relationships drawn from statistical analysis are an accurate reflection of the real world. Internal validity is the extent to which the effects detected in the study are a reflection of reality rather than a result of the effects of extraneous variables. Construct validity refers to the fit between the conceptual and operational definitions of variables. External validity refers to the extent to which study findings can be generalized beyond the sample used in the study.

Four common types of quantitative designs are used in nursing: descriptive, correlational, quasi-experimental, and experimental. Descriptive studies are designed to gain more information about variables within a particular field of study. Their purpose is to provide a picture of situations as they naturally happen. No manipulation of variables is involved. Descriptive designs vary in level of complexity; some contain only two variables, whereas others include multiple variables. Correlational studies examine relationships between variables. The researcher may seek to describe a relationship, predict relationships among variables, or test the relationships proposed by a theoretical proposition.

The purpose of quasi-experimental and experimental designs is to examine causality. The power of the design to accomplish this purpose depends on how well the actual effects of the experimental treatment (the independent variable) can be detected by measurement of the dependent variable. Threats to validity are controlled through selection of subjects, manipulation of the treatment, and reliable measurement of variables. Experimental designs, with their strict control of variance, are the most powerful method of examining causality. Quasi-experimental designs were developed to provide alternative means for examining causality in situations not conducive to experimental controls. The three essential elements of experimental research are: (1) the random assignment of subjects to groups; (2) the researcher's manipulation of the independent variable; and (3) the researcher's control of the experimental situation and setting, including a control or comparison group.

The purpose of design is to maximize the possibility of obtaining valid answers to research questions or hypotheses. In most studies comparisons are the basis of obtaining valid answers. A good design provides the subjects, the setting, and the protocol within which these comparisons can be clearly examined. Critiquing a design involves examining the study's environment, sample, treatment, and measurement.

In critiquing the study, it is important to identify variables not included in the design (extraneous variables) that could explain some of the variance in measurement of the study variables. In a good design the effect of these variables on variance is controlled. Outcomes research was developed to examine the end results of patient care. Those promoting outcomes research demand that providers justify the selection of patient care interventions and systems of care based on evidence of improved patient lives and increased cost effectiveness.

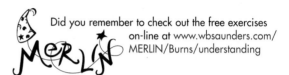

Did you remember to check out the free exercises on-line at www.wbsaunders.com/ MERLIN/Burns/understanding

REFERENCES

Beck, C. T. (1994). Replication strategies for nursing research. *Image: Journal of Nursing Scholarship, 26*(3), 191–194.

Berger, A. M., & Walker, S. N. (2001). An explanatory model of fatigue in women receiving adjuvant breast cancer chemotherapy. *Nursing Research, 50*(1), 42–52.

Burns, N., & Grove, S. K. (2001). *The practice of nursing research: Conduct, critique and utilization* (4th ed.). Philadelphia: Saunders.

Clark, J., & Lang, N. (1992). Nursing's next advance: An internal classification for nursing practice. *International Nursing Review, 39*(4), 109–111, 128.

Cook, T. D., & Campbell, D. T. (1979). *Quasi-experimentation: Design and analysis issues for field settings.* Chicago: Rand McNally.

Dormire, S. L. (1992). *Human agency perspectives in adolescent motherhood: Self-esteem and socio-cultural variables.* Unpublished doctoral dissertation. University of Florida Gainsville.

Dormire, S. L., & Yarandi, H. (2001). Predictors of risk for adolescent childbearing. *Applied Nursing Research, 14*(2), 81–86.

Earl, M. L., Jackson, M. M., & Rickman, L. S. (2001). Improved rates of compliance with hand antisepsis guidelines: A three-phase observational study. *American Journal of Nursing, 101*(3), 26–33.

Egan, E. C., Snyder, M., & Burns, K. R. (1992). Intervention studies in nursing: Is the effect due to the independent variable? *Nursing Outlook, 40*(4), 187–190.

Fetter, M. S., et al. (1989). Randomized clinical trials: Issues for researchers. *Nursing Research, 38*(2), 117–120.

Fisher, R. A. (1935). *The design of experiments.* New York: Hafner.

Haller, K. B., & Reynolds, M. A. (1986). Using research in practice: A case for replication in nursing—part two. *Western Journal of Nursing Research, 8*(2), 249–252.

Hollingshead, A. (1975). *Four factor index of social status,* New Haven: Yale University Press.

Johnson, J. E., Fieler, V. K., Wlasowicz, G. S., Mitchell, M. L., & Jones, L. S. (1997). The effects of nursing care guided by self-regulation theory on coping with radiation therapy. *Oncology Nursing Forum, 24*(6), 1041–1050.

Kelly, K. C., Huber, D. G., Johnson, M., McCloskey, J. C., & Maas, M. (1994). The Medical Outcomes Study: A nursing perspective. *Journal of Professional Nursing, 10*(4), 209–216.

Lennie, T. A., Christman, S. K., & Jadack, R. A. (2001). Educational needs and altered eating habits following a total laryngectomy. *Oncology Nursing Forum, 28*(4), 667–674.

Lillard, J., & McFann, C. L. (1990). A marital crisis: For better or worse…hospice involvement. *Hospice Journal—Physical, Psychosocial & Pastoral Care of the Dying, 6*(2), 95–109.

Littlefield, V. M., Chang, A., & Adams, B. N. (1990). Participation in alternative care: Relationship to anxiety, depression, and hostility. *Research in Nursing & Health, 13*(1), 17–25.

Martin, P. A. (1995). More replication studies needed. *Applied Nursing Research, 8*(2), 102–103.

Mimnaugh, L., Winegar, M., Mabrey, Y., & Davis, J. E. (1999). Sensations experienced during removal of tubes in acute postoperative patients. *Applied Nursing Research, 12*(2), 78–85.

Monahan, R. S. (1991). Potential outcomes of clinical experience. *Journal of Nursing Education, 30*(4), 176–181.

Olsen, D. L. et al. (2001). The effect of aloe vera gel/mild soap versus mild soap alone in preventing skin reactions in patients undergoing radiation therapy. *Oncology Nursing Forum, 28*(3), 543–547.

Parker, G., Tupling, H., & Brown, L. B. (1979). A parental bonding instrument. *British Journal of Medical Psychology, 52,* 1–10.

Rew, L., Taylor-Seehafer, M., Thomas, N. Y., & Yockey, R. D. (2001). Correlates of resilience in homeless adolescents. *Journal of Nursing Scholarship, 33*(1), 33–40.

Ropka, M. E. (1996). Commentary [on Diarrhea associated with nasogastric feedings by Reese, Means, Hanrahan, Clearman, Colwill, & Dawson]. *Oncology Nursing Forum, 23*(1), 66–68.

Rosenberg, M. (1965). *Society and the adolescent self-image.* Princeton, NJ: Princeton University Press.

Sheahan, S. L. (2000). Documentation of health risks and health promotion counseling by emergency department nurse practitioners and physicians. *Journal of Nursing Scholarship, 32*(3), 245–250.

Spector, P. E. (1981). *Research designs.* Beverly Hills, CA: Sage.

Tauton, R. L. (1989). Replication: Key to research application. *Dimensions of Critical Care Nursing, 8*(3), 156–158.

Tyzenhouse, P. S. (1981). Technical notes: The nursing clinical trial. *Western Journal of Nursing Research, 3*(1), 102–109.

U.S. Dept. Of Health and Human Services. (1991). *Healthy People 2000, National health promotion and disease prevention objectives.* Publication (PHS) 91-50213. Washington, DC: Author.

U.S. Department of Health and Human Services. (2000). *Healthy People 2010.* Washington, D.C.: U.S. Dept. of Health and Human Services: For sale by the U.S. G.P.O., Supt of Docs., [2000].

U.S. Preventive Services Task Force. (1996). *Guide to clinical preventive services* (2nd ed.). Alexandria, VA: International Medical Publishing.

Waltz, C. F., & Bausell, R. B. (1981). *Nursing research: Design, statistics and computer analysis.* Philadelphia: Davis.

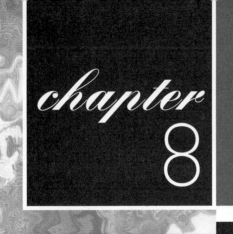

chapter 8

Populations and Samples

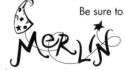

Be sure to check out the free exercises on-line at
www.wbsaunders.com/MERLIN/Burns/
understanding

OUTLINE—cont'd

OBJECTIVES

Completing this chapter should enable you to:
1. Describe sampling theory, including the following concepts: sample, population, subject, target population, elements of the population, sample criteria, sampling frame, sampling plan, accessible population, representativeness, statistics, precision, sampling error, and systematic bias.
2. Describe probability and nonprobability sampling methods.
3. Differentiate probability from nonprobability sampling methods in published studies.
4. Describe the sampling methods used in qualitative research.
5. Examine the elements that influence the decision of sample size in quantitative and qualitative studies.
6. Explain the purposes of power analysis.
7. Critique the sample size in quantitative and qualitative studies.
8. Critique the sample section in published quantitative and qualitative nursing studies.

RELEVANT TERMS

Accessible population
Cluster sampling
Comparison group
Control group
Convenience sampling
Effect size
Element
Exclusion criteria
Generalization
Inclusion criteria
Multistage sampling
Network or snowball sampling
Nonprobability sampling
Population
Power
Power analysis
Probability sampling
Purposive sampling

Quota sampling
Random sampling
Random variation
Refusal rate
Representativeness
Sample mortality
Sample size
Sampling
Sampling or eligibility criteria
Sampling frame
Sampling plan
Saturation of data
Simple random sampling
Stratified random sampling
Subjects
Systematic sampling
Systematic variation
Target population

Students often enter the field of research with preconceived notions about samples and sampling. Many of these notions are acquired through exposure to television advertisements, public opinion polls, market researchers in shopping centers, and newspaper reports of research findings. A television commercial boasts that four of five doctors recommend a particular product; a newscaster announces that John Jones is predicted to win the senate election by a margin of 10%; a newspaper reports that researchers have now shown that aggressive treatment of hypertension to maintain a blood pressure of 130/80 or lower significantly reduces the risk for stroke.

All of these examples use sampling techniques. However, some of the outcomes are more valid than others. The differences in validity are due in part to the sampling techniques used, since sampling is a key element of research methodology. Thus in critiquing a published study, the sampling method used by the researchers should be identified and its adequacy evaluated. The sampling procedure is usually described in the methods section of a published research report. To judge its adequacy, it is necessary to understand some of the principles of sampling theory. This chapter discusses sampling theory and concepts; sampling plans, both probability and non-probability; sample size in quantitative and qualitative studies; and the adequacy of a sample in quantitative and qualitative studies.

SAMPLING THEORY

Sampling involves selecting a group of people, events, behaviors, or other elements with which to conduct a study. A sampling plan defines the selection process and the sample defines the selected group of people (or elements). Samples are expected to represent a population of people. The population might be all individuals who have diabetes, all patients who have abdominal surgery, or all individuals who receive care from a nurse practitioner. However, in most cases it would be impossible for a researcher to study an entire population. Sampling theory was developed to determine the most effective way to acquire a sample that would accurately reflect the population under study. Key concepts of sampling theory include elements, populations, sampling or eligibility criteria, representativeness, sampling frames, and sampling plans. The following sections explain the meaning of these concepts. In later sections these concepts are used to explain a variety of sampling techniques.

Elements and Populations

An individual unit of a population is called an *element*. An element can be a person, event, experience, behavior, or any other single unit of a study. The elements of the study could be the experience of homelessness in a large city or the event of using iced or room-temperature injectant to measure cardiac output in a critical care unit. When elements are persons, they are referred to as *subjects*. The subjects might be patients with hypertension who were seen in primary care clinics. The sample is selected to represent the population of hypertensive patients. The *population,* sometimes referred to as the *target population,* is the entire set of individuals (or elements) who (that) met the sampling criteria (defined in the next section). When studying the effect of relaxation on hypertension, the sampling criteria might be patients who are 18 years of age or older and were diagnosed with hypertension in the last three months. An *accessible population* is the portion of the target population to which the researcher has reasonable access. The accessible population might be all hypertensive patients seen in primary care clinics within a city, a section of a city, or one clinic.

The sample is obtained from the accessible population, and findings are generalized to the target population. *Generalization* involves extending the findings from the sample under study to the larger population. The extent of the generalization is influenced by the quality of the study and the consistency of the study's findings with the findings from previous research in this area. If a study were of high quality with findings that are consistent with previous research, then the researchers would have confidence in generalizing their findings from their sample to the target population. For example, the findings from the study of hypertensive patients in one clinic might be generalized to the target population of all adult patients with hypertension seen in primary care clinics. With this information, a nurse can decide whether it is appropriate to use these findings clinically in caring for the same type of patients.

 In critiquing a study, you need to identify the subjects or elements, accessible population, and target population of the study and evaluate the appropriateness of the generalization. The following questions might provide you assistance during a critique of these aspects in the sample section of a study.

1. Who (or what) were the subjects (or elements) in the study?
2. Who (or what) was the accessible population?
3. Who (or what) was the target population?
4. Were the sample and population appropriate for study purpose and design?
5. What generalizations did the researchers make? Were these generalizations appropriate based on the quality of the study and the consistency of the study findings with previous research?

Sampling or Eligibility Criteria

Sampling criteria, also referred to as *eligibility criteria,* include the list of characteristics essential for eligibility or membership in the target population. For example, researchers might study the effect of preoperative teaching on the outcome length of hospital stay following abdominal surgery. In this study the sampling criteria might include: (1) being at least 18 years old, (2) having the ability to speak and read English at the sixth-grade level, and (3) having no history of previous surgeries. The sample is selected from the accessible population that meets these sampling criteria. Sampling criteria for a study might consist of inclusion criteria, exclusion criteria, or both. *Inclusion criteria* are those characteristics that the subject or element must possess to be part of the target population. In the example the inclusion criteria are individuals over 18 years of age who can speak and read English at the sixth-grade level.

Exclusion criteria are those characteristics that can cause a person or element to be excluded from the target population. For example, any subjects with a history of previous surgeries would be excluded from the preoperative teaching study.

When the study is completed, the findings are generalized from the sample to the target population that meets the sampling criteria. The sampling criteria may be narrowly defined to make the sample as homogeneous (or similar) as possible or to control for extraneous variables. The criteria might be broadly defined to ensure that the study sample is a heterogeneous population with a broad range of values on the variables being studied. If the sampling or eligibility criteria are narrow and restrictive, the researcher may have difficulty finding subjects who meet the criteria and may not be able to obtain a sufficiently large sample from the accessible population.

In discussing the generalization of findings in a published research report, researchers sometimes attempt to generalize beyond the sampling criteria. The researcher may contend that the sample was limited by the sampling criteria only for convenience in conducting the study but that the findings really apply to a larger population. Using the example preoperative teaching study, the sample may have been limited to subjects who speak and read English because the preoperative teaching would be performed in English and because one of the measurement instruments required that subjects be able to read English at the sixth-grade level. However, the researcher may believe that the findings can be generalized to non–English-speaking individuals. Practicing nurses need to consider carefully the implications of using these findings with non–English-speaking populations. Perhaps these populations, because they come from another culture, might not have responded to the teaching in the same way as other populations.

Generalizing to people unable to read English at the sixth-grade level might also be inappropriate. Poorly educated people might respond differently than other groups to the preoperative teaching. Subjects unable to read at the sixth-grade level might not be able to read or comprehend written material given to them. They might be reluctant to ask questions when they did not understand something. Many of them may have difficulty organizing their ideas and would not be able to express them to another person. They might try to conceal their lack of understanding, making it difficult to clarify misconceptions. Thus the preoperative teaching program developed for a more educated population may be unlikely to alter the postoperative outcome or length of hospital stay of members of a poorly educated population.

The researchers also limited the population to individuals who had no previous surgery because they would have the least knowledge of the postoperative experience and how they might best care for themselves. To test differences among groups, the most extreme groups are selected so that the differences are as great as possible, and the statistical procedures are most likely to determine a difference. In this hypothetical study of preoperative teaching, one group would have either standard care or the small amount of teaching the hospital routinely provides, and the other group would receive the preoperative teaching treatment. Thus the researchers would expect that the patients' knowledge of how to take care of themselves after surgery would be limited in the standard care group and their length of stay longer. In the treatment group, the researchers could control the subjects' knowledge about how to take care of themselves after surgery by providing the information through a structured preoperative teaching program. The researchers would hypothesize that the subjects will use the information to take better care of themselves after surgery, which would result in a shorter hospital stay.

However, the researchers might argue that the findings can be generalized to patients who have had previous surgery. The effect of the preoperative teaching on patients with past surgical experience might be less than the effect on subjects without past surgical experience, because experienced patients might already know some of the information taught. However, the experienced patients might also be able to use the information to take better care of themselves after surgery and thus shorten their hospital stay. Therefore the researchers' claim that the findings can be generalized to patients who have had previous surgery may be justified. However, researchers need to be very cautious not to generalize beyond their sampling criteria, unless there is a sound rationale for this based on the findings from previous research.

In critiquing a study, you need to address the following questions:

1. What are the sampling or eligibility criteria in the study?
2. Are inclusion sampling criteria, exclusion sampling criteria, or both used to determine the target population?
3. Are sampling criteria appropriate for the study problem, purpose, and design?
4. Is the study sample homogeneous or heterogeneous?
5. What are the limitations of the study based on the sampling criteria?
6. In examining the study conclusions, did the researcher generalize beyond the sampling criteria? The logic of the generalizations that were made in the study should be critiqued.

Lyon and Munro (2001) studied the disease severity and symptoms of depression in Black Americans infected with the human immunodeficiency virus (HIV) and defined their sampling or eligibility criteria as follows:

"Data for this study were collected from 79 HIV-infected Black adults, who sought routine health care services through a University-based clinic that serves as a regional referral center in a small city in the Southeastern United States…. Inclusion criteria for the study included (1) an HIV-seropositive diagnosis, (2) an immunological panel drawn the date of primary data collection, (3) physical ability to comfortably endure filling out the questionnaire packet, (4) age greater than 18 years, and (5) willingness to allow chart access for the investigator to obtain laboratory data. Exclusion criteria included (1) diagnosis of dementia or other significant psychiatric disease (excluding depression), (2) central nervous system involvement of disease, as determined by chart review and/or investigator screening using a score of 19 or less on the Cognitive Capacity Screening Examination.... (3) initiation of significant change in antiretroviral medication in the month preceding data collection for the study, and/or (4) current or previous protease inhibitor use." (p. 5)

Lyon and Munro's (2001) inclusion and exclusion sampling criteria precisely designated the characteristics of the subjects who comprised the target population. These sampling criteria were probably narrowly defined by the researchers to promote the selection of a homogeneous sample of adult Black Americans with a diagnosis of HIV, documented by lab tests. These sampling criteria are supportive of the study purpose, which was to expand the understanding of depression and its relationship to HIV disease severity in a selected culture, Black Americans. The exclusion criteria, dementia, other psychiatric diseases, and central nervous system involvement with HIV disease, were implemented to prevent these extraneous variables from influencing the subjects' responses to the study measurement tools. The significant change in antiretroviral medication in the last month and the use of protease inhibitor were controlled to decrease the influence of the severity of the HIV disease on the study variables. These sampling criteria limit generalization of the study findings but studying this sample provides information on a very understudied population of Black Americans with HIV.

Lyon and Munro's (2001) sample included 79 subjects, which is somewhat small for a descriptive-correlational study. However, 79 subjects might be considered an adequate sample size, when studying such a specific target population. These researchers did not attempt to generalize their findings beyond the sample studied. Thus they made no claim that their findings would apply to all HIV-infected Black Americans. The researchers did identify the following implications for practice: "there is a significant unmet need for identification and treatment of depressive symptoms among Blacks receiving routine care for HIV disease.... Because depression is amenable to treatment, identifying depressive symptoms is an important part of clinical assessment" (Lyon & Munro, 2001, p. 9). They also identified the need for further research by stating that:

"the elevated level of depressive symptoms in this sample indicates a need for future research that specifically addresses depressive disorders in Black men and women living with HIV disease. Given that elevated depressive symptoms were not associated with either HIV disease stage, demographic variables, or laboratory markers, other factors need to be explored that may be associated with, or predictive of depressive symptoms in Blacks living with HIV disease." (p. 9)

Representativeness

Representativeness means that the sample, the accessible population, and the target population are alike in as many ways as possible. Representativeness needs to be evaluated in terms of the setting, characteristics of the subjects, and distribution of values on variables measured in the study. Individuals seeking care in a particular setting may be different from those who would seek care for the same problem in other settings or from those who choose to use self-care to manage their problems. The setting can influence representativeness in a variety of ways. Studies conducted in private hospitals usually exclude the poor. Other settings may exclude the older adults or the undereducated. Those who do not have access to care are usually excluded from studies. Subjects in research centers and the care they receive are different from patients and the care they receive in community hospitals, public hospitals, veterans' hospitals, or rural hospitals. People living in rural settings may respond differently to a health situation than those who live in urban settings. Obese individuals who chose to enter a program to lose weight may differ from those who did not enter such a program. Thus gathering subjects across a variety of settings provides a more representative sample of the target population than limiting the study to a single setting.

A sample should be representative in terms of characteristics such as age, gender, ethnicity, income, and education, which often influence study variables. These are examples of demographic or attribute variables that might be selected by the researchers for examination in their study. The data collected on the demographic variables are analyzed to produce the sample characteristics, which are used to provide a picture of the sample. For example, the sample characteristics in the preoperative teaching study might have been that the mean age of the subjects was 55 (SD=5.6), the majority were female (65%), and they had varied ethnic backgrounds (45% Caucasian, 25% African American, 23% Hispanic, and 7% other). The sample characteristics should be representative of the characteristics of the population. If the study includes groups, the subjects in the groups should have comparable demographic characteristics. Chapter 3 contains a more detailed discussion of demographic variables and sample characteristics.

The sample should be representative, relative to the variables being examined in the study. For example, if the study examined attitudes toward acquired immunodeficiency syndrome (AIDS), the sample should be representative of the distribution of attitudes toward AIDS that exist in the specified population. If a study involved blood pressures of patients in a surgical recovery room, the blood pressures of subjects should be representative of those usually noted in a surgical recovery unit.

Measurement values should also be representative. Measurement values in a study are expected to vary randomly among subjects. *Random variation* is the expected difference in values that occurs when different subjects from the same sample are examined. The difference is random because some values will be higher and others lower than the average (mean) population value. As sample size increases, random variation decreases, improving representativeness.

Systematic variation, or systematic bias—a serious concern in sampling—is a consequence of selecting subjects whose measurement values differ in some specific way from those of the population. This difference is usually expressed as a difference in the average (or mean) values between the sample and the population. Because the subjects have something in common, their values tend to be similar to those of others in the sample but different in some way from those of the population as a whole. These values do not vary randomly around the population mean. Most of the variation from the mean is in the same direction; it is systematic. For example, the sample mean may be higher than the mean of the target population. Increasing the sample size has no effect on systematic variation.

If all the subjects in a study examining some type of knowledge have an intelligence quotient (IQ) above 120, then all of their test scores in the study are likely to be higher than the mean IQ of a population (100) that includes individuals with a wide variation in IQ scores. The IQs of the subjects would introduce a systematic bias. When a systematic bias occurs in an experimental study, it can lead the researcher to think that the treatment has made a difference, when in actuality the values would have been different even without the treatment.

The probability of systematic variation increases when the sampling process is not random. However, even in a random sample, systematic variation can occur when a large number of the potential subjects declines participation. The greater the number declining participation, the greater the possibility of a systematic bias. In published studies researchers might identify a *refusal rate,* which is the percentage of subjects that declined to participate in the study, and the subjects' rationales for not participating. For example, in their study of predictors of acute coronary syndromes in younger and older patients, Milner, Funk, Richards, Vaccarino, and Krumholz (2001), stated that the refusal rate for participation in their study was less than 1%. This low rate of refusal to participate in this study made the sample more representative of the population.

Systematic variation may also occur in studies with sample mortality or attrition. *Sample mortality* is the withdrawal or loss of subjects from a study. Systematic variation is greatest when a high number of subjects withdraw from the study before data collection is completed or when a large number of subjects withdraw from one group but not the other(s) in the study. In studies involving a treatment, subjects in the control group who do not receive the treatment may be more likely to withdraw from the study. Sample mortality or attrition should be reported in the published study.

 In critiquing a published study, you need to evaluate the representativeness of the sample by addressing the following questions.

1. Are the demographic characteristics of the sample comparable to the target population? The researcher may provide information about the target population in the literature review. Otherwise, in making a judgment, there are limitations about what is known about the target population.

2. Are the mean sample values of the study variables comparable to the values of the target population, as determined from previous research?

Continued

3. What is the sample mortality? Does the author provide information on characteristics of subjects who left the study and why the subjects left? If the author does not directly report this information, it might be found by comparing the number of subjects originally included in the study with the number used in reporting statistical results.

4. What are the possibilities of systematic bias in the setting and characteristics of the sample, and the ranges of values on measured variables? The number and characteristics of persons who declined to participate in the study should be determined. As the number of subjects who decline to participate increases, the probability of systematic bias increases. Subjects who decline may be different in important ways from those who agree to participate.

Example Critique of Representativeness

Pellino (1997) conducted a study of the relationships between patient attitudes, subjective norms, perceived control, and analgesic use following elective orthopedic surgery. She described her sampling method, refusal rate, and sample mortality as follows.

"Adults scheduled for elective orthopedic surgery were recruited from the outpatient practices of 32 orthopedic surgeons in two cities in the Midwest. Patients were excluded if they had a known history of drug or alcohol abuse. Two hundred and forty patients were approached and 172 patients agreed to participate (a 70% recruitment rate) [30% refusal rate]. Reasons for not participating included time constraints, the questionnaire was too long, and being overwhelmed by the prospect of having surgery. Complete data were available for 137 subjects who returned the postoperative questionnaire and had no missing data on critical variable(s). Subjects who used over two standard deviations more than the mean of the group for medication intake were dropped ($n = 2$).

The 69 women and 68 men who completed the study had an average age of 51.9 (SD = 16.1) years (range = 18-87 years). Subjects reported completing an average of 13.3 (SD = 2.6) years of education (range 6-23 years) and a middle economic status [M = 2.87; range = 1 (lower) to 5 (upper)]. A variety of orthopedic disorders (such as degenerative joint disease, scoliosis, and trauma) and procedures (such as total joint replacements, spinal fusions, and ligament reconstructions) were represented in the sample. The majority of patients ($n = 103$) had PCA [patient-controlled analgesia] ordered; intramuscular (IM), oral, or epidural analgesia was ordered as the primary pain medication for 34 patients." (p. 99)

In this study the sampling criteria identified subjects as adults scheduled for elective orthopedic surgery. Exclusion criteria included a known history of drug or alcohol abuse. Given the focus of the study on analgesic use, this exclusion seems appropriate since persons with a history of drug or alcohol abuse might be different from others in their analgesic use, increasing the risk of bias in the sample. Selecting patients with a variety of diagnoses and procedures provides a heterogeneous sample, which allows generalization to a larger target population. Accessing subjects from the outpatient practices of 32 orthopedic surgeons decreases the bias that could occur from recruiting patients at a single surgical facility. However, this sampling strategy excludes patients who are financially unable to access this type of outpatient practice. Thus the results cannot be generalized to low-income patients without further study. No ethnic description of subjects is provided. Since the literature provides evidence of cultural differences in attitudes, expression, and management of pain, this seems like a serious omission. Because of the lack of information provided about the sample, it is not possible to determine whether or not the findings can be generalized to various ethnic groups. The study had a refusal rate of 30% and a mortality rate of 20%, since 35 of the 172 who agreed to participate in the study withdrew. Both the refusal rate and sample mortality probably resulted in systematic variation that reduced the representativeness of the sample.

Random Sampling

From a sampling theory perspective each individual in the population should have an opportunity to be selected for the sample. One method of providing this opportunity is referred to as *random sampling.* The purpose of random sampling is to increase the extent to which the sample is representative of the target population. However, random sampling must take place in an accessible population that is representative of the target population. It is rarely possible to obtain a random sample for clinical nursing studies because of informed consent requirements. Those who volunteer to participate in a study may differ in important ways from those not willing to participate. (Methods of achieving random samples are described later in the chapter.) The use of the term *control group* is limited to those studies using random sampling methods. If nonrandom methods are used for sample selection, the group not receiving a treatment is referred to as a *comparison group* because there is an increased possibility of preexisting differences between the experimental and comparison groups.

Sampling Frames

For each person in the accessible population to have an opportunity for selection in the sample, each person in the population must be identified. To accomplish this, a list of every member of the population must be acquired, using the sampling criteria to define eligibility. This list is referred to as the *sampling frame.* Subjects are then selected from the sampling frame using a sampling plan.

Sampling Plans

A *sampling plan* outlines strategies used to obtain a sample for a study. Like a design, a sampling plan is not specific to a study. The plan is designed to increase representativeness and decrease systematic bias. The sampling plan may use probability (random) or nonprobability (nonrandom) sampling methods.

In critiquing a study, you need to be able to identify and describe the sampling plan the researcher used. You need to use critical reasoning skills to answer the following questions:

1. Has the researcher successfully implemented the sampling plan?
2. How effective is the sampling plan in achieving representativeness?
3. In what ways is the sample not representative?
4. Are there possibilities for biases in the sample?
5. Were subjects selected from a sampling frame?
6. Is random sampling used?
7. Are control groups or comparison groups used in the study?

PROBABILITY SAMPLING METHODS

Probability sampling methods have been developed to increase the representativeness of the sample. In *probability sampling,* every member (element) of the population has a probability higher than zero of being selected for the sample. To achieve this probability, the sample is obtained randomly. All the subsets of the population, which may differ from each other but contribute to the parameters of the population, have a chance to be represented in the sample. There is less opportunity for systematic bias when subjects are selected randomly, although it is possible for a systematic bias to occur by chance. Without random sampling strategies, the researchers, who have a vested interest in the study, could tend (consciously or unconsciously) to select subjects whose conditions or behaviors are consistent with the study hypotheses. The researchers could decide that person X would be a better subject for the study than person Y. In addition, the researchers could exclude a subset of people from being selected as subjects because they do not agree with them, do not like them, or find them hard to deal with. Potential subjects could be excluded because they are too sick, not sick enough, coping too well, not coping adequately, uncooperative, or noncompliant. By using random sampling, researchers leave the selection to chance and thus increase the validity of their studies. Four sampling designs have been developed to achieve probability sampling: simple random sampling, stratified random sampling, cluster sampling, and systematic sampling.

Simple Random Sampling

Simple random sampling is the most basic of the probability sampling plans, and it is achieved by randomly selecting elements from the sampling frame. Random selec-

TABLE 8-1

SECTION FROM A RANDOM NUMBERS TABLE

06	84	10	22	56	72	25	70	69	43
07	63	10	34	66	39	54	02	33	85
03	19	63	93	72	52	13	30	44	40
77	32	69	58	25	15	55	38	19	62
20	01	94	54	66	88	43	91	34	28

tion can be accomplished in a variety of ways, limited only by the imagination of the researcher. If the sampling frame is small, names can be written on slips of paper, placed in a container, mixed well, and then drawn out one at a time until the desired sample size has been reached. The most common method of random selection is to use a table of random numbers. A section from a random numbers table is presented in Table 8-1. To use a table of random numbers, the researcher places a pencil or finger on the table with the eyes closed. That number is the starting place. Then, moving the pencil or finger up, down, right, or left, numbers are used in order until the desired sample size is obtained. Table 8-1 could be used in the following way to select 5 subjects from a population of 100. If the pencil was initially placed on 58 in Table 8-1, which is the fourth column from the left and the fourth row down, and then moved across the columns to the right, the subject numbers would be 58, 25, 15, 55, and 38. Table 8-1 is useful only when the population number is less than 100. However, tables and computer programs are available for selecting larger populations. A large Table of Random Numbers is available in Appendix A of Burns and Grove (2001, p. 760).

Shelton (2001) used simple random sampling to study the emotional disorders in young offenders in the Maryland Juvenile Justice System. She examined the "psychopathology and level of functioning in a random sample of 312 committed and detained youth (60 females, 252 males)" (p. 259). Shelton (2001) described her sampling method as follows.

"This cross-sectional design was used to randomly sample all youth in 15 detention and committed juvenile justice facilities in Maryland over a 4-month period in 1996. Twenty-five percent of male youth in facilities during the time of data collection were randomly sampled. All female youth (n = 60) were sampled because of their small number. This 60% to 40% split was consistent with proportions in the system between committed and detention programs." (p. 260)

The sampling frame was all youth who were in 15 detention and committed juvenile justice facilities in Maryland over a 4-month period. The sampling plan involved the random selection of 25% of the males from the sampling frame. Shel-

Continued

ton (2001) did not discuss the refusal rate, which might have been zero. Data were collected and analyzed on all subjects, indicating that sample mortality was zero. Thus the simple random sampling method used in this study probably provided a representative sample of both committed and detained youth in the Maryland Juvenile Justice System.

Stratified Random Sampling

Stratified random sampling is used in situations in which the researcher knows some of the variables in the population that are critical for achieving representativeness. Variables commonly used for stratification include age, gender, ethnicity, socioeconomic status, diagnosis, geographic region, type of institution, type of care, and site of care. Stratification ensures that all levels of the identified variables will be adequately represented in the sample. With stratification the researcher can use a smaller sample size to achieve the same degree of representativeness, relative to the stratified variable that would result from a large sample acquired through simple random sampling. One disadvantage is that a large population must be available from which to select subjects.

If the researcher used stratification, categories (strata) of the variables selected for stratification need to be defined in the published report. For example, using ethnicity for stratification, the researcher might have defined four strata: Caucasian, African American, Mexican American, and other. The population might have been 60% Caucasian, 20% African American, 15% Mexican American, and 5% other. The researcher might have selected a random sample for each stratum equivalent to the target population proportions of that stratum. Alternatively, equal numbers of subjects might have been randomly selected for each stratum. For example, if age was used to stratify a sample of 100 subjects, the researcher might have obtained 25 subjects age 18 to 34, 25 subjects aged 35 to 50, 25 subjects aged 51 to 66, and 25 subjects over age 66.

Uphold, Lenz, and Soeken (2000) used stratified random sampling to study the "social support transactions between professional and nonprofessional women and their mothers" (p. 447). The following text describes their sampling procedure.

"A stratified, random sampling procedure was used to select participants. Computer printouts which listed all full-time, permanent, female clerical workers and faculty members were obtained from the personnel directors of two campuses of a large statewide university system.... Because there was no way of determining demographic characteristics of potential participants before collecting the data, a decision was made to send questionnaires to all women who were selected by the sampling procedure, then to exclude from analysis the women who were less than 25 years of age and women who had severely ill or demented mothers.

> A table of random numbers was used to select the desired number of women from each job category. From the printout, 470 nonprofessional women (i.e., clerical workers) and 470 professional women (i.e., faculty members) or a total of 940 university employees were selected.
>
> A total of 620 women or 66% of the original sample returned the questionnaire. Of these 620 respondents, six women were eliminated because they failed to complete the questionnaire correctly and 239 women were eliminated because of failure to meet the study criteria. Twenty-four women were eliminated because of their age, 16 women were eliminated because of their mothers' health conditions, and 199 women were eliminated because they did not have a living, elderly dyad member. The final sample consisted of 210 faculty members and 165 clerical workers, or a total of 375 respondents." (p. 451)
>
> From the universities' personnel directors, Uphold and colleagues (2000) obtained computerized lists of nonprofessional and professional women that clearly identified the study's sampling frame or a list of every potential subject in the accessible population. The researchers also identified the random selection process and the stratification of subjects into two categories, nonprofessional and professional women. The sample has a potential for bias since the two groups of women were unequal (210 professional women and 165 nonprofessional women). However, the final sample was large (375 subjects) and the 66% return rate for questionnaires is strong, which increase the representativeness of the sample in this study.

Cluster Sampling

In *cluster sampling,* a sampling frame is developed that includes a list of all the states, cities, institutions, or organizations with which elements of the identified population would be linked. A randomized sample of these states, cities, institutions, or organizations would then be used in the study. In some cases, this randomized selection continues through several stages and is then referred to as *multistage sampling.* For example, the researcher might first randomly select states and then randomly select cities within the sampled states. Then hospitals within the randomly selected cities might be randomly selected. Within the hospitals, nursing units might be randomly selected. At this level, all the patients on the nursing unit who fit the criteria for the study might be included, or patients could be randomly selected.

Cluster sampling is used in two situations. The first is one in which the researcher considers it necessary to obtain a geographically dispersed sample but realizes that a simple random sample would be prohibitive in terms of travel time and cost. The second situation is one in which the individual elements making up the population are not known, thus preventing the development of a sampling frame. For example, there is no list of all individuals in the United States who have had open-heart surgery. In such a case it is often possible to obtain lists of institutions or organizations with which the elements of interest are associated and randomly select institutions from which subjects could be acquired.

> Golding (1996) used multistage probability sampling in her study, "Sexual Assault History and Limitations in Physical Functioning in Two General Population Samples." The following text describes her sampling technique.
>
> "Respondents were selected using multistage area probability sampling from household residents 18 years of age and older at each site. The Los Angeles sample was selected to represent adults in two mental health catchment areas in Los Angeles County, one of which was 83% Latino and the other 21% Latino. The Latino residents were largely of Mexican cultural or ethnic origin…. The North Carolina sample was selected to represent adults in two mental health catchment areas in North Carolina, one consisting of Durham County, which is primarily urban, and the other four contiguous rural counties." (p. 34)
>
> The author used pooled data obtained from two sites of a five-site program initiated by the National Institute of Mental Health (NIMH). Information provided about the sampling method is sparse. The researcher does not provide a rationale for the use of multistage sampling or reasons for choosing the selected sites. Although the author indicates that this is a probability sample, she does not indicate how the sites or subjects were randomly chosen. There is some indication that the original study may have intentionally chosen one area with a large Hispanic population, but no mention is made of a similar effort to include other minority groups. There also appeared to be an effort to include both urban and rural sites. There is insufficient information to judge the adequacy of the sampling plan.

Systematic Sampling

Systematic sampling can be conducted when an ordered list of all members of the population is available. The process involves selecting every kth individual on the list, using a starting point selected randomly. If the initial starting point is not random, the sample is not a probability sample. To use this design, the researcher must know the number of elements in the population and the size of the sample desired. The population size is divided by the desired sample size, giving k, the size of the gap between elements selected from the list. For example, if the population size is $N = 1200$ and the desired sample size is $n = 100$, then $k = 12$. Every 12th person on the list would be included in the sample. This value is obtained by using the following formula: $k = 1200 \div 100 = 12$. Some argue that this procedure does not truly give each element an opportunity to be included in the sample; it provides a random but not equal chance for inclusion.

Tolle, Tilden, Rosenfeld, and Hickman (2000) used systematic sampling in their study, "Family Reports of Barriers to Optimal Care of the Dying." They described their sampling plan as follows.

"After approval of Institutional Review Boards at both the University and the Oregon Health Division, death certificates for all Oregon deaths occurring in the 14 months between November 1996 and December 1997 were systematically randomly sampled, excluding decedents under the age of 18 years and deaths attributable to suicide, homicide, accident or those undergoing medical examiner review. Out of a sampling frame of $N = 24,074$, the systematic random sample yielded 1458 death certificates. Although the name of a family contact is listed on each death certificate, Oregon death certificates do not list an address or telephone number for family contacts. As a result, case finding for family contacts was unsuccessful for 44% of the sample. Using newspaper obituaries and published telephone directories, a total of 816 family contacts were located, of whom 59% ($n = 475$) agreed to participate.... Of those who refused, the most frequent reason mentioned for not participating was that talking about the death would be too painful." (p. 311)

The systematic sampling plan used by Tolle and colleagues (2000) has both strengths and weaknesses. Because their sampling frame was 24,074 death certificates and their desired sample size was 1458, the researchers systematically selected every 16th death certificate to identify families for inclusion in their study. Two potential areas of bias are that 44% of the families of the originally selected 1458 death certificates could not be contacted. Of the 816 families contacted, 41% refused to participate. Those families who could not be contacted or refused to participate might be different in some way from those who did participate, which decreases the sample's representativeness of the population. However, the representativeness of the sample is strengthened by the sample size, $n = 475$, and the use of a probability sampling method.

NONPROBABILITY SAMPLING METHODS USED IN QUANTITATIVE RESEARCH

In *nonprobability sampling,* not every element of the population has an opportunity for selection in the sample. Although this approach decreases a sample's representativeness of a population, it is commonly used in nursing studies. In an analysis of nursing studies published in six nursing journals from 1977 to 1986, only 9% used random sampling (Moody et al., 1988). Since this trend continues today, many of the nursing studies use nonprobability sampling methods. Thus nurses should be able to discriminate among the various nonprobability sampling plans used in nursing research. Each plan addresses a different research need. The four nonprobability sampling plans used most frequently in nursing research are: convenience sampling, quota sampling, purposive sampling, and network sampling. Convenience sampling and quota sampling are often used in quantitative studies. Purposive sampling and network sampling are used more frequently in qualitative research and will be discussed later in this chapter.

Convenience Sampling

Convenience sampling (also called "accidental sampling") is considered a poor approach because it provides little opportunity to control for biases; subjects are included in the study merely because they happened to be in the right place at the right time. A classroom of students, patients who attend a clinic on a specific day, subjects who attend a support group, patients currently admitted to a hospital with a specific diagnosis or nursing problem, and every fifth person who enters the emergency room on a given day are examples of convenience samples. Available subjects are simply entered into the study until the desired sample size is reached. Multiple biases may exist in the sample, some of which may be subtle and unrecognized. However, serious biases are not always present in convenience samples.

Convenience samples are inexpensive, accessible, and usually less time-consuming than other types of samples. They provide means to conduct studies on topics that cannot be examined with probability sampling. However, this type of sampling should be used in quantitative studies only when it is not possible to obtain a sample by other means.

Most quasi-experimental studies and clinical trials in both medicine and nursing use convenience sampling. As a component of the study design, subjects are randomly assigned to groups. This random assignment to groups, which is not a sampling method, does not alter the risk of biases resulting from convenience sampling. With these potential biases and the narrowly defined sampling criteria used to select subjects in most clinical trials, representativeness of the sample is a concern.

In critiquing a study using a convenience sample, you need to judge the representativeness of the sample by addressing the following questions.
1. Could the researcher have used another sampling method to improve study validity given the circumstances of the study?
2. Did the researcher identify and describe the known biases in the sampling plan?
3. Were the steps taken to increase the representativeness of the sample explained?

Song and Lee (2001) conducted a quasi-experimental study to "determine the effects of a 12-week cardiac rehabilitation exercise program on the motivation and lifestyle of persons recovering from a recent heart attack or cardiac-related procedures" (p. 200). The researchers conducted their study with a convenience sample and described their sampling plan as follows.

"A convenient sample of 114 adults was selected and divided evenly into 2 groups. The sampling procedure required that the prospective subjects met the following criteria: (1) diagnosed with myocardial infarction (MI) or angina, or having undergone cardiac-related procedures such as CABG (coronary artery bypass graft) surgery or PTCA (percutaneous transluminal coronary angioplasty); (2) able to participate in cardiac rehabilitation exercise program for more than 8 weeks (for the exercise group) with an attendance rate of more than 70%; and (3) classified as being a low to intermediate risk for a recurrent cardiac event secondary to the prescribed exercise, according to the risk stratification procedure." (pp. 201–202)

Four cardiac rehabilitation centers in Northeast Ohio provided a 12-week exercise program that was based on recommendations made by the American Heart Association.... The subjects in the exercise program were recruited on the first day of the program.... The subjects in the comparison group were contacted by phone 8 to 10 weeks after they were discharged. (p. 202)

A total of 133 subjects (70 for the exercise group and 63 for the comparison group) participated in the study for the pretest measure, and 57 subjects for each group were available after 12 weeks for the post-test. The dropout rate from the cardiac rehabilitation program for the sample was 12%, which was much lower than the rate (20% to 50%) reported in previous studies.

The age of the subjects ranged from 40 to 81 years, with a mean age of 64.6 years for the exercise group (SD, 10.4) and 64.0 years for the comparison group (SD, 7.6). The majority of the subjects were white (96%) and married (76%). Women made up about 35% of the total sample, which was close to the reported ratio of the population who had undergone cardiac-related procedures.... Compared with the comparison group, significantly more persons in the exercise group had completed college or held graduate degrees (F = 12.5, P < .05) and earned higher annual incomes (F = 14.6, P < .05). No significant differences were found between the groups in other demographic characteristics." (p. 204)

Song and Lee (2001) attempted to make the sample as representative of the accessible population as possible by recruiting a large sample of 114 subjects from four rehabilitation centers. The attrition rate of 12% was compared to previous research and found to be minimal for this type of study. The percent of females in the sample was consistent with the target population. The researchers also compared the demographic variables of the experimental group with those of the comparison group and noted significant differences related to education and income. These differences were controlled by the use of selected statistical analysis techniques. Another source of bias was the self-selection of subjects into the experimental and comparison groups rather than the random assignment of subjects to groups. The researchers identified and described this bias by stating:

Continued

"Random assignment of subjects to the 2 groups was neither feasible nor ethically acceptable in this study because the outpatient cardiac rehabilitation program has been routinely recommended for its beneficial effects. Consequently sample bias in the study may have contributed to nonsignificant group differences on the post-test, even with statistical control." (Song & Lee, 2001, p. 207)

Convenience sampling can be strengthened, as in this study, but still has a potential for bias that can influence study outcomes and decrease the sample's representativeness of the target population.

Quota Sampling

Quota sampling uses a convenience sampling technique with an added feature—a strategy to ensure the inclusion of subject types who are likely to be underrepresented in the convenience sample, such as females, minority groups, and those individuals who are elderly, poor, rich, or undereducated. The goal of quota sampling is to replicate the proportions of subgroups present in the population. The technique is similar to that used in stratified random sampling. Quota sampling requires that the researcher be able to identify subgroups in the target population that are important for achieving representativeness in the problem being studied. In addition, the researcher must determine what proportion of the target population each identified subgroup represents. Quota sampling offers an improvement over convenience sampling and tends to decrease potential biases.

In critiquing a study using a quota sampling method, you need to use critical thinking to judge the adequacy of the subgroups selected in improving the representativeness of the sample. You might ask the following questions:
1. Were the subgroups selected appropriate for the study purpose?
2. Were the proportions assigned to each subgroup reflective of the target population?

Milner, Funk, Richards, Vaccarino, and Krumholz (2001) used quota sampling in their study of the symptoms that are predictors of acute coronary syndromes (ACS), including unstable angina and acute myocardial infarction (MI), in younger and older patients. They described their sampling plan as follows.

"The study was conducted in the ED [emergency department] of a 900-bed regional cardiac referral center in New England. Patients were approached if they were > 45 years of age and reported at least one typical or atypical symptom suggestive of ACS.... A total of 536 patients met study criteria and were approached for participation. Of these, 531 patients agreed to participate (< 1% refusal rate). Patients were stratified into two age groups, > 70 years (n = 208) and < 70 years (n = 323). Age 70 was selected as the cut-off based on previous research which demonstrated that presentation

with typical symptoms is less common in individuals over 70 years of age."
(p. 235)

Milner and colleagues (2001) selected a convenience sample of 531 subjects, who were stratified into two subgroups: under 70 years of age and over 70 years of age. The sample size and the stratification of subjects into subgroups based on previous research increase the representativeness of the sample. However, a potential bias exists since the subgroups were of unequal size, with one group having 115 more subjects than the other group.

CRITIQUING SAMPLE SIZE IN QUANTITATIVE STUDIES

One of the most troublesome questions that arise during the critique of a study is whether the sample size was adequate. If the study was designed to make comparisons and significant differences were found, the *sample size*, or number of subjects participating in the study, was adequate. Questions about the adequacy of the sample size occur only when no significance was found. Thus when critiquing a quantitative study in which no significance was found in at least one of the hypotheses or research questions, the adequacy of the sample size should be evaluated. Is there really no difference or relationship? Or is there a difference or relationship that was not found because of inadequacies in the research methods?

Currently, the adequacy of the sample size is evaluated using a *power analysis*. *Power* is the capacity of the study to detect differences or relationships that actually exist in the population. Expressed another way, it is the capacity to correctly reject a null hypothesis. The minimum acceptable level of power for a study is 0.8 (Cohen, 1988). This power level results in a 20% chance of a Type II error, in which the study fails to detect existing effects (differences or relationships). An increasing number of researchers are performing a power analysis before the conduct of their study to determine an adequate sample size. The results of this analysis are usually included in the sample section of the published study. Researchers should also perform a power analysis to evaluate the adequacy of their sample size for all nonsignificant findings and include this in the discussion section of their published study.

Nurse researchers have only recently begun using power analysis to evaluate sample size. Polit and Sherman (1990) evaluated the sample size of 62 studies published in 1989 in *Nursing Research* and *Research in Nursing & Health*. They found that most of the studies examined had inadequate sample sizes for making comparisons between groups. The studies needed an average of 218 subjects per group to have a power level of 0.8. Therefore, in most of these studies, the risk of a Type II error was extremely high. A power analysis was performed in only one of the studies to determine the adequacy of the sample size.

Other factors that influence the adequacy of sample size (because they affect power) include effect size, type of study, number of variables, sensitivity of the measurement tools, and data analysis techniques. In critiquing the adequacy of the sample size, the influence of all of these factors should be considered.

Effect Size

The effect is the presence of the phenomenon examined in a study. *Effect size* is the extent to which the null hypothesis is false. In a study in which two populations are compared, the null hypothesis states that the difference between the two populations is zero. However, if the null hypothesis were false, there would be an effect. If the null hypothesis is false, it is false to some degree; this is the effect size (Cohen, 1988). The statistical test tells you that there is a difference between groups. The effect size tells you how much this difference is.

When the effect size is large (e.g., considerable difference between groups), detecting it is easy and requires only a small sample; when the effect size is small (e.g., only a small difference between groups), detecting it is more difficult and requires larger samples. Broadly, a small effect size would be about 0.2, a medium effect size 0.5, and a large effect size 0.8 (Cohen, 1988). Effect size is smaller with a small sample, and thus effects are more difficult to detect. Increasing the sample size also increases the effect size, making it more likely that the effect will be detected.

In the nursing studies examined by Polit and Sherman (1990), 52.7% of the effect sizes computed were small. These researchers found that in nursing studies, for small effects, average power was less than 0.3. Thus there was less than a 30% probability that acceptance of the null hypothesis was correct. In most cases, this was due to an insufficient sample size. Even when the effect size was moderate, the average power in the nursing studies examined was only 0.7. The nursing studies reached an acceptable level of power only when the effect size was large, and 11% of these studies were underpowered. Only 15% of the studies had sufficient power for all of their analyses.

Types of Quantitative Studies

Descriptive studies (particularly those using survey questionnaires) and correlational studies often require very large samples. In these studies, multiple variables may be examined, and extraneous variables are likely to affect subject response(s) to the variables under study. Statistical comparisons are often made on multiple subgroups in the sample, requiring that an adequate sample be available for each subgroup being analyzed. Quasi-experimental and experimental studies use smaller samples more often than descriptive and correlational studies do. As control in the study increases, the sample size can decrease and still approximate the population. Instruments in these studies tend to be more refined, thus increasing precision. Designs that use blocking or stratification usually increase the total sample size required. Designs that use matched pairs of subjects have increased power and thus require a smaller sample (Burns & Grove, 2001).

Number of Variables

As the number of variables under study increases, the sample size needed may increase. Including variables such as age, gender, ethnicity, and education in the data analyses can increase the sample size needed to detect differences between groups. Using them only to describe the sample does not cause a problem in terms of power. A number of the studies analyzed by Polit and Sherman (1990) had sufficient sample size for the primary analyses but failed to plan for analyses involving subgroups, such as analyzing the data by age category or ethnic group. The inclusion of multiple dependent variables also increases the sample size needed.

Measurement Sensitivity

Well-developed instruments measure phenomena with precision. A thermometer, for example, measures body temperature precisely. Tools measuring psychosocial variables tend to be less precise. However, a tool that is reliable and valid measures more precisely than a tool that is less well developed. Variance tends to be higher in a less well-developed tool than in one that is well developed. For example, if anxiety was being measured and the actual anxiety score of several subjects was 80, measures ranging from 70 to 90 might be obtained with a less well-developed tool. There is much more variation from the true score than when a well-developed tool is used, which would tend to show a score closer to the actual score of 80 for each subject. As variance in instrument scores increases, the sample size needed to obtain significance increases. Measurement sensitivity is discussed further in Chapter 9.

Data Analysis Techniques

Data analysis techniques vary in their ability to detect differences in the data. Statisticians refer to this as the "power of the statistical analysis." There is also an interaction between the measurement sensitivity and the power of the data analysis technique. The power of the analysis technique increases as precision in measurement increases. Larger samples are needed when the power of the planned statistical analysis is weak.

For some statistical procedures, such as the *t*-test and ANOVA (analysis of variances), equal group sizes will increase power because the effect size is maximized. The more unbalanced the group sizes are, the smaller the effect size is. Therefore in unbalanced groups, the total sample size must be larger (Kraemer & Theimann, 1987). The chi-square test is the weakest of the statistical tests and requires very large sample sizes to achieve acceptable levels of power. As the number of categories increases, the sample size increases. Also, if there are small numbers in some of the categories, the sample size must be increased.

Berger and Walker (2001) studied fatigue in women receiving chemotherapy for breast cancer and provided the following detailed description of their sample size.

"Sample size was determined by power analysis for multiple regression. Power analysis (Cohen, 1988), based on a maximum of 16 variables entered

Continued

in one regression equation, level of significance set at 0.05, and a medium effect size of 0.30, indicated that [a] sample of 60 subjects would produce a power of 0.80. To allow for 15% attrition, 72 subjects were recruited from the offices of medical oncologists who received referrals from surgeons affiliated with the hospitals in the study.... Seventy-seven eligible women were identified, 5 declined to participate, and 12 withdrew before completing the study, leaving a sample of 60.... Nine of the 12 women who withdrew were not married, resulting in the possibility of sample bias." (p. 45)

Berger and Walker (2001) provided an excellent description of how they achieved their final sample size. The original sample size was based on a power analysis that included a power of 0.8, alpha or level of significance of 0.05, and an effect size of 0.3, which is a small effect size. The researchers also identified the number of variables (16) and analysis technique (regression analysis) implemented in the study. They recruited enough subjects to give a sample size large enough to allow for attrition, and they examined the type of subjects who withdrew from the study. This enabled them to identify the potential sample bias related to unmarried women.

CRITIQUING THE ADEQUACY OF THE SAMPLE IN QUANTITATIVE STUDIES

In critiquing the sample of quantitative studies, you need to address the following questions:

1. Are the sampling inclusion criteria, sampling exclusion criteria, or both clearly identified and appropriate?
2. Is the sample size identified? If groups were included in the study, is the sample size for each group discussed?
3. Is a power analysis reported?
4. Is the refusal rate and sample mortality addressed? If the refusal rate or mortality is high, does the researcher provide rationales for these?
5. Are the characteristics of the sample detailed?
6. Is the sampling plan adequate to achieve a representative sample?
7. Is the sample representative of the accessible and target populations?
8. What was the possibility of Type II error?
9. Are the potential biases in the sample discussed?
10. If groups were used, were the groups equivalent?
11. Does the researcher(s) define the target population to which the findings are generalized?

SAMPLING IN QUALITATIVE RESEARCH

Qualitative research is conducted to gain insights and discover meaning about a particular experience, situation, cultural element, or historical event (Burns & Grove, 2001). The intent of qualitative research is an in-depth understanding of a purposefully selected sample and not the generalization of the findings from a randomly selected sample to a target population, as in quantitative research. Thus in qualitative research, experiences, events, and incidents are more the focus of sampling than people (Sandelowski, 1995). The researcher attempts to select subjects who are able to provide extensive information about the experience or event being studied. For example, if the goal of the study was to describe the phenomenon of living with chronic pain, the researcher would purposefully select those subjects who were articulate and reflective, had a history of chronic pain, and were willing to share their chronic pain experience (Coyne, 1997). Two common sampling methods used in qualitative research are purposive sampling and snowball sampling. These sampling methods enable the researcher to select the specific subjects who will provide the most extensive information about the phenomenon, event, or situation being studied (Clifford, 1997). The sample selection process can have a profound effect on the quality of the research and should be described in enough depth to promote the interpretation of the findings and the replication of the study.

Purposive Sampling

Purposive sampling, sometimes referred to as "judgmental, theoretical, or selective sampling," involves the conscious selection by the researcher of certain subjects, elements, events, or incidents to include in the study. Efforts might be made to include typical or atypical subjects or situations. The researcher might select subjects who are of various ages, those who have differences in diagnoses or severity of illness, or those who received an ineffective treatment rather than an effective treatment for their illness. This sampling plan has been criticized because it is difficult to evaluate the precision of the researcher's judgment. Thus researchers need to indicate the characteristics that they desire in subjects and provide a rationale for selecting these types of subjects to obtain essential data for their study. In qualitative research this sampling method seems to be the best way to gain insight into a new area of study or to obtain in-depth understanding of a complex experience or event.

 In critiquing a qualitative study using a purposive sampling method, the characteristics for which subjects were purposively selected should be identified. You need to use critical reasoning to answer the following questions.

1. What rationale does the researcher(s) give for selecting those characteristics?
2. Does the rationale seem logical to you?
3. Does (do) the researcher(s) provide information on how subjects were determined to have the characteristics selected?
4. Does the researcher describe his or her sampling plan in sufficient detail?

Scott-Findlay and Chalmers (2001) conducted an ethnographic study to describe "rural families' perspectives on having a child with cancer." (p. 205) They described their sample as follows.

"Families in the study were recruited from the pediatric oncology clinic at the provincial cancer treatment center through the pediatric oncology nurse clinician. Purposive sampling was used to obtain the rural sample and was guided by the principles of adequacy and appropriateness.... Families involved in the study included those with children who were at various points in the cancer experience; for example, those newly diagnosed, in remission, with recurrent disease, and with advanced disease. No families with a child in the palliative stage were included.

Ten families (25 family members) participated in the study.... The purposive sampling procedure was successful in including a range in the children's ages, diagnoses, and length of time since diagnosis." (p. 207)

Scott-Findlay and Chalmers (2001) clearly identified their use of a purposive sampling plan to obtain a sample of rural families, who have children diagnosed with cancer. Purposive sampling enabled the researchers to gain rich descriptions of the families' experiences and perspectives and to include families of children of various ages, diagnoses, and length of illness.

Network Sampling

Network sampling, sometimes referred to as *snowball sampling* holds promise for locating subjects who would be difficult or impossible to obtain in other ways or who had not been previously identified for study. Network sampling takes advantage of social networks and the fact that friends tend to have characteristics in common. When the researcher has found a few subjects with the necessary criteria, he or she asks their assistance in getting in touch with others with similar characteristics. The first few subjects are often obtained through a convenience sampling method and the sample size is expanded using network sampling. This sampling method is used in quantitative studies, but is more commonly used in qualitative studies. In qualitative research, network sampling is an effective strategy for identifying subjects who can provide the greatest insight and essential information about an experience or event that is being studied. This strategy is also particularly useful for finding subjects in socially devalued populations such as those who are dependent on alcohol, abuse children, commit sexual offenses, are addicted to drugs, or commit criminal acts. These individuals are seldom willing to make themselves known. Other groups, such as widows, grieving siblings, or those successful at lifestyle changes, can be located using this strategy. These individuals are outside the existing health care system and are difficult to find.

In critiquing a study using a network or snowball sampling plan, you might address the following questions:
1. Are the networks used to obtain the sample identified?
2. Were adequate and appropriate subjects identified using the network sampling plan?
3. Did the subjects provide the rich depth of data needed to address the study purpose?

Coté-Arsenault and Morrison-Beedy (2001) conducted a phenomenological study entitled "Women's Voices Reflecting Changed Expectations for Pregnancy after Perinatal Loss." They described the sampling plan for their study as follows.

"Following IRB [institutional review board] approval, a snowball sampling approach was used to recruit women who had experienced at least one perinatal loss and a minimum of one subsequent pregnancy. Recruitment was accomplished using various sources: personal contacts, the local perinatal loss support group, and flyers placed within the university community and local community health settings.... The sample consisted of 21 women with diverse pregnancy and loss histories.

The diversity of childbearing experiences was extensive, encompassing one woman who was currently pregnant, a woman who had given birth 14 weeks before, and women whose last birth was more than two decades prior to this study. The women had experienced from 1 to 7 losses which occurred throughout the three trimesters of pregnancy and at birth. All currently had living children." (p. 241)

The researchers clearly identified the networks (personal contacts, loss support group, and flyers) that were used to recruit subjects. This sampling plan successfully identified women with diverse childbearing experiences, who provided detailed data on the expectations for pregnancy after perinatal loss.

CRITIQUING SAMPLE SIZE IN QUALITATIVE STUDIES

In quantitative research, the sample size must be large enough to identify relationships among variables or to determine differences between groups. The larger the sample, the greater the power to detect relationships and differences. However, in qualitative research, the focus is on the quality of information obtained from the person, situation, or event sampled rather than the size of the sample (Sandelowski, 1995). The sample size and sampling plan are determined by the purpose of the study. The depth of information that is obtained and needed to gain insight into a phenomenon, describe a cultural element, develop a theory, or understand a historical event determines the number of people, sites, artifacts, or documents sampled. The sample size can be too small when the data collected lacks adequate depth or richness. Thus an inadequate sample size can reduce the quality and credibility of the research findings. Many qualitative researchers use purposive sampling plans to select the specific subjects, events, or situations that they believe will provide them with the rich data needed to gain insights and discover new meaning in an area of study.

The number of participants in a qualitative study is adequate when saturation of information is achieved in the study area. *Saturation of data* occurs when additional sampling provides no new information, only redundancy of previous collected data. Important factors that need to be considered in determining sample size to achieve saturation of data are: (1) scope of the study, (2) nature of the topic, (3) quality of the data, and (4) design of the study (Morse, 2000).

Scope of the Study

If the scope of the study is broad, then extensive data will be needed to address the study purpose and it will take longer to reach saturation. Thus studies with a broad scope will require more sampling of participants, events, or documents than would a study with a narrow scope (Morse, 2000). A study that has a clear focus and provides focused data collection usually has richer, more credible findings. Qualitative studies should be critiqued to determine if the sample size was adequate for the identified scope of the study.

Nature of the Topic

If the topic of study is clear and easily discussed by the subjects, then fewer subjects are needed to obtain the essential data. If the topic is difficult to define and awkward for people to discuss, then an increased number of participants will probably be needed to achieve data saturation (Morse, 2000). For example, a phenomenological study of the experience of an adult living with a history of child sexual abuse is a very sensitive, complex topic to investigate. This type of topic would probably require increased participants and interview time to collect essential data. Published studies should be critiqued to determine if the sample size was adequate based on the complexity and sensitivity of the topic studied.

Quality of the Data

The quality of information obtained from an interview, observation, or document review influences the sample size. When the quality and richness of the data are high, few participants are needed to achieve saturation of data in the area of study. Quality data are best obtained from articulate, well-informed, and communicative participants (Sandelowski, 1995). These participants are able to share more rich data in a clear and concise manner. In addition, participants who have more time to be interviewed usually provide data with greater depth and breadth. Qualitative studies require the critique of: the quality of the participants, events, or document; the richness of the data collected; and the adequacy of the sample based on the findings obtained.

Study Design

Some studies are designed to increase the number of interviews with participants. When more interviews are conducted with a person, better quality data are collected. For example, a study design that included an interview both before and after an event would produce more data than a single interview. Designs that involve interviewing a family rather than an individual produce more data than an interview with a single subject. In critiquing a qualitative study, the adequacy of the sample size for the design of the study should be determined.

CRITIQUING THE ADEQUACY OF THE SAMPLE IN QUALITATIVE STUDIES

In critiquing the sample of qualitative studies, you need to use critical reasoning to address the following questions.

1. Are the sampling inclusion criteria, sampling exclusion criteria, or both appropriate?
2. Is the sampling plan adequate to address the purpose of the study? If purposive sampling was used, does the researcher provide a rationale for the sample selection process? If network sampling was used, does the researcher identify the networks used to obtain the sample and provide a rationale for these?
3. Is the sample size adequate, based on the scope of the study, nature of the topic, quality of the data, and study design?
4. Are the sample refusal rate and the participant mortality rate for the study discussed?
5. Are the characteristics of the sample adequately described?
6. Does the researcher discuss the quality of the study participants? Were the participants articulate, well-informed, and willing to share information relevant to the study topic?
7. Did the sample produce saturation of data in the area of the study?
8. Does the researcher identify the study setting?

O'Brien (2001) conducted a qualitative study to "examine the experience of providing long-term home care for the child who is technology dependent from the family's viewpoint" (p. 14). Technology dependence was defined as the child being dependent on a medical device to compensate for a loss of vital body function and the need for ongoing nursing care to avert death or further disability. O'Brien (2001) described her sample as follows.

"A purposive sample [sampling plan] of 15 families [sample size], which included a child who was technology dependent was obtained through

Continued

family response to an introductory letter about the study distributed by health care agencies, social service agencies, and parent support groups [participant selection process]. The child who was technology dependent was 3 to 12 years of age, had been dependent on technology and living at home for at least 1 year, and was medically stable at the time of the study [sample inclusion criteria]. The sample selection continued until there was evidence of thick data description and no new data were being obtained [saturation of data]. A total of 11 mothers and 4 parent couples (mother and father) were interviewed [description of the participants], and all chose to be interviewed in their homes [setting]. One family who had originally indicated interest in the study decided not to participate because of the ongoing issues related to the pending adoption of the child who was technology dependent [refusal rate].

The demographic characteristics of the children who were technology dependent and their families varied considerably [quality of the data]. One exception was race: All of the parents were European-American, and all of the children who were technology dependent were also European-American with the exception of one African-American child [sample characteristics]." (p. 14)

O'Brien (2001) provided extensive detail of her sample and sampling plan that is quoted above. The article also included three additional paragraphs that detailed the characteristics of the sample and the quality of the study participants that were not quoted in this text. The focus of the purposive sampling plan was addressed, with a limited rationale for selecting this sampling plan. The sample size of 15 seemed adequate, since saturation of data was achieved by interviewing these families. The scope of the study, nature of the topic, quality of the data, and study design were addressed and seemed to support the sample size obtained. The refusal rate was minimal, one family out of 16 families approached, with no participant mortality. The setting of the study was identified as the home and described in more detail with the discussion of the participants and sample characteristics.

SUMMARY

Sampling involves selecting a group of people, events, behaviors, or other elements with which to conduct a study. Sampling defines the process of making the selections; sample defines the selected group of elements. Sampling theory was developed to determine the most effective way of acquiring a sample that would accurately reflect the population under study. Important concepts in sampling theory include population, population elements, sampling criteria, representativeness, randomization, sampling frame, and sampling plan.

In quantitative research a sampling plan is developed to increase representativeness, de-

crease systematic bias, and decrease sampling error. The two main types of sampling plans are probability and nonprobability. Probability sampling plans have been developed to ensure some degree of precision in estimating the population values. Thus probability samples reduce sampling error. To obtain a probability sample, the researcher must know every element in the population. A sampling frame must be developed and the sample randomly selected from the sampling frame. Four sampling designs have been developed to achieve probability sampling: simple random sampling, stratified random sampling, cluster sampling, and systematic sampling.

In nonprobability sampling, not every element of the population has an opportunity for selection in the sample. There is no sampling frame. Several types of nonprobability sampling designs exist and each addresses a different research need. The four nonprobability designs discussed in this chapter are convenience sampling, quota sampling, purposive sampling, and network sampling. Convenience sampling and quota sampling are frequently used in quantitative research. Purposive sampling and network sampling are more commonly used in qualitative research.

A major concern in critiquing the sampling procedure in quantitative research is the evaluation of the adequacy of the sample size. Factors that must be considered in making decisions about sample size include the type of study, number of variables, sensitivity of the measurement tools, data analysis techniques, and expected effect size. Detailed guidelines are provided for conducting a critique of the sample section of a quantitative study.

Qualitative research is conducted to gain insights and discover meaning about a particular experience, situation, cultural element, or historical event. The intent is to gain an in-depth understanding of a purposefully selected sample and not to generalize the findings from a randomly selected sample to a target population, as in quantitative research. Thus experiences, events, and incidents are more the focus of sampling than people. The researcher attempts to select subjects who are able to provide extensive information about the experience or event being studied. Most qualitative studies use purposive sampling that involves the conscious selection of certain subjects or elements by the researcher for inclusion in the study. A high-quality subject is a person who is articulate, well informed on the research topic, and willing to share his or her knowledge. Network sampling is also used in qualitative research to gain insight into subjects who are difficult to locate or have not been previously identified for study.

In qualitative research, the focus is on the quality of information obtained from the person, situation, or event sampled rather than the size of the sample. The sample size and sampling plan are determined by the purpose of the study. The number of participants in a qualitative study is adequate when saturation of information is achieved in the study area. Saturation of data occurs when additional sampling provides no new information, only redundancy of previous collected data. Important factors that need to be considered in determining sample size to achieve saturation of data are: (1) scope of the study, (2) nature of the topic, (3) quality of the data collected, and (4) design of the study. The chapter concludes with detailed guidelines to conduct a critique of the sample section of a qualitative study.

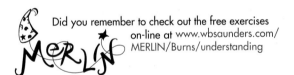 Did you remember to check out the free exercises on-line at www.wbsaunders.com/ MERLIN/Burns/understanding

REFERENCES

Berger, A. M., & Walker, S. N. (2001). An explanatory model of fatigue in women receiving adjuvant breast cancer chemotherapy. *Nursing Research, 50*(1), 42–52.

Burns, N., & Grove, S. K. (2001). *The practice of nursing research: Conduct, critique, and utilization* (4th ed.). Philadelphia: Saunders.

Clifford, C. (1997). *Qualitative research methodology in nursing and healthcare.* New York: Churchill Livingstone.

Cohen, J. (1988). *Statistical power analysis for the behavioral sciences* (2nd ed.). New York: Academic Press.

Coté-Arsenault, D., & Morrison-Beedy, D. (2001). Women's voices reflecting changed expectations for pregnancy after perinatal loss. *Journal of Nursing Scholarship, 33*(3), 239–244.

Coyne, I. T. (1997). Sampling in qualitative research. Purposeful and theoretical sampling: Merging or clear boundaries. *Journal of Advanced Nursing, 26*(3), 623–630.

Golding, J. M. (1996). Sexual assault history and limitations in physical functioning in two general population samples. *Research in Nursing & Health, 19*(1), 33–44.

Kraemer, H. C., & Theimann, S. (1987). *How many subjects? Statistical power analysis in research.* Newbury Park, CA: Sage.

Lyon, D. E., & Munro, C. (2001). Disease severity and symptoms of depression in black Americans infected with HIV. *Applied Nursing Research, 14*(1), 3–10.

Milner, K. A., Funk, M., Richards, S., Vaccarino, V., & Krumholz, H. M. (2001). Symptom predictors of acute coronary syndromes in younger and older patients. *Nursing Research, 50*(4), 233–241.

Moody, L. E., Wilson, M. E., Smyth, K., Schwartz, R., Tittle, M., & Van Cott, M. L. (1988). Analysis of a decade of nursing practice research: 1977-1986. *Nursing Research, 37*(6), 374–379.

Morse, J. M. (2000). Determining sample size. *Qualitative Health Research, 10*(1), 3–5.

O'Brien, M. E. (2001). Living in a house of cards: Family experiences with long-term childhood technology dependence. *Journal of Pediatric Nursing, 16*(1), 13–22.

Pellino, T. A. (1997). Relationships between patient attitudes, subjective norms, perceived control, and analgesic use following elective orthopedic surgery. *Research in Nursing & Health, 20*(2), 97–105.

Polit, D. F., & Sherman, R. E. (1990). Statistical power in nursing research. *Nursing Research, 39*(6), 365–369.

Sandelowski, M. (1995). Focus on qualitative methods: Sample size in qualitative research. *Research in Nursing & Health, 18*(2), 179–183.

Scott-Findlay, S., & Chalmers, K. (2001). Rural families' perspectives on having a child with cancer. *Journal of Pediatric Oncology Nursing, 18*(5), 205–216.

Shelton, D. (2001). Emotional disorders in young offenders. *Journal of Nursing Scholarship, 33*(3), 259–263.

Song, R., & Lee, H. (2001). Effects of a 12-week cardiac rehabilitation exercise program on motivation and health-promoting lifestyle. *Heart & Lung, 30*(3), 200–209.

Tolle, S. W., Tilden, V. P., Rosenfeld, A. G., & Hickman, S. E. (2000). Family reports of barriers to optimal care of the dying. *Nursing Research, 49*(6), 310–317.

Uphold, C. R., Lenz, E. R., & Soeken, K. L. (2000). Social support transactions between professional and nonprofessional women and their mothers. *Research in Nursing & Health, 23*(6), 447–460.

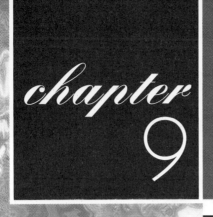

chapter 9

Measurement and Data Collection in Research

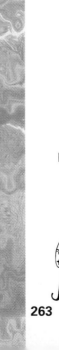
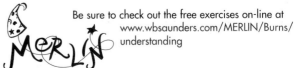

Be sure to check out the free exercises on-line at
www.wbsaunders.com/MERLIN/Burns/
understanding

OUTLINE—cont'd

Maintaining Controls
Protecting Study Integrity
Solving Problems
Serendipity

OBJECTIVES

Completing this chapter should enable you to:
1. Use measurement theory and the relevant concepts (directness of measurement, measurement error, levels of measurement, reliability, and validity) in critiquing published studies.
2. Identify possible sources of measurement error in published studies.
3. Critique the levels of measurement (nominal, ordinal, interval, and ratio) used in published studies.
4. Identify the aspects of reliability (stability, equivalence, and homogeneity) and the extent of reliability of measurement techniques reported in published studies.
5. Determine the types and extent of validity of measurement techniques reported in published studies.
6. Critique the reliability and validity of physiological measures used in published studies.
7. Examine the measurement approaches (physiological measures, observations, interviews, questionnaires, and scales) used in published studies.
8. Critique the measurement section in a research article.
9. Critique the data collection section in a research article.

RELEVANT TERMS

Accuracy
Content-related validity
Data collection
Direct measures
Equivalence
Error in physiological measures
Focus groups
Homogeneity
Indirect measures
Interrater reliability
Interval-scale measurement
Interview
Levels of measurement
Likert scale
Measurement error

Nominal-scale measurement
Observational measurement
Ordinal-scale measurement
Physiological measurement
Precision
Questionnaire
Random error
Rating scale
Ratio-scale measurement
Reliability
Scale
Selectivity
Semantic differential scale
Sensitivity
Serendipity

RELEVANT TERMS—cont'd

Split-half reliability
Stability
Structured interview
Systematic error
Test-retest reliability

True score
Unstructured interview
Validity
Visual analogue scale

The purpose of measurement is to produce trustworthy data that can be used in statistical analyses. In critiquing a published study, you must judge the trustworthiness of the measurement methods used in the study. To produce trustworthy measures, rules have been established to ensure that values or categories will be assigned consistently from one subject (or event) to another and, eventually, if the measurement strategy is found to be meaningful, from one study to another. The rules of measurement established for research are similar to those used in nursing practice. For example, when pouring a liquid medication, the rule is that the measuring container must be placed at eye level. This ensures accuracy and consistency in the dose of medication. When measuring abdominal girth to detect changes in ascites, the skin on the abdomen is marked to ensure that the measure is always taken the same distance below the umbilicus. Using this method, any change in measurement can be attributed to a change in ascites rather than to an inadvertent change in the measurement site. Understanding the logic of measurement is important for critiquing the adequacy of measurement methods in a nursing study. This chapter includes a discussion of some of the concepts of measurement theory, measurement strategies in nursing, and the process of data collection.

CONCEPTS OF MEASUREMENT THEORY

Measurement theory guides the development and use of measurement methods. The following section discusses some of the basic concepts of measurement theory, including directness of measurement, measurement error, levels of measurement, reliability, and validity.

Directness of Measurement

To measure, the researcher must first identify the object, characteristic, or element to be measured. In some cases, identifying the object to measure and measurement strategy to use is quite simple and straightforward, such as when the researcher measures a person's height or wrist circumference. These are referred to as *direct measures.* Direct measures of concrete elements such as height, weight, temperature, time, space, movement, heart rate, and respiration are commonly used in nursing. Technology is available to measure many bodily functions and biological and chemical characteristics. The focus of measurement in these instances is on the precision of measurement. Nurses are also experienced in gathering direct measures of attribute or demographic variables such as age, gender, ethnic origin, diagnosis, marital status, income, and education.

However, in many cases in nursing research, the characteristic the researcher needs to measure is an abstract idea, such as stress, caring, coping, anxiety, compliance, or pain. When abstract concepts are measured, *indirect measures,* indicators or attributes of the concept, are used to represent the abstraction. For example, indicators of coping might be the frequency or accuracy of problem identification, the speed or effectiveness of problem resolution, level of optimism, and types of self-actualization behaviors. Rarely, if ever, can a single measurement strategy measure all aspects of an abstract concept.

 In critiquing a study, you need to determine the variables that were measured and identify the methods used to measure each variable. Determine whether the type of measurement is direct or indirect.

Measurement Error

The ideal, perfect measure is referred to as the "true measure." However, error is inherent in any measurement strategy. *Measurement error* is the difference between the *true score* and what is actually measured. The amount of error varies between measurements. Thus there may be considerable error in one measurement and very little in the next. Measurement error exists in both direct and indirect measures and can be random or systematic. With direct measures, both the object and the measurement are visible. Direct measures, which are generally expected to be highly accurate, are subject to error. For example, a weight scale may not be accurate, a precisely calibrated thermometer may decrease in precision with use, or a tape measure may not be held at exactly the same tightness.

With indirect measures, one cannot directly see the object being measured. For example, you cannot see hope. You may see behavior or hear words that you think represent hope. But hope is a feeling that is not always recognized or clearly expressed by the individual. The measure of hope is usually a scale that is intended to reflect the amount of hope an individual feels. The scale gives us numerical values of the extent of hope, based on the individual's responses to the scale. Efforts to measure concepts such as hope usually result in measuring only part of the concept. Sometimes measures may identify one aspect of the concept but may also include other elements that are not part of the concept. For example, an instrument designed to measure anxiety might also measure aspects of fear.

Two types of error are of concern in measurement: random error and systematic error. The difference between random and systematic error is the direction of the error. In *random error,* the difference between the measured value and the true value is without pattern or direction (random). In one measurement, the actual value obtained may be lower than the true value; whereas in the next measurement, the actual value obtained may be higher than the true value. A number of situations can occur during the measurement process that can result in random error. For example, the person taking the measurements may not use the same procedure every time; a subject completing a paper-and-pencil scale may accidentally mark the wrong column; or the person entering the data into a computer may punch the wrong key. The purpose of measuring is to estimate the true value, usually by combining a number of values and calculating an average. Thus an average value, such as the mean, is an estimate of the true value. As the number of random errors increases, the precision of the estimate decreases.

Measurement error that is not random is referred to as systematic error. In *systematic error,* the variation in measurement values from the calculated average is primarily in the same direction. For example, most of the variation may be higher or lower than the average we calculated. Systematic error occurs because something else is being measured in addition to the concept. A scale that always shows a weight that is 2 pounds more than the true weight would cause systematic error. All of the measured weights would be high, and as a result the mean would be higher than it would be if an accurate scale had been used. Some systematic error occurs in almost any measure. Because of the importance of this type of error in a study, researchers spend considerable time and effort refining their measuring instruments to minimize systematic error.

In critiquing a published study, you will not be able to judge the extent of measurement error directly. However, you may find clues to the amount of error in the published report. For example, if the researcher has described the method of measurement in great detail, and provided evidence of accuracy and consistency of measurement, the probability of error should be reduced. If weight scales are recalibrated periodically during data collection, error should be reduced. Measurement should be more precise if the researcher has used a well-developed, reliable, and valid paper-and-pencil scale, instead of a newly developed scale.

Accuracy of measurement is important in both research and clinical practice. Craft and Moss (1996) discuss error in the assessment of infant emesis volume.

"Liquid amounts are particularly difficult to verify because of the instability of the configuration from event to event. When visualized, the variety in edges, colors, and direction of the liquid in each occurrence makes a template for comparison difficult.

Liquid volumes in the form of emesis are often estimated in nurseries and pediatric units at hospitals. The smaller the patient, the more crucial is accurate fluid output assessment. Infants demand the accurate estimation of fluid loss, and measures to increase accuracy in visual processing are needed. The emesis of infants is particularly difficult to estimate because the infant cannot verbalize the presence of nausea, which would help nurses anticipate vomiting. Therefore nurses are often unable to preweight bibs, spit cloths, or bed linen, or to catch the fluid in a container for objective measurement. (p. 3)

The non-experimental study was conducted using 109 subjects who had a large range of experience in assessing infant emesis volume. Practicing pediatric nurses were invited to participate in the study by displaying

Continued

posters on pediatric and neonatal areas in a large university hospital. Nursing students from the university also were invited to participate.

Because the purpose of this study was to determine the accuracy of assessing infant emesis volume, a realistic situation was provided, using displays of actual formula volumes on receiving blankets that were all folded to one eighth of their original size. Subjects were asked to write down the correct volume perceived and to state whether they had picked up the blanket to evaluate the weight of the display.

Twenty receiving blankets were used as displays. The amounts of formula to be poured on the blankets was [sic] randomly selected by writing amounts on slips of paper.... The subjects were read the following scenario: 'You have just fed Timmy 50 ML of formula before he vomits. You are to determine how much he has vomited.' Subjects began at display 1 and walked to display 20, writing down their volume estimations.

Absolute accuracy was defined as subject choosing the exact number of milliliters corresponding to what was measured and poured on the display.... The investigators were concerned about the small number of displays that were assessed accurately. This small number necessitated a change from analyzing accuracy to analyzing relative error. Relative error was determined by the range of milliliter chosen on either side of the exact amount.... The findings showed that novice subjects, or students, overestimated an average of 1% of the correct volume, whereas more experienced subjects underestimated an average of 16% of the volume. Subjects who stated they were unsure of what method they used underestimated an average of 60%, and subjects who said they used 'experience' as a method underestimated an average of 50% of the correct volume.

Thus, the amount of error in judging amounts of emesis is high, and is problematic both clinically and in nursing studies. Experience alone does not increase accuracy although teaching a method for estimating volume is related to accuracy in judgments about volume." (p. 4)

Levels of Measurement

The traditional *levels of measurement* were developed by Stevens in 1946. Stevens organized the rules for assigning numbers to objects so that a hierarchy in measurement was established. The levels of measurement from low to high are nominal, ordinal, interval, and ratio.

Nominal-scale measurement
Nominal-scale measurement is the lowest of the four measurement categories. It is used when data can be organized into categories of a defined property, but the categories cannot be compared. For example, you might categorize people by diagnosis. However, you cannot say that the category "kidney stone" is higher than the category "peptic ulcer," or that "ovarian cyst" is closer to "kidney stone" than to "peptic ulcer." The categories differ in quality but not quantity. Therefore one cannot say that

subject A possesses more of the property being categorized than does subject B. (Rule: The categories must not be orderable.) Categories must be established in such a way that a datum will fit into only one of the categories. (Rule: The categories must be exclusive.) All the data must fit into the established categories. (Rule: The categories must be exhaustive.) Data such as gender, ethnicity, marital status, and diagnoses are examples of nominal data.

Ordinal-scale measurement

With *ordinal-scale measurement,* data are assigned to categories that can be ranked. To rank data, one category is judged to be (or is ranked) higher or lower, or better or worse than another category. Rules govern how the data are ranked. As with nominal data, the categories must be exclusive and exhaustive. With ordinal data, the quantity can also be identified. For example, if you were measuring intensity of pain, you could identify different levels of pain. You would develop categories that ranked these different levels of pain, such as excruciating, severe, moderate, mild, and no pain. However, when using categories of ordinal measurement, there is no certainty that the intervals between the ranked categories are equal. A greater difference might exist between mild and moderate pain than between excruciating and severe pain. Therefore ordinal data are considered to have unequal intervals.

Many scales used in nursing research are ordinal levels of measurement. For example, one could rank degrees of coping, levels of mobility, ability to provide self-care, or daily amount of exercise on an ordinal scale. Using daily exercise, the scale could be 0 = no exercise, 1 = moderate exercise with no sweating, 2 = exercise to the point of sweating, 3 = strenuous exercise with sweating for at least 30 minutes a day, and 4 = strenuous exercise with sweating for at least 1 hour per day. The measurement is ordinal because we cannot claim that equal distances exist between the rankings. There may be a greater difference between the ranks of 1 and 2 than there is between the ranks of 2 and 3.

Interval-scale measurement

Interval-scale measurement uses interval scales, which have equal numerical distances between intervals. These scales follow the rules of mutually exclusive categories, exhaustive categories, and rank ordering and are assumed to be a continuum of values. Thus the magnitude of the attribute can be more precisely defined. However, it is not possible to provide the absolute amount of the attribute because there is no zero point on the interval scale. Temperature is the most commonly used example of an interval scale. The difference between the temperatures of 70° and 80° is the same as the difference between the temperatures of 30° and 40°. Changes in temperature can be precisely measured. However, a temperature of 0° does not indicate the absence of temperature.

Ratio-scale measurement

Ratio-scale measurement is the highest form of measurement and meets all the rules of other forms of measurement: mutually exclusive categories, exhaustive categories, ordered ranks, equally spaced intervals, and a continuum of values. In addition, ratio-level measures have absolute zero points. Weight, length, and volume are commonly used as examples of ratio scales. All three have absolute zero points, at which a value of zero indicates the absence of the property being measured; zero weight means the absence of weight. Because of the absolute zero point, such statements as "object A weighs twice as much as object B" or "container A holds three times as much as container B" can be justified.

In critiquing a published study, you need to determine the level of each measurement used in the study. In some studies, the researcher will indicate the level of measurement used. In others, you will need to determine the level of measurement from the description of the measurement method used.

In the study titled "Perceptions of Health and Their Relationship to Symptoms in African American Women with Type 2 Diabetes," Stover, Skelly, Holditch-Davis, and Dunn (2001) described their approach to measuring symptoms related to diabetes as follows.

"At this point, the research assistant reviewed with the study subjects the symptoms they had reported and asked, 'Which ones do you think could be caused by diabetes?' Subject answers were coded as 'yes,' 'no,' 'uncertain,' and 'do not know.' For the purposes of analysis, the categories of 'uncertain' and 'do not know' were collapsed into a single category." (p. 74)

This measure has the characteristics of a nominal scale. The scale responses are categories of "yes," "no," "uncertain," and "do not know," which cannot be ranked.

Reliability

Reliability is concerned with the consistency of the measurement technique. For example, if a scale is being used to weigh a subject, the scale should indicate the same weight each time the subject steps on and off the scale. A scale that did not show the same weight every time would be unreliable.

Reliability testing is a measure of the amount of random error in the measurement technique. It takes into account such characteristics as dependability, consistency, accuracy, and comparability. Because all measurement techniques contain some random error, reliability exists in degrees and is usually expressed as a form of correlation coefficient, with a coefficient of 1.00 indicating perfect reliability and a coefficient of 0.00 indicating no reliability. A reliability of 0.80 is considered the lowest acceptable coefficient for a well-developed measurement tool. For a newly developed instrument, a reliability of 0.70 is considered acceptable (Burns & Grove, 2001). Estimates of reliability are specific to the sample being tested. Thus high reliability values reported for an established instrument do not guarantee that reliability will

be satisfactory in another sample or with a different population. Therefore reliability testing should be performed on each instrument used in a study before other statistical analyses are performed. The results of reliability tests should be included in published reports of the study. Reliability testing focuses on three aspects of reliability: stability, equivalence, and homogeneity.

Stability

Stability is an assessment of the consistency of repeated measures. The most commonly used stability test is *test-retest reliability*. This measure of reliability is generally used with physical measures, technological measures, and paper-and-pencil scales. Use of the technique requires an assumption that the factor to be measured remains the same at the two testing times and that any change in the value or score is a consequence of random error. A high correlation coefficient between the test and the retest indicates high reliability.

> In Defloor and De Schuijmer's (2001) study evaluating the effectiveness of four operating-table mattresses in preventing pressure ulcers, a method was needed to measure the degree to which each mattress reduced pressure. The Ergocheck system (ABW, Hamburg, Germany) was used for this purpose. The authors describe how this instrument measures pressure as follows:
>
> "This system consists of a measuring mat containing 684 sensors, positioned at a distance of three cm. Each of these sensors has a diameter of 0.4 cm, is filled with air, and linked to a pressure transducer by means of a polyvinyl chloride (PVC) air tube. Pressure exerted on a sensor is accompanied by a displacement of air through the air channel. This displacement of air is converted into a digital signal by the pressure transducer. The signals of each separate sensor were registered on a computer system. The Ergocheck® allows not only measurement of the pressure on each sensor, but also measurement of the size of the whole contact surface. The measuring sheet is very flexible, so the influence on the pressure-reducing properties of the mattresses tested is minimal (Willems, 1995).
>
> The system was standardized prior to every measurement and with every manipulation of the measuring mat. The reported measuring error is between 1.7 and 3.7% ± 2.5% on the entire measuring sheet (Defloor, 2000).
>
> Interface pressure measurements in the supine position were done twice for each test subject. The test-retest reliability was high (.99; p < .001)." (p. 137)
>
> The authors found that "the foam mattress and the gel mattress seem to have little or no pressure-reducing effect; the polyurethane mattress and the polyether mattress reduce interface pressure significantly better (p < .001); but none of the mattresses reduce pressure sufficiently to prevent the occurrence of pressure ulcers" (p. 134).

Equivalence

Equivalence, or *interrater reliability,* is an assessment of the agreement between measurements made by two or more observers who have measured the same event. Interrater reliability values should be reported in any study in which observational data are collected or judgments are made by two or more data gatherers. Two or more raters independently observe and record the same event using the data collection procedure developed for the study, or the same rater observes and records an event on two occasions. Every data collector used in the study should be tested for interrater reliability. There is no absolute value below which interrater reliability is unacceptable. However, any value below 0.80 (80%) should generate serious concern about the reliability of the data. A value of 0.90 (90%) is more desirable. The numerical reliability value should be reported in published studies.

> In a study of adolescent parent-infant interactions, Letourneau (2001) reported interrater reliability of the observational measures of parent-infant interaction, using NCATS (nursing child assessment teaching scale) and NCAFS (nursing child assessment feeding scale). The measures and findings related to reliability were described in the published study as follows.
>
> "Mothers and babies were videotaped in a laboratory setting during feeding and teaching interactions at 7 to 9 weeks postpartum and again at 11 to 13 weeks postpartum. A certified instructor taught one data coder, blind to participants' group assignments, to score the tapes according to the NCAFS and NCATS protocols. Before coding the dependent variables of NCAFS and NCATS, the data coder achieved interrater reliability of greater than or equal to 90% with videotapes previously scored by the University of Washington, Nursing Child Assessment Satellite Training (NCAST) program. As a check on intrarater reliability, a random numbers table was used to select 6 of the 31 NCAFS and 6 of the 31 NCATS for rescoring. The mean intrarater reliability was 95.3% (range = 90% to 99%) for the NCAFS and 94.0% (range = 90% to 97%) for the NCATS." (pp. 56–57)
>
> The study found that an intervention called "Keys to Caregiving" was effective in improving adolescent mothers' interactions with their infants. The measurement methods used were carefully developed and have well-documented reliability and validity. The author carefully trained coders who observed behavior, and also measured interrater reliability of the coders.

Homogeneity

Tests of instrument *homogeneity* are used primarily with paper-and-pencil tests and address the correlation of various items within the instrument. The original approach to determining homogeneity was *split-half reliability,* which was a method of assessing test-retest reliability without administering the test twice. Instead, the instrument items were split in half, and a correlational procedure was performed between the two halves. The Spearman-Brown correlation formula has generally been used for this procedure (Burns & Grove, 2001).

More recently, testing the homogeneity of all the items in the instrument has been considered a better approach to determining reliability. This procedure examines the extent to which all items in the instrument consistently measure the construct. It is a test of internal consistency. The statistical procedure used for this process is Cronbach's alpha coefficient. If the coefficient is 1.00, each item in the instrument is consistently measuring the same thing. When this occurs, one might question the need for more than one item. A slightly lower coefficient (0.80 to 0.90) indicates that the instrument will provide fine discrimination in the levels of the construct.

In a study examining types of social support available for homeless women and the impact of social support on psychosocial resources, health and health behaviors, and use of health services, Nyamathi, Leake, Keenan, and Gelberg (2000) measured social support using five items from the RAND Course of Homelessness Study (Burnam & Koegel, 1989). These five items were tested for reliability using Cronbach's alpha coefficient.

"These items elicit information about how often respondents had friends, family, or partners available to offer them a good time, provide them with food or a place to stay, listen to them talk about themselves or their problems, accompany them to an appointment to provide moral support, and show their love and care. The original 19-item instrument demonstrated high convergent and discriminant validity and internal consistency reliability coefficients ranging from 0.91 to 0.97 for the four subscales (Sherbourne & Stewart, 1991). Women were asked to respond to these five items first to describe their substance-using sources of support, and then again to describe their substance-nonusing support sources. The women were asked to exclude professionals such as nurses, caseworkers, and social workers, from their reporting. Responses were scored on a 5-point Likert scale ranging from 1 (none of the time) to 5 (all of the time). Women without a given source of support were assigned a score of 1. Means for the five items were computed for substance-using and substance-nonusing support sources and used to form two scales measuring level of support from friends, family, and partners who did and did not use alcohol or drugs. Internal consistency for the two scales, as measured by Cronbach's alpha, was 0.93 for support from substance users and 0.97 for support from substance nonusers." (p. 320)

The study found that

"[a]s compared with those who have little or no support, women whose support included substance nonusers reported better psychosocial profiles and somewhat greater use of health services. Support from substance

Continued

nonusers only was associated with better health behaviors and greater use of health services. Support from substance users only was essentially equivalent to not having support. Modifying the social networks of homeless women appears to be associated with improved mental health outcomes, less risky health behaviors, and greater use of health services." (p. 318)

This carefully designed study developed reliable and valid means to measure sources of support for homeless substance-using women. Their excellent measure can be applied to clinical practice by allowing nurses to assess available resources needed by the client to move toward healthy behaviors.

In critiquing a study, you need to determine the method used to evaluate reliability, and identify the reliability value. Using this information, the adequacy of reliability should be judged for each measurement method used in the study. In some studies, the author will not report the reliability. In others, the author may state that the reliability has been reported to be acceptable in previous studies. If reliability values are not provided for these previous studies, there is little information on which to judge previous reliability and none on which to judge reliability in the study being reported. This does not mean that the reliability is poor; it simply means that there is not sufficient information to judge the adequacy of measurement reliability in the study.

Validity

The *validity* (sometimes referred to as "construct validity") of an instrument is a determination of how well the instrument reflects the abstract construct (or concept) being examined (Berk, 1990; Rew, Stuppy, & Becker, 1988). Validity, like reliability, is not an all-or-nothing phenomenon; it is measured on a continuum. No instrument is completely valid. Thus one determines the degree of validity of a measure rather than whether validity exists. Validity will vary from one sample to another and from one situation to another; therefore validity testing evaluates the use of an instrument for a specific group or purpose, rather than the instrument itself. An instrument may be valid in one situation but not in another.

Several sources that provide evidence of validity are described in this section: content, contrasting groups, convergence, divergence, discriminant analysis, prediction of future events, prediction of concurrent events, and successive verification of validity (information obtained from repeated use of the same method of measurement).

Content-related validity. *Content-related validity* is the extent to which the method of measurement includes all the major elements relevant to the concept being measured. In reporting content-related validity, the researcher may cite sources from the literature, seek feedback from individuals who might be subjects in a study using the measurement, or seek feedback from individuals who are considered experts at measuring the concept. These experts may complete a form called the Content Validity Index

(CVI), which evaluates the validity of the method of measurement. In this case, the researcher reports a numerical value for the level of content-related validity.

Evidence of validity from contrasting groups or known groups. Evidence of validity can be obtained by identifying groups who are expected to have contrasting scores on the instrument. The researcher selects samples from at least two such groups. For example, the researcher might measure hope in newly married individuals and in hospitalized suicidal individuals. If the groups' responses are significantly different in the expected directions, the researcher reports it as evidence of the validity of the instrument.

Evidence of validity from examining convergence. Evidence of validity can be obtained by comparing the instrument that will be used with other instruments that measure the same concept. This type of comparison is particularly important for newly developed instruments. To evaluate convergent validity, the researcher administers all of the selected instruments concurrently to a sample of subjects. Then statistical analyses are performed to determine how closely related the scores are. The statistical result would be a value (r) ranging from -1 to $+1$. If the convergent measures are closely related, the validity of each instrument is strengthened.

Evidence of validity from examining divergence. Evidence of validity can be obtained from instruments that measure a concept opposite to the concept measured by the newly developed instrument. For example, if the newly developed instrument is a measure of hope, the researcher would search for an instrument that measured hope-lessness. The researcher would then administer the two instruments to a single sample of subjects. Statistical analyses (usually correlation) would be performed to determine the extent to which measures from the two instruments were opposite each other (were negatively correlated). The statistical result would be a correlational value (r) ranging from -1 to $+1$. If the divergent measure was negatively correlated with other measures, validity for each of the instruments would be strengthened.

Evidence of validity from discriminant analysis. Evidence of validity can be obtained if instruments have been developed to measure concepts closely related to the concept measured by the newly developed instrument. For example, two instruments might measure the closely related concepts of coping and adaptation. The researcher would administer the two instruments to a single sample and then perform statistical analyses to test the ability of both instruments to discriminate between two concepts that are closely related.

Evidence of validity from prediction of future events. Evidence of validity can be obtained by testing the ability of the instrument to predict future performance or attitudes based on instrument scores. For example, nurse researchers might determine whether a scale that measures health-related behaviors can predict the future health status of individuals.

Evidence of validity from prediction of concurrent events. Evidence of validity can be obtained by examining whether the value of one measure can be predicted from the measurement of another concept. For example, one might be able to predict the self-esteem score of an individual who had a high score on an instrument that measured coping.

Successive verification of validity. Evidence of validity can be obtained by successive verification, or repeated use of the instrument. Each time a researcher uses the instrument, more knowledge is gained about its validity. When a researcher uses the instrument, information on validity is reported from previous studies, as well as from the new study. Thus with each successive study, the validity of the instrument is further verified.

In critiquing a study, you need to judge the validity of the measures that were used. However, you cannot consider validity apart from reliability. If a measurement method does not have acceptable reliability, its validity becomes a moot issue. Unfortunately, not all published studies include information on the validity and reliability of instruments. Selby-Harrington, Mehta, Jutsum, Riportella-Muller, and Quade (1994) found that 47% of a random sample of 55 nursing studies published in 1989 had no evidence of validity for any data collection instruments, 36% had no evidence of reliability, and 29% had no evidence of either validity or reliability. Content validity was addressed in only 27% of the studies.

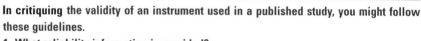

In critiquing the validity of an instrument used in a published study, you might follow these guidelines.
1. What reliability information is provided?
2. Does the author include reports of the validity of the instrument from previous studies? Unfortunately, in some cases, the researcher will simply state that previous research has found validity of the measurement method to be acceptable. This statement does not provide the information you need to judge validity. In this case, you would simply state that you had insufficient information, other than the author's statement that the validity was acceptable, on which to judge validity.
3. Did the author perform pilot studies to examine the validity of the instrument?
4. In the discussion of findings near the end of the report, did the researcher report the use of data from the present study to examine instrument validity?

In a study titled "Changes in well-being of women cancer survivors following a survivor weekend experience," Rutledge and Raymon (2001) report reliability and validity information on an instrument used to measure quality of life in women who have breast cancer.

"Quality of Life-Breast Cancer (QOL-BC) (Ferrell et al., 1996) was a newly developed instrument based on the reliable and valid Quality of Life-Cancer Survivors (QOL-CS) Tool (Ferrell, Dow, Leigh, et al., 1995). The 46-item QOL-BC included items dealing with issues of concern to breast cancer survivors. Items represent the four domains of QOL: psychological well-being (22 items), physical well-being (8 items), social well-being (9 items), and spiritual well-being (7 items).... Individual items, subscale, and total QOL responses ranged from 0-10. Higher scores indicated better QOL. Documented reliability and validity of the QOL-CS included test-retest reliability over two weeks (r = 0.89), internal consistency reliability using Cronbach's alpha coefficient (subscale scores, 0.81 - 0.93), content validity with a panel of QOL researchers and oncology nurses, and both convergent and divergent validity with known groups (Ferrell, Dow, & Grant, 1995). In the current study, alpha reliabilities for the well-being subscales pretreat (N = 59) were physical (0.78), psychological (0.93), social (0.87), and spiritual (0.71) and for total QOL it was 0.95." (p. 87)

Conclusions: "The Healing Odyssey Retreats enhanced women cancer survivors' total QOL-BC specifically their well-being in four dimensions" (p. 85).

Critique

The information given about the tool provides the reader with sufficient information to critique the reliability and validity of the tool. The QOL-BC was first described in the literature in 1996 (Ferrell, Grant, Funk, Garcia, Otis-Green, & Schaffner, 1996) and is based on a broader tool measuring quality of life of cancer survivors. New items were added that are of specific concern to breast cancer survivors. The validity testing reported addresses the use of QOL-CS, not QOL-BC, which is the tool used in the study. QOL-BC was tested, but numeric results of the testing were not reported by Rutledge and Raymon (2001). However, references are provided for readers who want to obtain specific results of validity testing. The effect of the added items on validity apparently has not yet been addressed. Reliability of subscales and total score in the present study are high. The authors report item analyses in the discussion of the study findings.

RELIABILITY AND VALIDITY OF PHYSIOLOGICAL MEASURES

Reliability and validity of physiological and biochemical measures tend not to be reported in published studies. The assumption is made, which is not always correct, that routine physiological measures are valid and reliable. The most common physiological measures used in nursing studies are blood pressure, heart rate, weight, and body temperature. These measures are often obtained from the patient's record, with no consideration of their accuracy. Researchers using physiological measures should provide evidence of the validity of their measures. Gift and Soeken (1988) identify five terms that are critical to evaluation of physiological measures: accuracy, selectivity, precision, sensitivity, and error.

Accuracy. *Accuracy* is comparable to validity in that evidence of content-related validity addresses the extent to which the instrument measured the concept defined in the study. Thus it is an evaluation of the adequacy of the operational definition. For example, arterial blood gases may be a more accurate measure of oxygen saturation than is pulse oxymetry.

Selectivity. *"Selectivity,* an element of accuracy, is the ability to identify correctly the signal under study and to distinguish it from other signals" (Gift & Soeken, 1988, p. 129). For example, on an electrocardiogram, electrical signals coming from the myocardium can be distinguished from similar signals coming from skeletal muscles. Content validity of biochemical measures can be determined by contacting experts in the laboratory procedure or the manufacturer of the physiological equipment and asking them to judge the appropriateness of the measure for the concept being measured.

Precision. *Precision* is the degree of consistency or reproducibility of measurements using physiological instruments. Thus precision is comparable to reliability. The reliability of most physiological instruments is determined by the manufacturer and is part of quality control testing. Recalibration of mechanical equipment is used in many physiological studies to maintain precision. Because of fluctuations in most physiological measures, test-retest reliability is inappropriate.

Sensitivity. *"Sensitivity* of physiologic measures is related to the amount of change of a parameter that can be measured precisely" (Gift & Soeken, 1988, p. 130). If changes are expected to be very small, the instrument must be highly sensitive to detect the changes. For example, a bathroom scale is not sufficiently sensitive to detect very small changes in weight. The stability of the instrument is also related to sensitivity. Stability may be judged in terms of the ability of the system to resume a steady state after a disturbance in input. For example, does a scale return to zero quickly after a weight is removed (return to a steady state), or does an unsteady state affect the measurement of the next item placed on it? For electrical systems, this is referred to as "freedom from drift" (Gift & Soeken, 1988).

Error in physiological measures. Error has a number of sources in physiological measures. Environmental factors such as temperature, barometric pressure, and static electricity can alter measurements. Variations in operation of equipment can occur as a result of operation by different users, changes in supplies, changes in procedures, or any combination of these factors. Machine error may be related to calibration or to the stability of the machine. Electrical signals transmitted from the machine can result in misinterpretation (Gift & Soeken, 1988).

Biological variability in biochemical measures can occur because of factors such as age, gender, body size, diurnal rhythms, and seasonal cycles. Thus variations may be caused by the patients' eating habits, drug use, exercise schedule, and stress level. Materials, equipment, procedures, and personnel used to perform measures can cause errors. Errors can also occur in the recording of measurement values.

In critiquing a study, you need to judge the adequacy of accuracy, selectivity, precision, and sensitivity of any physiological measures used in the study. However, it is important to remember that initial attempts to measure a physiological element important to nursing practice are likely to be less valid than those that have been refined in several studies. Much work is needed to clarify specific elements of physiological assessment in nursing practice; the use of physiological measures in research requires even more rigor than those used in nursing practice.

Engle and Graney (2000) used the Total Pulse Amplitude in a study of the biobehavioral effects of therapeutic touch (TT). One effect of TT is relaxation, which occurs because of responses of the autonomic nervous system. How are changes in the autonomic nervous system measured? These authors used a very sensitive physiological measure of blood flow of small arteries in the deep dermal layers of the skin in the extremities. This blood flow, affected by the sympathetic autonomic nervous system, is referred to as pulse amplitude. A higher total pulse amplitude is correlated with vasodilation, and a lower amplitude is correlated with vasoconstriction.

The authors describe the measurement as follows:

"Medasonics™ infrared light sensor was lightly taped to the pad of the third finger of the left hand. To prevent arm movement (Goetz, 1940), the participant's arm was stabilized by placing the arm fully extended and palm upward on a 45-degree tilt board using Hartwig and colleagues (1994) protocol. An 8-channel Grass™ polygraph and integrator channel converted signals from the sensor into uniform composite wave forms up to 40 mm in height to represent pulsation.... The average of three total pulse amplitude wave form measurements, calculated at the beginning, middle, and end of each time period, was used for data analysis. Test-retest reliability of this measurement protocol for total pulse amplitude for vasoconstriction with ice water has been estimated to be r = .90 for healthy, middle-aged volunteers (Hartwig et al., 1994)." (p. 289)

A critique of the measurement of Total Pulse Amplitude follows.

ACCURACY. Accuracy, the extent to which the instrument measures autonomic responses (used as a proxy for relaxation), is unclear. When compared to the value before TT, the Total Pulse Amplitude changed significantly after TT. The authors expected that TT would cause vasodilation; but instead they found that vasoconstriction occurred in response to the TT. The authors speculated that "vasodilation may have occurred in subjects' mesenteric plexus, the area directly under the TT therapist's hands, with a corresponding reflex vasoconstriction in subjects' peripheral circulation" (pp. 291–292). The effect was present in the subjects that received TT, but not in subjects who were in the mimic therapeutic touch group. Other variables examined, such as mean arterial blood pressure, pulse rate, and skin temperature, were not affected by TT.

SELECTIVITY. The instrument is highly selective in distinguishing total pulse amplitude from other signals, such as blood pressure, pulse rate, and skin temperature.

PRECISION. No information is provided on testing the precision of Total Pulse Amplitude calibration.

SENSITIVITY. The description of the measurement method suggests that the instrument is very sensitive. However, specific information on the amount of change that can be measured is not provided.

Continued

MEASUREMENT STRATEGIES IN NURSING

Nursing studies examine a wide variety of phenomena and thus require an extensive array of measurement tools. Many nursing phenomena have not been examined because no one has thought of a way to measure them. This has implications for both clinical practice and research. This section describes some of the most common measurement approaches used in nursing research, including physiological measurement, observational measurement, interviews, focus groups, questionnaires, and scales.

Physiological Measurements

Because of measurement problems, physiological nursing research has lagged behind studies of the psychosocial dimensions of nursing practice. Some of the first physiological nursing studies examined basic care activities, such as mouth care; decubitus care; the effect of preoperative teaching on postoperative recovery; and infection control related to urinary bladder catheterization, intravenous therapy, and tracheotomy care. Even at this fairly simple level, developing valid methods to measure the variables of interest was difficult and required considerable time and expense. For example, how does one measure changes in a decubitus ulcer? What criteria can be used to determine the effectiveness of a mouth-care regimen? Creativity and attention to detail are needed to develop effective physiological measurement strategies.

An increased need for means to measure the outcomes of nursing care has also generated more nursing studies that include physiological measures. The outcome of interest may be the outcome of all nursing care received for a particular care episode or the outcome of a particular nursing intervention. An important focus of *physiological measurement* is finding means to quantify changes either directly or indirectly that occur in physiological variables in nursing practice. This upsurge of interest in outcome measures has broadened the base of physiological research beyond nurse physiologists to include nurse clinicians. The number of nursing studies including physiological measures has increased dramatically in recent years. The detailed description of physiological measures in a research report should include the exact procedures followed and specific descriptions of equipment used in measurement, as can be seen from some of the following examples.

There are a variety of approaches to obtaining physiological measures. Some measurements are relatively easy to make and are an extension of the measurement methods used in nursing practice, such as those used to obtain weight and blood pressure. Other measurements are not difficult to make, but the method requires an imaginative approach. For example, some phenomena are traditionally only observed in clinical practice, but not measured. Some physiological measures are obtained using self-report or paper-and-pencil scales.

Covey, Larson, Alex, Wirtz, and Langbein (1999) used self-report to obtain information on symptoms of perceived breathlessness (RPB) and leg fatigue (RPLF) of subjects during exercise.

"Subjects rated symptoms of perceived breathlessness (RPB) and leg fatigue (RPLF) during the last 10 seconds of each minute of exercise using the Borg Category-Ratio Scale (Borg, 1982). Subjects were introduced to the scale before the exercise test, and directions were given verbatim according to a script. The Borg scale is a vertical numeric scale with a range of 0 to 10 and is anchored with descriptors beside many of the numbers (range, *nothing at all to maximal*)." (p. 11)

Data on physiological parameters are sometimes obtained with observational data collection methods.

Algase, Kupferschmid, Beel-Bates, and Beattie (1997) measured wandering behavior of cognitively impaired elders using observational methods. The following is a description of their observational methods.

"Ambulation cycles were measured using time-study techniques. Observers recorded time of onset and cessation for each ambulation episode on the Datamyte 1010 (Allen-Bradley, Minnetonka, MN). The Datamyte 1010 is a portable terminal with programmable clock, solid-state memory, and storage capacity to 64K characters in computer-readable format. Each locomoting phase was also coded for impetus (self- or other-directed starts) and pattern (direct, lapping, pacing, or random).

Data were downloaded directly to a microprocessor for analysis. Cycle period was computed as the time elapsed from the onset of one ambulation episode to the onset of the next. Locomoting phase duration was the time elapsed from the onset of an episode of locomotion to its cessation; nonlocomoting phase was the time elapsed from the cessation of an episode of locomotion to the onset of the next episode. Percent-of-cycle-locomoting was the locomoting phase divided by the cycle period (x 100). All ambulation episodes were observed, but only those coded as self-initiated were analyzed. Of those, lapping, pacing, and random patterns were considered wandering, while the direct pattern was not." (p. 174)

Measurement of physiological variables can be either direct or indirect. Direct measures are more valid. Norman, Gadaleta, and Griffin (1991) used both direct and indirect measures of blood pressure in their study. The measurement of arterial pressure waveforms through an arterial catheter provides a direct measure of blood pressure, whereas use of a stethoscope and sphygmomanometer provides an indirect measure.

> Kotzer (1990) describes a creative method of indirectly measuring physiological parameters of preverbal infants.
>
> "Heart rate, respirations and mobility are monitored through passive-motion sensors embedded in a mattress that fits into the infant's bassinet. The data are fed directly into a computer where the physiological record is analyzed and categorized into quiet sleep, active sleep, transitions, indeterminant, awake, and crying." (p. 50)

Sometimes, physiological measures are obtained from laboratory or x-ray results. If so, the same detailed description of the process of obtaining the values to be included in the study is expected.

> Metheny et al. (1999) used a measure of bilirubin content in their study of pH and concentration of bilirubin in feeding tube aspirates as predictors of tube placement. The following is a description of the process for analyzing bilirubin content of aspirate from a feeding tube.
>
> "pH was measured by Beckman pHI 10 pH meters (Beckman Instruments, Inc., Fullerton, CA), accurate to two decimal places. Specimens were centrifuged and then assayed for bilirubin content in a research laboratory using a kit for the measurement of total bilirubin in serum (SIGMA Diagnostics, procedure #552, St. Louis, MO). The determination of bilirubin in this assay (a modification of the procedure described by Hillmann and Beyer, 1967) is based on its reaction with diazotized chloroaniline to form a colored product that is proportional to the bilirubin concentration. Absorbance measurements were made at 540 nm on a UV/VIS Lambda 2 spectrometer (Perkin Elmer Corp, Analytical Instruments, Norwalk, CT). Before each analysis, the spectrophotometer was calibrated with standard bilirubin solutions (SIGMA Diagnostics). Results were reported in milligrams per deciliter (mg/dl)." (p. 192)

The authors found that the mean pH levels in the lung (7.73) and in the intestine (7.35) were significantly higher than the mean pH level in the stomach (3.90). Mean bilirubin levels were significantly lower in the lung (0.08 mg/dl) and stomach (1.28 mg/dl) than in the intestine (12.73 mg/dl). By coupling the two values, a correct prediction of the location of the feeding tube could be made.

The authors provide excellent detail of the laboratory analysis of pH and measurement of bilirubin content. The report indicates the accuracy of the measurement of pH, the frequency of recalibration of the spectrometer, and the precision of results reported in milligrams per deciliter.

In critiquing physiological measures, you might ask the following questions.
1. Is the method of measurement clearly described?
2. Is the method of measurement direct or indirect?
3. How accurate, precise, selective, and sensitive is the measure?

Observational Measurements

Although *observational measurement* is most commonly used in qualitative research, it is used to some extent in all types of studies. Unstructured observations involve spontaneously observing and recording what is seen. Although unstructured observations give the observer freedom, there is a risk that objectivity will be lost and a possibility that the observer may not remember all the details of the observed event. In structured observational measurement, the researcher carefully defines what is to be observed and how the observations are to be made, recorded, and coded. In most cases a category system is developed for organizing and sorting the behaviors or events being observed. Checklists are often used to indicate whether or not a behavior occurred. Rating scales allow the observer to rate the behavior or event. This provides more information for analysis than dichotomous data, which indicate only whether or not the behavior occurred.

Observation tends to be more subjective than other types of measurement and thus is often considered less credible. However, in many cases this approach is the only way to obtain important data for nursing's body of knowledge. As with any means of measurement, consistency is very important; thus reporting interrater reliability is essential.

Holditch-Davis et al. (2001) used observational methods to record mother-infant interactions in a study of parental caregiving and developmental outcomes of infants of mothers with HIV. The observations were made during home visits, when the infants were 12, 18, and 24 months of age. Data were collected during periods when the infant was awake and not due for a feeding.

"During the 1-hour observation, the occurrences of 17 maternal and 12 infant behaviors during each 10-second period were recorded onto paper, using a one-zero sampling method. The end of each 10-second period was signaled audibly to the observer through an earphone from a small electronic timer (Holditch-Davis & Thoman, 1988; Miller & Holditch-Davis, 1992; Tesh & Holditch-Davis, 1997). Five mother variables were used in this study: negative (directing negative affect toward the child), positive (directing positive affect toward the child), play with child, talk, and interaction (talking to, touching, gesturing toward, or playing with child). To adjust for variations in the lengths of observations, these variables were measured as percentages of the total observation. The percentages were calculated by dividing the number of 10-second periods during which a behavior occurred by the number of 10-second periods in the observation.

Continued

Four observers conducted the observations. Before beginning observations, each observer achieved interrater reliability of at least 85% exact agreement on occurrences by coding live observations on volunteer children or study participants along with an investigator who was experienced in behavioral observation. It took 3 to 6 months of practice before initial reliability was achieved. Ongoing interrater reliability for the observation was assessed approximately every other observation throughout the study by having two observers score an observation together. Cohen's kappas were 0.75 for negative, 0.90 for positive, 0.85 for play, 0.85 for talk, and 0.82 for interaction." (p. 7–8)

The authors found that mental development and adaptive behavior decreased as the child grew older. Infants who changed primary caregiver had lower motor and adaptive behavior. More positive attention and more negative control were associated with higher mental, motor, and adaptive behavior.

Holditch-Davis, et al (2001) clearly identified and defined the observations to be recorded. The frequency of observations was timed electronically at 10-second intervals for 1 hour. The techniques for recording observations are carefully described. Observers were trained for a 3 to 6 month period before initiating the study and then trained repeatedly during the data collection period. Interrater reliability was high, indicating that the observational training was very successful. The observer recorded observations every 10 seconds onto paper, using the codes written on the paper, and indicating a 1 if the coded behavior was occurring and 0 if it was not. This allowed the observer to record multiple behaviors during the 10 seconds.

In critiquing observational measures, you might ask the following questions.
1. Is the object of observation clearly identified and defined?
2. Is interrater reliability described?
3. Are the techniques for recording observations described?

Interviews

An *interview* involves verbal communication between the researcher and the subject during which information is provided to the researcher. Although this measurement strategy is most commonly used in qualitative and descriptive studies, it can also be used in other types of studies. A variety of approaches can be used to conduct an interview, ranging from a totally *unstructured interview,* in which the content is completely controlled by the subject, to a *structured interview,* in which the content is similar to a questionnaire, with the possible responses to questions carefully designed by the researcher.

Unstructured interviews may be initiated by asking a broad question, such as "Describe for me your experience with.... " After the interview has begun, the role of the interviewer is to encourage the subject to continue talking, using techniques such as nodding the head or making sounds that indicate interest. In some cases, the subject may be encouraged to elaborate further on a particular dimension of the topic of discussion.

During structured interviews, the researcher uses strategies to control the content of the interview. Questions the interviewer asks are designed by the researcher before the initiation of data collection, and the order of the questions is specified. In some cases the interviewer can elaborate on the meaning of the question or to modify the way in which the question is asked so that the subject can understand it better. In more structured interviews, the interviewer is required to ask the question precisely as it has been designed.

Because nurses frequently use interviewing techniques in nursing assessment, the dynamics of interviewing are familiar; however, using the technique for measurement in research requires greater sophistication. Interviewing is a flexible technique that allows the researcher to explore meaning in greater depth than can be obtained with other techniques. Interpersonal skills can be used to facilitate cooperation and elicit more information. Since there is a higher response rate to interviews than to questionnaires, interviewing often allows a more representative sample to be obtained. Interviewing allows collection of data from subjects who are unable or unlikely to complete questionnaires, such as those who are very ill or whose ability to read, write, and express themselves is marginal.

Interviews are a form of self-report, and it must be assumed that the information provided is accurate. Because of time and costs, sample size is usually limited. Subject bias is always a threat to the validity of the findings, as is inconsistency in data collection from one subject to another.

Hatton (1997) conducted interviews to gather data for a study titled "Managing health problems among homeless women with children in a transitional shelter." She describes the data-gathering process as follows.

"[T]he investigator conducted 30 in-depth, semi-structured interviews with a convenience sample of women living in transitional housing. The sample was 13 Latina, 11 White, and 6 African American women. The typical respondent was age 20 to 30. The investigator interviewed each woman at least once, and, in most cases, obtained additional data from later informal conversations. Questions during the interviews included: How is your health? What makes you say you are healthy or unhealthy? Do you have any current concerns about particular diseases? What will you do about these? Have you ever had a sickness that lasted for a long time? When was the last time you went to a health care provider—such as a nurse or doctor? Each question was explored in further detail with the investigator asking

Continued

how respondents perceived various symptoms, how their severity was managed, and how they decided on various treatments.

An interpreter assisted during the interviews with Spanish-speaking women ($n = 10$). The researcher familiarized the interpreter, who had considerable experience translating, with the overall purpose of the study. After each interview, the researcher and interpreter held debriefing sessions to review what each woman said and to discuss its meaning.

Interviews lasted from 30 minutes to 2 hours depending on the client's desire to talk with the researcher and the woman's busy schedule that included responsibilities for child rearing. All but two of the respondents had children. The two women without children were pregnant. At the beginning of the study, the investigator audiotaped the interviews and transcribed them verbatim ($n = 7$). As the study proceeded, however, women commented that they did not want their interviews audiotaped because they discussed problems they considered shameful. As Vredevoe, Shuler, and Woo (1992) have noted, disclosure can be a methodological problem when doing research among the homeless. Thus, during the latter part of the study, the investigator did not audiotape the interviews but took extensive notes that were later transcribed ($n = 23$)." (p. 34)

In critiquing interview methods of measurement in studies, you might ask the following questions.

1. Do the interview questions address concerns expressed in the research problem?
2. Are the interview questions relevant for the research purpose and objectives, questions, or hypotheses?
3. Does the design of the questions tend to bias subjects' responses?
4. Does the sequence of questions tend to bias subjects' responses?

Focus Groups

The use of focus groups is a relatively recent strategy in nursing studies, beginning in the late 1980s. However, they have been in use in other fields for a long time. The technique serves several purposes in nursing research. Focus groups are used to study qualitative issues, analyze policy, assess consumer satisfaction, evaluate quality of care, examine the effectiveness of public health programs, make professional decisions, develop instruments, explore patient-care problems, develop effective interventions and education programs, study various patient populations, and gather data for participatory research projects. A study using focus groups usually includes between 1 and 50 groups.

Focus groups are designed to obtain the participants' perceptions of a narrow subject in a setting that is permissive and non-threatening. One of the assumptions underlying the use of focus groups is that the group dynamics can encourage people to express and clarify their views in ways that are less likely to occur in a one-to-one interview. The group may give a sense of "safety in numbers" to those wary of researchers or those who are anxious. Many different forms of communication are used in focus groups, including teasing, arguing, joking, and telling anecdotes. Nonverbal approaches, such as gesturing, facial expressions, and other body language, are used as well. Everyday forms of communication may tell us as much, if not more, about what people know or experience. Recruiting the appropriate participants for each of the focus groups is critical. Recruitment is the most common source of failure in research using focus groups. Each focus group should include 6 to 10 participants. Fewer participants tend to result in inadequate discussion. In most cases, participants should be unknown to each other. However, when targeting professional groups such as clinical nurses or nurse educators, this is usually not possible. The researcher may use purposive sampling, in which individuals known to have the desired expertise are sought. In other cases, participants may be sought through the media, posters, or advertisements.

Segmentation is the process of sorting participants into focus groups with common characteristics. Selecting participants who are similar to each other, in lifestyle or experiences, views, and characteristics facilitate more open discussion. Validity is increased by conducting multiple focus groups with participants of differing characteristics in separate groups. These characteristics might be age, gender, social class, ethnicity, culture, life style, or health status. In some cases, groups may be naturally occurring, such as several individuals who work together.

Selecting effective moderators is as critical as selecting appropriate participants. The moderator must be successful at encouraging participants to talk about the topic. In some cases a moderator and assistant moderator should be included. A successful moderator encourages participants to interact with one another, formulate ideas, and draw out cognitive structures not previously articulated. Moderators should remain neutral and nonjudgmental. If the topic is sensitive, the moderators should be able to put the participant at ease. This may be accomplished by using a moderator who shares certain characteristics with the group's participants.

The setting for the focus group should be relaxed, with space for each participant to sit comfortably in a circle and maintain eye contact with all other participants. The group should meet in a room with good acoustics, so that a high-quality tape recording of the session can be made. Sessions usually last 1 to 2 hours, although some may extend to an entire afternoon or continue to a series of meetings.

Data collected from focus groups are analyzed the same way as data collected from qualitative studies. However, data from focus groups are complex; analysis is required at several levels: across responses given by the same individual, among individuals in the same group, and among different groups. It is important to attend to the degree of consensus and interest in the topics generated in the discussion. Analysis of deviance and of minority opinions is important. Paying attention to the context within which statements were made is critical to the analysis (Morgan, 1995).

Jones and Broome (2001) conducted focus groups with African-American adolescents to obtain recommendations for strategies that could enhance recruitment and retention in intervention studies. They describe their process as follows:

"Fifteen African American adolescents, ages 13 to 17 years, participated in this study. Adolescents attended one of three focus groups, which varied by size, gender, and type of chronic condition. The three focus groups consisted of adolescents who were well (n = 7), had sickle cell disease (SCD, n = 5), or diabetes (n = 3). The well group (WG) of adolescents without any known health problem or illness served as a comparison group. The groups consisted of adolescents diagnosed with SCD, and adolescents in the diabetes group (DG) all had Type I insulin-dependent diabetes. The teens with SCD were recruited because the large intervention study to be implemented later was developed for teens with a chronic pain condition. The teens with diabetes were targeted to compare their responses with those teens that were well and those with SCD to determine whether their concerns were disease focused or could be generalized to adolescents with a chronic health condition.

A structured focus group interview guide was developed that included 15 questions that elicited adolescents' ideas about strategies, perceptions, and concerns related to recruitment and retention of adolescents into research. The interview guide was an important factor in controlling variability across the three focus group discussions. Questions elicited adolescents' perceptions and recommendations about potential symptom management interventions (self-management of a disease, art, relaxation, and imagery), class structure and content, teacher characteristics, and specific incentives/disincentives. Probe questions were included to gain more specific and detailed information (e.g., to clarify a statement such as 'someone who can speak our language').

Each focus group discussion was audiotaped and transcribed. Audiotapes were erased by the investigator after they have been listened to, transcribed, and the accuracy of transcribed content validated. Confidentiality of transcribed data was addressed by using adolescents' first names only. After each focus group session the investigator also recorded field notes that documented her thoughts, impressions, and events capturing the context and the processes of the group." (pp. 90–91)

After analyzing the data, the authors summarized their findings.

"Important factors to consider in 'getting adolescents there' included straightforward communication about how they or others would benefit from the research, what would be expected of them, incentives, and accessing them where they 'were'.... Suggestions for keeping teens interested in a research study included honest, open communication between the investigators, the teen and their parents, incentives, and allowing for exercise of choice and active involvement in the research intervention.... Employing honest and respectful communication strategies with the teens, showing respect for their contributions and a willingness to listen were viewed as critical to keeping them coming back.... The adolescents also thought investigators need to recognize the potential for family problems (e.g., lack of transportation or the need for a teen to babysit) that might interfere with their attendance." (pp. 92–93)

In critiquing a focus group study, you need to consider the following questions:

1. What was the aim of the focus group?
2. Was the group size appropriate for the focus group method?
3. Was the group sufficiently homogeneous to speak candidly?
4. Was the moderator successful in keeping the discussion focused?
5. Was the aim of the focus group achieved?
6. Did the conclusions appear to be a valid representation of the discussion?
7. Were minority positions identified and explored?

Questionnaires

A *questionnaire* is a printed self-report form designed to elicit information through written or verbal responses of the subject. Questionnaires are sometimes referred to as surveys, and a study using a questionnaire may be referred to as survey research. The information obtained from questionnaires is similar to that obtained by an interview, but the questions tend to have less depth. The subject is not permitted to elaborate on responses or ask for clarification of questions, and the data collector cannot use probing strategies. However, questions are presented in a consistent manner to each subject, and there is less opportunity for bias than in an interview. Questionnaires are often used in descriptive studies to gather a broad spectrum of information from subjects, such as facts about the subject; facts about persons, events, or situations known by the subject; or beliefs, attitudes, opinions, knowledge, or intentions of the subject. Like interviews, questionnaires can have various structures. Some questionnaires ask open-ended questions, which require written responses from the subject. Other questionnaires ask closed-ended questions, which only have answers selected by the researcher. A recent modification is the use of computers to gather questionnaire data (Saris, 1991).

Stotts, Henderson, and Burns (1988) used a questionnaire to examine smoking patterns of nurses in the state of Texas. Items from that questionnaire are shown in Fig. 9-1.

Although questionnaires can be distributed to very large samples, either directly or through the mail, the response rate to questionnaires is generally lower than that

1. Do you currently smoke cigarettes?
   a. No
   b. Yes

2. How old were you when you started smoking?
   a. Under 15 years   e. 18 years   h. 21 years
   b. 15 years   f. 19 years   i. 22 years
   c. 16 years   g. 20 years   j. Over 22 years
   d. 17 years

3. Before entering your basic (GENERIC) nursing education program, on average, about how many cigarettes a day did you smoke?
   a. Did not smoke at all   d. 15 to 24 cigarettes per day
   b. Did not smoke every day   e. 25 to 39 cigarettes per day
   c. Less than 15 cigarettes per day   f. 40 or more cigarettes per day

4. During your basic (GENERIC) nursing education program, on average, about how many cigarettes a day did you smoke?
   a. Did not smoke at all   d. 15 to 24 cigarettes per day
   b. Did not smoke every day   e. 25 to 39 cigarettes per day
   c. Less than 15 cigarettes per day   f. 40 or more cigarettes per day

5. How many organized programs have you attended to help you quit smoking?
   a. None   d. Three   g. Six
   b. One   e. Four   h. Seven
   c. Two   f. Five   i. More than seven

6. What is the longest single period you have stopped smoking?
   a. Have never stopped   e. More than 1 month but less than 1 year
   b. Less than a day   f. More than 1 year but less than 3 years
   c. Less than a week   g. 3 years or more
   d. Less than a month

7. Aside from what you think you actually could do, which would you most like to do?
   a. Quit smoking   d. Not sure at this time
   b. Cut down   e. Smoke as much as now
   c. Cut down just a little

Fig. 9-1   Examples of items from a smoking questionnaire.

of other forms of self-report, particularly if the questionnaires are mailed. If the response rate is lower than 50%, the representativeness of the sample is seriously in question. The response rate for mailed questionnaires is usually small (25% to 30%), so the researcher is frequently unable to obtain a representative sample, even with random sampling methods. Respondents commonly fail to mark responses to all the questions, especially on long questionnaires. This can threaten the validity of the instrument.

In critiquing a published study that used a questionnaire, you need to evaluate the adequacy of the questionnaire to measure the concepts important to the study (content-related validity evidence). In most studies, only a brief description of the questionnaire is provided. Usually, the questionnaire itself will not be available for you to examine in the published report. Compare the description of the contents of the questionnaire with the conceptual definitions the questions are intended to reflect. Search for information on content-related validity. If the CVI (Content Validity Index, see pp. 274–275) was used, the value obtained should be reported.

With most questionnaires, researchers analyze data at the level of individual items, rather than adding the items together and analyzing the total scores. Responses to items are usually measured at the nominal or ordinal level. Because individual items may address a variety of topics associated with the research area, attempting to determine reliability by using tests of homogeneity may not be logical.

Kaas, Dehn, Dahl, Frank, Markley, and Hebert (2000) used a questionnaire in their study titled "View of Prescriptive Practice Collaboration: Perspectives of Psychiatric-Mental Health Clinical Nurse Specialists [CNS] and Psychiatrists." They describe the questionnaire as follows.

"A 34-item questionnaire was developed by the investigators to identify the characteristics, role activities, responsibilities, outcomes, and satisfaction of collaboration between the CNSs and psychiatrists. Demographic information included age, gender, work setting, psychiatric subspecialty, certification, number of years as a clinician, number of years as a prescriber (CNS), and number of years using a collaborative prescribing agreement. An expert panel of 5 advanced practice psychiatric nurses with prescriptive authority and 2 collaborating psychiatrists reviewed the survey for content validity and ease in answering. For each question, subjects were given a list of responses and asked to check off their choices. Respondents were asked to identify the characteristics of the collaborative practice in which they were currently engaged. Satisfaction was measured using a Likert scale with 1 being very dissatisfied and 5 being very satisfied." (p. 225)

Findings: "Good communication, trust, shared goals for patient outcomes, shared professional values, and respect for clinical competency were identified as important characteristics for effective collaboration. CNSs identified increased professional growth and job satisfaction as professional benefits, while psychiatrists reported shared workload responsibilities" (p. 222).

Scales

The *scale,* a form of self-report, is a more precise means of measuring phenomena than the questionnaire. Most scales measure psychosocial variables. However, scaling techniques can be used to obtain self-reports on physiological variables such as pain, nausea, or functional capacity. The various items on most scales are summed to obtain a single score. These are referred to as "summated scales." Fewer random and systematic errors occur when the total score of a scale is used. The various items in a scale increase the dimensions of the concept that are reflected in the instrument. The types of scales described in the following text include rating scales, Likert scales, semantic differential scales, and visual analogue scales.

Rating scales

Rating scales are the crudest form of measure using scaling techniques. A *rating scale* lists an ordered series of categories of a variable and is assumed to be based on an underlying continuum. A numerical value is assigned to each category. The subtlety of the distinctions among categories varies with the scale. Rating scales are commonly used by the general public. In conversations, one can hear statements such as, "On a scale of one to ten, I would rank that…. This type of scale is often used in observational measurement to guide data collection. Burns (1974) used the rating scale in Fig. 9-2 to examine differences in communication among nurses and both cancer patients and other medical-surgical patients.

---

1. Nurses come into my room
   a. Rarely
   b. Sometimes
   c. Whenever I call them
   d. Frequently just to speak or check on me
2. I would *like* nurses to come into my room
   a. Rarely
   b. Sometimes
   c. Whenever I call them
   d. Frequently just to speak or check on me
3. When a nurse enters my room, he/she usually
   a. Talks very little
   b. Tries to talk about things I do not wish to discuss
   c. Talks only about casual things
   d. Is willing to listen or discuss what concerns me
4. When a nurse enters my room, I would *prefer* that he/she
   a. Talk very little
   b. Talk only when necessary
   c. Talk only about casual things
   d. Be willing to listen or discuss what concerns me
5. When a nurse talks with me, he/she usually seems
   a. Not interested
   b. In a hurry
   c. Polite but distant
   d. Caring for me as a person

Fig. 9-2   A rating scale used to measure the nature of nurse-patient communications.

6. When a nurse talks with me, I would *prefer* that he/she be
   a. Not interested
   b. In a hurry
   c. Polite but distant
   d. Caring for me as a person

7. When a nurse talks with me, he/she usually
   a. Stands in the doorway
   b. Stands at the foot of the bed
   c. Stands at the side of the bed
   d. Sits beside the bed

8. When a nurse talks with me, I would *prefer* that he/she
   a. Stand in the doorway
   b. Stand at the foot of the bed
   c. Stand at the side of the bed
   d. Sit beside the bed

9. When a nurse talks with me, he/she is
   a. Strictly business
   b. Casual
   c. Friendly but does not talk about feelings
   d. Open to talking about things I worry or think about

10. When a nurse talks with me, I would *prefer* that he/she keep the conversation
    a. Strictly business
    b. Casual
    c. Friendly but not talk about feelings
    d. Open to talk about things I worry or think about

11. Nurses talk with me about things important to me
    a. Rarely
    b. Sometimes
    c. Frequently
    d. As often as I need to talk

12. I would *like* for the nurse to talk with me about things important to me
    a. Rarely
    b. Sometimes
    c. Frequently
    d. As often as I need to talk

13. The nurse looks me in the eye when he/she talks with me
    a. Rarely
    b. Sometimes
    c. Frequently
    d. Very frequently

14. I would *prefer* that the nurse look me in the eye when he/she talks with me
    a. Rarely
    b. Sometimes
    c. Frequently
    d. Very frequently

Fig. 9-2—cont'd

Continued

15. When a nurse talks to me, he/she touches me
    a. Rarely
    b. Sometimes
    c. Frequently
    d. Very frequently

16. When a nurse talks to me, I would *prefer* that he/she touches me
    a. Rarely
    b. Sometimes
    c. Frequently
    d. Very frequently

17. My feelings about nurses talking to me are which of the following?
    a. They should do their work well and otherwise leave me alone.
    b. They may talk if they need to; it does not bother me.
    c. I enjoy talking with the nurses.
    d. When the nurse lets me talk with him/her about things important to me, I feel that he/she cares for me as a person.

On question 18, please mark as many answers as you wish.

18. I would like to feel free to talk with the nurse about my
    a. Illness
    b. Future
    c. Financial problems
    d. Feelings about myself
    e. Feelings about my family
    f. Life up to this time

Fig. 9-2—cont'd   A rating scale used to measure the nature of nurse-patient communications.

Lenz and Perkins (2000) used a rating scale to measure functional health in their study titled "Coronary Artery Bypass Graft Surgery Patients and Their Family Member Caregivers: Outcomes of a Family-Focused Staged Psychoeducational Intervention." Their description of the rating scale is as follows.

"The patient's functional health status was measured using the COOP charts (Nelson, Wasson, & Kirk, 1987), a standardized, 10-item pictorial self-report instrument. For each aspect of functioning, the subject rates himself/herself on a 5-point scale in which higher values reflect poorer functional status. The measure has physical (fitness, daily activities, and pain items) and emotional (feelings, social activities, and quality-of-life items) subscales, as well as a total score that ranges from 10 to 50. The instrument developers reported test-retest reliability alpha values ranging from .73 to .98. Both convergent and divergent validity have been satisfactory in multiple populations; however the COOP charts have sacrificed both sensitivity and specificity in the interest of brevity and ease of administration (Nelson, Landgraf, Hays, Wasson, & Kirk, 1990; Wasson et al., 1992). The internal consistency of the scale ranged from .63 to .81 in the study sample of patients." (p. 145)

Findings: "Differences in the number of self-reported complications/symptoms were not in the predicted direction. Improvement occurred in clinical, functional, and emotional outcomes; however, several symptoms, such as fatigue and pain, persisted. Family caregivers reported more depressive symptoms than patients preoperatively and at later stages of recovery." (p. 142)

In critiquing a rating scale, you might ask the following questions.
1. Is the instrument clearly described?
2. Are the techniques that were used to administer and score the scale provided?
3. Is information about validity and reliability of the scale described from previous studies?
4. Is information about validity and reliability of the scale described for the present sample?
5. If the scale was developed for the study, was the instrument development process described?

Likert scales

The *Likert scale,* which was designed to measure the opinion or attitude of a subject, contains a number of declarative statements with a scale after each statement. The Likert scale is the most commonly used scaling technique. The original version of the scale consisted of five categories. However, the number of categories may range from four to seven. Values are placed on each response, with a value of 1 on the most negative response and a value of 5 on the most positive response (Nunnally & Berenstein, 1994). Response choices on a Likert scale most commonly address agreement, evaluation, or frequency. Agreement responses may include options such as strongly agree, agree, uncertain, disagree, and strongly disagree. Evaluation responses ask the respondent for a categorical rating along a good to bad continuum, such as positive to negative or excellent to terrible. Categorical options may include such responses as rarely, seldom, sometimes, occasionally, and usually. The values from each item are summed to provide a total score. Fig. 9-3 illustrates the form used for this type of scale.

Badger, McNiece, and Gagan (2000) used a Likert-type scale to measure depression in their study of the incidence of depression, need for services, and use of services in vulnerable populations. The following is a description of their instrument.

"[Depression] was measured using the 20-item Center for Epidemiological Studies-Depression Scale (CES-D) (Radloff, 1977). The CES-D has been

Continued

used in both general and clinical populations to measure the frequency and severity of depression symptomatology. Participants were asked to rate each depressive symptom experienced in the past week on a 4-point Likert-type scale, ranging from 0 (rarely or none of the time) to 3 (most or all of the time). Scores are then summed and range from 0 to 60, with higher scores reflecting greater depressive symptoms. Although scores >16 are typically used to indicate significant depressive symptoms, in this study the more conservative criterion of >27 was used. The more conservative score is recommended when the participants have multiple chronic illnesses or disabling conditions (Schulberg et al., 1985). Adequate reliability and validity with other community samples have been established (Davidson, Feldman, & Crawford, 1994: Schulberg et al., 1985). Cronbach's alpha in this study was .92." (p. 29)

Findings: "Significant differences were found between the 2 groups for predisposing characteristics, enabling characteristics, need for care, service use, and satisfaction with services." (p. 173)

	Strongly Disagree	Disagree	Uncertain	Agree	Strongly Agree
People with cancer almost always die					
Chemotherapy is very effective in treating cancer					
We are close to finding a cure for cancer					
I would work next to a person with cancer					
Nurses take good care of patients with cancer					

Fig. 9-3   Example of items that could be included in a Likert scale.

In critiquing a Likert scale, you might ask the following questions:
1. Is the instrument clearly described?
2. Are the techniques needed to complete and score the scale provided?
3. Is information about validity and reliability of the scale described from previous studies?
4. Is information about reliability and validity of the scale described for the present sample?
5. If the scale was developed for the study, is the instrument development process described?

Semantic differential scales

The *semantic differential scale* measures attitudes and beliefs. A semantic differential scale consists of two opposite adjectives with a 7-point scale between them. The subject is asked to select one point on the scale that best describes his or her view of the concept being examined. Values of 1 to 7 are assigned to each space, with 1 being the most negative response and 7 being the most positive. The placement of negative responses to the left or right of the scale should be randomly varied to avoid global responses (in which the subject places checks in the same column of each scale item). Values that are reversed are transposed before the values are added. The values for the scales are summed to obtain one score for each subject. Burns (1981, 1983) developed a semantic differential scale that uses descriptive phrases to measure beliefs about cancer. Fig. 9-4 includes descriptive phrases from this 23-item scale.

In critiquing a semantic differential, you might ask the following questions.
1. Is the instrument clearly described?
2. Are the techniques to administer and score the scale provided?
3. Is information about validity and reliability of the scale described from previous studies?
4. Is information about validity and reliability of the scale described for the present sample?
5. If the scale was developed for the study, is the instrument development process described?

CANCER

Certain death |___|___|___|___|___|___|___| Being cured

Punishment |___|___|___|___|___|___|___| No punishment

Painless |___|___|___|___|___|___|___| Severe, constant untreatable pain

Abandoned |___|___|___|___|___|___|___| Cared for

Fig. 9-4 Example of items from the Burns Cancer Beliefs Scales.

No pain └──┘ Pain as bad as it
                                                                    can possibly be

Fig. 9-5   Example of a visual analogue scale.

Visual analogue scales

The *visual analogue scale* is a line that is 100 mm long, with right angle stops at either end. The line may be oriented horizontally or vertically. Bipolar anchors are placed beyond either end of the line. These end anchors should include the entire range of sensations possible for the phenomenon being measured (e.g., all and none, best and worst, no pain and most severe pain).

The subject is asked to place a mark through the line to indicate the intensity of the stimulus. A ruler is then used to measure the distance between the left end of the line and the subject's mark. This measure is the value of the stimulus. The visual analogue scale has been used to measure pain, mood, anxiety, alertness, craving for cigarettes, quality of sleep, attitudes toward environmental conditions, functional abilities, and severity of clinical symptoms (Wewers & Lowe, 1990). An example of a visual analogue scale is shown in Fig. 9-5.

Strategies commonly used to evaluate the reliability of scales are not useful for visual analogue scales. Because these scales are used to measure phenomena that are erratic over time, test-retest reliability is inappropriate; and because each scale contains a single item, other methods of determining reliability cannot be used.

In critiquing a visual analogue scale, you might ask the following questions.
1. Is the instrument clearly described?
2. Are the techniques needed to administer and score the scale provided?
3. Is information about validity of the scale described from previous studies?
4. Is information about validity of the scale described for the present sample?
5. If the scale was developed for the study, is the instrument development process described?

PROCESS OF DATA COLLECTION

Data collection is the process of acquiring the subjects and collecting the data for the study. The actual steps of collecting the data are specific to each study and depend on the research design and measurement techniques. During the data collection period, the researcher focuses on obtaining subjects, training data collectors, collecting data in a consistent way, maintaining research controls, protecting the integrity (or validity) of the study, and solving problems that threaten to disrupt the study.

The researcher should describe the data collection process in the published study. The strategies used to approach potential subjects who meet the sampling criteria should be clear. The number and characteristics of subjects who decline to participate in the study should be reported. The approach used to perform measurements, and the time and setting at which measurements are taken should be described. The result should be a step-by-step description of exactly how, where, and in what sequence the data were collected.

In many studies, data collection forms are used to gather data. These forms may be used to record data from the patient record, or to ask the subject for such information as demographic data. The form itself is not a measurement tool. In many cases, each item on these forms is a separate measurement. Thus the researcher should report the source of information and describe the method and level of measurement of each item on the form. An example of a data collection form is shown in Fig. 9-6.

Data Collection Tasks

During either quantitative or qualitative research, the investigator performs five tasks during the data collection process. These tasks are interrelated and run concurrently rather than in sequence. The tasks include selecting subjects, collecting data in a consistent way, maintaining research controls as indicated in the study design, protecting the integrity (or validity) of the study, and solving problems that threaten to disrupt the study.

Recruiting subjects

Subjects may be recruited only at the initiation of data collection or throughout the data collection period. The design of the study determines the method of selecting subjects. Recruiting the number of subjects originally planned is critical because data analysis and interpretation of findings depend on having an adequate sample size. Factors related to subject recruitment and selection should be continually examined to determine possible biases in the sample obtained.

Recruiting subjects for research is becoming more difficult for a variety of reasons, including the following: (1) an increasing number of nurses are conducting research, (2) clinical agencies are placing constraints on the time staff nurses can be released from patient care for research activities, (3) patients are being protected from participating in too many investigations, and (4) access to patients is being limited so that agency personnel can use these patients for their own research (Cronenwett, 1986). Thus in the future, nurse researchers should be creative and persistent in recruiting adequate numbers of subjects. In recruiting subjects, researchers have found that direct contact with potential subjects is the most effective method, telephone contact is less effective, and mail contact is least effective. Direct contact in small groups is usually more effective for subject recruitment than contact in large groups (Crosby, Ventura, Finnick, Lohr, & Feldman, 1991). The researcher must determine the most effective recruitment approach based on the purpose of the study, the type and number of subjects required, and the design of the study.

Maintaining Consistency

The key to accurate data collection in any study is consistency. Consistency involves maintaining the data collection pattern for each collection event as it was developed in the research plan. A good plan will facilitate consistency and maintain the validity of the study. However, developing a consistent plan is easier than implementing it. Deviations, even if they are minor, should be noted and evaluated for their impact

DATA COLLECTION FORM

Subject identification number _____   Date _____

A. Age _____   B. Gender: ❑ Male ❑ Female

C. Weight _____ pounds   D. Height _____ inches

E. Surgical diagnosis _____

F. Surgery date _____   Time _____

G. Narcotics order after surgery _____

_____

H. Narcotic administration:
      Date   Time   Type of narcotic   Dose
    1.
    2.
    3.
    4.
    5.

I. Patient instructed on Pain Scale: Date _____ Time _____

    Comments:

J. Type of treatment: ❑ TENS   ❑ Placebo-TENS   ❑ No treatment control

K. Treatment implemented: Date _____   Time _____

    Comments:

L. Dressing change: Date _____   Time _____

    Hours since surgery _____

M. Score on Visual Analogue Pain Scale _____

    Date _____   Time _____

Data collector's name _____

    Comments:

Fig. 9-6 Hypothetical data collection form for Hargreaves and Lander's (1989) study, "The use of transelectrical nerve stimulation (TENS) for management of postoperative pain.

on the interpretation of the findings. When data collectors are used in a study, they should be trained to note deviations during the data collection process.

Maintaining controls

Research controls should be built into the plan, to minimize the influence of intervening forces on study findings. Maintenance of these controls is essential; many controls are not natural in a field setting, and maintaining them is not easy. In some cases the controls slip without the researcher realizing it. In addition to maintaining the controls identified in the plan, the researcher needs to continually look for previously unidentified, extraneous variables that might have an impact on the data being collected. This type of variable is often specific to a study and tends to become apparent during the data collection period. The extraneous variables identified during data collection must be considered during data analysis and interpretation. These variables should also be noted in the research report, so that future researchers can be aware of and attempt to control them.

Protecting study integrity

Maintaining consistency and controls during subject selection and data collection protects the integrity or validity of the study. In addition, the integrity of the study should be considered in a broad context. To accomplish this, the researcher should view the process of data collection as a whole, instead of examining single elements of data collection. Changes in one small component of data collection can modify other elements and thus alter the entire process in ways that threaten the validity of the outcomes.

> Harrison, Wells, Fisher, and Prince (1996) conducted a study to evaluate evidence of the effectiveness of practice guidelines for the prediction and prevention of pressure ulcers. They used a Demographic and Clinical Profile Form to capture information about age and sex of the subjects, length of hospital stay, reason for admission, diagnosis of medical problem, use of pressure relief devices, and type of nursing unit the subject was treated in. The Prevalence Grid was used to identify 20 sites to assess skin integrity. If ulcers were present, a staging classification system was used to categorize ulcers from Stage I to Stage IV. The Braden Scale (Bergstrom, Braden, Laguzza, & Holman, 1987) was used to assess the risk of pressure ulcers. The authors described their data collection procedure as follows.
>
> "A survey team of 23 registered nurses conducted a head-to-toe skin assessment and administered the Braden Scale to consenting subjects. The surveyors were prepared through an education workshop that included an orientation to the study purpose and procedures, the use of data collection instruments, and a theoretical and practical 'hands-on' component to stage ulcers and conduct risk assessment. The training films developed by

Continued

Bergstrom and Braden were included in the workshop format. Reliability was assessed on a range of known cases where team members went to clinical areas, staged ulcers, and then had these assessments checked by a clinical expert (enterostomal therapist).

On prevalence day [days of the week selected to assess skin integrity of all subjects], the surveyors were divided into four data collection teams plus a validation team. Each had a team leader who was not directly involved in data collection to attend to administrative tasks, such as tracking admissions and discharges, and deploying surveyors. The team members were assigned to clinically familiar areas (e.g., critical care nurses to critical care areas) but not to their home units where they would know the patients. The enterostomal therapist was on call at all times if the surveyors required a second opinion on an assessment of ulcer stage.

The validation team, [composed] of two registered nurse surveyors, reassessed a randomly selected subsample of 10% of the prevalence population to assess reliability. Correlation of the survey team and validation team on total Braden scores was calculated using Pearson's product moment correlation. Correlation of the survey team and validation team assessments was $r = 0.87$. The degree of association indicates a strong relationship between assessments.

The surveyors conducted a full skin examination and administered the Braden Scale for risk assessment on prevalence day. The risk assessment was completed using the chart, plan of care, clinical assessment, and consultation with the patient's assigned nurse to complete the data collection. The Braden Scale was administered in this manner because it closely emulates the way in which clinical staff would use such a scale if implemented institution-wide.

To determine the Braden Scale's accuracy in the setting, the same data (full skin assessment and administration of the Braden Scale) was collected in a 20-week follow-up on a Monday-Wednesday-Friday schedule by a subsample of the surveyors. They had no information of the subjects' prior risk scores, and with the number of surveyors, computer calculation of total scores, and the large number of patients in the study, the likelihood of bias by remembering an assessment was minimal.

To evaluate the Braden Scale and the risk cut-off scores, the sensitivity (i.e., percentage of all subjects who developed a pressure ulcer and were so predicted by the scale), specificity (i.e., percentage of all subjects who did not develop pressure ulcers and were so predicted by the scale), positive predictive value (i.e., percentage of subjects who were predicted to be at risk and did develop a pressure ulcer), and the negative predictive value (i.e., percentage of subjects who were predicted to be at low risk and did not develop a pressure ulcer) were calculated. The calculations are well described by Bergstrom, Demuth, and Braden (1987)." (pp. 12–13)

As can be seen in the report, Harrison and colleagues (1996) took careful steps to maintain the rigor of their data collection plan. They built in multiple cross-checks and avoided biases by not assessing patients they had personally cared for. The reliability of the skin assessments were validated by a second assessment team that crosschecked measures of 10% of the sample.

Solving problems

Problems can be perceived either as a frustration or as a challenge. The fact that the problem occurred is not as important as the success of problem resolution. Therefore the final and perhaps most important task of the data collection period may be problem resolution. Little has been written in the scientific literature about the problems encountered by nurse researchers. The research reports often read as though everything went smoothly. The implication is that good researchers have no problems, which is not true. Research journals generally do not provide sufficient space to allow description of the problems encountered, and this gives a false impression to the inexperienced researcher. A more realistic picture can be obtained through personal discussions with researchers about the data collection process.

 In critiquing the data collection process of a published study, you might follow these guidelines.
1. Is the way subjects were obtained described and evaluated?
2. Are the procedures for data collection described and evaluated?
3. Do the descriptions of the data collection process identify possible threats to validity?
4. Is the training of data collectors described and evaluated?
5. Is the use of data collection forms identified and evaluated?

Serendipity

Serendipity is the accidental discovery of something useful or valuable. During the data collection phase of studies, researchers often become aware of elements or relationships that they had not previously identified. Therefore in some published studies the researcher has gathered data, made observations, or recorded events that were not originally planned. These new-found aspects may or may not be closely related to the planned study. Because the researcher is focused on close observation, other elements in the situation can come into clearer focus and take on new meaning. Serendipitous findings are important for the development of new insights in nursing, and they can lead to new areas of research that generate knowledge.

SUMMARY

The purpose of measurement is to produce trustworthy evidence that can be used in evaluating the outcomes of research. The rules of measurement ensure that the assignment of values or categories is performed consistently from one subject (or event) to another and, eventually, if the measurement strategy is found to be meaningful, from one study to another. Measurement begins by clarifying the object, characteristic, or element to be measured. Direct measurement is the measurement of concrete factors such as height or wrist circumference. Indirect measurement is used to measure abstract concepts such as stress, caring, coping, anxiety, compliance, and pain. Measurement error is the difference between the actual value and the measured value.

The levels of measurement from low to high are nominal, ordinal, interval, and ratio. Nominal-scale measurement is used when data can be organized into categories of a defined property, but the categories cannot be compared. Data that can be measured at the ordinal-scale level can be assigned to categories of an attribute that can be ranked. In addition to following the rules of mutually exclusive categories, exhaustive categories, and rank ordering, interval scales have equal numerical distance between intervals of the scale. Ratio-level measures are the highest form of measure and meet all the rules of other forms of measures. In addition, ratio-level measures have absolute zero points.

Reliability in measurement is concerned with the consistency of the measurement technique. Reliability testing is considered a measure of the amount of random error in the measurement technique. Reliability testing focuses on three aspects of reliability: stability, equivalence, and homogeneity. The validity of an instrument is a determination of the extent to which the instrument reflects the abstract concept being examined. Validity, like reliability, is not an all-or-nothing phenomenon; it is a matter of degree. No instrument is completely valid. Validity, or construct validity, is considered a single broad method of evaluating measurements. Validity testing assesses the use of an instrument for a specific group or purpose, rather than the instrument itself. An instrument may be valid in one situation, but not valid in another. There are a number of ways to assess the validity of an instrument. Reliability and validity of physiological and biochemical measures tend not to be reported in published studies. Researchers often erroneously assume that routine physiological measures are valid and reliable. Evaluation of physiological measures requires a different perspective than does evaluation of behavioral measures.

Nursing studies require an extensive array of measurement tools. Common measurement approaches used in nursing research include physiological measures, observation, interviews, questionnaires, and scales. Many questions in nursing research require the measurement of physiological dimensions. Measurements of physiological variables can be either direct or indirect. Many physiological measures require the use of specialized equipment; some require laboratory analysis. When publishing the results of a physiological study, the measurement technique should be described in great detail.

Observational measurement may be unstructured or structured. In structured observational studies, category systems should be developed. Checklists or rating scales are developed from the category systems and are used to guide data collection. Interviews involve verbal communication between the researcher and the subject, during which information is provided to the researcher. A questionnaire is a printed self-report form designed to elicit information through written responses of the subject. Scales, a form of self-report, are a more precise means of measuring phenomena than questionnaires. A rating scale lists an ordered series of categories for a variable; the scale is assumed to be based on an underlying continuum. The Likert scale is designed to determine the opinion or attitude of a subject and contains a number of declarative statements, with a scale after each statement. A semantic differential scale consists of two opposite adjectives with a 7-point scale between them. The visual analogue scale is a line that is 100 mm long, with a right-angle stop at either end. Adjectives expressing the opposite extremes of psychosocial or behavioral responses (e.g., pain, mood, or anxiety) are placed beyond either end of the line.

The researcher performs five tasks during the process of data collection: (1) obtaining subjects, (2) collecting data in a consistent way, (3) maintaining research controls, (4) protecting the integrity (or validity) of the study, and (5) solving problems that threaten to disrupt the study. It is important to critique the description of the data collection process for threats to validity. During data collection, the researcher may make an accidental discovery of valuable information unrelated to the planned study; this is called serendipity.

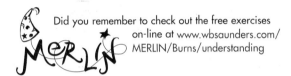

Did you remember to check out the free exercises on-line at www.wbsaunders.com/ MERLIN/Burns/understanding

REFERENCES

Algase, D. L., Kupferschmid, B., Beel-Bates, C. A., & Beattie, E. R. (1997). Estimates of stability of daily wandering behavior among cognitively impaired long-term care residents. *Nursing Research, 46*(3), 172–178.

Badger, T. A., McNiece, C., & Gagan, M. J. (2000). Depression, service need, and use in vulnerable populations. *Archives of Psychiatric Nursing, 14*(4), 173–182.

Bergstrom, N., Braden, B. H., Laguzza, A., & Holman, V. (1987). The Braden Scale for predicting pressure sore risk. *Nursing Research, 36*(4), 205–210.

Bergstrom, N., Demuth, P. J., & Braden, B. J. (1987). A clinical trial of the Braden Scale for predicting pressure sore risk. *Nursing Clinics of North America, 22*(2), 417–428.

Berk, R. A. (1990). Importance of expert judgment in content-related validity evidence. *Western Journal of Nursing Research, 12*(5), 659–671.

Borg, G. A. (1982). Psychophysical bases of perceived exertion. *Medicine and Science in Sports and Exercise, 14*(5), 377–381.

Burnam, M. A., & Koegel, P. (1989). *The course of homelessness among the seriously mentally ill.* An NIMH funded proposal, Rockville, MD.

Burns, N. (1974). *Nurse-patient communication with the advanced cancer patient.* Unpublished master's thesis, Texas Woman's University, Dallas.

Burns, N. (1981). *Evaluation of a supportive-expressive group for families of cancer patients.* Unpublished doctoral dissertation, Texas Woman's University, Denton.

Burns, N. (1983). *Development of the Burns cancer beliefs scale.* Proceedings of the American Cancer Society Third West Coast Cancer Nursing Research Conference Proceedings, 308–329.

Burns, N., & Grove, S. K. (2001). *The practice of nursing research: Conduct, critique, and utilization* (4th ed.). Philadelphia: Saunders.

Covey, M. K., Larson, J. L., Alex, C. G., Wirtz, S., & Langbein, W. E. (1999). Test-retest reliability of symptom-limited cycle ergometer tests in patients with chronic obstructive pulmonary disease. *Nursing Research, 48*(1), 9–19.

Craft, M. J., & Moss, J. (1996). Accuracy of infant emesis volume assessment. *Applied Nursing Research, 9*(1), 2–8.

Cronenwett, L. (1986). Research reflections: Access to research subjects. *Journal of Nursing Administration, 16*(1), 8–9.

Crosby, F., Ventura, M. R., Finnick, M., Lohr, G., & Feldman, M. J. (1991). Enhancing subject recruitment for nursing research. *Clinical Nurse Specialist, 5*(1), 25–30.

Davidson, H., Feldman, P. H., & Crawford, S. (1994). Measuring depressive symptoms in the frail elderly. *Journal of Gerontology B Psychological Sciences and Social Sciences, 49*(4), P159–P184.

Defloor, T. (2000). The effect of position and mattress on interface pressure. *Applied Nursing Research, 13*(1), 2–11.

Defloor, T., & De Schuijmer, J. D. S. (2001). Preventing pressure ulcers: An evaluation of four operating-table mattresses. *Applied Nursing Research, 13*(3), 134–141.

Engle, V. F., & Graney, M. J. (2000). Biobehavioral effects of therapeutic touch. *Journal of Nursing Scholarship, 32*(3), 287–293.

Ferrell, B. R., Dow, K. H., & Grant, M. (1995). Measurement of quality of life in cancer survivors. *Quality of Life Research, 4,* 523–531.

Ferrell, B. R., Dow, K. H., Leigh, S., Ly, J., & Gulasekaram, P. (1995). Quality of life in long-term cancer survivors. *Oncology Nursing Forum, 22*(6), 915–922.

Ferrell, B. R., Grant, M., Funk, B., Garcia, N., Otis-Green, S., & Schaffner, M. L. J. (1996). Quality of life in breast cancer. *Cancer Practice, 4,* 331–340.

Gift, A. G., & Soeken, K. L. (1988). Assessment of physiologic instruments. *Heart & Lung, 17*(2), 128–133.

Goetz, R. H. (1940). Plethysmography of the skin in the investigation of peripheral vascular diseases. *British Journal of Surgery, 27,* 506–520.

Hargreaves, A., & Lander, J. (1989). Use of transcutaneous electrical nerve stimulation for postoperative pain. *Nursing Research, 38*(3), 159–161.

Harrison, M. B., Wells, G., Fisher, A., & Prince, M. (1996). Practice guidelines for the prediction and prevention of pressure ulcers: Evaluating the evidence. *Applied Nursing Research, 9*(1), 9–17.

Hartwig, M. S., Hathaway, D. K., Cardoso, S. S., & Gaber, A. O. (1994). Reliability and validity of cardiovascular and vasomotor autonomic function tests. *Diabetes Care, 17*(12), 1433–1434.

Hatton, D. C. (1997). Managing health problems among homeless women with children in a transitional shelter. *Image: Journal of Nursing Scholarship, 29*(1), 33–37.

Hillmann, G., & Beyer, G. (1967). [Rapid diazo method for determination of total bilirubin with a combined reagent.] [In German] *Zeitschrift für Klinische Chemie und Klinische Biochemie, 5*(2), 92–93.

Holditch-Davis, D., Miles, M. S., Burchinal, M., O'Donnell, K., McKinney, R., & Lim, W. (2001). Parental caregiving and developmental outcomes of infants of mothers with HIV. *Nursing Research, 50*(1), 5–14.

Holditch-Davis, D., & Thoman, E. (1988). The early social environment of premature and full term infants. *Early Human Development, 17*(2–3), 221–232.

Jones, R. C., & Broome, M. E. (2001). Focus groups with African American adolescents: Enhancing recruitment and retention in intervention studies. *Journal of Pediatric Nursing, 16*(2), 88–96.

Kaas, M. J., Dehn, D., Dahl, D., Frank, K., Markley, J., & Hebert, P. (2000). A view of prescriptive practice collaboration: Perspectives of psychiatric-mental health clinical nurse specialists and psychiatrists. *Archives of Psychiatric Nursing, 14*(5), 222–234.

Kotzer, A. M. (1990). Creative strategies for pediatric nursing research: Data collection. *Journal of Pediatric Nursing, 5*(1), 50–53.

Lenz, E. R., & Perkins, S. (2000). Coronary artery bypass graft surgery patients and their family member caregivers: Outcomes of a family-focused staged psychoeducational intervention. *Applied Nursing Research, 13*(3), 142–150.

Letourneau, N. (2001). Improving adolescent parent-infant interactions: A pilot study. *Journal of Pediatric Nursing, 16*(1), 2001.

Metheny, N. A., Stewart, B. J., Smith, L., Yan, H., Diebold, M., & Clouse, R. E. (1999). pH and concentration of bilirubin in feeding tube aspirates as predictors of tube placement. *Nursing Research, 48*(4), 189–197.

Miller, D. B., & Holditch-Davis, D. (1992). Interactions of parents and nurses with high-risk preterm infants. *Research in Nursing & Health, 15*(3), 187–197.

Morgan, D. L. (1995). Why things (sometimes) go wrong in focus groups. *Qualitative Health Research, 5*(4), 516–523.

Nelson, E. C., Landgraf, J. M., Hays, R. D., Wasson, J. H., & Kirk, J. W. (1990). The functional status of patients: How can it be measured in physicians' offices? *Medical Care, 28*(12), 1111–1126.

Nelson, E. C., Wasson, J. H., & Kirk, J. W. (1987). Assessment of function in routine clinical practice: Description of the COOP chart method and preliminary findings. *Journal of Chronic Disease, 49*(Suppl. 1), 55S–63S.

Norman, E., Gadaleta, D., & Griffin, C. C. (1991). An evaluation of three blood pressure methods in a stabilized acute trauma population. *Nursing Research, 40*(2), 86–89.

Nunnally, J. C., & Bernstein, I. H. (1994). *Psychometric theory* (3rd ed.). New York: McGraw-Hill.

Nyamathi, A., Leake, B., Keenan, C., & Gelberg, L. (2000). Type of social support among homeless women: Its impact on psychosocial resources, health and health behaviors, and use of health services. *Nursing Research, 49*(6), 318–326.

Radloff, L. S. (1977). The CES-D scale: A self report depression scale for research in the general population. *Applied Psychological Measures, 1,* 385–394.

Rew, L., Stuppy, D., & Becker, H. (1988). Construct validity in instrument development: A vital link between nursing practice, research, and theory. *Advances in Nursing Science, 10*(4), 10–22.

Rutledge, D. N., & Raymon, N. J. (2001). Changes in well-being of women cancer survivors following a survivor weekend experience. *Oncology Nursing Forum, 28*(1), 85–91.

Saris, W. E. (1991). *Computer-assisted interviewing.* Newbury Park, CA: Sage.

Schulberg, H. C., Saul, M., McClelland, M., Ganguli, M., Christy, W., Frank, R. (1985). Assessing depression in primary medical and psychiatric practices. *Archives of General Psychiatry, 42*(12), 1164–1170.

Selby-Harrington, M. L., Mehta, S. M., Jutsum, V., Riportella-Muller, R., & Quade, D. (1994). Reporting of instrument validity and reliability in selected clinical nursing journals, 1989. *Journal of Professional Nursing, 10*(1), 47–56.

Sherbourne, C. D., & Stewart, A. L. (1991). The MOS social support survey. *Social Science and Medicine, 32*(6), 705–714.

Stevens, S. S. (1946). On the theory of scales of measurement. *Science, 103*(2684), 677–680.

Stotts, C., Henderson, A., & Burns, N. (1988). *Health exemplar? Nurses, nursing students and smoking behavior.* XIII World Conference on Health Education Proceedings, Houston, TX, August 28–September 2.

Stover, J. C., Skelly, A. H., Holditch-Davis, D., & Dunn, P. F. (2001). Perceptions of health and their relationship to symptoms in African American women with type 2 diabetes. *Applied Nursing Research, 14*(2), 72–80.

Tesh, E. M., & Holditch-Davis, D. (1997). Home Inventory and NCATS: Relation to mother and child behaviors during naturalistic observations. *Research in Nursing & Health, 20*(4), 295–307.

Vredevoe, D. L., Shuler, P., & Woo, M. (1992). The homeless population. *Western Journal of Nursing Research, 14*(6), 731–740.

Wasson, J., Keller, A., Rubenstein, L., Hays, R., Nelson, E., Johnson, D., & The Dartmouth Primary COOP Project (1992). Benefits and obstacles of health status assessment in ambulatory settings, *Medical Care, 30*(5, Suppl.), MS42–MS49.

Wewers, M. E., & Lowe, N. K. (1990). A critical review of visual analogue scales in the measurement of clinical phenomena. *Research in Nursing & Health, 13*(4), 227–236.

Willems, P. (1995). Het Drukreducerend Effect Van Schulmrummer Matrassen [The pressure reducing effect of foam mattresses]. *Verpleegwetenschap K. U. Leuven.*

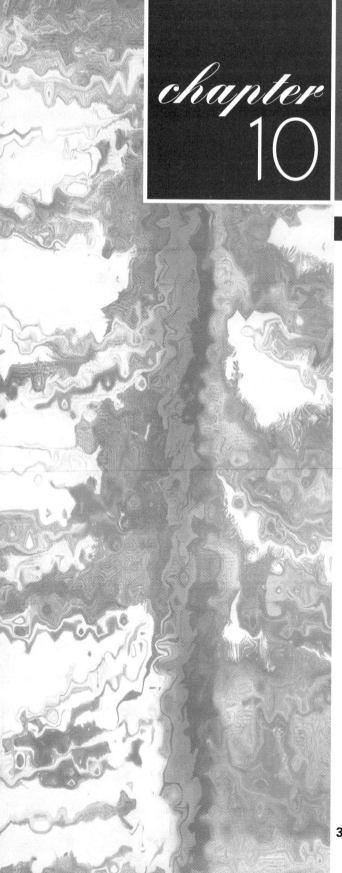

chapter 10

Understanding Statistics in Research

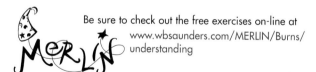

Be sure to check out the free exercises on-line at
www.wbsaunders.com/MERLIN/Burns/
understanding

OBJECTIVES

Completing this chapter should enable you to:
1. Identify the purposes of statistical analysis.
2. Describe the process of data analysis: (a) preparing the data for analysis; (b) describing the sample; (c) testing the reliability of the measurement methods; (d) conducting exploratory analysis of the data; (e) conducting confirmatory analyses guided by objectives, questions, or hypotheses; and (f) conducting posthoc analyses.
3. Differentiate probability theory from decision theory.
4. Describe the process of inferring from a sample to a population.
5. Discuss the distribution of the normal curve.
6. Compare and contrast Type I and Type II errors.
7. Differentiate a one-tailed test of significance from a two-tailed test of significance.
8. Compare the clinical and the statistical significance of findings.
9. Differentiate the ungrouped frequency distribution from the grouped frequency distribution.
10. Describe the three measures of central tendency (mean, median, and mode).
11. Discuss the purpose of measures of dispersion.
12. Discuss the purposes and interpretation of results of chi-square analysis, *t*-test, analysis of variance, Pearson's correlation, and regression analysis.
13. Critique the use of chi-square analysis, *t*-test, analysis of variance, Pearson's correlation, and regression analysis in published studies.
14. Describe the five types of results obtained from quasi-experimental and experimental studies that are interpreted within a decision theory framework: (a) significant and predicted results, (b) nonsignificant results, (c) significant and unpredicted results, (d) mixed results, and (e) unexpected results.
15. Differentiate the results, findings, and conclusions in a study.
16. Critique findings for statistical significance and practical significance in a study.
17. Identify the following elements of a research report: findings, conclusions, significance of findings, generalization of findings, implications, and suggestions for further study.
18. Given a study, critique the results, findings, conclusions, generalizations, implications, and suggestions for further study.

RELEVANT TERMS

Analysis of covariance
Analysis of variance
Between-group variance
Bivariate correlation
Chi-square test of independence

Clinical significance
Coefficient of multiple determination
Conclusions
Confirmatory analysis
Correlation matrix

Decision theory

Degrees of freedom

Dependent groups

Descriptive statistics

Effect size

Empirical generalizations

Explained variance

Exploratory analysis

Factor

Factor analysis

Findings

Frequency distribution

Generalization

Grouped frequency distribution

Implications

Independent groups

Inference

Level of significance

Line of best fit

Mean

Measure of dispersion

Measures of central tendency

Median

Mixed results

Mode

Multiple regression

Negative relationship

Nonsignificant results

Normal curve

One-tailed test of significance

Outliers

Pearson's product-moment correlation

Percentage distributions

Positive relationship

Posthoc analyses

Power

Power analysis

Probability theory

Range

Regression analysis

Scatterplot

Significant and unpredicted results

Significant results

Standard deviation

Standardized scores

Statistical significance

Symmetrical

Total variance

t-Test

Two-tailed test of significance

Type I error

Type II error

Unexpected results

Unexplained variance

Ungrouped frequency distribution

Variance

Within-group variance

X axis

Y axis

Z-score

The expectation that the practice of nursing be evidence-based has made it more important that clinical nurses acquire skills in reading and evaluating the results of statistical tests. Nurses probably have more anxiety about statistical results and data analysis than they do about any other aspect of the research process. We hope this chapter will dispel some of that anxiety and facilitate critique of studies. The statistical information in this chapter is provided from the perspective of reading, understanding, and critiquing published studies, rather than from that of selecting statistical procedures or performing statistical analyses. To critique a quantitative study, you need to be able to (1) identify the statistical procedures used; (2) judge whether these procedures were appropriate for the hypotheses, questions, or objectives of the study, and for the level of measurement of the variables; (3) comprehend the discussion of data analysis results in the study; (4) judge whether the author's interpretation of the results is appropriate; and (5) evaluate the clinical significance of the findings.

The chapter begins with a discussion of some of the more pragmatic aspects of quantitative data analysis procedures: the purposes of statistical analysis and the process of performing data analysis. The reasoning behind statistics is explained, and some of the more common statistical procedures used to describe variables, examine relationships, and predict and test causal hypotheses are introduced. The chapter concludes with strategies for judging statistical suitability and evaluating the interpretation of statistical outcomes.

PROCESS OF DATA ANALYSIS

Statistical procedures are used to examine the numerical data gathered in a study. In critiquing a study, it may be helpful to understand the process the researcher uses to perform data analyses. There are several stages in the quantitative data analysis process: (1) preparing the data for analysis; (2) describing the sample; (3) testing the reliability of measurement methods; (4) conducting exploratory analysis of the data; (5) conducting confirmatory analysis guided by the hypotheses, questions, or objectives; and (6) conducting posthoc analysis. Although not all of these stages are equally reflected in the final published report of the study, they all contribute to the insights that can be gained from analysis of the data.

Preparing the Data for Analysis

Except in very small studies, researchers almost always use computers for data analyses. The first step of the process is entering the data into the computer. The researcher uses a systematic plan for data entry designed to reduce errors during the entry phase. After entry, the data are "cleaned." This process is time intensive and tedious but essential for ensuring accuracy of the data. If the data file is small enough, every datum on the printout is cross-checked with the original datum for accuracy. Otherwise, data points are randomly checked for accuracy. All identified errors are corrected. Missing data points are identified. If the information can be obtained, the missing data are entered into the data file. If enough data are missing for certain variables, the researcher may have to determine whether there are sufficient data to perform analyses using those variables. In some cases, subjects must be excluded from an analysis because data that is considered essential to that analysis is missing.

 In critiquing a study, search for information on the amount of missing data and clues to the accuracy of the data.

Describing the Sample

Next, the researcher obtains as complete a picture of the sample as possible. First, frequencies of descriptive variables related to the sample are obtained. Estimates of central tendency (such as the mean) and dispersion (such as the standard deviation) of variables relevant to the sample are calculated. Variables relevant to the sample might include age, education level, health status, gender, and ethnicity. If the study includes more than one group (e.g., treatment group and control group), the researcher might compare the various groups in relation to these variables. For example, it might be important to know whether the age distribution of the various groups was similar. If the groups being compared are not equivalent in ways important to the study, the groups cannot justifiably be compared through statistical procedures. Thus the researcher must decide whether to continue the analysis process.

In critiquing a study, you need to judge the representativeness of the sample and the equivalence of groups that are compared in the statistical analyses.

Testing the Reliability of Measurement

After describing the sample, the researcher examines the reliability of the measurement methods used in the study. Reliability of observational or physiological measures may have been determined during the data collection phase, but will be noted again at this point. If paper-and-pencil scales were used to collect data, Cronbach's alpha will be performed on the scale items. If Cronbach's alpha coefficient is unacceptably low (below .70), the researcher must decide whether to analyze the data collected with the instrument.

In critiquing a study, search for information on the reliability of measures used to gather data for the analyses.

Conducting Exploratory Analyses

The next step, *exploratory analysis,* is used to examine all of the data descriptively. This step will be discussed in more detail in this chapter, in the section "Using Statistics to Describe." The researcher should become as familiar as possible with the nature of the data obtained on variables that will be used to test hypotheses, research questions, or objectives. Data on each variable are examined using measures of central tendency and dispersion to determine the nature of variation in the data and to identify *outliers,* which are subjects or data points with extreme values that seem unlike the rest of the sample. The most valuable insights from a study often come from careful examination of outliers (Tukey, 1977). In many studies, relationships among variables and differences between groups are explored using statistical procedures that are also used in confirmatory studies. However, when these procedures are used for exploratory purposes, the results are not generalized to a larger population. The results are used to give a better understanding of the data.

In critiquing a study, examine the values obtained for the study variables. Do they appear to be representative of values you would expect to find in the population under study? Is the full range of values for each variable represented in the data? What is the nature of outliers in the sample? Is it likely that data from outliers affected the results of the analyses? Are analyses used for exploratory or confirmatory purposes?

Conducting Confirmatory Analyses

Confirmatory analysis is performed to confirm expectations regarding the data that are expressed as hypotheses, questions, or objectives. When confirmatory analyses are performed, the findings are generalized from the sample to appropriate populations. Statistical procedures designed for the purpose of making inferences (inferential statistical procedures) are used. To justify generalization of the results of confirmatory analyses, a rigorous research methodology is needed, including a strong research design, reliable and valid measurement methods, and a large sample size.

In critiquing a study, identify the confirmatory analyses performed. Is the research methodology sufficiently rigorous to warrant using confirmatory analyses?

Conducting Posthoc Analyses

Some statistical analyses, such as chi-square analysis and analysis of variance (ANOVA), are used to test for differences among groups in studies including more than two groups. These statistical procedures indicate significant differences among groups but do not specify which groups are different. For example, a study might examine the proportion of the sample in four occupational groups who smoked to determine differences in smoking behavior among the groups. Chi-square analysis or ANOVA might show significant differences among the groups, but the researcher would not be able to determine which groups were different. In these studies, when significant differences are found, *posthoc analyses* are performed after the initial statistical analysis to identify which groups are significantly different.

In critiquing a study, you need to identify the specific posthoc analyses that were done. These should be indicated in the research report.

REASONING BEHIND STATISTICS

One reason that nurses tend to avoid statistics is that many were taught only the mathematical procedures of calculating statistical equations, with little or no explanation of the logic behind those procedures or the meaning of the results. Computation is a mechanical process usually performed by a computer, and information about the calculation procedure is not necessary to begin understanding statistical results. We will approach data analysis with the goal of enhancing the reader's understanding of the statistical analysis process. This understanding can then be used to critique data analysis techniques in the results section of research reports.

A brief explanation of some concepts that are commonly used in statistical theory is presented. The concepts include probability theory, decision theory, hypothesis testing, level of significance, inference, generalization, the normal curve, tailedness, Type I and Type II errors, power, and degrees of freedom. For a more extensive discussion of these topics, see Burns and Grove (2001).

Probability Theory

Probability theory, which is deductive, is used to explain the extent of a relationship, the probability that an event will occur in a given situation, or the probability that an event can be accurately predicted. The researcher might want to know the probability that a particular outcome will result from a nursing action. For example, the researcher might want to know how likely it is that urinary catheterization during hospitalization will lead to a bladder infection after discharge from the hospital. The researcher might want to know the probability that subjects in the experimental group are members of the same larger population from which the control group subjects were taken. Probability is expressed as a lowercase letter p, with values expressed as percentages or as a decimal value ranging from 0 to 1. For example, if the probability is 0.23, then it is expressed as $p = 0.23$. This means that there is a 23% probability that a particular outcome (such as a bladder infection) will occur. Probability values can be expressed as less than a probability value, such as 0.05, expressed as $p < 0.05$. (The symbol $<$ means "less than.") The researcher could state in a research report the finding that the probability that the experimental group subjects were members of the same larger population as the control group subjects was less than or equal to 5% (≤ 0.05). Probability values are often stated with the results of statistical analyses. In critiquing studies, it is useful to recognize these symbols and understand what they mean.

Decision Theory, Hypothesis Testing, and Level of Significance

Decision theory, which is inductive, assumes that all of the groups in a study (e.g., experimental and control groups) used to test a particular hypothesis are components of the same population relative to the variables under study. This expectation (or assumption) is traditionally expressed as a null hypothesis, which states that there is no difference between (or among) the groups in a study, in terms of the variables included in the hypothesis. It is up to the researcher to provide evidence that there really is a difference between the groups. For example, the researcher might hypothesize that there is no difference in the frequency of urinary tract infections that occurred after discharge from the hospital in patients who were catheterized during hospitalization, compared with those who were not catheterized. To test the assumption of no difference, a cutoff point is selected before data collection. The cutoff point, referred to as alpha (α), or the *level of significance,* is the probability level at which the results of statistical analysis are judged to indicate a statistically significant difference between the groups. The level of significance selected for most nursing studies is 0.05. This means that if the level of significance found in the statistical analysis is ≤ 0.05, the experimental and control groups are considered to be significantly different (members of different populations). In some studies, the more rigorous level of significance of 0.01 may be chosen. In some studies, this may be written as $\alpha = 0.01$, particularly in tables and figures.

Decision theory requires that the cutoff point selected for a study be absolute. Absolute means that even if the value obtained is only a fraction above the cutoff point, the samples are considered to be from the same population, and *no* meaning can be attributed to the differences. Thus it is inappropriate when using decision theory to state that the findings *approached* significance at the 0.051 level if the alpha level was set at 0.05. Using decision theory rules, this finding indicates that the groups tested are not significantly different, and the null hypothesis is not rejected. On the other hand, once the level of significance has been set at 0.05 by the researcher, if the analysis reveals a significant difference of 0.001, this result is not considered more significant than the 0.05 originally proposed (Slakter, Wu, & Suzaki-Slakter, 1991). The level of significance is dichotomous, which means that the difference is either significant or not significant; there are no degrees of significance. However, some individuals, not realizing that their reasoning has shifted from decision theory to probability theory, indicate in their research report that the 0.001 result makes the findings more significant than if they had obtained only a 0.05 level of significance. The researcher might state that the findings are "highly" significant, which is unacceptable from the perspective of decision theory.

From the perspective of probability theory, there is considerable difference in the risk of occurrence of a Type II error when the probability is between 0.05 and 0.001. If $p = 0.001$, the probability that the two groups are components of the same population is 1 in 1000, compared with $p = 0.05$, which indicates that the probability of the groups belonging to the same population is 5 in 100. In other words, if $p = 0.05$, then in 5 times out of 100, groups with statistical values such as those found in these statistical analyses are actually members of the same population, and the conclusion that the groups are different is erroneous.

In computer analysis the probability value obtained from each data analysis (e.g., $p = 0.03$ or $p = 0.07$) is frequently provided on the printout and is often reported by the researcher in the published study, along with the level of significance set before data analysis was done. In summary, the probability *(p)* value reveals the risk of a

Type II error. The alpha (α) value reveals whether the probability value for a particular analysis met the cutoff point for deciding whether there is a significant difference between or among groups.

In critiquing a study, you need to identify the level of significance and determine whether the findings show significant differences. You need to judge the risk of a Type II error. (Type I and Type II errors are defined and discussed later in the section entitled Type I and Type II Errors.)

Inference and Generalization

An *inference* is a conclusion or judgment based on evidence. Statistical inferences are made cautiously and with great care. The decision theory rules used to interpret the results of statistical procedures increase the probability that inferences are accurate. A *generalization* is the application of information that has been acquired from a specific instance to a general situation. Generalizing requires making an inference; both require the use of inductive reasoning. Inductively, an inference is made from a specific case and extended to a general truth, from a part to the whole, from the concrete to the abstract, and from the known to the unknown. In research, an inference is made from the study findings obtained from a specific sample and applied to a more general population, using the results from statistical analyses. Thus the researcher might conclude in a research report that a significant difference was found in the number of urinary tract infections found between two samples, one in which the subjects had been catheterized during hospitalization, and one in which the subjects had not. In addition, the researcher would conclude that this difference could be expected in all patients who had been cared for in hospitals. The findings are generalized from the sample in the study to all previously hospitalized patients. Statisticians and researchers can never prove something using inference; they can never be certain that their inferences and generalizations are correct. For example, the researcher's generalization of the incidence of urinary tract infection may not have been carefully thought out; the findings may have been generalized over too broad a population. It is possible that in the more general population, there is no difference in the incidence of urinary tract infection that is based on whether the patient was catheterized.

In critiquing a study, you must judge whether generalizations made by the researcher are justified based on the study results.

Normal Curve

The theoretical *normal curve* is an expression of statistical theory (Fig. 10-1). A normal curve is a theoretical frequency distribution of all *possible* values in a population;

however, no *real* distribution exactly fits the normal curve. The idea of the normal curve was developed by an 18-year-old mathematician, Johann Gauss, in 1795. He found that data from variables (e.g., the mean of each sample) measured repeatedly in many samples from the same population can be combined into one large sample. From this large sample, a more accurate representation can be developed of the pattern of the curve in that population than is possible with only one sample. Surprisingly, in most cases the curve is similar, regardless of the specific variables examined or the population studied.

Levels of significance and probability are based on the logic of the normal curve. The normal curve presented in Fig. 10-1 shows the distribution of values for a single population. Note that 95.5% of the values are within 2 standard deviations of the mean, ranging from −2 to +2 standard deviations. (Standard deviations are defined and discussed in this chapter, in the section titled "Using Statistics to Describe.") Thus there is approximately a 95% probability that a given measured value (e.g., the mean of a group) would fall within 2 standard deviations of the mean of the population, and there is a 5% probability that the value would fall in the tails of the normal curve (the extreme ends of the normal curve, below −2 standard deviations [2.5%] or above +2 standard deviations [2.5%]). If the groups being compared were from the same population (not significantly different), you would expect the value (e.g., the mean) of each group to fall within the 95% range of values on the normal curve. If the groups were from (significantly) different populations, you would expect one of the group values to be outside the 95% range of values. A statistical

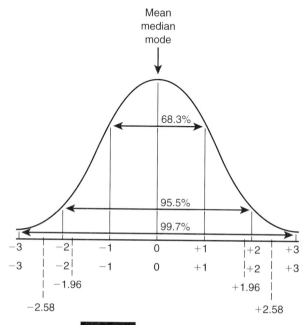

Fig. 10-1 The normal curve.

analysis performed to determine differences between or among groups, using a level of significance set at 0.05, would test that expectation. If the statistical test demonstrates a significant difference (the value of one group does not fall within the 95% range of values), the groups are considered to belong to different populations. However, in 5% of the statistical tests, the value of one of the groups can be expected to fall outside the 95% range of values but still belong to the same population (a Type I error).

Tailedness

Nondirectional hypotheses usually assume that an extreme score (obtained because the group with the extreme score did not belong to the same population) can occur in either tail of the normal curve (Fig. 10-2). The analysis of a nondirectional hypothesis is called a *two-tailed test of significance*. In a *one-tailed test of significance*, the hypothesis is directional, and extreme statistical values that occur on a single tail of the curve are of interest (see Chapter 3 for discussion of directional and nondirectional hypotheses). The hypothesis states that the extreme score is higher or lower than that of 95% of the population, indicating that the sample with the extreme score is not a member of the same population. In this case, 5% of statistical values that are considered significant will be in one tail, rather than two. Extreme statistical values occurring in the other tail of the curve are not considered significantly different. In Fig. 10-3, which shows a one-tailed figure, the portion of the curve in which statistical values will be considered significant is the right tail. Developing a one-tailed hypothesis requires that the researcher have sufficient knowledge of the variables to predict whether the difference will be in the tail above the mean or in the tail below the mean. One-tailed statistical tests are uniformly more powerful than two-tailed tests, decreasing the possibility of a Type II error.

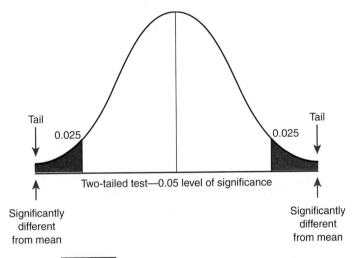

Fig. 10-2 The two-tailed test of significance.

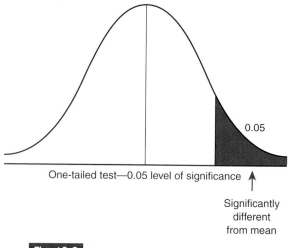

0.05

One-tailed test—0.05 level of significance

Significantly
different
from mean

Fig. 10-3   The one-tailed test of significance.

In critiquing a study, determine whether there are one-tailed or two-tailed hypotheses. If the researcher states a one-tailed hypothesis, judge whether there is sufficient knowledge on which to base a one-tailed statistical test.

Type I and Type II Errors

According to decision theory, two types of error can occur when a researcher is deciding what the result of a statistical test means: Type I and Type II. A *Type I error* occurs when the null hypothesis is rejected when it is true (e.g., when the results indicate that there is a significant difference, when, in reality, there is not). The risk of a Type I error is indicated by the level of significance. There is a greater risk of a Type I error with a 0.05 level of significance than with a 0.01 level of significance. As the level of significance becomes more extreme, the risk of a Type I error decreases, as illustrated in Fig. 10-4.

A *Type II error* occurs when the null hypothesis is regarded as true, but it is false. For example, the statistical analyses might indicate that there were not significant differences between groups, but in reality the groups were different. There is a greater risk of a Type II error when the level of significance is 0.01 than when it is 0.05. However, Type II errors are often caused by flaws in the research methods. In nursing research, many studies are conducted with small samples and with instruments that do not precisely measure the variables under study. In many nursing situations, multiple variables interact to cause differences within populations. However, when only a few of the interacting variables are examined, small differences may be overlooked, which can lead to the false conclusion that there are no differences between the samples. Thus the risk of a Type II error is high in many nursing studies.

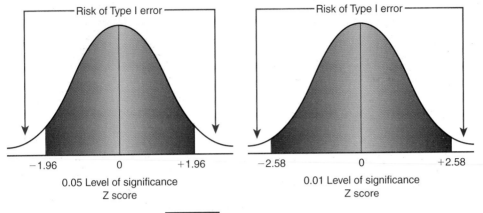

Fig. 10-4 Risk of Type I error.

In critiquing a study, evaluate the risk of a Type I or Type II error.

Power: Controlling the Risk of a Type II Error

Power is the probability that a statistical test will detect a significant difference that exists. The risk of a Type II error can be determined using *power analysis.* Cohen (1988) has identified four parameters of a power analysis: the level of significance, sample size, power, and effect size. If three of the four are known, the fourth can be calculated using power analysis formulas. The minimum acceptable power level is 0.80. The researcher determines the sample size and the level of significance. *Effect size* is "the degree to which the phenomenon is present in the population, or the degree to which the null hypothesis is false" (Cohen, 1988, pp. 9–10). For example, if changes in anxiety level were measured in a group of patients before surgery, with the first measurement taken when the patients were at home, and the second taken just before surgery, effect size would be large if a great change in anxiety occurred in the group between the two time periods. If the effect of a preoperative teaching program on the level of anxiety was measured, the effect size would be the difference in the posttest level of anxiety in the experimental group compared with that in the control group. If only a small change in the level of anxiety was expected, the effect size would be small. In most nursing studies, only small effect sizes can be expected. This small effect size occurs because nursing studies tend to use samples that are small, study designs in which threats are not tightly controlled, and measurement methods that measure only large changes. The power level should be reported in studies that fail to reject the null hypothesis (or have nonsignificant findings). If the power level is below 0.80, you should question the validity of nonsignificant findings.

In critiquing a study, look for reports of the effect size and the power level.

Degrees of Freedom

The concept of *degrees of freedom* (df) is important for calculating statistical procedures and interpreting the results using statistical tables. However, df is difficult to explain because of the complex mathematics involved. Degrees of freedom involve the freedom of a score's value to vary given the other existing scores' values and the established sum of these scores. Degrees of freedom are often reported with statistical results.

USING STATISTICS TO DESCRIBE

In any study in which the data are numerical, data analysis begins with *descriptive statistics* (also called "summary statistics"). For some descriptive studies, data analyses are limited to descriptive statistics. For other studies, descriptive statistics are used primarily to describe the characteristics of the sample from which the data were collected and to describe values obtained from the measurement of variables. Descriptive statistics presented in this text include frequency distributions, measures of central tendency, measures of dispersion, and standardized scores.

Frequency Distributions

Frequency distribution is usually the first method used to organize the data for examination. There are two types of frequency distributions: ungrouped and grouped.

Ungrouped frequency distributions

Most studies have some categorical data that are presented in the form of an *ungrouped frequency distribution,* in which a table is developed to display all numerical values obtained for a particular variable. This approach is generally used on discrete rather than continuous data. Examples of data commonly organized in this manner include gender, ethnicity, marital status, diagnostic category of study subjects, and values obtained from the measurement of variables. In Table 10-1, LoBiondo-Wood, Williams, Wood, and Shaw (1997) present the ungrouped frequency of subject characteristics in their study of the impact of liver transplantation on quality of life.

Grouped frequency distributions

Grouped frequency distributions are used when continuous variables, such as age, are being examined. Many measures taken during data collection, including body temperature, vital lung capacity, weight, scale scores, and time, are measured using a

TABLE 10-1

SUBJECT CHARACTERISTICS

VARIABLE	n	PERCENTAGE
Gender		
Male	19	46.3
Female	22	53.7
Marital status		
Single	4	9.8
Married	32	78.0
Divorced	4	9.8
Widowed	1	2.4
Education		
High school	18	43.9
Attended/completed college	12	29.3
Attended/completed graduate school	10	24.4
Income—family		
Below $20,000	14	34.4
$20,001–$30,000	6	14.6
$30,001–$40,000	7	17.1
$40,001–$50,000	5	12.2
$50,001–$60,000	3	7.3
Above $60,000	3	7.3
Diagnosis		
Cirrhosis	24	58.5
Primary biliary cirrhosis	8	19.5
Primary sclerosing cholangitis	7	17.1
Secondary biliary cirrhosis	1	2.4
Malignancy	1	2.4
Occupation		
Unemployed	20	48.8
Laborer	6	14.6
Semiskilled	2	4.9
Skilled	1	2.4
Clerical	2	4.9
Semiprofessional	2	4.9
Minor/lesser professional	6	14.6
Professional	3	7.3

From LoBiondo-Wood, G., Williams, L., Wood, R. P., & Shaw, B. W. (1997). Impact of liver transplantation on quality of life: A longitudinal perspective. *Applied Nursing Research, 10*(1), 29, with permission.

continuous scale. Any method of grouping results in loss of information. For example, if age is grouped, a breakdown into two groups, under 65 years of age and over 65 years of age, provides less information about the data than groupings of 10-year age spans. As with levels of measurement, rules have been established to guide classification systems. There should be at least 6 but not more than 20 groups. The classes established must be exhaustive; each datum must fit into one of the identified classes. The classes must be exclusive; each datum must fit into only one. A common mistake occurs when the ranges contain overlaps that would allow a datum to fit into more than one class. For example, the researcher might have classified age ranges as 20 to 30, 30 to 40, 40 to 50, and so on. In this case, subjects aged 30, 40, and so on could have been classified into more than one class. The range of each class must be equivalent; with age, for example, if 10 years is the range, each class must include 10 years of ages. This rule is violated in some cases to allow the first and last categories to be open-ended and worded to include all scores above or below a specified point. In Table 10-1, "Income" is a grouped frequency.

Percentage distributions

Percentage distributions indicate the percentage of the sample whose scores fall into a specific group and the number of scores in that group. Percentage distributions are particularly useful for comparing the present data with findings from other studies that have different sample sizes. The percentage distribution is provided for each variable in Table 10-1. A cumulative distribution is a type of percentage distribution in which the percentages and frequencies of scores are summed, as one moves from the top of the table to the bottom. Thus the bottom category would have a cumulative frequency equivalent to the sample size and a cumulative percentage of 100 (Table 10-2). Frequency distributions are also displayed using tables or graphs (e.g., pie charts, bar charts, histograms, and frequency polygons). Graphic displays of the grouped frequency distribution of data from Table 10-2 are presented in Fig. 10-5.

Measures of Central Tendency

A measure of central tendency is frequently referred to as an "average," which is a lay term not commonly used in statistics because it is vague. The measures of central tendency are the most concise statement of the nature of the data; the three that are

---

TABLE 10-2

EXAMPLE OF A CUMULATIVE FREQUENCY TABLE

SCORE	FREQUENCY	PERCENT	CUMULATIVE FREQUENCY (f)	CUMULATIVE PERCENT
1	4	8	4	8
3	6	12	10	20
4	8	16	18	36
5	14	28	32	64
7	8	16	40	80
8	6	12	46	92
9	4	8	$n=50$	100

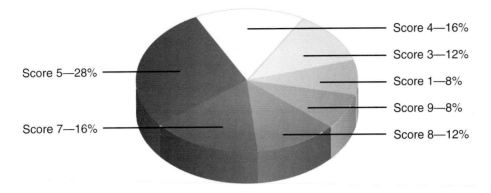

Score 4—16%
Score 3—12%
Score 5—28%
Score 1—8%
Score 9—8%
Score 7—16%
Score 8—12%

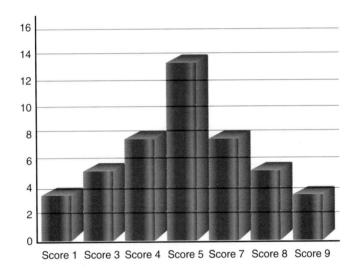

Score 1 Score 3 Score 4 Score 5 Score 7 Score 8 Score 9

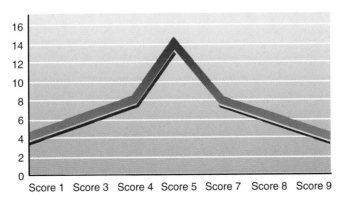

Score 1 Score 3 Score 4 Score 5 Score 7 Score 8 Score 9

Fig. 10-5 Commonly used graphic displays of frequencies distribution.

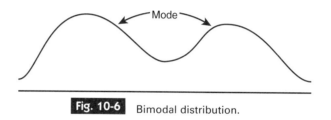

Fig. 10-6   Bimodal distribution.

commonly used in statistical analyses are the mode, median, and mean. For a data set that has a normal distribution, these values are equal (see Fig. 10-1); however, they are usually different for data obtained from real samples.

Mode

The *mode* is the numerical value or score that occurs with greatest frequency; it does not necessarily indicate the center of the data set. The mode can be determined by examination of an ungrouped frequency distribution of the data. In Table 10-2, the mode is the score of 5, which occurred 14 times in the data set. The mode can be used to describe the typical subject or to identify the most frequently occurring value on a scale item. The mode is the appropriate measure of central tendency for nominal data. A data set can have more than one mode. If two modes exist, the data set is referred to as "bimodal," as illustrated in Fig. 10-6. More than two modes would be multimodal.

Median

The *median* is the score at the exact center of the ungrouped frequency distribution— the 50th percentile. The median is obtained by rank ordering the scores. If the number of scores is uneven, exactly 50% of the scores are above the median and 50% are below it. If the number of scores is even, the median is the average of the two middle scores; thus the median may not be one of the scores in the data set. Unlike the mean, the median is not affected by extreme scores in the data (outliers). The median is the most appropriate measure of central tendency for ordinal data. The median for the data in Table 10-2 is 5.

Mean

The most commonly used measure of central tendency is the mean. The *mean* is the sum of the scores divided by the number of scores being summed. Thus, like the median, the mean may not be a member of the data set. The mean is the appropriate measure of central tendency for interval and ratio level data. The mean for the data in Table 10-2 is 5.28.

Measures of Dispersion

Measures of dispersion, or variability, are measures of individual differences of the members of the sample. They give some indication of how scores in a sample are dispersed around the mean. These measures provide information about the data that is not available from measures of central tendency. They indicate how different the scores are, or the extent to which individual scores deviate from one another. If the individual scores are similar, measures of variability are small, and the sample is relatively homogeneous, or similar, in terms of those scores. A heterogeneous sample has a wide variation in scores. The measures of dispersion most commonly used are range, variance, and standard deviation. Standardized scores may be used to express measures of dispersion. Scatterplots are frequently used to illustrate the dispersion in the data.

Range

The simplest measure of dispersion is the *range*, which is obtained by subtracting the lowest score from the highest score. The range for the scores in Table 10-2 is calculated as follows: $9 - 1 = 8$. The range is a difference score, which uses only the two extreme scores for the comparison. It is a very crude measure and is sensitive to outliers.

Variance

The *variance* is calculated with a mathematical equation. The numerical value obtained from the calculation depends on the measurement scale used; the calculated variance value has no absolute value and can be compared only with data obtained using similar measures. Generally, however, the larger the variance value, the greater the dispersion of scores. The variance for the data in Table 10-2 is 4.94.

Standard deviation

The *standard deviation* is the square root of the variance. Just as the mean is the average value, the standard deviation is the average difference (deviation) value. The standard deviation provides a measure of the average deviation of a value from the mean in that particular sample. It indicates the degree of error that would be made if the mean alone were used to interpret the data. In the normal curve, 68% of the value will be within 1 standard deviation above or below the mean, 95% will be within 2 standard deviations above or below the mean, and 99% will be within 3 standard deviations above or below the mean (see Fig. 10-1).

The standard deviation for the data in Table 10-2 is 2.22. Because we know that the mean is 5.28, we can determine that the value of a subject 1 standard deviation below the mean would be $5.28 - 2.22$ (3.06). The value of a subject 1 standard deviation above the mean would be $5.28 + 2.22$ (7.50). Thus we know that approximately 68% of the sample (and perhaps the population from which it was derived) can be expected to have values in the range of 3.06 to 7.50. Extending this calculation further, the value of a subject 2 standard deviations above the mean would be $5.28 + 2.22 + 2.22 = (9.72)$. Using this strategy, the entire distribution of values can be estimated. The value of a single individual can be compared with the values of the total sample. Standard deviation is an important measure, both for understanding dispersion within a distribution and for interpreting the relationship of a particular value to the distribution.

Standardized scores

Because of differences in the characteristics of various distributions, comparing a value in one distribution with a value in another is difficult. Let us say, for example, that you wanted to compare test scores from two classroom examinations. The highest possible score in one test was 100 and in the other 70; the scores would be difficult to compare. To facilitate this comparison, a mechanism was developed to transform raw scores into *standardized scores*. Numbers that make sense only within the framework of measurements used within a specific study are transformed into numbers (standardized scores) that have a more general meaning. Transformation into standardized scores allows an easy conceptual grasp of the meaning of the score. A common standardized score is called a *Z-score*. It expresses deviations from the mean (difference scores) in terms of standard deviation units (see Fig. 10-1). A score that falls above the mean will have a positive Z-score, whereas a score that falls below the mean will have a negative Z-score. The mean expressed as a Z-score is zero. The standard deviation is equal to the Z-score. Thus a Z-score of 2 indicates that the score from which it was obtained is 2 standard deviations above the mean. A Z-score of -0.5 indicates that the score was 0.5 standard deviations below the mean.

Scatterplots

A *scatterplot* has two scales: horizontal and vertical. Each scale is referred to as an axis. The vertical scale is called the *Y axis;* the horizontal scale is the *X axis*. A scatterplot can be used to illustrate the dispersion of values on a variable. In this case, the X axis would represent the possible values of the variable. The Y axis would represent the number of times each value of the variable occurred in the sample. Scatterplots can also be used to illustrate the relationship between values on one variable and values on another. In this case, each axis would represent one variable. For example, if a graph was developed to illustrate the relationship between the number of days a patient was hospitalized and the stage of the patient's decubitus ulcer, the horizontal axis might represent days and the vertical axis decubitus ulcer stage. For each unit or subject, there is a value for X and a value for Y. The point at which the values of X and Y for a single subject intersect is plotted on the graph (Fig. 10-7). When the values for each subject in the sample have been plotted, the degree of relationship between the variables is revealed (Fig. 10-8).

Understanding Descriptive Statistical Results

In a published study, descriptive statistics are often reported in the text of the results section, usually as part of the description of the sample. It is also important to report the values obtained on study variables, as well as the measures of central tendency and dispersion of each variable. In some studies, descriptive statistics may be summarized in a table. Schmelzer, Case, Chappell, and Wright (2000) used a table to report descriptive statistics in a study that compared the effectiveness of two enema solutions. The results of descriptive analysis of these data are presented in Table 10-3.

Descriptive statistics can also be used to describe differences between either groups or variables. Examining differences between variables also reflects their relatedness. From a descriptive perspective of descriptive analyses, the purpose is not to test for causality but rather to describe their differentness. One statistical procedure used for this purpose is the chi-square test.

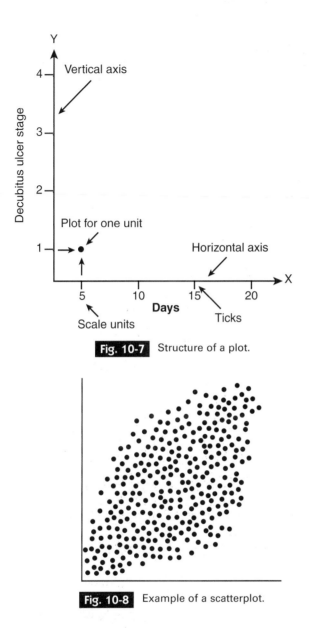

Fig. 10-7   Structure of a plot.

Fig. 10-8   Example of a scatterplot.

Chi-Square Test of Independence

The *chi-square test of independence* determines whether two variables are independent or related; the test can be used with nominal or ordinal data. The procedure examines the frequencies of observed values and compares them with the frequencies that would be expected if the data categories were independent of each other. The procedure is not very powerful; thus the risk of a Type II error is high, and large samples are needed to reduce this risk. Therefore, most studies using this procedure place little importance on results in which no differences are found. Researchers frequently perform multiple chi-square tests in a sample. However, results are generally presented only when a chi-square analysis shows a significant difference.

TABLE 10-3

COMPARISON OF ENEMA INSTILLED, NET OUTPUT, PEG CONCENTRATION, AND PERCENT OF PEG RECOVERY

	ENEMA INSTILLED (g)	NET OUTPUT[a] (g)	PEG [PEG][b] (g/L)	RECOVERY[c]
Tap water group (n = 12)	M: 939 SD: 70 Range: 723 to 980[d]	M: −175.3 SD: 185.6 Range: −556 to +147	M: 1.7 SD: 0.45	68%
Soapsuds group (n = 13)	M: 918 SD: 202 Range: 400 to 976[e]	M: +10.5 SD: 106.1 Range: −205 to +173	M: 1.4 SD: 0.35	72%
Statistical significance (α = 0.05)	No significant difference (α = 0.05)	t = −3.039 df = 17 p = 0.007	No significant difference (α = 0.05)	No significant difference

[a]Weight of enema returns minus weight of enema instilled.
[b]Concentration of a PEG marker in the enema returns.
[c]Percentage of original polyethylene glycol marker added to the enema that was recovered in the enema returns.
[d]One man retained less than 900 g total tap water; he retained 723 g.
[e]Four people retained less than 900 g of soapsuds enema. Two women received 400 g and 718 g, and two men received 448 g and 794 g of solution.

df, Degrees of freedom; *M,* mean; *p,* probability; *PEG,* polyethylene glycol 3350; *SD,* standard deviation; *t,* t-test.

From Schmelzer, M., Case, P., Chappell, S. M., & Wright, K. B. (2000). Colonic cleansing, fluid absorption, and discomfort following tap water and soapsuds enemas. *Applied Nursing Research, 13*(2), 88.

Interpreting results

The result of the mathematical calculation is a chi-square statistic, which is compared with the chi-square values in a statistical table. If the value of the statistic is equal to or greater than the value identified in the chi-square statistical table (Burns & Grove, 2001, p. 768 for statistical table), the researcher can conclude that there are significant differences between the two variables. The exact location of specific differences among categories of variables cannot be determined from this analysis. Posthoc analyses can be used to identify the categories where the differences lie. In some published studies, the researchers discuss the results as if they knew where the differences were without having performed posthoc analyses. Readers should view these reports with skepticism.

In a published study, chi-square test results may be reported in the text of the results section. In a study examining depression, service needs, and service use in vulnerable populations, Badger, McNiece, and Gagan (2000) compared enabling characteristics that assist or inhibit individuals seeking health care. For the analysis, subjects were assigned to one of two groups: depressed individuals and nondepressed individuals. A 0.05 level of significance was set for the study. The authors report their findings as follows.

"There were significant differences between the 2 groups for work status (χ^2 [4] = 18.10, p = 0.001). More depressed participants (70%) were disabled compared to nondepressed participants (43%). There were also fewer retirees among depressed participants." (p. 178)

Often the first reaction to a sentence such as the previous one by those unfamiliar with reading statistical results is panic. The next reaction might be to avoid looking at the sentence and skip to the next one. Maybe it will make more sense. However, a sentence such as this provides a great deal of information in a small amount of space. Rather than trying to take in the entire sentence in one glance, examine the component parts first. In the component, "(χ^2 [4] = 18.10, p = 0.001)," the author is using chi-square (χ^2) analysis to compare the depressed and nondepressed groups. The author provides the df (df = 4), so that the reader can validate the accuracy of the results using a statistical chi-square table (Burns & Grove, 2001, p. 768). The numerical value after the first equal sign, 18.10, is the chi-square value obtained from calculating the chi-square equation (probably using a computer). This value has no inherent meaning other than to determine significance on a statistical table. As noted earlier, the symbol p is the abbreviation for probability. The groups were significantly different because p = 0.001, which is below the cutoff point of 0.05. The phrase also indicates that the probability is equal to 0.001 (0.1% or 1 in a 1000) that these groups come from the same population.

Chi-square results are sometimes provided within a table. Fitch, Gray, Franssen, and Johnson (2000) used a table and text, to report chi-square test results from their study. Table 10-4 indicates the results of chi-square analyses examining differences in the adequacy of help received for a variety of problems in two groups of men, all of whom had prostate cancer. One group was composed of men who had not had a recurrence of cancer, and the other group was composed of men who had. The following text discusses the results presented in Table 10-4.

"Table 10-4 provides the percentage of men in each group who indicated that they had received adequate help for the most frequently identified problems they experienced. For the entire sample of men who had experienced a particular problem since their diagnosis, approximately two-thirds indicated that they had received adequate help for their problems with side effects (56%) and pain (60%). Approximately one-third (37%) reported that they received adequate help for problems with incontinence, whereas one-fourth or less received adequate help related to fear of dying (25%), anger (22%), and sexual function (19%). A higher percentage of men with recurrent disease reported receiving adequate help with pain (72% versus 28%, χ^2 = 5.9, df = 1, p <0.001)." (p. 1258)

TABLE 10-4

PROBLEMS IDENTIFIED SINCE DIAGNOSIS

PROBLEM CITED	NO RECURRENT DISEASE (n = 845)	RECURRENT DISEASE (n = 120)	WHOLE GROUP (n = 965)
Sexual function	49%	56%	50%
Side effects*	32%	60%	35%
Incontinence	25%	29%	25%
Anger[†]	12%	26%	14%
Fear of dying	13%	18%	14%
Pain[‡]	12%	30%	14%
Getting around	8%	20%	9%
Diet	5%	13%	6%
Self blame/guilt	5%	9%	6%
Feeling isolated	5%	12%	6%
Change in family relationships	4%	12%	4%
Household responsibilities	4%	9%	5%
Get to out-of-town appointments	4%	7%	5%
Change in friend relationship	4%	9%	5%
Bathing	4%	8%	5%
Social relations	4%	15%	5%
Feeling stigmatized	3%	5%	4%
Financial	3%	8%	4%
Get to in-town appointments	3%	7%	3%
Feeling discriminated against	2%	3%	2%
Dressing	2%	10%	3%
Loss of employment	2%	9%	3%

*$p < 0.001$; [†]$p < 0.01$; [‡]$p < 0.005$.

USING STATISTICS TO EXAMINE RELATIONSHIPS

Correlational analyses are performed to identify relationships between or among variables. The purpose of the analysis may be to describe relationships between variables, clarify the relationships among theoretical concepts, or assist in identifying possible causal relationships, which can then be tested by causal analyses. All the data for the analysis should have been obtained from a single population from which values were available on all variables to be examined in a correlational analysis. Data measured at the interval level provides the best information on the nature of the relationship. However, analysis procedures are available for most levels of measurement. Data for a correlational analysis should also span the full range of possible values on each variable used in the analysis. For example, if values for a particular variable could range from a low of 1 to a high of 9, each of the values from 1 to 9 should be found in subjects in the data set. If all or most of the values are in the middle of that scoring range (4, 5, and 6) and few or none have extreme values, a full understanding of the relationship cannot be obtained from the analysis. Thus large samples with diverse scores are desirable for correlational analyses.

Pearson's Product-Moment Correlation

Pearson's product-moment correlation is a parametric test used to determine relationships among variables. *Bivariate correlation* measures the extent of relationship between two variables. Data are collected from a single sample, and measures of the two variables to be examined must be available for each subject in the data set. Less commonly, data are obtained from two related subjects, such as breast cancer incidence in mothers and daughters. Correlational analysis provides two pieces of information about the data: the nature of a relationship (positive or negative) between the two variables and the magnitude (or strength) of the relationship. Scatterplots are sometimes presented to illustrate the relationship graphically. The outcomes of correlational analyses are symmetrical rather than asymmetrical. *Symmetrical* means that there is no indication from the analysis of the direction of the relationship. One cannot say from the analysis that variable A leads to or causes variable B, or that B causes A.

Interpreting results

The outcome of the Pearson product-moment correlation analysis is a correlation coefficient (r) value between -1 and $+1$. This r value indicates the degree of relationship between the two variables. A value of 0 indicates no relationship. A value of -1 indicates a perfect negative (inverse) correlation. In a *negative relationship,* a high score on one variable is correlated with a low score on the other variable. A value of $+1$ indicates a perfect positive relationship. In a *positive relationship,* a high score on one variable is correlated with a high score on the other variable. A positive correlation also exists when a low score on one variable is correlated with a low score on the other variable. The variables vary or change in the same direction, either increasing or decreasing together. As the negative or positive values of r approach 0, the strength of the relationship decreases. Traditionally, an r value of 0.1 to 0.3 is considered a weak relationship; a value between 0.4 and 0.5 is a moderate relationship; and the r value is above 0.5, it is considered a strong relationship (Burns & Grove, 2001). However, this interpretation of the r value depends to a great extent on the variables being examined and the situation in which they were measured. Therefore interpretation requires some judgment on the part of the researcher.

When Pearson's correlation coefficient is squared (r^2), the resulting number is the percentage of variance explained by the relationship. Even when two variables are related, values of the two variables will not be a perfect match. For example, if two variables show a strong positive relationship, a high score on one variable can be expected to be associated with a high score on the other variable. However, a subject who has the highest score on one value will not necessarily have the highest score on the other variable. Thus r^2 indicates the variance that is known by correlating two variables. There will be some variation in the relationship between values for the two variables for individual subjects. Some of the variation in values is explained by the relationship between the two variables. This is called *explained variance.* The amount of explained variation is indicated by r^2 and is expressed as a percentage. The author might state that the relationship of the two variables, as expressed by r^2, explained 43% of the variance of scores in the two variables. However, part of the variation is the result of things other than the relationship. This is called *unexplained variance.* In the example provided 57% of the variation in scores is due to something other than the relationship studied, perhaps variables not examined in the study. A strong correlation has less unexplained variance than a weak correlation.

There has been a tendency to disregard weak correlations in nursing research. This could result in overlooking a relationship that might have some meaning within nursing knowledge if the relationship was examined in the context of other variables. This situation, which is similar to a Type II error, commonly occurs for three reasons. First, many nursing measurements are not powerful enough to detect fine discriminations. Some instruments may not detect extreme scores, and a relationship may be stronger than indicated by the crude measures available. Second, correlational studies must have a wide range of scores for relationships to be detected. If the study scores are homogeneous or the sample is small, relationships that exist in the population may not show up as clearly in the sample. Third, in many cases, bivariate analysis does not provide a clear picture of the dynamics in the situation. A number of variables can be linked through weak correlations, but together they provide increased insight into situations of interest. Statistical procedures (such as regression analysis) are available for examining the relationships among multiple variables simultaneously.

Testing the significance of a correlation coefficient

Before inferring that the sample correlation coefficient applies to the population from which the sample was taken, statistical analysis must be performed to determine whether the coefficient is significantly different from zero (no correlation). With a small sample, a very high correlation coefficient can be nonsignificant. With a very large sample, the correlation coefficient can be statistically significant when the degree of association is too small to be clinically significant. Therefore when judging the significance of the coefficient, both the size of the coefficient and its statistical significance should be considered.

Lyon and Munro (2001) reported the results of correlations in a study of disease severity and symptoms of depression in Black Americans infected with HIV. In the study, five measures were correlated: HIV RNA viral load (measures the number of human immunodeficiency viral particles in plasma), CD4+ T-lymphocyte count (crucial control cells in the acquired immune response), CDC (Center[s] for Disease Control [and Prevention]) stage of disease (1993 Revised Classification System for HIV Infection), number of years the subject had been HIV-seropositive, and the CES-D (Center for Epidemiologic Studies Depression Scale) score. The results were reported as follows:

"Of the HIV disease severity measures, viral load was the only laboratory or clinical indicator that was correlated with depressive symptoms at a statistically significant level. CD4+ T-lymphocyte counts were not associated with depressive symptom[s] nor was CDC HIV stage. There was no trend in the data consistent with a higher frequency of depressive symptoms according to time of known HIV-seropositivity or at certain potential crisis points such as initial diagnosis or at late-stage immune compromise. Depressive symptoms were prominent at all levels of HIV disease." (p. 7)

Tables are sometimes used to report the results of correlations, particularly when several variables have been correlated.

Lyon and Munro (2001) presented their findings in a table. Correlational results for a number of variables presented in table form are referred to as a *correlation matrix*. The numbers from the variables listed on the left side of the table indicate the same variables as the numbers across the top of the table. For example the variable "CDC stage" is number 3, both on the left side and at the top. The blank spaces in the table are typical of a correlational matrix. A blank space is present just to the right of variable 1, viral load, and below the number 1. This space indicates the relationship between variable 1 and variable 1, which will always be a perfect relationship of +1. By tradition, this space is left blank rather than showing the perfect relationship value of +1. The spaces that show the relationship of each of the other variables to itself are also blank. There are also other blanks in this table. For example, variable 3, CDC state (on the left), has a blank in the first column, which should show the value between variables 1 and 3. The value that should be shown here can be found on the first line of variable 1 (viral load) under 3. This value is 0.217. For each one of the variables, there are two places on the matrix that the same value could be given. These unseen values are referred to as mirror images and are left blank to keep the table as simple as possible. You can determine the percentage of variance explained by each relationship by squaring the values shown in Table 10-5. For example, viral load explained 4.95% of the variance in the relationship with CD4+ count.

TABLE 10-5

INTERCORRELATIONS AMONG HIV DISEASE MEASURES AND DEPRESSIVE SYMPTOMS

	1	2	3	4	5
1. Viral load		−0.225	0.217	0.262[a]	0.252[a]
2. CD4+			−0.589[b]	−0.078	0.075
3. CDC stage				0.060	−0.09
4. Years HIV+					0.054
5. CES-D score					

[a]Correlation is significant at the 0.05 level (two-tailed).
[b]Correlation is significant at the 0.01 level (two-tailed).

CDC, Centers for Disease Control and Prevention; *CES-D*, Center for Epidemiologic Studies Depression Scale; *HIV*, human immunodeficiency virus.

Factor Analysis

Factor analysis examines interrelationships among large numbers of variables and disentangles those relationships to identify clusters of variables that are most closely linked. Intellectually, you might do this by identifying categories and sorting the variables according to your judgment of the most appropriate category. Factor analysis sorts the variables into categories according to how closely related they are to the other variables. Closely related variables are grouped together into a *factor*. Several factors may be identified within a data set. Once the factors have been identified mathematically, the researcher must interpret the results by explaining why the analysis grouped the variables in a specific way. Statistical results will indicate the amount of variance in the data set that can be explained by a particular factor, and the amount of variance in the factor that can be explained by a particular variable. Factor analysis aids in the identification of theoretical constructs; it is also used to confirm the accuracy of a theoretically developed construct. For example, a theorist might state that the concept (or construct) of "hope" consisted of the following elements: (1) anticipation of the future, (2) belief that things will work out for the best, and (3) optimism. Ways could be developed to measure these three elements, and a factor analysis could be conducted on the data to determine whether subject responses clustered into these three groupings. Factor analysis is frequently used in the process of developing measurement instruments, particularly those related to psychological variables, such as attitudes, beliefs, values, and opinions. The instrument operationalizes a theoretical construct. Factor analysis can also be used to sort out meaning from large numbers of questions on survey instruments.

USING STATISTICS TO PREDICT

The ability to predict future events is becoming increasingly important in our society. We are interested in predicting who will win the football game, what the weather will be like next week, or what stocks are likely to rise in the near future. In nursing practice, as in the rest of society, the capacity to predict is crucial. For example, we would like to be able to predict the length of a hospital stay for patients with illnesses of different severity, as well as the response of patients with a variety of characteristics to nursing interventions. We need to know what factors play an important role in a patient's response to rehabilitation. Predictive analyses are based on probability theory rather than decision theory. Prediction is one approach to examining causal relationships between or among variables.

Regression Analysis

Regression analysis is used to predict the value of one variable when we know the value of one or more other variables. The variable to be predicted in a regression analysis is referred to as the dependent variable. The dependent variable is usually measured at the interval level. The goal of the analysis is to explain as much of the variance in the dependent variable as possible. In regression analysis, variables used to predict values of the dependent variable are referred to as independent variables. If there is more than one independent variable, the analysis is referred to as *multiple regression.* In regression analysis, the symbol for the dependent variable is Y, and the symbol for the independent variable(s) is X. Scatterplots and a bivariate correlation matrix are often developed before regression analysis to examine the relationships that exist in the variables. The purpose of the regression analysis is to develop a *line of best fit* that will best reflect the values on the scatterplot. The line of best fit is often illustrated as an overlay on the

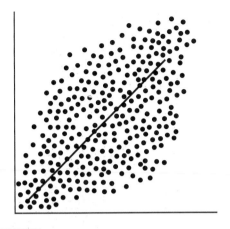

Fig. 10-9 Overlay of scatterplot and best-fit line.

scatterplot (Fig. 10-9). Many types of regression analyses have been developed to analyze various types of data. One type, logistic regression, was developed to predict values of a dependent variable measured at the ordinal level. Logistic regression is being used with increasing frequency in nursing studies.

Interpreting results

The outcome of a regression analysis is the regression coefficient R. When R is squared (R^2), it indicates the amount of variance in the data that is explained by the equation. When more than one independent variable is being used to predict values of the dependent variable, R^2 is sometimes referred to as the *coefficient of multiple determination*. The test statistic used to determine the significance of a regression coefficient may be t or F. Small sample sizes decrease the possibility of obtaining statistical significance. Values for R^2, t, and F are reported with the results of a regression analysis. The calculated coefficient values may also be expressed as an equation. Many studies using regression analysis are complex, including multiple independent variables and involving more than one regression procedure. Understanding the discussion of complex results requires reading each sentence carefully for comprehension before proceeding to the next sentence.

Craft and Moss (1996) used regression analysis in their study of how accurately the volume of infant emesis could be assessed. In their study, carefully measured amounts of baby formula were poured on receiving blankets. Nurses and nursing students were asked to estimate the volume poured on each of 20 receiving blankets. Each nurse examined the blankets in the same order so that the researchers could determine if accuracy changed as the number of blankets examined by each nurse increased. Error was calculated as the difference between the volume actually poured on the blanket and the volume estimated by the nurse. The authors report the results of the regression analysis as follows:

Continued

"Analysis with stepwise multiple regression using relative error per subject as the dependent measure showed that subject practice status (student versus practicing nurse), the nature of subject clinical experience, and number of displays assessed for weight accounted for a significant proportion of variance (Table 10-6). Nurses from large newborn nurseries underestimated 23% to 30%, whereas nurses from units with sick toddlers had a lower percentage of underestimation ($M = -0.13$). These data show that the nature of experience, rather than the length of experience, could be important. Only a small portion of the variance ($R^2 = .19$) in mean relative error per subject was accounted for by the variables studied, indicating the need for further study of other variables that must also influence the accuracy of visual assessment in emesis volume determination." (p. 6)

TABLE 10-6

STEPWISE MULTIPLE REGRESSION OF INDEPENDENT VARIABLES ON MEAN RELATIVE ERROR

VARIABLE	R	R^2	R^2 INCREASE	F	p
Subject practice (student versus practicing nurse)	0.26	0.07	0.07	7.55	0.007
Nature of clinical practice	0.36	0.13	0.06	7.53	0.001
Number of displays assessed for weight	0.36	0.19	0.06	7.21	0.001

From Craft, M. J., & Moss, J. (1996). Accuracy of infant emesis volume assessment. *Applied Nursing Research, 9*(1), 6, with permission.

USING STATISTICS TO EXAMINE CAUSALITY

Causality is a way of knowing that one thing causes another. Because they can be used to understand the effects of interventions, statistical procedures that examine causality are critical to the development of nursing science. These statistics examine causality by testing for significant differences between or among groups.

t-Tests

One of the most common analyses used to test for significant differences between two samples is the *t-test*. A variety of *t*-tests have been developed for various types of samples. Frequently, researchers misuse the *t*-test by using multiple *t*-tests to examine differences in various aspects of data collected in a study. When this is done, there is an escalation of significance that increases the risk of a Type I error. Bonferroni's procedure, which controls for the escalation of significance, may be used when multiple t-tests must be performed on different aspects of the same data.

Interpreting results

The result of the mathematical calculation is a t statistic. This statistic is compared with the t values in a statistical table (see Burns & Grove, 2001, p. 763). The table is used to identify the critical value of t. If the computed statistic is greater than or equal to the critical value, the groups are significantly different.

> Stover, Skelly, Holditch-Davis, and Dunn (2001) used a t-test to compare subjects who reported symptoms with subjects who did not report symptoms. The SF-20, a measure of symptoms and other health perceptions, was used. They reported the results of the t-test in the text as follows.
>
> "The mean of each of the 6 subscales of the SF-20 [a measure of health perceptions] were compared [between] subjects reporting symptoms and those that did not using student t tests. Mental health is the first column across the top of Table 10-7. The t values, degrees of freedom, and p values are shown in the last three rows of the table (bottom three lines of the left column). On average, African American women with Type 2 diabetes and symptoms of upper and lower neuropathy and/or peripheral vascular disease rated their perceptions of general health, physical role, social functioning, and bodily pain as poorer, compared with subjects without these symptoms." (p. 65)

TABLE 10-7

SF-20 AND SYMPTOMS OF UPPER OR LOWER NEUROPATHY OR PERIPHERAL VASCULAR DISEASE IN THE PAST 2 WEEKS

	n	SUBSCALE OF THE SF-20 MENTAL HEALTH	GENERAL HEALTH	PHYSICAL FUNCTION	ROLE FUNCTION	SOCIAL FUNCTION	BODILY PAIN
Subjects with no symptoms in past 2 weeks	29 (SD)	60.1 (6.5)	45.5 (27.2)	78.7 (23.5)	74.1 (41.3)	83.5 (28.8)	62.8 (29.1)
Subjects with symptoms in past 2 weeks	46 (SD)	57.7 (9.0)	29.8 (21.6)	50.0 (34.6)	41.3 (47.5)	63.0 (35.0)	49.1 (26.9)
t values		1.3	2.6	4.3	3.1	2.6	2.1
Degrees of freedom		71.6	49.8	72.5	65.6	67.8	56.1
p values		18.0	<0.01	<0.01	<0.01	<0.01	<0.05

From Stover, J. C., Skelly, A. H., Holditch-Davis, D., & Dunn, P. F. (2001). Perceptions of health and their relationship to symptoms in African American women with type 2 diabetes. *Applied Nursing Research, 14*(2), 76.

Because they provided a table (see Table 10-7) with the statistical results, these were not provided in the text. If the results of comparing mental health, for example, had been presented in text, the discussion would have been presented as follows: There was no significant difference in mental health ($t = 1.3$, $df = 71.6$, $p = 0.18$) between subjects who did not report symptoms in the past 2 weeks and subjects who did.

The phrase ($t = 1.3$, $df = 71.6$, $p = 0.18$) tells you that the value of t was 1.3, the df was 71.6, and the results were not significant, since $p = 0.18$ is above the 0.05 cutoff. The t value, 1.3, has no meaning other than to determine the level of significance on a statistical table. In Table 10-7 the authors provide the mean (M) and standard deviation (SD) for each variable, the t value, and the p value. Providing this information allows another researcher to check the accuracy of the analyses reported in the study, to perform a power analysis, or to use the data in a meta-analysis. Because the authors used more than one t-test to examine data in the same sample, there is an increased risk of a Type I error. Researchers would have less Type I error if they had analyzed their data using the Bonferroni procedure for multiple t-tests.

Analysis of Variance

Analysis of variance (ANOVA) tests for differences between means. ANOVA is more flexible than other analyses, because it can be used to examine data from two or more groups. There are many types of ANOVA, some developed for analysis of data from complex experimental designs, such as those using blocking or repeated measures. Rather than focusing just on differences between means, ANOVA tests for differences in variance. One source of variance is the variance within each group, because individual scores in the group will vary from the group mean. This variance is referred to as the *within-group variance.* Another source of variation is variation of the group means around the grand mean, which is referred to as the *between-group variance.* One could assume that if all the samples were drawn from the same population, there would be little difference in these two sources of variance. When these two types of variance are combined, they are referred to as the *total variance.* The test for ANOVA is always one-tailed.

Interpreting results

The results of an ANOVA are reported as an F statistic. The F distribution table is used to determine the level of significance of the F statistic. (See F statistical tables, Burns & Grove, 2001, pp. 764-767.) If the F statistic is equal to or greater than the appropriate table value, there is a significant difference between the groups. If only two groups are being examined, the location of a significant difference is clear. However, if more than two groups are under study, it is not possible to determine from the ANOVA where the significant differences lie. One cannot assume that all the groups examined are significantly different. Therefore posthoc analyses are conducted to determine the location of the differences among groups. The frequently used posthoc tests are Bonferroni's procedure, Newman-Keuls' test, Tukey's Honestly Significantly Different (HSD) test, Scheffé's test, and Dunnett's test (Burns & Grove, 2001).

In their study of perceptions of health and their relationship to symptoms in African American women with Type 2 diabetes, Stover and colleagues (2001) also reported the results of an ANOVA to determine the effects of the number of complications reported by the subjects. The authors report their findings as follows:

"To determine the effects of the number of complications, we placed subjects into three groups according to the number of complications listed in their medical records (specifically, nephropathy, retinopathy, neuropathy, peripheral vascular disease [PVD], and amputation) and then compared these groups using one-way analysis of variance (ANOVAs) for each subscale" (p. 75). The three groups were (1) no complications, (2) one complication, and (3) more than one complication. The subscales of the SF-20 used were mental health, general health, physical function, role function, social function, and bodily pain. "A significant difference was found in the mean perceived bodily pain scores of subjects with varied number of complications using one-way ANOVA ($F[2,72] = 4.2; p = 0.02$)" (p. 75). F is the statistic reported when reporting ANOVA; (2,72) are the df. The value 4.2 is the statistical F value obtained from the analysis; $p = 0.02$ is the probability that the groups are different. "We then calculated the Tukey's Honest Square Difference posthoc analysis, which showed that individuals with two or more of the provider-defined complications experienced more pain than individual[s] with only 1 complication" (p. 77).

Sometimes, ANOVA results are reported in a table. Froman and Owen (1997) used a table to report the results of an ANOVA in their study on the validity of the AIDS Attitude Scale. They proposed that pediatric nurses would have more positive attitudes (higher empathy, lower avoidance) than nurses caring for adults. They administered the instrument to 28 pediatric nurses and 36 nurses caring for adults. Half of each group worked in an intensive care unit (ICU), and the other half worked on a floor setting. Table 10-8 presents their findings in an ANOVA summary table. The three sources of variance analyzed in ANOVA (between groups, within groups, and total) are given, as are the df for each source of variance. The sum of squares (SS) and mean square (MS) values, which are used in the process of performing an ANOVA, are provided. With these values, an individual could recalculate the F value to verify its accuracy. The p value is indicated by an asterisk beside the F value if the value is significant at the 0.05 level. Two ANOVAs were performed, one with Avoidance as the dependent variable and one with Empathy as the dependent variable. The authors discuss their results as follows.

TABLE 10-8

ANOVA SUMMARIES FOR AVOIDANCE AND EMPATHY

DEPENDENT VARIABLE	SOURCE	SS	df	MS	F
Avoidance	Patient age	0.01	1	0.01	0.02
	Intensity	1.07	1	1.07	2.19
	Age × intensity	2.02	1	2.02	4.14*
	Error	29.25	60	0.49	
Empathy	Patient age	0.59	1	0.59	1.63
	Intensity	0.79	1	0.79	2.19
	Age × intensity	1.96	1	1.96	5.43*
	Error	21.66	60	0.36	

*$p = < 0.05$.

From Froman, R. D., & Owen, S. V. (1997). Further validation of the AIDS Attitude Scale. *Research in Nursing & Health, 10*(2), 166. ©1997. Reprinted by permission of John Wiley and Sons, Inc.

"The results of the ANOVAs conducted...reveal a more complex relationship than had been expected, showing a joint effect of intensity of care and patient age on attitude. With further consideration, this finding is understandable in the context of construct validity. Nurses caring for children, regardless of their own risk of exposure, maintain similarly therapeutic and accepting attitudes. These attitudes are adequately sturdy and young patients are sufficiently attractive to counteract influences on attitude that might result from increased risks associated with ICU care. Nurses caring for noncritically ill adults (those experiencing illnesses requiring hospitalization but not fully debilitated) hold similar attitudes. Nurses in the non-ICU setting are likely to interact with their adult AIDS patients and know them as individuals. It is only the combination of adult patients and ICU setting, with its assumed advanced illness condition, that is associated with notably negative attitudes. In discussing these findings with practicing nurses they were not surprised at such results. Their interpretation, put simply, was that adult AIDS patients in ICU settings are repellent as a result of many diseases associated with AIDS (e.g., Kaposi's sarcoma, pneumocystic pneumonia). They are usually uncommunicative either because of apparatus (i.e., ventilator) or disease processes. Given these characteristics, the adult ICU AIDS patients lose opportunity to elicit the accepting attitudes that pediatric patients or alert adult patients experience." (Froman & Owen, 1997, p. 167)

Analysis of Covariance

Analysis of covariance (ANCOVA) allows the researcher to examine the effect of a treatment apart from the effect of one or more potentially confounding variables (see Chapter 3 for a discussion of confounding variables). Potentially confounding variables that are commonly of concern include pretest scores, age, education, social class, and anxiety level. These variables would be confounding if they were not measured and if their effects on study variables were not statistically removed by performing regression analysis before performing ANOVA. This strategy removes the effect of differences among groups that is due to a confounding variable. Once this effect is removed, the effect of the treatment can be examined more precisely. This technique is sometimes used as a method of statistical control when it is not possible to design the study so that potentially confounding variables are controlled. However, control through careful planning of the design is more effective than statistical control.

ANCOVA may be used in pretest-posttest designs in which differences occur in groups on the pretest. For example, individuals who achieve low scores on a pretest tend to have lower scores on the posttest than those whose pretest scores were higher, even if the treatment had a significant effect on posttest scores. Conversely, if an individual achieves a high pretest score, it is doubtful that the posttest will indicate a strong change as a result of the treatment. ANCOVA maximizes the capacity to detect differences in such cases.

JUDGING STATISTICAL SUITABILITY

Multiple factors are involved in determining the suitability of a statistical procedure for a particular study. These include the study's: (1) purpose; (2) hypotheses, questions, or objectives; (3) design; and (4) level of measurement. Determining the suitability of various statistical procedures for a particular study is not straightforward. Regrettably, there is not usually one "right" statistical procedure for a particular study.

 In critiquing suitability, you must not only be familiar with the statistical procedure used in the study but must also be able to compare that procedure with others that could have been used, perhaps to greater advantage. You must judge whether the procedure was performed appropriately and the results interpreted correctly.

Evaluating statistical procedures requires that you make a number of judgments about the nature of the data and what the researcher wanted to know. You need to determine (1) whether the data for analysis were treated as nominal, ordinal, or interval; (2) how many groups were in the study; and (3) whether the groups were dependent or independent. In *independent groups,* the selection of one subject is totally unrelated to the selection of other subjects. For example, if subjects are randomly assigned to treatment and control groups, the groups are independent. In *dependent*

groups, subjects or observations selected for data collection are related in some way to the selection of other subjects or observations. For example, if subjects serve as their own control by using the pretest as a control, the observations (and therefore the groups) are dependent. Also, if matched pairs of subjects are used for control and treatment groups, the observations are dependent. For example, in a study of twins, one twin might be placed in the control group and the other in the treatment group. Because they are twins, they are matched on several variables.

One approach to judging the appropriateness of an analysis technique for a critique is to use an algorithm, which directs you by gradually narrowing the number of appropriate statistical procedures as you make judgments about the nature of the study and the data. An algorithm that has been helpful in judging the appropriateness of statistical procedures is presented in Fig. 10-10. This algorithm identifies four factors related to the appropriateness of a statistical procedure: the research question, level of measurement, design, and type of sample. To use the algorithm in Fig. 10-10, you would (1) determine whether the research question focuses on differences (I) or associations (relationships) (II), (2) determine the level of measurement (A, B, or C), (3) select the design listed that most closely fits the study you are critiquing (1, 2, or 3), and (4) determine whether the study samples are independent (a), dependent (b), or mixed (c). The lines on the algorithm are followed through each selection to identify the appropriate statistical procedure.

INTERPRETING STATISTICAL OUTCOMES

To be useful, the evidence from data analysis should be carefully examined, organized, and given meaning. Evaluating the entire research process, organizing the meaning of the results, and forecasting the usefulness of the findings, all of which are involved in interpretation, require high-level intellectual processes. In this segment of a study, the researcher translates the results of analysis into findings and then interprets them by attaching meaning to the findings.

Within the process of interpretation are several intellectual activities that can be isolated and explored, including examining evidence, forming conclusions, considering implications, exploring the significance of the findings, generalizing the findings, and suggesting further studies. This information is usually included in the final section of published studies, which is often entitled "Discussion."

Types of Results

Interpretation of results from quasi-experimental and experimental studies is traditionally based on decision theory, with five possible results: (1) significant results that agree with those predicted by the researcher, (2) nonsignificant results, (3) significant results that are opposite those predicted by the researcher, (4) mixed results, and (5) unexpected results. In critiquing a study, you need to identify which types of results were presented in the study.

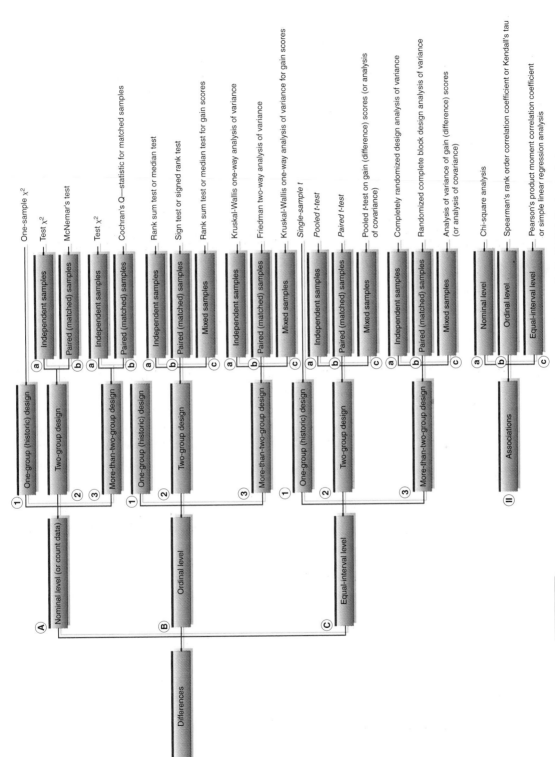

Fig. 10-10 Algorithm for choosing a statistical test. *(From Knapp, R. B. [1985].* Basic statistics for nurses. *Albany, NY: Delmar. Reproduced by permission.)*

Significant and predicted results

Significant results agree with those predicted by the researcher and support the logical links developed by the researcher between the framework, questions, variables, and measurement tools. However, you need to consider the possibility of alternative explanations for the positive findings. What other elements could possibly have led to the significant results?

Nonsignificant results

Nonsignificant (or inconclusive) *results,* often referred to as "negative results," could be a true reflection of reality. In this case the reasoning of the researcher or the theory used by the researcher to develop the hypothesis is in error. If so, the negative findings are an important addition to the body of knowledge. But the results could also stem from a Type II error due to inappropriate methods, a biased sample, a small sample, problems with internal validity, inadequate measurement, weak statistical measures, or faulty analysis. If so, the reported results could introduce faulty information into the body of knowledge (Angell, 1989). Negative results do not mean that no relationships exist among the variables. Negative results only indicate that the study failed to find any. Nonsignificant results provide no evidence of either the truth or the falsity of the hypothesis.

Significant and unpredicted results

Significant and unpredicted results are the opposite of those predicted by the researcher and indicate that flaws are present in the logic of both the researcher and the theory being tested. However, if the results are valid, they are an important addition to the body of knowledge. An example would be a study in which social support and ego strength were proposed to be positively correlated. If the study showed that high social support was correlated with low ego strength, the result would be opposite that predicted.

Mixed results

Mixed results are probably the most common outcome of studies. In this case, one variable may uphold predicted characteristics, whereas another does not; or two dependent measures of the same variable may show opposite results. These differences may be due to methodology problems, such as differing reliability or sensitivity of two methods of measuring variables. The mixed results may also indicate that existing theory should be modified.

Unexpected results

Unexpected results are usually relationships found between variables that were not hypothesized and not predicted from the framework being used. Most researchers examine as many elements of data as possible, in addition to those directed by the questions. These findings can be useful in the modification of existing theory and in the development of both new theories and later studies. In addition, serendipitous results are important evidence for developing the implications of the study. However, serendipitous results must be interpreted carefully, because the study was not designed to examine these results.

Findings

Results in a study are translated and interpreted; then they become *findings,* which are a consequence of evaluating evidence. Although much of the process of developing findings from results occurs in the mind of the researcher, evidence of the thinking can be found in published research reports.

 In critiquing a study, you need to identify the findings and evaluate the linkages between statistical results and the findings expressed by the researcher.

In their study, "Perceptions of Health and Their Relationship to Symptoms in African American Women with Type 2 Diabetes," Stover and colleagues (2001) present the following results and findings.

Results

"The most common symptoms that the subjects experienced in the preceding two weeks were headache, abdominal pain, dizziness, fatigue, and knee pain. There were no subjects who were asymptomatic. The range of symptoms per subject was from 1 to 12 with a mean of 4 symptoms." (p. 75)

"The mean general health score for all subjects was 35.9% (SD of 24.9%), based on a scale of 0 to 100. The mean physical functioning score was 61.1% (SD 33.7%), role functioning was 54% (SD 47.8%) and social functioning was 70.9% (SD 34.1%). The mean mental health score was 70.9% (SD 22.8%) and the mean pain score was 54.4% (SD of 28.4%). Perception of health scores were found to be generally lower than those previously reported in chronically ill and non-chronically ill subjects." (p. 76)

"On average, African American women with Type 2 diabetes and symptoms of upper and lower neuropathy and/or peripheral vascular disease rated their perceptions of general health, physical role, social functioning, and bodily pain as poorer, compared with subjects without these symptoms. African American women with symptoms of visual change rated their mental health, general health, role functioning, and bodily pain perceptions poorer than the ratings of subjects without these symptoms. Visual change (retinopathy) was the only variable we analyzed that had a statistically significant relationship to mental health perception." (p. 77)

"A significant difference was found in the mean perceived bodily pain scores of subjects with varied number of complications…. We also found a significantly lower physical functioning score in subjects with peripheral vascular disease (PVD) when compared with subjects without PVD. There were no other significant differences in the mean scores of the SF-20 by complication type…. We found a significant relationship between age at diagnosis and mean scores on both the general health and social functioning subscales." (p. 77)

Findings

"The major finding of this study is that African American women with Type 2 diabetes have poorer perceptions of their health status when compared with other women with chronic illnesses. These women also have a poorer perception of health when compared with other individuals with diabetes as noted in previous studies (Glasgow et al, 1997; Stewart et al, 1989). This finding may reflect the symptoms they were experiencing." (p. 78) As can be seen in this example, the findings are related to findings from previous research and theoretical literature.

Conclusions

Conclusions are a synthesis of the findings. In forming conclusions, the researcher uses logical reasoning, creates a meaningful whole from pieces of information obtained through data analysis and findings from previous studies, remains receptive to subtle clues in the data, and considers alternative explanations of the data. One of the risks in developing conclusions is going beyond the data, or forming conclusions that are not warranted by the data. This occurs more frequently in published studies than one would like to believe.

In critiquing a study, you need to identify the conclusions and judge whether they are warranted by the data.

Stover and colleagues (2001) concluded that "Data show that African American women with Type 2 diabetes have a wide variety of symptoms and poor perceptions of their general health and physical functioning" (p. 72).

Considering Implications

Implications are the meanings of conclusions from scientific research for the body of nursing knowledge, theory, and practice. Implications are based on but are more specific than conclusions, and they provide specific suggestions for implementing the findings. For example, the researcher might suggest how nursing practice should be modified. If a study indicated that a specific solution was effective in decreasing stomatitis, the implications would state how the care of patients with stomatitis should be modified.

In critiquing a study, you need to identify the implications indicated by the researcher. In addition, you may be able to identify implications not considered by the author.

A study by Stover and colleagues (2001) suggested these implications:

"Although quality of life is often an elusive concept to define and/or describe, there is some evidence that symptom distress and quality of life are linked (Germino, 1987). Our findings indicate that individuals with diabetes experience frequent symptoms that influence how they appraise the quality of their lives. Patients live with symptoms (e.g., toe pain, foot numbness) and understand symptoms more readily than the more abstract concepts of glycosylated hemoglobin and target blood sugar ranges. Health care providers need to address symptoms with as much attention and concern as is paid to 'object data,' such as blood glucose levels and cardiograms. As health care providers, we need to re-evaluate the content of the information we provide when educating patients. Improved self-care practices can be presented as a strategy for symptom relief. More emphasis needs to be placed on helping patients differentiate among their current or past pattern of symptoms and increasing their repertoire of strategies to assess their problems and identify patterns of change in serious symptoms. Effective symptom-focused diabetes care has the potential to improve the quality of life for persons with diabetes." p. 79

Exploring the Significance of Findings

The significance of a study is associated with its importance to the nursing body of knowledge. Significance is not a dichotomous characteristic because studies contribute in varying degrees to the body of knowledge. Significance may be associated with the amount of variance explained, the degree of control in the study design to eliminate unexplained variance, or the ability to detect statistically significant differences. To the extent possible at the time the study is reported, the researcher is expected to clarify the significance.

A few studies, referred to as "landmark studies," become important reference points in the discipline (Johnson, 1972; Lindeman & Van Aernam, 1971; Passos & Brand, 1966; Williams, 1972). The true importance of a particular study may not become apparent for years after publication. However, there are some characteristics associated with the significance of studies. Significant studies make an important difference in peoples' lives; it is possible to generalize the findings far beyond the study sample so that the findings have the potential of affecting large numbers of people. The implications of significant studies go beyond concrete facts to abstractions and lead to the generation of theory or revisions of existing theory. A very significant study has implications for one or more disciplines in addition to nursing. The study is accepted by others in the discipline and is frequently referenced in the literature. Over a period of time, the significance of a study is measured by the number of studies it generates.

In critiquing a study, you need to judge the significance of the study and indicate factors that make it significant.

Clinical Significance

The findings of a study can have statistical significance but not clinical significance. *Clinical significance* is related to the practical importance of the findings. However, there is no common agreement in nursing about how to evaluate the clinical significance of a finding. The effect size can be used to determine clinical significance. For example, one group of patients might have a body temperature 0.1° F higher than that of another group. Data analysis might indicate that the two groups are statistically significantly different, but the findings have no clinical significance. The difference is not sufficiently important to warrant changing patient care. However, in many studies, it is difficult to judge how much change would constitute clinical significance. In studies testing the effectiveness of a treatment, clinical significance could be judged based on the proportion of subjects who showed improvement or the extent to which subjects returned to normal functioning. But how much improvement would subjects need to demonstrate for the findings to be considered clinically significant? There are also questions about who should judge clinical significance: the patients and their families, the clinician, the researcher, or society at large. At this point in the development of nursing knowledge, clinical significance is ultimately a value judgment (LeFort, 1993).

 In critiquing a study, you need to evaluate its clinical significance.

Generalizing the Findings

Generalization extends the implications of the findings from the sample studied to a larger population. The findings may be extended from the situation studied to a larger situation. For example, if the study was conducted on diabetic patients, it may be possible to generalize the findings to persons with other illnesses or to well individuals. In the study by Stover and colleagues (2001) the authors cautioned that "[b]ecause this was an exploratory study and we did not perform a correction for multiple tests, it is possible that an isolated finding might be due to chance and need to be confirmed" (p. 79). In such a study it would be unwise to suggest generalization of the findings without further confirmatory studies.

How far can generalizations be made? From a very narrow perspective, one cannot really generalize from the sample on which the study was conducted; any other sample is likely to be different in some way. Those with a conservative view consider generalization particularly risky if the sample was not randomly selected. According to Kerlinger and Lee (1999), unless special precautions are taken and efforts made, the research results are frequently not representative and thus not generalizable. Most nurse researchers are not this conservative in making generalizations.

Empirical generalizations are based on accumulated evidence from many studies and are important for the verification of theoretical statements or the development of new theory. Empirical generalizations are the base of a science and contribute to scientific conceptualization. Nursing has few empirical generalizations at this time.

 In critiquing a study, you need to determine the populations to which the researcher has generalized and judge the appropriateness of the generalization. You may be able to identify other populations to which the findings should be generalized.

Suggesting Further Studies

In every study, the researcher gains knowledge and experience that can be used to design a better study next time. Therefore, the researcher will often make suggestions for future studies that emerge logically from the present study. Recommendations for further study may include replications or repeating the design with a different or larger sample. Recommendations may also include the formation of hypotheses to further test the framework in use.

 In critiquing a study, you need to identify the researcher's recommendations for future research. You may be able to make additional recommendations.

Stover and colleagues (2001) made the following recommendations for future research:

"In subsequent investigations, it will be important to obtain information on descriptors of the symptom experience to provide a better basis for interventions. In this initial attempt to look at symptoms and their relationship to perceptions of health and functioning in African American women with Type 2 diabetes, we did not attempt to address the severity, frequency, or duration of their symptoms. We also did not investigate the

Continued

amount of distress caused by these symptoms (the physical or mental anguish or suffering that results from the experience of a symptom occurrence) (Rhodes & Watson, 1987) or the measures participants used to control and/or alleviate their symptoms. Diabetes is a chronic disorder that necessitates lifelong commitment to an often complex self-care regimen. Associated with diabetes is the potential for long-term complications that often significantly affect an individual's quality of life." (p. 79)

SUMMARY

In critiquing a quantitative study, you should: (1) identify the statistical procedures used; (2) judge whether these statistical procedures were appropriate for the hypotheses, questions, or objectives of the study and to the data available for analysis; (3) comprehend the discussion of data analysis results; (4) judge whether the author's interpretation of the results is appropriate; and (5) evaluate the clinical significance of the findings. There are several stages to quantitative data analysis: (1) preparing the data for analysis; (2) describing the sample; (3) testing the reliability of measurement methods; (4) conducting exploratory analysis of the data; (5) conducting confirmatory analyses guided by the hypotheses, questions, or objectives; and (6) conducting posthoc analyses.

You need to understand the concepts of statistical theory to critique research effectively. Probability theory, which is deductive, is used to explain a relationship, the probability of an event's occurring in a given situation, or the probability of accurately predicting an event. Decision theory, which is inductive, assumes that all of the groups in a study (such as experimental and control groups) used to test a particular hypothesis are components of the same population in relation to the variables under study. The researcher must provide evidence that there is a difference between the groups.

To test the assumption of no difference, a cutoff point is selected before data collection. The cutoff point, referred to as alpha (α), or the level of significance, is the probability level at which the results of statistical analysis are judged to indicate a statistically significant difference between the groups. A statistical inference is a conclusion or judgment based on evidence. A generalization is the application of information that has been acquired from a specific instance to a general situation. In research, one infers from the study findings obtained from a specific sample to a more general population, using information obtained through statistical analyses.

The normal curve is a theoretical frequency distribution of all possible values in a population. Levels of significance and probability are based on the logic of the normal curve. Hypotheses usually assume that extreme scores, which fall in the tails of the normal curve, result because the group with the extreme score does not belong to the same population. A Type I error occurs when the null hypothesis is rejected when it is true; the risk of a Type I error is indicated by the level of significance. A Type II error occurs when the null hypothesis is accepted when it is false. Type II errors are often a consequence of flaws in the research methods. Power is the probability that a statistical test will detect a significant difference that exists. The risk of a Type II error can be determined using power analysis. Degrees of freedom involve the freedom of a score's value to vary given the other existing scores' values and the established sum of these scores. Degrees of freedom are often indicated in reporting statistical results.

Summary statistics include frequency distributions, measures of central tendency, and measures of dispersion. Statistical procedures frequently used to address research questions or test hypotheses include Pearson's product-moment correlation that tests for relationships; the chi-square test of independence, *t*-test, analysis of variance, which tests for differences, and regression analysis, which tests prediction.

Judging statistical suitability in a critique requires that you be familiar with the statistical procedure used in the study. You must judge whether the procedure was performed appropriately and the results interpreted correctly. In the discussion section of the research report, the researcher examines evidence, forms conclusions, considers implications, explores the significance of the findings, generalizes the findings, and suggests further studies. In critiquing a study, you need to evaluate the appropriateness of the researcher's discussion.

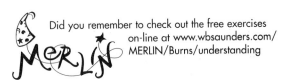 Did you remember to check out the free exercises on-line at www.wbsaunders.com/ MERLIN/Burns/understanding

REFERENCES

Angell, M. (1989). Negative studies. *New England Journal of Medicine, 321*(7), 464–466.

Badger, R. A., McNiece, C., & Gagan, M. J. (2000). Depression, service need, and use in vulnerable populations. *Archives of Psychiatric Nursing, 14*(4), 173–182.

Burns, N., & Grove, S. K. (2001). *The practice of nursing research: Conduct, critique, and utilization* (4th ed.). Philadelphia: Saunders.

Cohen, J. (1988). *Statistical power analysis for the behavioral sciences* (2nd ed.). New York: Academic Press.

Craft, M. J., & Moss, J. (1996). Accuracy of infant emesis volume assessment. *Applied Nursing Research, 9*(1), 2–8.

Fitch, M. I., Gray, R., Franssen, E., & Johnson, B. (2000). Men's perspectives on the impact of prostate cancer: Implications for oncology nurses. *Oncology Nursing Forum, 27*(8), 1255–1263.

Froman, R. D., & Owen, S. V. (1997). Further validation of the AIDS Attitude Scale. *Research in Nursing & Health, 20*(2), 161–167.

Germino, B. B. (1987). Symptom distress and quality of life. *Seminars in Oncology Nursing, 3*(4), 299–302.

Glasgow, R., Dryfoos, J., Ruggiero, L., Chobanin, L., & Eakin, E. (1997). Quality of life and associated characteristics in a large national sample of adults with diabetes. *Diabetes Care, 20*(4), 562–567.

Johnson, J. E. (1972). Effects of structuring patients' expectations on their reactions to threatening events. *Nursing Research, 21*(6), 499–503.

Kerlinger, F. N., & Lee, H. B. (1999). *Foundations of behavioral research.* New York: Harcourt Brace.

Knapp, R. B., (1985). *Basic statistics for nurses.* Albany, NY: Delmar.

LeFort, S. M. (1993). The statistical versus clinical significance debate. *Image: Journal of Nursing Scholarship, 25*(1), 57–62.

Lindeman, C. A., & Van Aernam, B. (1971). Nursing intervention with the presurgical patient: The effects of structured and unstructured preoperative teaching. *Nursing Research, 20*(4), 319–332.

LoBiondo-Wood, G., Williams, L., Wood, R. P., & Shaw, B. W. (1997). Impact of liver transplantation on quality of life: A longitudinal perspective. *Applied Nursing Research, 10*(1), 27–32.

Lyon, D. E., & Munro, C. (2001). Disease severity and symptoms of depression in Black Americans infected with HIV. *Applied Nursing Research, 14*(1), 3–10.

Passos, J. Y., & Brand, L. M. (1966). Effects of agents used for oral hygiene. *Nursing Research, 15*(3), 196–202.

Rhodes, V. A., & Watson, P. M. (Eds.). (1987). Symptom Distress. *Seminars in Oncology Nursing, 3*(4), 299–302.

Schmelzer, M., Case, P., Chappell, S. M., & Wright, K. B. (2000). Colonic cleansing, fluid absorption, and discomfort following tap water and soapsuds enemas. *Applied Nursing Research, 13*(2), 83–91.

Slakter, M. H., Wu, Y. B., & Suzaki-Slakter, N. S. (1991). *, **, and ***, statistical nonsense at the 0.00000 level. *Nursing Research, 40*(4), 248–249.

Stewart, A. L., Greenfield, S., Hayes, R. D., Wells, K., Rogers, W. H., Berry, S. D., McGlynn, E. A., & Ware, J. E. (1989). Functional status and well-being of patients with chronic conditions. *Journal of the American Medical Association, 262*(7), 907–913.

Stover, J. C., Skelly, A. H., Holditch-Davis, D., & Dunn, P. F. (2001). Perceptions of health and their relationship to symptoms in African American Women with Type 2 diabetes. *Applied Nursing Research, 14*(2), 72–80.

Tukey, J. W. (1977). *Exploratory data analysis.* Reading, MA: Addison-Wesley.

Williams, A. (1972). A study of factors contributing to skin breakdown. *Nursing Research, 21*(3), 238–243.

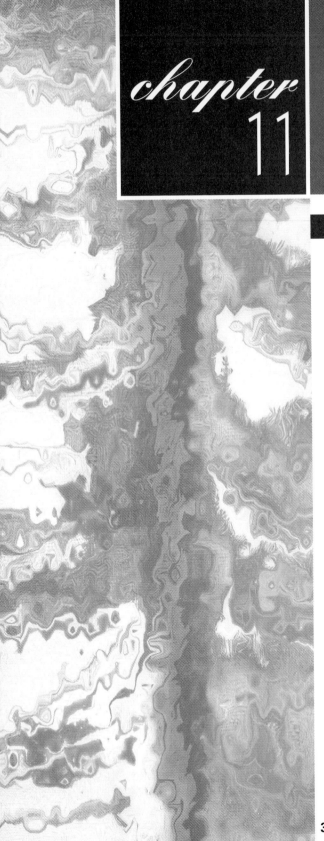

chapter 11

Introduction to Qualitative Research

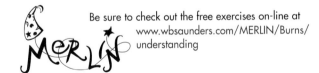

Be sure to check out the free exercises on-line at
www.wbsaunders.com/MERLIN/Burns/
understanding

OUTLINE—cont'd

OBJECTIVES

Completing this chapter should enable you to:
 1. Describe the scientific rigor associated with qualitative research.
 2. Differentiate the purposes of the four types of qualitative research.
 3. Examine the research processes used in phenomenological, grounded theory, ethnographic, and historical research.
 4. Describe the use of a decision trail, a qualitative research strategy.
 5. Examine the data collection issues for a qualitative study, including the relationships between the researcher and the participants and the reflections of the researcher on the meaning of the data.

RELEVANT TERMS

Auditability
Bracketing
Coding
Decision trail
Emic approach
Ethnographic research
Ethnonursing research
Etic approach
External criticism
Grounded theory research
Historical research

Internal criticism
Phenomenological research
Primary source
Qualitative research
Reflexive thought
Researcher-participant relationships
Rigor
Secondary source
Storytakers
Storytelling

Qualitative research is a systematic, subjective approach used to describe life experiences and give them meaning (Leininger, 1985; Munhall, 1989; Munhall, 2001; Silva & Rothbart, 1984). Qualitative research is not a new idea in the social or behavioral sciences (Baumrind, 1980; Glaser & Strauss, 1967; Kaplan, 1964; Scheffler, 1967). However, the nursing community's interest in qualitative research is relatively recent, beginning in the late 1970s.

The terminology and the methods of reasoning used in qualitative research differ from those used in more traditional quantitative research methods and reflect alternative philosophical orientations. The specific philosophical orientation of each approach directs the research method. Although each qualitative approach is unique, there are many commonalities.

In this chapter, we introduce some of the qualitative research approaches commonly used in nursing and their contributions to nursing knowledge. To facilitate comprehension of these methods, the logic underlying the qualitative approach is explored. A general overview of the following qualitative approaches is presented: phenomenological research, grounded theory research, ethnographic research, and historical research. The methods used to collect, analyze, and interpret qualitative data are described. The content should provide a background for you in reading and comprehending published qualitative studies and applying study findings to your clinical practice.

LOGIC OF QUALITATIVE RESEARCH

Qualitative research focuses on understanding the whole, which is consistent with the holistic philosophy of nursing (Baer, 1979; Leininger, 1985; Ludemann, 1979; Munhall, 1982b, 1989, 2001). Within a holistic framework, qualitative research explores the depth, richness, and complexity inherent in phenomena. In addition, qualitative research is useful in understanding such human experiences as pain, caring, powerlessness, and comfort.

The qualitative approaches are based on a world view that has the following beliefs:

1. There is not a single reality.
2. Reality, based on perceptions, is different for each person and changes over time.
3. What we know has meaning only within a given situation or context.

The reasoning process used in qualitative research involves putting pieces together perceptually to construct a whole picture. From this process, meaning is produced. However, many different meanings are possible, because perception varies from person to person (Munhall, 2001).

Frameworks are used in a different sense in qualitative research than they are in quantitative studies, because the goal is not theory testing. Nonetheless, each type of qualitative research is guided by a particular philosophical stance. The philosophy directs the questions that are asked, the observations that are made, and the approach that is used to interpret data (Munhall, 1982a, 1988, 1989). These philosophical bases and their associated research methods, developed outside of nursing, are undergoing evolutionary changes within nursing.

The data from qualitative studies are subjective and incorporate the perceptions and beliefs of the researcher and the participants (Eisner, 1981; Leininger, 1985). The findings from a qualitative study lead to understanding a phenomenon in a particular situation and are not generalized in the same way that quantitative studies are.

However, understanding the meanings of a phenomenon in a particular situation gives insights that can be applied more broadly. The insights from qualitative studies can guide nursing practice and aid in the important process of theory development for building nursing knowledge (Schwartz-Barcott & Kim, 1986).

Morse (1999b) describes the reaction of a colleague to her qualitative research project:

"Once a colleague, who specialized in the effects of smoking on health, came knocking on my door to 'see what I was up to.' He was mildly interested in qualitative research, but when I showed him a video clip that I was analyzing, he was aghast: 'You study that!' the chaos of the scene—a cluster of physicians and nurses providing trauma care to a critically injured patient—was beyond his definition of researchable problems and far beyond his conceptualization of research. The scene was not only 'uncontrolled' in his eyes, but it was such a crowded shouting mass that it was difficult to even ascertain what was going on. The video showed a number of physicians hunched over a gurney so that one could not see the patient, who, as evidenced from the loud cries, sobs, and pleading, was a young child. Over these cries, caregivers were shouting instructions or calling out results of their examinations for recording or the information of others. Yet, despite this bedlam, one could hear the nurse's voice, interrupting the child's cries, soothing, consoling, reassuring, and coaching." (p. 393)

Dr. Morse has been delineating comfort since 1989 with the objective of improving nursing care. She says, "Comfort has always been somewhere in the heart of nursing, but little attention has been given to its investigation" (Morse, 1999b, p. 394). During this period of study, she explored the meaning of comfort, conducted an ethnographic study exploring the context of comfort, and conducted a grounded theory study examining the process of comforting. She discovered that nursing's theoretical base and existing body of knowledge about comfort is grossly inadequate. At the time of this published paper, Morse (1999b) had received funding for the previous 8 years of research and had just received funding for the next 5 years. Her work is highly valued by the Canadian government and by clinical nurses who await her findings.

With the current emphasis on evidence-based practice and the need to focus on testing nursing interventions, it is possible that the use of qualitative studies might decline. However, as Green and Britten (1998) suggest:

"Qualitative research may seem unscientific and anecdotal to many medical scientists. However, as the critics of evidence-based medicine are quick to point out, medicine itself is more than the application of scientific rules. Clinical experience, based on personal observation, reflection, and judgment, is also needed to translate scientific results into treatment of individual patients. Personal experience is often characterised as being anecdotal, ungeneralisable, and a poor basis for making scientific decisions. However, it is often a more powerful persuader than scientific publication in changing clinical practice as illustrated by the occasional series 'A patient who changed my practice' in the *British Medical Journal.*" (p. 1230)

Qualitative research provides a process through which nurses can examine a phenomenon outside of traditional views. The earliest and perhaps most dramatic demonstration of the influence qualitative research can have on nursing practice was the 4-year study conducted by Glaser and Strauss (1965, 1968, 1971), who initiated the use of grounded theory research methods for health-related studies. Their study, which described the social environment of dying patients in hospitals, was reported in three books: *Awareness of Dying* (Glaser & Strauss, 1965), *Time for Dying* (Glaser & Strauss, 1968), and *Status Passage* (Glaser & Strauss, 1971). At the time Glaser and Strauss were conducting their studies, the traditional view was that people could not cope with knowing that they were dying. The environment of care was designed to protect the patient from that knowledge. Glaser and Strauss (1965, 1968, 1971) examined what that protective social environment meant for the patient. This study changed the perception of nurses, who saw that the traditional care of the dying created loneliness and isolation, rather than protection. Nurses began to see the patient in a new light, and changed their methods of patient care. Kübler-Ross (1969), perhaps influenced by the work of Glaser and Strauss, began her studies of the dying, using an approach similar to that of phenomenology. From this new orientation to care for the dying, hospice care developed. Now more than 30 years later the environment of care for the dying has changed.

APPROACHES TO QUALITATIVE RESEARCH

Four common approaches to qualitative research used in nursing are presented in this chapter: phenomenological, grounded theory, ethnographic, and historical. In some ways, these approaches differ greatly. Ethnographic and historical research are broad and are the accepted methodologies for a discipline. The worldview of phenomenology is more unique and is controversial. However, in each approach, the purpose is to examine meaning, and the unit of analysis is a word or phrase rather than a numerical value.

Each of these four approaches is based on a philosophical orientation that influences the interpretation of the data. Thus it is critical to understand the philosophy on which the method is based. Each approach is discussed in relation to its philosophical orientation and nursing knowledge, and a nursing study is provided to illustrate each methodology.

Phenomenological Research

Phenomenology is both a philosophy and a research method. The purpose of *phenomenological research* is to describe experiences as they are lived, in phenomenological terms, to capture the "lived experience" of study participants. The philosophical positions taken by phenomenological researchers are very different from the positions that are common in nursing culture and research traditions, and thus they are difficult to understand. However, discussions of this philosophical stance, appearing more frequently in the nursing literature, are introducing these ideas to a broader audience (Anderson, 1989; Leonard, 1989; Munhall, 1989; Salsberry, Smith, & Boyd, 1989).

Philosophical orientation

Phenomenologists view the person as integrated with the environment. The world shapes the self, and the self shapes the world. Reality is considered subjective; thus an experience is unique to the individual. Even the reality of the researcher's experiences during data collection and analysis is considered subjective. "Truth is an interpretation of some phenomenon; the more shared that interpretation is, the more factual it seems to be, yet it remains temporal and cultural" (Munhall, 1989, p. 22). Heideggerian phenomenologists believe that the person is a self within a body. Thus the person is referred to as embodied. "Our bodies provide the possibility for the concrete actions of self in the world" (Leonard, 1989, p. 48). The person has a world that is "the meaningful set of relationships, practices, and language that we have by virtue of being born into a culture" (Leonard, 1989, p. 43). The person is situated as a consequence of being shaped by his or her world and thus is constrained in the ability to establish meanings by language, culture, history, purposes, and values. The term situated as used in phenomenology is not familiar. Situated means that the place of a person in the world shapes them in ways that limit their thinking and behavior. Each person has only situated freedom, not total freedom. A person's world is so pervasive that it is generally not noticed unless some disruption occurs. Not only is the world of each person different, but each person's concerns are qualitatively different. The body, world, and concerns, which are unique to each person, are the context within which that person can be understood. The person experiences *being* within the framework of time. This is referred to as being-in-time. The past and the future influence the now and thus are part of being-in-time (Leonard, 1989).

Nursing knowledge and phenomenological research

Phenomenology is the philosophical base for three nursing theories: Parse's (1981) "Theory of Man-Living-Health," Paterson and Zderad's (1976) "Theory of Humanistic Nursing," and Watson's (1985) "Theory of Caring." The broad research question that phenomenologists ask is, What is the meaning of one's lived experience? Being a person is self-interpreting; therefore, the only reliable source of information to answer this question is the person. Understanding human behavior or experience, which is a central concern of nursing, requires that the person interpret the action or experience for the researcher; the researcher must then interpret the explanation provided by the person. Boyd (2001) suggests that the long-range goal should be that of "making phenomenology work well for us in nursing research—that is, of extrapolating nursing research methodology from phenomenology. Phenomenology invites this kind of effort and insists on an openness that can protect such ideas about method from being reduced to dogma." (p. 93)

Example Study

One of the most significant nursing studies conducted using the phenomenological method is Benner's (1984) work, a critical description of nursing practice presented in the book, *From Novice to Expert: Excellence and Power in Clinical Nursing Practice.* This study was funded by a grant from the Department of Health and Human Services, Division of Nursing, at a time when external funding for qualitative research was almost unheard of.

Benner (1984) explored the experience of clinical practice. The researcher develops a research question, which involves the consideration of two factors (expressed as questions): "(1) What are the necessary and sufficient constituents of this feeling or experience? (2) What does the existence of this feeling or experience indicate concerning the nature of the human being?" (Omery, 1983, p. 55). Benner's research question was whether there were "distinguishable, characteristic differences in the novice's and expert's descriptions of the same clinical incident. If so, how could these differences, if identifiable from the nurses' descriptions of the incidents, be accounted for or understood?" (Benner, 1984, p. 14).

Benner (1984) conducted paired interviews with both beginning and expert nurses. Twenty-one pairs of nurses were selected from three hospitals in which preceptors were used to orient new graduates. Each member of the pair, one a preceptor and one a new graduate, was interviewed separately about patient-care situations they had experienced together. Interviews and participant observation were conducted with additional nurses, including 51 experienced nurse clinicians, 11 new nursing graduates, and 5 senior nursing students. Individual interviews, small group interviews, and participant observation were conducted at six hospitals. Before the interviews, participants were given written explanations of the kinds of clinical descriptions of interest to the researchers. Interviews were recorded on tape and transcribed.

Benner's (1984) data analysis was an interpretative strategy based on Heideggerian phenomenology. She describes the procedure as follows*:

"The interviews and participant-observer records were read independently by the research team members, and interpretations of the data were compared and consensually validated. Each interpretation was accepted only if there was agreement in labeling and interpreting the major competency demonstrated and only if it was effective in describing skilled practice." (p. 16)

---

*From Benner, P. (1984). *From novice to expert: Excellence and power in clinical nursing practice.* Menlo Park, CA: Addison-Wesley. Reprinted by permission.

Continued

Benner's (1984) structural explanation of her findings was presented as five stages of gaining experience in clinical practice, which describe the nurse in a particular clinical situation as a novice, an advanced beginner, competent, proficient, or expert. The stages identified are based on the "Dreyfus Model of Skill Acquisition."

Stage 1: Novice

"Beginners have had no experience of the situations in which they are expected to perform. To give them entry to these situations and allow them to gain the experience so necessary for skill development, they are taught about the situations in terms of objective attributes such as weight, intake and output, temperature, blood pressure, pulse, and other such objectifiable, measurable parameters of a patient's conditions—features of the task that can be recognized without situational experiences. Novices are also taught context-free rules to guide action in respect to different attributes." (pp. 20–21)

Stage 2: Advanced Beginner

"Advanced beginners are ones who can demonstrate marginally acceptable performance, ones who have coped with enough real situations to note (or to have pointed out to them by a mentor) the recurring meaningful situational components…. Aspects, in contrast to the measurable, context-free attributes or the procedural lists of things to do that are learned and used by the beginner, require prior experience in actual situations for recognitions. Aspects include overall, global characteristics that can be identified only through prior experience." (p. 22)

Stage 3: Competent

"Competence, typified by the nurse who has been on the job in the same or similar situations two to three years, develops when the nurse begins to see his or her actions in terms of long-range goals or plans of which he or she is consciously aware. The plan dictates which attributes and aspects of the current and contemplated future situation are to be considered most important and those which can be ignored. Hence, for the competent nurse, a plan establishes a perspective, and the plan is based on considerable conscious, abstract, analytic contemplation of the problem." (p. 26)

Stage 4: Proficient

"Characteristically, the proficient performer perceives situations as wholes rather than in terms of aspects, and performance is guided by maxims. Maxims are cryptic instructions passed on by experts. Maxims make sense only if the person already has a deep understanding of the situation. (p. 10) Perception is the key word here. The perspective is *not* thought out but 'presents itself' based upon experience and recent events. Proficient nurses understand a situation as a whole because they perceive its meaning in terms of long-term goals." (p. 27)

Stage 5: Expert

"The expert performer no longer relies on an analytic principle (rule, guideline, maxim) to connect her or his understanding of the situation to an appropriate action. The expert nurse, with an enormous background of experience, now has an intuitive grasp of each situation and zeros in on the accurate region of the problem without wasteful consideration of a large range of unfruitful, alternative diagnoses and solutions." (p. 32)

Benner (1984) also identified seven domains of practice: (1) the helping role, (2) the teaching-coaching function, (3) the diagnostic and patient-monitoring function, (4) effective management of rapidly changing situations, (5) administering and monitoring therapeutic interventions and regimens, (6) monitoring and ensuring the quality of health-care practices, and (7) organizational and work-role competencies. Nursing competencies representative of each domain were identified.

Grounded Theory Research

Grounded theory research is an inductive technique that emerged from the discipline of sociology. The term *grounded* means that the theory that developed from the research has its roots in the data from which it was derived.

Philosophical orientation

Grounded theory is based on symbolic interaction theory, which holds many views in common with phenomenology. George Herbert Mead (1934), a social psychologist, was a leader in the development of symbolic interaction theory. Symbolic interaction theory explores how people define reality and how their beliefs are related to their actions. Reality is created by attaching meanings to situations. Meaning is expressed in such symbols as words, religious objects, and clothing. These symbolic meanings are the basis for actions and interactions. However, symbolic meanings are different for each individual, and we cannot completely know the symbolic meanings of another individual. In social life, meanings are shared by groups and are communicated to new members through socialization processes. Group life is based on consensus and shared meanings. Interaction may lead to redefinition and new meanings and can result in the redefinition of self. Because of its theoretical importance, the interaction is the focus of observation in grounded theory research (Chenitz & Swanson, 1986).

Grounded theory has been used most frequently to study areas in which little previous research has been conducted and to gain a new viewpoint in familiar areas of research. However, because of the high quality of theory generated through this method, further theory testing is not usually needed to enhance its usefulness.

Nursing knowledge and grounded theory research

Artinian (1988) has identified four qualitative modes of nursing inquiry within grounded theory: descriptive mode, discovery mode, emergent fit mode, and intervention mode. Each mode is used for different purposes: The descriptive mode provides rich detail and must precede all other modes. This mode, ideal for the beginning researcher, answers such questions as: What is going on? How are activities organized? What roles are evident? What are the steps in a process? What does a patient do in a particular setting? The discovery mode leads to the identification of patterns in life experiences of individuals and relates the patterns to each other. Through this mode a theory of social process referred to as substantive theory is developed; the theory explains a particular social world. The emergent fit mode is used when substantive theory has been developed to extend or refine this existing theory. This mode enables the researcher to focus on a selected portion of the theory, to build on previous work, or to establish a research program around a particular social process. The intervention mode is used to test the relationships in the substantive theory. The fundamental question for this mode is: How can I make something happen in a way that brings about new and desired states of affairs? This mode demands deep involvement on the part of the researcher and practitioner.

Example Study

One significant study using a grounded theory approach that is relevant to clinical nursing practice is Fagerhaugh and Strauss's (1977) study of the politics of pain management. This study emerged from the previous work of Glaser and Strauss in the care of the dying (Glaser & Strauss, 1965, 1968; Strauss & Glaser, 1970) and chronically ill (Strauss, 1975; Strauss et al., 1984). The study of pain involved 5 researchers and 2 years of systematic observations in 20 wards, 2 clinics, and 9 hospitals. The purposes of the study were to do the following: (1) develop an approach to pain management that was radically different from established approaches and (2) develop a substantive theory about what happens in hospitals when people are confronted with pain and attempt to deal with it (Fagerhaugh & Strauss, 1977, p. 13). The research questions were, "Under what conditions is pain encountered by staff?" and "How will it be handled?" (Fagerhaugh & Strauss, 1977, p. 13).

In their study on pain, Fagerhaugh and Strauss (1977) observed a variety of situations in which pain was a common phenomenon. The areas studied included an intensive care unit for severe burns, a cardiac care unit, an obstetrics ward, a physical rehabilitation unit, a neurology and neurosurgery unit, a routine surgery unit, a medical ward, an x-ray department, an emergency department, a kidney transplant unit, and a cancer ward. The following excerpt is from the report of the grounded theory study on pain. It focuses on a description of the sampling process and demonstrates the care and detailed thought that must go into the development of sampling categories.

"On all these wards we made 'internal comparisons' along the theoretical dimensions. That is, we continued our theory-directed sampling: for instance, high-pain regimens versus low-pain regimens; experienced inflicters of regimen pain versus new inflicters; delivering mothers who had the fathers supporting their efforts to endure pain versus those who had no such supporting or controlling agents. Meanwhile, we were also looking at an activity that spanned separate wards and which would maximize variables as they related to pain infliction. We followed a number of personnel who drew blood from patients. We observed some who were very experienced, some who were not; some who were able to work in a leisurely fashion, some who were not; some who met 'first-time' patients, others who met patients very experienced at this particular procedure; some who encountered patients with much ongoing pain and some who did not; some who had recently had experiences with accusations of incompetence and some who had not." (p. 308)

The core categories that evolved in the study were pain work, pain trajectories, legitimation, balancing, and accountability. Pain work was further classified into nurses relieving pain, nurses handling pain expression, nurses diagnosing the meaning of pain, nurses inflicting pain, nurses minimizing or preventing pain, patients enduring pain, and the staff members' controlling their own reactions to the patient's response to pain. The patient's cooperation in the pain work and negotiation between the staff and the patient were identified as important factors. An example of negotiation is described by Glaser (1973) as follows:

"'This won't take long,' I said to her…. 'It's not going to hurt…. I think I can inject it right into the IV tubing and not have to stick you.' She looked unconvinced. 'Honestly I won't stick you unless I have to.'" (p. 130)

Pain trajectories were divided into expected and unexpected trajectories. For example, an expectant mother would have a very different pain trajectory from that experienced by a person with intractable back pain.

"An unexpected trajectory—unexpected for a given ward, that is—carries a potential for staff and patient disturbance and ward upset. Both the sentimental order and the work order of the ward are threatened…. Patients with an unexpected or atypical trajectory tend to be labeled as 'uncooperative' or 'difficult,' and relations between them and the staff are likely to grow progressively worse." (Fagerhaugh & Strauss, 1977, pp. 22-23)

The researchers also concluded that the pain trajectory was influenced by the patients' illnesses, their previous experience with pain, the medical care they were receiving, and their social history. The researchers observed that the nurs-

Continued

ing and medical staff seldom knew anything about the patient's pain trajectory other than what was currently occurring.

Assessing and legitimating pain was also an important factor. Staff often suspected that patients claimed to have more pain than they really had or that patients claimed they had pain when they really had none. This left patients in the position of attempting to convince the staff that they were actually having the pain they claimed to have (legitimating). The staff and patients were often involved in the process of balancing priorities during pain work. Decisions were based on what the staff considered to be most important.

> "The staff members may not always agree among themselves, and the balancing done by the patient may not agree with the staff's. Patient and staff may even opt for opposite choices, disagreeing over the value of living a bit longer versus enduring terrible pain. They may be balancing quite different considerations. The staff may be balancing more work versus quicker pain relief, while the patient may be balancing pride in not complaining about pain versus difficulty of enduring it without more medication." (p. 25)

In terms of accountability, the researchers found that staff members did not consider pain work a major priority, and they tended to be more concerned with controlling patients' expression of pain than the experience of pain.

Fagerhaugh and Strauss (1977) showed in their study that grounded theory research examines a much broader scope of dimensions than can be examined with quantitative research. The findings can be intuitively verified by the experiences of the reader. The clear, cohesive description of the phenomenon can allow greater understanding of the phenomenon and thus more control of nursing practice.

Fagerhaugh and Strauss (1977) concluded the following from their study.

> "Genuine accountability concerning pain work could only be instituted if the major authorities on given wards or clinics understood the importance of that accountability and its implications for patient care. They would then need to convert that understanding into a commitment that would bring about necessary changes in written and verbal communication systems. This kind of understanding and commitment can probably come about only after considerable nationwide discussion, such as now is taking place about terminal care, but that kind of discussion seems to lie far in the future." (p. 27)

Ethnographic Research

Ethnographic research was developed by anthropologists as a mechanism for studying cultures. The word "ethnographic" means "portrait of a people." Many nurses involved in this type of research obtained their doctoral preparation in anthropology and have used anthropological techniques to examine cultural issues of interest in nursing.

Philosophical orientation

The discipline of anthropology, which began about the same time nursing did (in the mid-nineteenth century), provides a means to understand people, including their ways of living, believing, and adapting to changing environmental circumstances. Culture, the most central concept to anthropology, is "a way of life belonging to a designated group of people…a blueprint for living which guides a particular group's thoughts, actions, and sentiments…all the accumulated ways a group of people solve problems, which are reflected in the people's language, dress, food, and a number of accumulated traditions and customs." (Leininger, 1970, pp. 48–49). The purpose of anthropological research is to describe a culture by examining these various cultural characteristics.

Anthropologists study a people's origins, past ways of living, and ways of surviving through time. "The Australian aborigine, who lives in a non-technological society and a harsh natural environment, is as important an area of study in furthering a broad understanding of man as is contemporary Western man, who lives in a highly technological modern world" (Leininger, 1970, p. 7). Anthropologists may study cultures in remote parts of the world, in modern cities, and in modern rural areas. By comparing these cultures, they gain insights that increase our ability to predict the future directions of cultures and the forces that guide their destinies or that may provide opportunities to influence the direction of cultural development (Leininger, 1970).

Culture is both material and nonmaterial. Material culture consists of all created objects associated with a given group. Nonmaterial culture consists of other aspects of culture, such as symbolic referents, the network of social relations, and the beliefs reflected in social and political institutions. Symbolic meaning, social customs, and beliefs cannot be touched or stored in a museum; thus they are not material, but they are essential elements of cultures. Cultures also have ideals that the people hold as desirable, even though they do not always live up to these standards. Anthropologists seek to discover the many parts of a whole culture and how these parts are interrelated so that a picture of the wholeness of the culture evolves (Leininger, 1970). Ethnographic research is used in nursing not only to increase ethnic cultural awareness but also to enhance the quality of health care for persons of all cultures. There are two basic research approaches in anthropology: emic and etic. The *emic approach* involves studying behaviors from within the culture; the *etic approach* involves studying behavior from outside the culture and examining similarities and differences across cultures.

Nursing knowledge and ethnographic research

A group of nurse scientists, influenced by Leininger's "Theory of Transcultural Nursing," (Leininger, 1985) has developed an ethnographic research strategy for nursing. They refer to this strategy as *ethnonursing research.* Ethnonursing "focuses mainly on observing and documenting interactions with people of how these daily life conditions and patterns are influencing human care, health, and nursing care practices" (Leininger, 1985, p. 238). However, a number of nurse anthropologists not associated with the ethnonursing orientation are also providing important contributions to the nursing body of knowledge.

Example Study

A study of how nurses define medication error titled "Rules outside the rules for administration of medication: A study in New South Wales, Australia" is used to explain ethnographic research (Baker, 1997). The purpose of this ethnomethodological study was to improve understanding of how nurses within the culture of hospital nursing practice define or redefine medication error.

In the brief literature review, Baker described Barker and McConnell's (1962) benchmark study reporting that the medication error rate of nurses was 1 in 10. The number of errors made was directly proportional to the number of medications administered by the nurse. These authors found that nurses were aware of only a few of the errors they made; of these recognized errors, they reported only a small number. Some studies found that as nurses became more experienced, they made fewer errors. Other studies indicated that experienced nurses made the same number of errors but reported fewer of them. A study by Frances (1980), which found that as nurses became more experienced, they seemed to redefine error, offered insight to Baker and raised a question that led her to conduct the present study: "If nurses do redefine error, what is the new definition?" (p. 155).

Baker (1997) spent 2 weeks in each of nine wards during morning, evening, and night shifts, and at times on weekends and public holidays. The total time spent in the wards was 18 weeks. She used participant observations, formal and informal interviews, written documents, and participation in shift reports. Some nurses did not wish to talk within the hospital, so arrangements were made to meet outside of the hospital. Shift reports proved to be a "rich source of data because nurses frequently account for their actions in asides during these formal reports" (p. 156). Baker discussed outcomes in three groups.

"The first group of findings are called situated and embodied logics. These are the practices adopted by nurses in order to accomplish certain goals in particular situations. Although they are situated, they and similar practices may be widespread. They include ways of managing the medication trolley, reading between lines of medication-order and administration sheets, and using the medication round for gathering information for other purposes. These situated and embodied logics help nurses to be orderly in the complex practice world.

> The second set of findings is called the criteria for redefinition of error. This is a set of criteria nurses use to decide whether an incident is a 'real' error. Of course every nurse is professionally obliged to report errors, but if an error can be redefined, a medication-related incident becomes a non-error that does not need to be reported and no guilt is attached to it.
>
> The third set of findings [was] serendipitous and included the other uses to which nurses turn institutional rules with the purpose of making their own lives orderly." (p. 156)
>
> The following criteria were used by nurses to decide whether incidents were errors.
> 1. If it's not my fault, it is not an error.
> 2. If everyone knows, it is not an error.
> 3. If you can put it right, it is not an error.
> 4. If a patient has needs that are more urgent than the accurate administration of medication, it is not an error.
> 5. A clerical error is not a medication error.
> 6. If an irregularity is carried out to prevent something worse, it is not an error.
>
> To validate her conclusions, Baker shared the results of her analyses with the nurses who had participated in the study. They agreed with Baker's findings.

Historical Research

Historical research examines events of the past. Many historians believe that the greatest value of historical knowledge is increased self-understanding; in addition, historical knowledge provides nurses with an increased understanding of their profession.

Philosophical orientation

History is a science that dates back to the beginnings of humankind. The primary questions of history are the following: Where have we come from? Who are we? and Where are we going? Although the questions do not change, the answers do.

One of the assumptions of historical philosophy is that "there is nothing new under the sun." Because of this assumption, the historian can search throughout history for generalizations. For example, one can ask, What causes wars? A historian could search throughout history for commonalities in various wars and develop a theoretical explanation of the causes of wars. The questions a historian asks, the factors a historian looks for throughout history, and the nature of the explanation a historian gives in a study are all based on a worldview (Heller, 1982). Another assumption of historical philosophy is that one can learn from the past. The philosophy of history is a search for wisdom in which the historian examines what has been, what is, and what ought to be. Historical philosophers have attempted to identify a developmental scheme for history to explain all events and structures as elements of the same social process.

Nursing knowledge and historical research

Christy (1978) asks, "How can we in nursing today possibly plan where we are going when we don't know where we have been nor how we got here?" (p. 9). One criterion of a profession is that there is knowledge of the history of the profession that is transmitted to those entering the profession. Until recently, historical nursing research has not been a valued activity, and few nurse researchers had the skills or desire to conduct it. Therefore our knowledge of our past is sketchy. However, there is now a growing interest in the field of historical nursing research (Sarnecky, 1990).

Lusk (1997) suggests the following:

> "Topics should be significant, with the potential to illuminate or place a new perspective on current questions, thus contributing to scholarly understanding. Topics should also be feasible in terms of data and resource availability. Finally, topics should be intriguing and capable of sustaining a researcher's interest." (p. 355)

Examples from Historical Nursing Research

The researcher may spend much time reading related literature before making a final decision about the precise topic. In her doctoral dissertation, Waring (1978) used historical research to examine the idea of the nurse experiencing a "calling" to practice nursing. She described the extensive process of developing a precise topic as follows:

> "Originally my idea was to pursue concepts in the area of Puritan social thought and to relate concepts such as altruism and self-sacrifice to nursing. Two years after the formulation of this first idea, I finally realized that the topic was too broad. Reaching that point was slow and arduous but quite essential to the development of my thinking and the prospectus that developed as an outcome. When I first began the process, it seemed that I might have to abandon the topic 'calling.' Now, since the clarification and tightening up of my title and the clarification of my study thesis, I open volumes fearing that I will find yet another reference, once overlooked. It is only recently that I have become convinced that there was a needle in the haystack and that I had indeed found it." (pp. 18–19) [Waring's original title was "American Nursing and the Concept of the Calling."]

Developing Research Questions

After the topic has been clearly defined, the researcher will identify the questions to be examined during the research process. These questions tend to be more general and analytical than those found in quantitative studies. Evans (1978), then a doctoral student, describes the research questions she developed for her historical study.

> "I propose to study the nursing student. Who was this living person inside the uniform? Where did she come from? What were her experiences as a nursing student? I use the word 'experience' in terms of the dictionary definition of 'living through.' What did she live through? What happened to her and how did she

respond, or react, as the case may be? What was her educational program like? We have a pretty good notion of what nurse educators and others thought about the educational program, but what about it from the students' point of view?

What were the functions of rituals and rites of passage such as bed check, morning inspection, and capping? What kind of person did the nursing student tend to become in order to successfully negotiate studenthood? What are the implications of this in terms of her own personal and professional development and the development of the profession at large?" (p. 16)

Developing an Inventory of Sources

The next step is to determine whether sources of data for the study are available. Many of the materials for historical research are contained in private archives in libraries or are privately owned. Written permission must be obtained to gain access to library archives. Private materials are often difficult to ferret out, and when they are discovered, access may again be a problem.

Historical materials in nursing, such as letters, memos, handwritten materials, and mementos of significant leaders in nursing, are being discarded because no one recognizes their value. The same is true of materials related to the history of institutions and agencies with which nursing has been involved. Christy (1978) states, "It seems obvious that interest in the preservation of historical materials will only be stimulated if there is a concomitant interest in the value of historical research" (p. 9). Sometimes when such material is found, it is in such poor condition that much of the data are unclear or completely lost. Christy (1978) describes one of her experiences in searching for historical data as follows:

"M. Adelaide Nutting and Isabel M. Stewart are two of the greatest leaders we have ever had, and their friends, acquaintances, and former students were persons of tremendous importance to developments in nursing and nursing education throughout the world. Since both of these women were historians, they saved letters, clippings, manuscripts—primary source materials of inestimable value. Their friends were from many walks of life: physicians, lawyers, social workers, philanthropists—supporters and nonsupporters of nursing and nursing interests. Miss Nutting and Miss Stewart crammed these documents into boxes, files, and whatever other receptacles were available and—unfortunately—some of these materials are this very day in those same old boxes.

When I began my research into the archives in 1966, the files were broken, rusty, and dilapidated. Many of the folders were so old and ill-tended that they fell apart in my hands, the ancient paper crumbled into dust before my eyes. My research was exhilaratingly stimulating, and appallingly depressing at the same time; stimulating due to the gold mine of data available, and depressing as I realized the lack of care provided for such priceless materials. In addition, there was little or no organization, and one had to go through each document, in each drawer, in each file, piece by piece.... The boxes and cartons were worse, for

Continued

> materials bearing absolutely no relationship to each other were simply piled, willy-nilly, one atop the other. Is it any wonder that it took me eighteen months of solid work to get through them?" (pp. 8–9)

Determining the Validity and Reliability of Data

The validity and reliability concerns in historical research are related to the sources from which data are collected. The most valued source of data is the primary source. A *primary source* is material most likely to shed true light on the information the researcher seeks. For example, material written by a person who experienced an event or letters and other mementos saved by the person being studied are primary source material. A *secondary source* is written by someone who previously read and summarized the primary source material. History books and textbooks are secondary source materials. Primary sources are considered more valid and reliable than secondary sources.

> "The presumption is that an eyewitness can give a more accurate account of an occurrence than a person not present. If the author was an eyewitness, he is considered a primary source. If the author has been told about the occurrence by someone else, the author is a secondary source. The further the author moves from an eyewitness account, the less reliable are his statements." (Christy, 1975, p. 191)

Historical researchers use primary sources whenever possible. The historical researcher must consider the validity and reliability of primary sources used in the study. To determine this, the researcher uses principles of historical criticism.

> "One does not merely pick up a copy of Grandmother's diary and gleefully assume that all the things Grandma wrote were the unvarnished facts. Grandmother's glasses may at times have been clouded, at other times rose-colored. The well-prepared researcher will scrutinize, criticize, and analyze before even accepting its having been written by Grandma! And even after the validity of the document is established, every attempt is made to uncover bias, prejudice, or just plain exaggeration on Grandmother's part. Healthy skepticism becomes a way of life for the serious historiographer." (Christy, 1978, p. 6)

Two strategies have been developed to determine the authenticity and accuracy of the source: external and internal criticism. External criticism is used to determine the validity of source material. The researcher needs to know where, when, why, and by whom a document was written. This may involve verifying the handwriting or determining the age of the paper on which it was written. Christy (1975) describes some difficulties she experienced in establishing the validity of documents.

"An interesting problem presented by early nursing leaders was their frugality. Nutting occasionally saved stationery from hotels, resorts, or steamship lines during vacation trips and used it at a later date. This required double checking as to her exact location at the time the letter was written. When she first went to Teachers College in 1907, she still wrote a few letters on Johns Hopkins stationery. I found this practice rather confusing in early stages of research." (p. 190)

Internal criticism is an examination of the reliability of the document. The researcher must determine possible biases of the author. To verify the accuracy of a statement, the researcher should have two independent sources that provide the same information. In addition, the researcher should ensure that he or she understands the statements made by the writer, because words and their meanings change across time and across cultures. It is also possible to read into a document a meaning not originally intended by the author. This is most likely to happen when one is seeking a particular meaning. Sometimes words can be taken out of context (Christy, 1975).

Collecting the Data

Data collection may require months or years of dedicated searching for pertinent material. Occasionally, one small source may open a door to an entire new field of facts. In addition, there is no clear, obvious end to data collection. By examining the research guide, the researcher must make the decision to discontinue collection of data. These facets of data collection are described by Newton (1965) as follows:

"The search for data takes the researcher into most unexpected nooks and corners and adds facet after facet to the original problem. It may last for months or years or a decade. Days and weeks may be fruitless and endless references may be devoid of pertinent material. Again, one minor reference will open the door to the gold mine of facts. The search becomes more exciting when others know of it and bring possible clues to the investigator. The researcher cultivates persistence, optimism, and patience in his long and sometimes discouraging quest. But one real 'find' spurs him on and he continues his search. Added to this skill is the training in the most meticulous recording of data with every detail complete, and the logical classification of the data." (p. 23)

Writing the Research Report

Historical research reports do not follow the traditional formalized style that is characteristic of much research. The studies are designed to attract the interest of the reader and may appear to be deceptively simple. The untrained eye may not recognize the extensive work that was required to write the paper. Christy (1975) explains as follows:

"The reader is never aware of the painstaking work, the careful attention to detail, nor the arduous pursuit of clues endured by the writer of history. Perhaps that is why so many nurses have failed to recognize historiography as a legitimate research endeavor. It looks so easy." (p. 192)

QUALITATIVE RESEARCH METHODOLOGY

This section presents a more detailed description of the methodologies commonly used in qualitative studies. In some ways the methods used are no different from those used in quantitative studies. The researcher must select a topic; state the problem or question; justify the significance of the study; design the study; identify sources of data, such as subjects; gain access to those sources of data; select subjects or other sources for study; gather data; describe, analyze, and interpret the data; and develop a written report of the results. There are, however, methods unique to qualitative studies and sometimes to specific types of qualitative research. Research reports of qualitative studies tend to focus on results and seldom clearly describe the methods used to reach the conclusions. However, understanding some of the unique methods used by qualitative researchers will help you appreciate the work involved in conducting such a study. This section describes how participants (subjects) are selected, and how data are collected, managed, and analyzed. The achievement of rigor in qualitative research will also be explored.

Selection of Participants (Subjects)

Subjects in qualitative studies are referred to as participants. Participants may volunteer to be involved in the study or be selected by the researcher because of their particular knowledge, experience, or views related to the study. Qualitative researchers use purposive sampling methods rather than probability or convenience sampling methods. The researcher may select individuals typical in relation to the phenomenon under study, or, to get diverse perspectives, the researcher might intentionally seek out individuals who are different in some way from other participants. The sampling technique of "snowballing," in which the researcher asks participants to suggest individuals known to them who could provide information useful to the study, is commonly used. Decisions regarding sample size are different from those in quantitative studies and are based on needs related to the purposes of the study. Usually the number of subjects is small relative to the number used in quantitative studies. In case studies, the researcher may use only one subject (Sandelowski, 1996). A study of 6 to 10 subjects is not unusual. However, studies seeking maximum variation to examine a complex phenomenon or to develop a theory may require larger samples. The decision to stop seeking new subjects is made when the researcher ceases learning new information (informational redundancy) or when theoretical ideas seem complete (theoretical saturation) (Sandelowski, 1995).

The historical researcher seeks sources of information about the event being studied. These sources may include individuals who have experienced the event. But in most cases the sources are written documents or films. The researcher develops an inventory of sources and determines the validity and reliability of data from those sources.

Researcher-participant relationships

One of the important differences between quantitative and qualitative research lies in the relationships between the researcher and the participants of the study. The nature of these *researcher-participant relationships* has an impact on the collection and interpretation of data. Participants in qualitative research are not research subjects in the usual sense of the word; they are colleagues. The researcher must have the support and confidence of these individuals to complete the research. Therefore maintaining these relationships is very important. In many qualitative studies the researcher observes social behavior and may interact socially with the participants.

In varying degrees the researcher influences the individuals being studied and, in turn, is influenced by them. The mere presence of the researcher may alter behavior in the setting. This involvement, considered a source of bias in quantitative research, is thought by qualitative researchers to be a natural and necessary element of the research process. The researcher's personality is a key factor in qualitative research. Skills in empathy and intuition are cultivated; the researcher must become closely involved in the subject's experience to interpret it. It is necessary for the researcher to be open to the perceptions of the participants rather than to attach his or her own meaning to the experience. Participants often assist in determining research questions, guiding data collection, and interpreting results. The ethnographic researcher must become very familiar with the culture being studied by active participation in it and by extensive questioning of participants. The process of becoming immersed in the culture involves gaining increasing familiarity with aspects of the culture, such as language; sociocultural norms; traditions; and other social dimensions, including family, communication patterns (verbal and nonverbal), religion, work patterns, and expression of emotion. Immersion also involves gradually increasing acceptance of the researcher into the culture. Although ethnographic researchers must be actively involved in the culture they are studying, they must avoid "going native," which will interfere with both data collection and analysis. In going native, the researcher becomes a part of the culture and loses all objectivity, along with the ability to observe clearly.

In addition to the role the qualitative researcher takes in the relationship, expectations of the study must be carefully considered. The researcher's aims and means need to be consistent with those of the participants. For example, if the researcher's desire is to change the behavior of the participants, this must also be their desire.

Data Collection Methods

The most common data collection methods used in qualitative studies are observing participants, interviewing participants, and examining written text. These three methods, as they are used in qualitative studies, are described in the following sections.

Observation

Observation is a fundamental method of gathering data for qualitative studies. The aim is to gather firsthand information in a naturally occurring situation. The researcher functions in the learning mode with the question, What is going on here? It is important for the researcher to look carefully and to listen. In most cases the activities being observed are routine for the participants. The researcher focuses on the details of the routine. The process of activities may be as important to note as the discrete events. Unexpected events occurring during routine activities may be significant and are carefully noted. As in any observation process, the qualitative researcher will attend to some aspects of the situation while disregarding others. The researcher's focus on particular aspects of the situation may increase as insights about "what is going on" occur (Silverman, 1993).

Historians may observe film, videotapes, photographs, or artistic representations of historical events. The historian must recognize that these sources are limited to information the photographer or artist selectively chooses to reveal. Important elements of the event may not have been photographed or may have been edited out. In some cases, film that has been edited out of finished products has been preserved and may be sought by historians. The breakdown of the Communist countries has provided a treasure trove of archived films that can be used to provide important historical insights into many aspects of people's lives, including health issues.

Various strategies may be used to record information about the observations. In some cases the researcher will take detailed handwritten notes while observing. In other cases the researcher may focus entirely on the observational experience to avoid missing something meaningful and may wait until after the observation period to make detailed notes. Another useful strategy is to videotape the events, so that careful observations and detailed notes can be taken at a later time.

Class exercise in qualitative observation. The class should be divided into groups. A familiar site, such as a grocery store checkout stand, a hospital lobby, or the university bookstore, should be selected by each group. Each member of the group should independently observe activities at the site, and take notes of the observations without discussing them with other group members. The notes should be saved for discussion and analysis during an exercise described later in the chapter.

Interviews

There are differences between interviews conducted for a qualitative study and those conducted for a quantitative study. In qualitative studies, the interview format is more likely to be open-ended. Although the researcher defines the focus of the interview, there is no fixed sequence of questions. The questions addressed in interviews tend to change as the researcher gains insights from previous interviews and observations. Respondents are allowed, even encouraged, to raise important issues not addressed by the researcher. In some cases groups of individuals, which may be referred to as focus groups, are interviewed.

During interviews for qualitative studies, the researcher and the participant are actively engaged in constructing a version of the world. The interview is performed so that a deep, mutual understanding is achieved. The researcher's goal is to obtain an authentic insight into the participant's experiences. Rather than occurring at a single point in time, dialogue between researcher and participant may continue at intervals across weeks or months. Having recurring interviews should decrease the problems associated with fleeting relationships, in which respondents may have little commitment to the study or may provide only the information they believe the researcher wishes to hear (Silverman, 1993). Wimpenny and Gass (2000) compare the interviewing process in phenomenological and grounded theory research, to determine differences in interview technique. They examined interview methods used in both approaches to qualitative research in studies published between 1995 and 1998. They found that many qualitative researchers did not explicitly describe their data collection methods. Wimpenny and Gass (2000) concluded that in phenomenological and grounded theory research the interview method was not clearly linked to the qualitative approach being used.

Historical researchers may interview individuals who were participants in or observers of historical events. The focus of the interview may be to validate available information about the event, uncover heretofore unknown details about the event, or obtain the views about the event from individuals who were not heard from previously. Historical events are generally considered to be constructed truths rather than factual. Individual perspectives on an event may provide additional insight into the event, but they are not expected to provide the truth of an event, which will never be known (and perhaps does not exist). Another strategy for collecting historical data is to interview individuals and construct their biographies. In addition, the personal histories of a number of individuals can be used to understand the evolving history of a region or institution.

Strategies used to record information from interviews include writing notes during the interview, writing detailed notes immediately after the interview, or recording the interview on tape.

Class exercise in qualitative interviewing. Each member of the class should interview an individual about his or her experiences with and perceptions of being in either a grocery store, a hospital lobby, or a university bookstore. Alternatively, each class member should interview an individual (faculty member, staff member, etc.) connected with the school of nursing to construct an oral history of the school. Data from the interviews should be recorded for reference in later exercises in this chapter.

Text as a source of qualitative data

In qualitative studies text is considered a rich source of data. The researcher may ask participants to write about a particular topic. In some cases these written narratives may be solicited by mail rather than in person. Text provided by participants may be a component of a larger study using a variety of sources of data. Text developed for other purposes, such as from patient records or procedure manuals, can be accessed for qualitative analysis. Published text from newspaper articles, magazine articles, books, or the Internet can be used as qualitative data. Transcriptions of recorded interviews are commonly used in qualitative studies. In historical research, written descriptions of historical events, letters, and documents related to the event may be accessed for analysis. A historical study might examine the changing pattern of nursing practice in a selected area or of a nursing procedure by examining nursing textbooks and journal articles that describe a particular practice at different times. Notes taken while reading written documents are important to the analysis process.

Class exercise in obtaining textual data for qualitative analysis. The class should select a topic related to health or patient care, such as asthma, diabetes, or weight loss. Each member of the class should search the Internet for chat lines or discussion groups related to the selected problem. Files of text written by individuals with the particular health problem should be printed or downloaded and saved for an analysis exercise later in the chapter.

Data Management

Qualitative data analysis occurs concurrently with data collection rather than sequentially, as in quantitative research. Therefore the researcher is attempting to simultaneously gather, manage, and interpret a growing bulk of data. Volumes of data are gathered during a qualitative study. The researcher must develop means of storing the data in an organized manner. Traditionally, qualitative data collection and analysis have been performed manually. The researcher records the data on small bits of paper or note cards that are then carefully coded, organized, and filed at the end of a day of gathering data. It is easy to lose data in the mass of paper. Keeping track of connections between various bits of data requires meticulous record keeping. Some qualitative researchers believe that a computer can be used to make management and analysis of qualitative data quicker and easier, without the risk of losing touch with the data. A computer assists such activities as processing, storing, retrieving, cataloging, and sorting, leaving the analysis up to the researcher.

Data Analysis

Qualitative data analysis occurs in three stages: description, analysis, and interpretation. The descriptive stage is more critical in qualitative studies than in quantitative ones. Researchers are encouraged to remain in the descriptive mode for as long as possible before moving on to analysis and interpretation. Because published qualitative studies tend not to describe the methodology in detail, many professionals believe that qualitative research is free-wheeling. According to Coffey and Atkinson (1996):

> "There still seem to be too many students and practitioners who believe implicitly that qualitative research can be done in a spirit of careless rapture, with no principled or disciplined thought whatsoever. They collect data with little thought for research problems and research design, and they think that they will know what to do with the data once those data are collected.... [When they begin analysis] they find that things are not quite so simple." (p. 11)

Description

In the initial phases of a qualitative study, the researcher needs to become familiar with the data. This may involve reading and rereading notes and transcripts, recalling observations and experiences, listening to audiotapes, and viewing videotapes until the researcher becomes immersed in the data. Audiotapes contain more than words; they contain feeling, emphasis, and nonverbal communication, which are as important to communication as words. In phenomenological research, this immersion in the data is referred to as dwelling with the data. The initial purpose of this immersion is to address the question, What is going on? An important methodological technique in grounded theory research is the constant comparative process, in which every piece of data is compared with every other piece.

During data analysis, a dynamic interaction occurs between the researcher self and the data, whether the data are communicated orally or in writing. During this process, referred to as *reflexive thought,* the researcher explores personal feelings and experiences that may influence the study and integrates this understanding into the study. The process requires a conscious self-awareness.

In a paper describing her experiences conducting a phenomenological study of caregiving behaviors, Drew (1989) describes the impact of relationships on her study as follows:

"A session with a person who had been willing to talk about his or her experiences with caregivers, and who had invested energy into the interview session, often generated for me a sense of doing something worthwhile, as well as a feeling that I would be competent to analyze the transcribed material in a meaningful way. This sense of competency dispelled any doubts about being an intruder. I became relaxed, unselfconscious, and more self-assured. However, an encounter with a person with blunt affect, abrupt answers, and a paucity of responses left me feeling awkward and self-conscious. A sense of doubt about the validity of my project encroached as I attempted to elicit that person's thoughts. At the time, my immediate reaction was to think that I had obtained nothing from these individuals, when in fact, as I was to discover later, the 'nothing' was something important that I was as yet unable to see.

It was at the point of discouragement about my interviewing skills that I became aware that I was mentally classifying interviews as either 'good' or 'bad,' depending on my emotional response to the subjects. Good interviews were those in which I felt effective as an interviewer and was able to facilitate the person's recounting of experiences with caregivers. I enjoyed the interaction and felt that we connected on some level that produced meaningful discussion about the topic of relationships between patient and caregiver.

Bad interviews, on the other hand, were those in which I could not seem to get subjects to talk about how they had experienced their caregivers. There seemed to be no questions that I could devise with which to explore feelings, either positive or negative, with them. They gave no indications of awareness of their feelings, or of feelings in others. Whereas the subjects of the good interviews were people I experienced as open, curious, and thoughtful, those

Continued

of the bad interviews were experienced as distrustful and elicited in me a sense of anxiety and frustration; it seemed I could not get through to them. I felt inadequate as an interviewer and was ready to discard these interviews. Frustration and anxiety arose because I felt that I was not getting the information that I needed for the study.

Subsequently, I discovered that my feelings of frustration and inadequacy were causing me to overlook data and that when I could put them aside, new data that were rich in meaning became apparent.... This discovery was a powerful experience for me, affecting my approach to subsequent interviews and influencing analysis of data thereafter." (pp. 433-434)*

*From Drew, N. (1989). The interviewer's experience as data in phenomenological research. *Western Journal of Nursing Research, 11*(4), 431–439. Reprinted with permission of Sage Publications, Inc.

In some phenomenological research this critical thinking leads to *bracketing*, which is used to help the researcher avoid misinterpreting the phenomenon as it is being experienced by the participants. Bracketing is suspending or laying aside what the researcher knows about the experience being studied (Oiler, 1982). Other phenomenologists, especially those using Heideggerian phenomenology, do not bracket, but they do identify beliefs, assumptions, and preconceptions about the research topic. These are put in writing at the beginning of the study for self-reflection and external review. These procedures are intended to facilitate openness and new insights.

Initial efforts at analysis focus on reducing the large volume of data acquired to facilitate examination. This may involve "selecting, focusing, simplifying, abstracting, and transforming the data" (Miles & Huberman, 1994, p. 10). During data reduction, the researcher begins to attach meaning to elements of the data; discovers classes of things, persons, events, and properties; and notes regularities in the setting or the people. The researcher then classifies the elements in the data, either by using an established classification system or by developing a new one.

Transcribing interviews. Tape-recorded interviews are generally transcribed word for word. Morse and Field (1995) provide the following instructions for transcribing a tape-recorded interview.

"Pauses should be indicated by using dashes, and ellipses should indicate gaps or prolonged pauses. All expressions, including exclamations, laughter, crying, and expletives, are included in the text and separated from the verbal text with square brackets. Type the interviews single-spaced with a blank line between each speaker. A generous margin on both sides of the page permits the left margin to be used for coding and the researcher's own critique of the interview style, and the right margin to be used for comments regarding the content.... Ensure that all pages are numbered sequentially and that each page is coded with the interview number and the participant's number." (p. 131)

The researcher should listen to recordings as soon as possible after an interview, listening to the voice tone, inflection, and pauses of the researcher and the participant, as well as to the content. While listening, the researcher is advised to read the written transcript of the tape and make notations of observations on the transcript (Morse & Field, 1995).

Codes and coding. *Coding* is a method of indexing or identifying categories in the data. A code is a symbol or abbreviation used to classify words or phrases in the data. Codes may be placed in the data when they are collected, entered into the computer, or when the data are examined at a later time. The purpose of coding is to facilitate the retrieval of data segments by coding category. Used in this manner, coding simplifies and reduces the data (Coffey & Atkinson, 1996; Miles & Huberman, 1994). Coffey and Atkinson (1996) point out that

> "...[t]he nature of qualitative data means that data relating to one particular topic are not found neatly bundled together at exactly the same spot in each interview (and field-notes usually have even less predictable organization). The ability to locate stretches of data that, at least ostensibly, are 'about' the same thing is a valuable aspect of data management." (p. 35)

Organizing data, selecting specific elements of the data for categories, and naming these categories will reflect the philosophical base of the study. Later in the study, coding may progress to the development of a taxonomy. For example, the researcher may develop a taxonomy of types of pain, types of patients, or types of patient education.

> Morse and Field (1995) suggest that when selecting elements of the data to code the researchers should note:
> "1. the kinds of things that are going on in the context being studied;
> 2. the forms a phenomenon takes; and
> 3. any variations within a phenomenon." (pp. 136-137)

Morse and Field (1995) suggest several innovative strategies for coding data. One approach is to use highlighter pens, with a different color for each major category. Another strategy, developed by Murdock (1971), is to assign each major category a number, which is inserted in the computerized text. Using this approach, a word or phrase in the text could easily have several codes indicated by numbers. Knafl and Webster (1988) suggest using colored markers, paper clips, index cards, or self-adhesive stickers to identify categories of data. Codes are often written in the margins. Then one can sort data by cutting the pages into sections according to codes. Each section can be taped or pasted onto an index card for filing. This procedure can be performed easily using computer programs for qualitative analysis, in which broad margins are available for coding. Computerized data can be sorted by code into separate files for each code, whereas identifiers such as data and source are retained.

Reflective remarks. While the researcher records notes, other thoughts or insights may emerge into his or her consciousness. These thoughts are generally included in the notes and are separated from the rest of the notes by ((double parentheses)). If needed, they may be extracted and used to construct memos later (Miles & Huberman, 1994).

Marginal remarks. As the notes are being reviewed, observations about them should be written immediately. These remarks are usually placed in the right-hand margin of the notes. The remarks often connect the notes with other parts of the data or suggest new interpretations. Reviewing notes can become boring, which is a signal that thinking has ceased. Making marginal notes assists the researcher in "retaining a thoughtful stance" (Miles & Huberman, 1994).

Data displays. One approach to describing qualitative data is data displays. Displays are highly condensed and are equivalent to the summary tables of statistical outcomes developed in quantitative research. These data displays allow the researcher to convey succinctly the main ideas of the research. Codes can be used to organize the display. The strategies for achieving displays are limited only by the imagination of the researcher. Displays can be developed relatively easily using computer spreadsheets, graphics programs, or desktop publishing programs. Miles and Huberman (1994) contains additional information on data displays.

Marsh (1990) used a process-oriented matrix to test conclusions and an emergent theory from a qualitative study that examined healthy lifestyle changes. Seven individuals who had made or were making lifestyle changes were interviewed, with a focus on the process of lifestyle change. Marsh's emergent theory describing the process of lifestyle change is as follows.

> "An individual, aware of the need and desiring to alter his or her life-style, makes one or more attempts to change over time. The attempts result in relapse. A self-monitoring process mediates between awareness of the individual's need to change and his or her relapses in the process of change. At some point tension mounts over the need to change. This tension, labeled 'readiness,' is characterized by a combination of personal and environmental variables, such as low self-esteem or support from significant others. Following readiness, the individual experiences a profound self-revelation. The revelation is characterized by a dramatic self-insight, a coming to as if shaken by a new understanding of reality. The revelation is followed by a belief system change about personal power, following which the individual makes and sustains a health life-style change. An individual who experiences no revelation remains in the initial pattern of attempted change and relapse. Revelation appeared to be the emerging core variable of the life-style change process." (p. 45)

To evaluate the trustworthiness of the emergent theory, all the data were examined for their fit in a matrix. Categories for the matrix were developed and decision rules established for inclusion of data within a category. Every subject was represented in the matrix. When a subject had made more than one lifestyle change, each change was represented separately in the matrix. The matrix is presented in Table 11-1 on pages 384–387.

Counting. Qualitative researchers tend to avoid the use of numbers. However, when judgments of qualities are made, counting occurs. In describing a pattern, the researcher may observe that a particular pattern occurs frequently or more often. Something is considered important or significant. These judgments are made in part by counting. If the researcher is counting, this should be recognized and planned. Counting can help researchers see what data they have, help them verify a hypothesis, and help them remain intellectually honest. Qualitative researchers work by insight and intuition; however, their conclusions can be wrong. It is easier to see confirming evidence than disconfirming evidence. Comparing insights by using numbers can be a good method of verification (Miles & Huberman, 1994).

Class exercise in describing qualitative research findings. Groups within the class should examine data obtained from observing, interviewing, and gathering textual data. Codes and remarks should be used to understand the content. A matrix should be developed with the codes. Results should be presented to the class, and similarities and differences in the findings of the class groups should be explored.

Analysis

Analysis goes beyond description, using methods to transform the data. Through this process, the researcher extends the data beyond the description. Using analysis, he or she identifies essential features and describes interrelationships among them (Wolcott, 1994). During analysis, the emphasis is on identifying themes and patterns in the data. Coding, used earlier for description, also can be used to expand, transform, and reconceptualize data, thus providing opportunities for more diverse analyses. Coffey and Atkinson (1996) suggest that by "reading through data extracts, one might discover particular events, key words, processes, or characters that capture the essence of a piece" (p. 31).

Memos are used to record insights or ideas related to notes, transcripts, or codes. Memos move the researcher toward theorizing and are conceptual rather than factual. They may link pieces of data or use a specific piece of data as an example of a concept. The memo may be written to someone else involved in the study or to oneself. It is important to value these insights and write them down quickly. Whenever an idea emerges, even if it is vague and not well thought out, it should be written down immediately. Although one might think that the idea is so clear in one's mind that it can be written later, the thought is often soon forgotten and cannot be retrieved. Memos should be dated, titled according to their key concept, and connected by codes to the field notes or forms that generated the thoughts (Miles & Huberman, 1994).

Storytelling. During observation and interviewing the researcher may record stories shared by participants. Banks-Wallace (1998) describes a story as "an event or series of events, encompassed by temporal or spatial boundaries, that are shared

TABLE **11-1**			

PROCESS-ORIENTED MATRIX OF LIFE-STYLE CHANGES

SUBJECT NO.	LIFE-STYLE CHANGE	PROBLEM AWARENESS	RELAPSE
1	Overeating*	In 8th grade, I was conscious of being overweight I need to do something for myself	I have no time to care for I have character defects I did not want to commit and fail
2	Overeating*	I feel uncomfortable and short of breath	I tried all new diets My spouse supported my failure, both have poor will power
	Alcohol	None	None
	Smoking	I have a bad cough	I made two failed attempts
3	Overeating*	Eating is a sin—I love it, I hate it At a group I was obsessive/compulsive over food	I had many, many failures Food controls me. I have little control I tried groups; I like the support but cannot keep with it

*Change currently being made. (Reprinted from *Advance in Nursing Science 12*(3), 51–52, with permission of Aspen Publishers, Inc. ©1990.)

TABLE **11-1**——CONT'D

PROCESS-ORIENTED MATRIX OF LIFE-STYLE CHANGES

SUBJECT NO.	LIFE-STYLE CHANGE	PROBLEM AWARENESS	RELAPSE
4	Overeating*	I was a fat slob and an introvert since I was a small child	I wanted a magic cure with no responsibility
5	Smoking*	I was tired of it It was a hassle	I have no one to share the problem with, no pats on back, no group support I am a failure
	Alcohol	I was sneaking I was hiding problem from family	None
6	Smoking*	I was thinking about change I feel scared, angry I need a focus My body and health are changing It is filthy I am ambivalent	I made it convenient I quit in past, started again I want others to help
7	Smoking*	It is expensive It is filthy I risk getting cancer of the mouth	I have made many attempts I am angry I do not want to give it up
	Alcohol	I was hiding bottles I was a closet drinker	I tried quitting for 6 years I only have myself to blame

change currently being made. (Reprinted from *Advance in Nursing Science 12*(3), 51–52, with permission of Aspen Publishers, Inc. ©1990.)

READINESS	REVELATION	BELIEF-SYSTEM CHANGE	BEHAVIORAL OUTCOME	PREDICT FUTURE OUTCOM
My husband was supportive I got a friend to go to a meeting with me People at group were honest I want to live Success of others in group was inspirational	I can use my power along with God's power to conquer the demon, overeating	I have strength in working with God; this gives me power, and I can use it	60-lb weight loss sustained for 4.5 months, confident of continued success	Will sust
I got help from spouse I got help from group	I realized, if that woman can do it, so can I	I no longer need to eat to be happy	75-lb weight loss sustained over 1 year	Will sus
I got support from spouse I have low self-esteem I got group support—I went willingly, with no expectations	It suddenly hit, "I didn't like me anymore"	I have personal power I find support in group	Alcohol abstinence	Will sus
My father's health was bad I had a bad cough I really wanted to quit	None	I can do it by myself (strength from alcohol problem)	Sustained smoking cessation for several years	Will sus
I have low self-esteem I am concerned for my child Group gives me hope and strength I have been depressed, I hate my life When I am okay, everything else is	None	None	Repeated relapses	Escalati readin

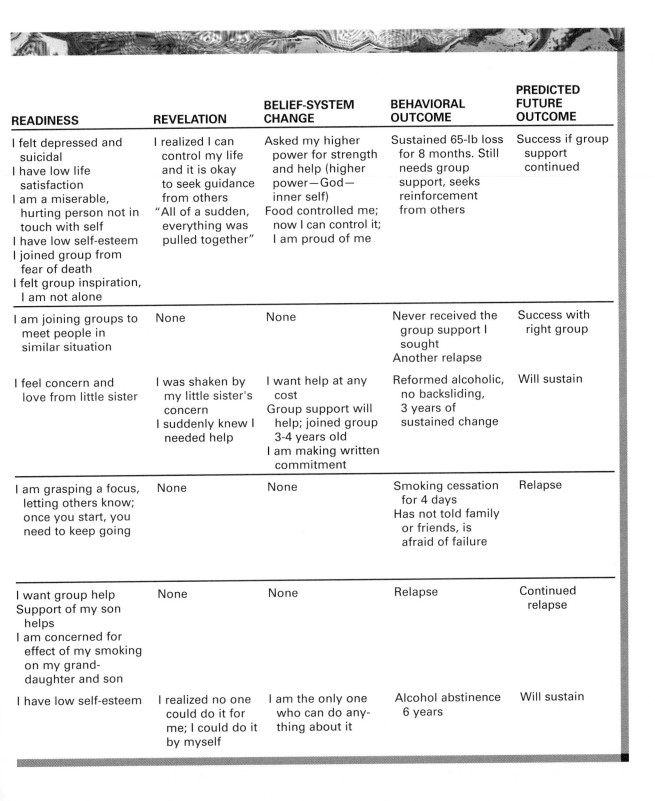

READINESS	REVELATION	BELIEF-SYSTEM CHANGE	BEHAVIORAL OUTCOME	PREDICTED FUTURE OUTCOME
I felt depressed and suicidal I have low life satisfaction I am a miserable, hurting person not in touch with self I have low self-esteem I joined group from fear of death I felt group inspiration, I am not alone	I realized I can control my life and it is okay to seek guidance from others "All of a sudden, everything was pulled together"	Asked my higher power for strength and help (higher power—God— inner self) Food controlled me; now I can control it; I am proud of me	Sustained 65-lb loss for 8 months. Still needs group support, seeks reinforcement from others	Success if group support continued
I am joining groups to meet people in similar situation	None	None	Never received the group support I sought Another relapse	Success with right group
I feel concern and love from little sister	I was shaken by my little sister's concern I suddenly knew I needed help	I want help at any cost Group support will help; joined group 3-4 years old I am making written commitment	Reformed alcoholic, no backsliding, 3 years of sustained change	Will sustain
I am grasping a focus, letting others know; once you start, you need to keep going	None	None	Smoking cessation for 4 days Has not told family or friends, is afraid of failure	Relapse
I want group help Support of my son helps I am concerned for effect of my smoking on my grand-daughter and son	None	None	Relapse	Continued relapse
I have low self-esteem	I realized no one could do it for me; I could do it by myself	I am the only one who can do any-thing about it	Alcohol abstinence 6 years	Will sustain

with others using an oral medium or sign language. *Storytelling* is the process or interaction used to share stories. People sharing a story (storytellers) and those listening to a story *(storytakers)* are the main elements of storytelling." (p. 17) Stories can promote understanding of a notable phenomenon. In some qualitative studies, the research may focus on gathering stories. Frank (2000) describes gathering narratives about illnesses. Gathering stories enables health-care providers to develop storytelling as a powerful means to increase insight and facilitate healthy behaviors of clients. For example, Nwoga (1997) studied how African-American mothers use storytelling to educate their adolescent daughters about their sexuality. The stories used by these mothers, captured by Nwoga, could be useful in assisting other mothers struggling to help their daughters deal with sexuality issues.

Coffey and Atkinson (1996) discuss the importance of capturing stories in qualitative studies.

"The story is an obvious way for social actors, in talking to strangers (e.g., the researcher), to retell key experiences and events. Stories serve a variety of functions. Social actors often remember and order their careers or memories as a series of narrative chronicles, that is, as [a] series of stories marked by key happenings. Similarly, stories and legends are told and retold by members of particular social groups or organizations as a way of passing on a cultural heritage or an organizational culture. Tales of success or tales of key leaders/personalities are familiar genres with which to maintain a collective sense of the culture of an organization. The use of atrocity stories and morality fables is also well documented within organizational and occupational settings. Stories of medical settings are especially well documented (Atkinson, 1992; Dingwall, 1977). Here tales of professional incompetence are used to give warning of 'what not to do' and what will happen if you commit mistakes…. Narratives are also a common genre from which to retell or come to terms with particularly sensitive or traumatic times and events." (p. 56)

Narrative analysis is a qualitative means of formally analyzing stories. Using this method, the researcher "unpacks" the structure of the story. A story includes a sequence of events with a beginning, a middle, and an end. Stories have their own logic and are temporal (Coffey & Atkinson, 1996; Denzin, 1989). The structures can also be used to determine how people tell stories, how they shape the events they describe, how they make a point, how they "package" events and react to them, and how they communicate their stories to audiences. The structure used for narrative analysis as identified by Coffey and Atkinson (1996, p. 58) is as follows:

Structure	Question
Abstract	What is this about?
Orientation	Who? What? When? Where?
Complication	Then what happened?
Evaluation	So what?
Result	What finally happened?
Coda	Finish narrative

The abstract initiates the narrative by summarizing the point of the story or stating the proposition the narrative will illustrate. The orientation provides an introduction to the major events central to the story. The complication continues the narrative, describing complications in the event that make it a story, taking the form, Then what happened? Evaluation is the point of the narrative, followed by the result, which gives the outcome or resolution of events. The coda ends the story and provides a transition to other topics.

The narrative analysis can focus on social action embedded in the text or can examine the effect of the story. Stories serve a purpose. They may make a point or be moralistic. They may be success stories, or may be a reminder of what not to do or how not to be, with guidance about how to avoid the fate described in the story. The purpose of the story can be the starting point for a more extensive narrative analysis. Narrative analysis may examine multiple stories of key life events and gain greater understanding of the impact of these events; it may assist in understanding the relationship between social processes and personal lives; or it may be used to understand cultural values, meanings, and personal experiences. Issues related to power, dominance, and opposition can be examined. Through stories, silenced groups can be given voice (Coffey & Atkinson, 1996).

Coding is not used in narrative analysis. Coding breaks data up into separate segments and is not useful in analyzing a story. The researcher can lose the sense that informants are providing an account or a narrative of events.

Qualitative researchers may choose to communicate the findings of their study as a story. A story can be a powerful way to make a point. A story can be presented from a variety of perspectives: following chronological order, following the order in which the story was originally presented, focusing on progressive issues, focusing only on a critical or key event in the story, describing the plot and characters as one would stage a play, following an analytical framework, providing versions of an event from the stories of several viewers, or presenting the story as one would write a mystery story, thus appealing to problem-solvers.

Interpretation

During interpretation, the researcher offers his or her interpretation of what is going on. The focus is on understanding and explaining it beyond what can be stated with certainty (Coffey & Atkinson, 1996; Wolcott, 1994). Interpretation may focus on the usefulness of the findings for clinical practice or may move toward theorizing.

As the study progresses, relationships among categories, participants, actions, and events begin to emerge. The researcher will develop hunches about relationships that can be used to formulate tentative propositions. Statements or propositions can be written on index cards and sorted into categories or entered into the computer (Miles & Huberman, 1994).

Using information in the matrix in Table 11-1, Marsh (1990) made the following interpretations:

"Subjects 1, 2, and 4 experienced revelation related to overeating, followed by a belief-system change. Each of these individuals had lost 60 to 75 pounds and had maintained the weight loss for 4.5 months to 1 year. Subject 3 experienced no revelation and had no success in weight loss. The matrix revealed patterns in the data that might have been overlooked." (p. 45)

For example, Marsh assumed that the belief-system change that occurred was a change in health beliefs. The matrix illustrated that the change was rather one of personal empowerment and involved beliefs about self, not about health.

As the data are collected and analyzed, the researcher gains increasing understanding of the dynamics in the process under study. This understanding might be considered a tentative theory. The first tentative theories are often vague and pieced together poorly; some are wrong. The best way to verify a tentative theory is to share it with others, particularly informants in the study situations. Informants have their own tentative theories, which have never been clearly expressed. The tentative theory needs to be expressed as a map. Developing a good map of the tentative theory is difficult and requires some hard work.

The validity of predictions developed in a tentative theory must be tested; however, finding effective ways to test them is difficult. Predictions are usually developed near the end of the study. Because the findings are often context-specific, the predictions must be tested on the same or a similar sample. One strategy suggested is to predict outcomes expected at 6 months after the study. Six months later, these predictions can be sent to informants who participated in the study. The informants can be asked to respond to the accuracy of (1) the predictions and (2) the explanation of why the predicted events were expected to occur (Miles & Huberman, 1994).

People may easily identify patterns, themes, and gestalts from their observations. It is often difficult to find *real* additional evidence of a pattern while remaining open to disconfirming evidence. Any identified pattern should be subjected to skepticism by the researcher and others (Miles & Huberman, 1994). Morse and Field (1995) state the following.

> "The researcher must distinguish between representative cases and anecdotal cases. Representative cases appear with regularity and encompass the range of behaviors described within a category. The anecdotal case appears infrequently and depicts a small range of events that are atypical of the larger group.... Negative cases are those episodes that clearly refute an emergent theory or proposition. Negative cases are important because they help to clarify additional causal properties that influence the phenomena under study (Denzin, 1978)." (p. 139)

Often during analysis, a conclusion seems plausible. It seems to fit; it makes good sense. When asked how he or she arrived at that point, the researcher may state that it "just feels right." These intuitive feelings are important in both qualitative and quantitative research. However, plausibility cannot stand alone. After plausibility must come systematic analysis. First, intuition occurs; then careful examination of the data is done to verify the validity of that intuition (Miles & Huberman, 1994).

Rigor in Qualitative Research

Scientific *rigor* is valued because it is associated with greater worth of research outcomes, and studies are critiqued as a means of judging rigor. Qualitative research methods have been criticized for lacking rigor; however, this criticism probably occurred because the rules developed to judge quantitative studies were also used to judge the rigor of qualitative studies. Morse (1999a), a well-known scholar in qualitative research methodology, stated the following in a discussion of validity and reliability of qualitative research:

> "I am puzzled why reliability and validity are not spoken about and have all but disappeared from the North American literature. According to my dictionary, they should be of utmost concern, relevant and right at the heart of any study. I agree, they have been operationalized very rigidly in quantitative texts, and these instructions are not pertinent to qualitative inquiry. But this does not mean that they should not be used and certainly should not stop them from being operationalized to meet the conditions and circumstances of qualitative inquiry." (p. 717)

Rigor needs to be defined differently for qualitative research because the desired outcome is different (Burns, 1989; Dzurec, 1989; Morse, 1989; Sandelowski, 1986). In quantitative research, rigor is reflected in narrowness, conciseness, and objectivity and leads to rigid adherence to research designs and precise statistical analyses. In qualitative research, rigor is associated with openness, scrupulous adherence to a philosophical perspective, thoroughness in collecting data, and consideration of all data in the subjective theory development phase. Evaluation of the rigor of a qualitative study is based, in part, on the logic of the emerging theory and the clarity with which it sheds light on the phenomenon studied. Lack of rigor in qualitative research is due to problems such as inconsistently applying the philosophy of the approach being used, failing to get away from older ideas, using poorly developed methods, not spending enough time collecting data, making poor observations, failing to give careful consideration to all data, and inadequately using data for theoretical development.

DECISION TRAILS

The credibility of qualitative data analysis has been seriously questioned in some cases by the larger scientific community. The concerns expressed are related to the inability to replicate the outcomes of a study, even when using the same data set. To respond to this concern, some qualitative researchers have attempted to develop strategies by which other researchers, using the same data, can follow the logic of the original researcher and arrive at the same conclusions. Miles and Huberman (1994) refer to this strategy as a *decision trail*; Guba and Lincoln (1982) refer to it as *auditability*.

Developing a decision trail requires that the researcher establish decision rules for categorizing data, arriving at ratings, or making judgments. A decision rule might say, for example, that a datum would be placed in a specific category if it met specified criteria. Another decision rule might say that an observed interaction would be considered an instance of an emerging theoretical explanation if it met specific criteria. A record is kept of all decision rules used in the analysis of data. All raw data are stored so that they are available for review if requested. As the analysis progresses, the researcher documents the data, the decision rules on which each decision was based, and the reasoning behind each decision. Thus evidence is retained to support the study conclusions and the emerging theory and is made available on request (Burns, 1989). However, Marshall (1984, 1985) cautioned against undermining the strengths of qualitative research with overly mechanistic data analysis. Marshall and Rossman (1989) expressed concern that efforts to increase validity will "filter out the unusual, the serendipitous—the puzzle that, if tended to and pursued, would provide a recasting of the entire research endeavor" (p. 113). Decision trails are not usually included as part of a published qualitative study. The author might state that a decision trail is available on request from the researcher.

SUMMARY

Qualitative research is a systematic, subjective approach used to describe life experiences and give them meaning. The terminology used in qualitative research and the methods of reasoning differ from those used in more traditional quantitative research methods and reflect different philosophical orientations. Qualitative research focuses on understanding the whole, which is consistent with the holistic philosophy of nursing. The qualitative approaches are based on a worldview that has the following beliefs: (1) there is not a single reality and (2) what we know has meaning only within a given situation or context.

Frameworks are used in a different sense in qualitative research than they are in quantitative studies, because the goal is not theory testing. Nonetheless, each type of qualitative research is guided by a particular philosophy. The data from qualitative studies are subjective, and incorporate the perceptions and beliefs of the researcher and the participants. Four common approaches to qualitative research used in nursing are presented in this chapter: phenomenological, grounded theory, ethnographic, and historical. The purpose of phenomenological research is to describe in phenomenological terms the experiences of the study participants, as they live them. Grounded theory research is based on symbolic interaction theory, which explores how people define reality and how their beliefs are related to their actions. Ethnographic studies are used to understand people: their ways of living, believing, and adapting to changing environmental circumstances. The primary questions of history are the following: Where have we come from? Who are we? and Where are we going?

In some ways the methods used in qualitative research are no different from those used in quantitative studies. The researcher must select a topic; state the problem or question; justify the significance of the study; design the study; identify sources of data such as subjects; gain access to those sources of data; select subjects or other sources for study; gather data; describe, analyze, and interpret the data; and develop a written report of their results. Some methods, however, are unique to all qualitative studies, and other methods are used with only specific types of qualitative research. Subjects in qualitative studies are referred to as participants. The relationship between the researcher and the individuals being studied is one of colleagues. The effectiveness of this relationship has an impact on the collection and interpretation of data. In many ways the researcher influences the individuals being studied and, in turn, is influenced by them. The researcher's aims need to be consistent with those of the participants. For example, if the researcher's desire is to change the behavior of the participants, this must also be their desire.

The most common data collection methods used in qualitative studies are observation, interviewing, and examination of textual data. Qualitative data analysis occurs concurrently with data collection rather than sequentially, as in quantitative research. Therefore the researcher is attempting to simultaneously gather, manage, and interpret data. Qualitative data analysis occurs in three stages: description, analysis, and interpretation. The descriptive stage is more critical in qualitative studies than in quantitative ones. Researchers are encouraged to remain in the descriptive mode as long as possible, before moving on to analysis and interpretation. In the initial phases of a qualitative study, the researcher needs to become familiar with the data. This may involve reading and rereading notes and transcripts, recalling observation and experiences, listening to audiotapes, and viewing videotapes until the researcher becomes immersed in the data. During data analysis, a dynamic interaction occurs between the researcher's self and the data, whether the data are communicated orally or in writing. During this process, referred to as reflexive thought, the researcher explores personal feelings and experiences that may influence the study and integrates this

understanding into the study. The process requires a conscious awareness of self.

Initial efforts of analysis are often focused on reducing the large volume of data to facilitate examination. Coding is used to index or identify categories in the data. One approach to describing qualitative data is data displays. Displays are highly condensed and are equivalent to the summary tables of statistical outcomes developed in quantitative research. Qualitative researchers tend to avoid the use of numbers. However, if the researcher is counting, this should be recognized and planned. Judgments in qualitative studies are made in part by counting. Analysis goes beyond description, using methods to transform the data. Through analysis the researcher identifies essential features, describes interrelationships among the data, and identifies the themes and patterns. Stories obtained during data gathering may be analyzed using narrative analysis. During interpretation, the researcher offers his or her interpretation of what is going on. The focus is on understanding the data and explaining it beyond what can be stated with certainty. Interpretation may focus on the usefulness of the findings for clinical practice or may move toward theorizing.

Qualitative research methods have been criticized for lack of rigor; however, this criticism was probably made because the rules developed to judge quantitative studies were also used to judge the rigor of qualitative studies. In qualitative research, rigor is associated with openness, scrupulous adherence to a philosophical perspective, thoroughness in collecting data, and consideration of all of the data in the subjective theory development phase. Evaluation of the rigor of a qualitative study is based, in part, on the logic of the emerging theory and the clarity with which it sheds light on the phenomenon studied.

In some cases, the credibility of qualitative data analysis has been questioned by members of the scientific community. The concerns expressed are related to the inability to replicate the outcomes of a study, even when using the same data set. To respond to the concern, some qualitative researchers have developed strategies called decision trails, by which other researchers, using the same data, can follow the logic of the original researcher and arrive at the same conclusions. Developing a decision trail requires that the researcher establish decision rules for categorizing data, arriving at ratings, or making judgments. As the analysis progresses, the researcher documents the data and the decision rules on which each decision was based and the reasoning that entered into each decision.

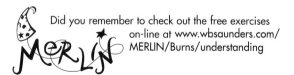

Did you remember to check out the free exercises on-line at www.wbsaunders.com/ MERLIN/Burns/understanding

REFERENCES

Anderson, J. M. (1989). The phenomenological perspective. In J. M. Morse (Ed.), *Qualitative nursing research: A contemporary dialogue* (pp. 15-26). Rockville, MD: Aspen.

Artinian, B. A. (1988). Qualitative modes of inquiry. *Western Journal of Nursing Research, 10*(2), 138–149.

Atkinson, P. (1992). The ethnography of a medical setting: Reading, writing and rhetoric. *Qualitative Health Research, 2*(4), 451–474.

Baer, E. D. (1979). Philosophy provides the rationale for nursing's multiple research directions. *Image, 11*(3), 72–74.

Baker, H. M. (1997). Rules outside the rules for administration of medication: A study in new South Wales, Australia. *Image: Journal of Nursing Scholarship, 29*(2), 155–158.

Banks-Wallace, J. (1998). Emancipatory potential of storytelling in a group. *Image: Journal of Nursing Scholarship, 30*(1), 17–22.

Barker, K., & McConnell, W. (1962). The problems of detecting medication errors in hospitals. *American Journal of Hospital Pharmacy, 19*(8), 360–369.

Baumrind, D. (1980). New directions in socialization research. *American Psychologist, 35*(7), 639–652.

Benner, P. (1984). *From novice to expert: Excellence and power in clinical nursing practice.* Menlo Park, CA: Addison-Wesley.

Boyd, C. O. (2001). Phenomenology: The method. In P. L. Munhall (Ed.), *Nursing research: A qualitative perspective* (pp. 93–122). Sudbury, MA: Jones & Bartlett.

Burns, N. (1989). Standards for qualitative research. *Nursing Science Quarterly, 2*(1), 44–52.

Chenitz, W. C., & Swanson, J. M. (1986). Qualitative research using grounded theory. In W. C. Chenitz & J. M. Swanson (Eds.), *From practice to grounded theory: Qualitative research in nursing* (pp. 3–15). Menlo Park, CA: Addison-Wesley.

Christy, T. E. (1975). The methodology of historical research: A brief introduction. *Nursing Research, 24*(3), 189–192.

Christy, T. E. (1978). The hope of history. In M. L. Fitzpatrick (Ed.), *Historical studies in nursing* (pp. 3–11). New York: Teachers College Press.

Coffey, A., & Atkinson, P. (1996). *Making sense of qualitative data.* Thousand Oaks, CA: Sage.

Denzin, N. K. (1978). *Sociological methods: A sourcebook* (2nd ed.). New York: McGraw-Hill.

Denzin, N. K. (1989). *Interpretive interactionism.* Newbury Park, CA: Sage.

Dingwall, R. (1977). Atrocity stories and professional relationships. *Sociology of Work and Occupations, 4*(4), 371–396.

Drew, N. (1989). The interviewer's experience as data in phenomenological research. *Western Journal of Nursing Research, 11*(4), 431–439.

Dzurec, L. C. (1989). The necessity and evolution of multiple paradigms for nursing research. *Advances in Nursing Science, 11*(4), 69–77.

Eisner, E. W. (1981). On the differences between scientific and artistic approaches to qualitative research. *Educational Researcher, 10*(4), 5–9.

Evans, J. C. (1978). Formulating an idea. In M. L. Fitzpatrick (Ed.), *Historical studies in nursing* (pp. 15–17). New York: Teachers College Press.

Fagerhaugh, S., & Strauss, A. (1977). *Politics of pain management: Staff-patient interaction.* Menlo Park, CA: Addison-Wesley.

Frances, G. (1980). Nurses' medication errors: A new perspective. *Supervisor Nurse, 11,* 11–13.

Frank, A. W. (2000). The standpoint of storyteller. *Qualitative Health Research, 10*(3), 354–365.

Glaser, B. G. (1973). *Ward four hundred two.* New York: George Braziller.

Glaser, B. G., & Strauss, A. (1965). *Awareness of dying.* Chicago: Aldine.

Glaser, B. G., & Strauss, A. (1967). *The discovery of grounded theory: Strategies for qualitative research.* Chicago: Aldine.

Glaser, B. G., & Strauss, A. (1968). *Time for dying.* Chicago: Aldine.

Glaser, B. G., & Strauss, A. (1971). *Status passage.* London: Routledge & Kegan Paul.

Green, J., & Britten, N. (1998). Qualitative research and evidence based medicine. *British Medical Journal (International), 316*(7139), 1230–1232.

Guba, E. G., & Lincoln, Y. S. (1982). *Effective evaluation.* Washington, DC: Jossey-Bass.

Heller, A. (1982). *A theory of history.* London: Routledge & Kegan Paul.

Kaplan, A. (1964). *The conduct of inquiry: Methodology for behavioral science.* New York: Chandler.

Knafl, K. A., & Webster, D. C. (1988). Managing and analyzing qualitative data: A description of tasks, techniques, and materials. *Western Journal of Nursing Research, 10*(2), 195–218.

Kübler-Ross, E. (1969). *On death and dying.* New York: Macmillan.

Leininger, M. M. (1970). *Nursing and anthropology: Two worlds to blend.* New York: Wiley.

Leininger, M. M. (1985). *Qualitative research methods in nursing.* Orlando, FL: Grune & Stratton.

Leonard, V. M. (1989). A Heideggerian phenomenologic perspective on the concept of the person. *Advances in Nursing Science, 11*(4), 40–55.

Ludemann, R. (1979). The paradoxical nature of nursing research. *Image, 11*(1), 2–8.

Lusk, B. (1997). Historical methodology for nursing research. *Image: Journal of Nursing Scholarship, 29*(4), 355–359.

Marsh, G. W. (1990). Refining an emergent life-style-change theory through matrix analysis. *Advances in Nursing Science, 12*(3), 41–52.

Marshall, C. (1984). Elites, bureaucrats, ostriches, and pussycats: Managing research in policy settings. *Anthropology and Education Quarterly, 15*(3), 235–251.

Marshall, C. (1985). Appropriate criteria of trustworthiness and goodness for qualitative research on education organizations. *Quality and Quantity, 19*(4), 353–373.

Marshall, C., & Rossman, G. B. (1989). *Designing qualitative research.* Newbury Park, CA: Sage.

Mead, G. H. (1934). *Mind, self and society,* Chicago: University of Chicago Press.

Miles, M. B., & Huberman, A. M. (1994). *Qualitative data analysis: An expanded sourcebook* (2nd ed.). Beverly Hills, CA: Sage.

Morse, J. M. (1989). Qualitative nursing research: A free-for-all? In J. M. Morse (Ed.), *Qualitative nursing research: A contemporary dialogue* (pp. 14–22). Rockville, MD: Aspen.

Morse, J. M. (1999a). Myth #93: Reliability and validity are not relevant to qualitative inquiry. *Qualitative Health Research, 9*(6), 717–718.

Morse, J. M. (1999b). Qualitative methods: The state of the art. *Qualitative Health Research, 9*(3), 393–406.

Morse, J. M., & Field, P. A. (1995). *Qualitative research methods for health professionals* (2nd ed.). Thousand Oaks, CA: Sage.

Munhall, P. L. (1982a). Nursing philosophy and nursing research: In apposition or opposition? *Nursing Research, 31*(3), 176–181.

Munhall, P. L. (1982b). Ethical juxtapositions in nursing research. *Topics in Clinical Nursing, 4*(1), 66–73.

Munhall, P. L. (1988). Ethical considerations in qualitative research. *Western Journal of Nursing Research, 10*(2), 150–162.

Munhall, P. L. (1989). Philosophical ponderings on qualitative research methods in nursing. *Nursing Science Quarterly, 2*(1), 20–28.

Munhall, P. L. (ed.) (2001). *Nursing research: A qualitative perspective.* Sudbury, MA: Jones & Bartlett.

Murdock, G. (1971). *Outline of cultural materials.* New Haven, CT: Human Relations Area Files Press.

Newton, M. E. (1965). The case for historical research. *Nursing Research, 14*(1), 20–26.

Nwoga, I. (1997). *Mother-daughter conversations related to sex-role socialization and adolescent pregnancy.* Ph.D. dissertation, The University of Florida.

Oiler, C. (1982). The phenomenological approach in nursing research. *Nursing Research, 31*(3), 178–181.

Omery, A. (1983). Phenomenology: A method for nursing research. *Advances in Nursing Science, 5*(2), 49–63.

Parse, R. R. (1981). *Man-living-health: A theory of nursing.* New York: Wiley.

Paterson, J. G., & Zderad, L. T. (1976). *Humanistic nursing.* New York: Wiley.

Salsberry, P. J., Smith, M. C., & Boyd, C. O. (1989). Dialogue on a research issue: Phenomenological research in nursing—Commentary and responses. *Nursing Science Quarterly, 2*(1), 9–19.

Sandelowski, M. (1986). The problem of rigor in qualitative research. *Advances in Nursing Science, 8*(3), 27–37.

Sandelowski, M. (1995). Sample size in qualitative research. *Research in Nursing & Health, 18*(2), 179–183.

Sandelowski, M. (1996). One is the liveliest number: The case orientation of qualitative research. *Research in Nursing & Health, 19*(6), 525–529.

Sarnecky, M. T. (1990). Historiography: A legitimate research methodology for nursing. *Advances in Nursing Science, 12*(4), 1–10.

Scheffler, I. (1967). *Science and subjectivity.* Indianapolis: Bobbs-Merrill.

Schwartz-Barcott, D., & Kim, H. S. (1986). A hybrid model for concept development. In P. L. Chinn (Ed.), *Nursing research methodology: Issues and implementation* (pp. 91–101). Rockville, MD: Aspen.

Silva, M. C., & Rothbart, D. (1984). An analysis of changing trends in philosophies of science on nursing theory development and testing. *Advances in Nursing Science, 6*(2), 1–13.

Silverman, D. (1993). *Interpreting qualitative data: Methods for analyzing talk, text and interaction.* Thousand Oaks, CA: Sage.

Strauss, A. L. (1975). *Chronic illness and quality of life.* St. Louis: Mosby.

Strauss, A. L., Corbin, J., Fagerhaugh, S., Glaser, B. G., Maines, D., Suczek, B., et. al. (1984). *Chronic illness and the quality of life* (2nd ed.). St. Louis: Mosby.

Strauss, A., & Glaser, B. G. (1970). *Anguish.* Mill Valley, CA: Sociology Press.

Waring, L. M. (1978). Developing the research prospectus. In M. L. Fitzpatrick (Ed.), *Historical studies in nursing* (pp. 18–20). New York: Teachers College Press.

Watson, J. (1985). *Nursing: Human science and human care: A theory of nursing.* Norwalk, CT: Appleton-Century-Crofts.

Wimpenny, P., & Gass, J. (2000). Interviewing in phenomenology and grounded theory: Is there a difference? *Journal of Advanced Nursing, 31*(6), 1485–1492.

Wolcott, H. F. (1994). *Transforming qualitative data: Description, analysis, and interpretation.* Thousand Oaks, CA: Sage.

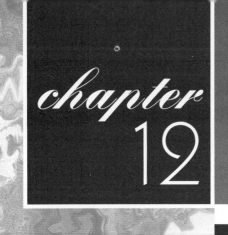

chapter 12

Critiquing Nursing Studies

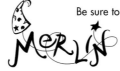

Be sure to check out the free exercises on-line at
www.wbsaunders.com/MERLIN/Burns/
understanding

OBJECTIVES

Completing this chapter should enable you to:
1. Define the term *intellectual research critique.*
2. Describe the basic guidelines that direct the conduct of a research critique.
3. Discuss the roles of different nurses in critiquing studies to identify evidence for use in practice.
4. Describe the four phases of quantitative research critique: comprehension, comparison, analysis, and evaluation.
5. Conduct a critique of a quantitative research report.
6. Explore the critique process for qualitative research.
7. Discuss the standards used in critiquing qualitative studies: descriptive vividness, methodological congruence, analytical preciseness, theoretical connectedness, and heuristic relevance.

RELEVANT TERMS

Analysis phase	Evaluation phase
Analytical preciseness	Heuristic relevance
Auditability	Intellectual research critique
Comparison phase	Methodological congruence
Comprehension phase	Rigor
Descriptive vividness	Theoretical connectedness
Critique	

Nursing is striving for evidence-based practice, which involves finding, critiquing, and applying scientific evidence in practice (Hamer & Collinson, 1999). Thus critiquing research is an essential step in moving toward a practice based on empirical evidence. However, the word *critique* is often linked with the word *criticize*, a term that is frequently viewed as negative. In the arts and sciences, critique takes on another meaning; it is associated with critical thinking and appraisal, which are tasks requiring carefully developed intellectual skills. This type of critique is sometimes referred to as an intellectual critique. An intellectual critique is directed at the element that is created, rather than at the creator. For example, one might conduct an intellectual critique of a work of art, an essay, or a study.

The idea of the intellectual critique was introduced early in this text and woven throughout the chapters. As each step of the research process was introduced, guide-

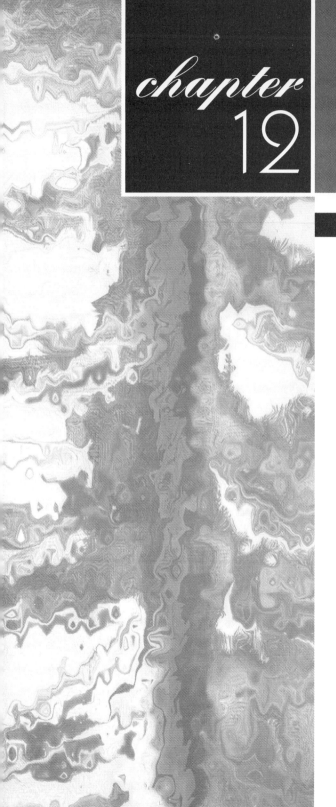

chapter 12

Critiquing Nursing Studies

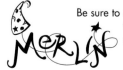

Be sure to check out the free exercises on-line at
www.wbsaunders.com/MERLIN/Burns/
understanding

OBJECTIVES

Completing this chapter should enable you to:
1. Define the term *intellectual research critique.*
2. Describe the basic guidelines that direct the conduct of a research critique.
3. Discuss the roles of different nurses in critiquing studies to identify evidence for use in practice.
4. Describe the four phases of quantitative research critique: comprehension, comparison, analysis, and evaluation.
5. Conduct a critique of a quantitative research report.
6. Explore the critique process for qualitative research.
7. Discuss the standards used in critiquing qualitative studies: descriptive vividness, methodological congruence, analytical preciseness, theoretical connectedness, and heuristic relevance.

RELEVANT TERMS

Analysis phase
Analytical preciseness
Auditability
Comparison phase
Comprehension phase
Descriptive vividness
Critique

Evaluation phase
Heuristic relevance
Intellectual research critique
Methodological congruence
Rigor
Theoretical connectedness

Nursing is striving for evidence-based practice, which involves finding, critiquing, and applying scientific evidence in practice (Hamer & Collinson, 1999). Thus critiquing research is an essential step in moving toward a practice based on empirical evidence. However, the word *critique* is often linked with the word *criticize*, a term that is frequently viewed as negative. In the arts and sciences, critique takes on another meaning; it is associated with critical thinking and appraisal, which are tasks requiring carefully developed intellectual skills. This type of critique is sometimes referred to as an intellectual critique. An intellectual critique is directed at the element that is created, rather than at the creator. For example, one might conduct an intellectual critique of a work of art, an essay, or a study.

The idea of the intellectual critique was introduced early in this text and woven throughout the chapters. As each step of the research process was introduced, guidelines were provided to direct the critique of that step in a research report. This chapter summarizes and builds on previous critique content and provides direction for conducting critiques of studies. The elements of intellectual critique of research used by nurses are described to assist you in determining the quality of empirical evidence generated by studies. In addition, the phases of critical thinking used to critique quantitative research (comprehension, comparison, analysis, and evaluation) are presented in detail. An example critique of a published quantitative study is provided. The chapter concludes with an introduction to the critique process for qualitative research.

EXAMINING THE ELEMENTS OF AN INTELLECTUAL RESEARCH CRITIQUE

An *intellectual research critique* is a careful, complete examination of a study, to judge its strengths, weaknesses, logical links, meaning, and significance. A quality study focuses on a significant problem, demonstrates sound methodology, produces credible findings, and is easily replicated by other researchers. Ultimately, the findings from several studies can be critiqued and synthesized to provide empirical evidence for use in practice (Brown, 1999).

In conducting an intellectual critique of a study, you need to address questions such as the following:

1. Was the research problem significant? Will it generate or refine knowledge for nursing practice?
2. What are the major strengths of the study?
3. What are the major weaknesses of the study?
4. Did the researchers use sound methodology?
5. Do the findings from the study accurately reflect reality? Are the findings credible?
6. What is the significance of the findings for nursing practice?
7. Are the findings consistent with those from previous studies?
8. Can the study be replicated by other researchers?

Answering these questions requires careful examination of the problem, purpose, literature review, framework, methods, results, and findings of the study.

The conduct of an intellectual critique involves applying some basic guidelines to assist you in answering the previous questions. The guidelines, presented in Table 12-1, stress the importance of critiquing the entire study and clearly, concisely, and objectively identifying the study's strengths and weaknesses. All studies have weaknesses or flaws; if all flawed studies were discarded, there would be no scientific evidence for use in practice. In fact science itself is flawed. Science does not completely or perfectly describe, explain, predict, and control reality. However, improved understanding and increased ability to predict and control phenomena depend on recognizing the flaws in studies and in science. Additional studies can then be planned to minimize the weaknesses of earlier studies.

TABLE 12-1

GUIDELINES FOR CONDUCTING A RESEARCH CRITIQUE

1. *Read and critique the entire study.* A research critique involves examining the quality of all steps of the research process.
2. *Examine the organization and presentation of the research report.* The report should be complete, concise, clearly presented, and logically organized. A study should not include excessive jargon that is difficult for students and practicing nurses to read. The references need to be complete and presented in a consistent format.
3. *Examine the significance of the problem studied for nursing practice.* The focus of nursing studies needs to be on significant practice problems if a sound knowledge base is to be developed for the profession.
4. *Identify the strengths and weaknesses of a study.* All studies have strengths and weaknesses, so attention must be given to all aspects of the study.
5. *Be objective and realistic in identifying the study's strengths and weaknesses.* Be balanced in your critique of a study. Try not to be overly critical in identifying a study's weaknesses or overly flattering in identifying the strengths.
6. *Provide specific examples of the strengths and weaknesses of a study.* Examples provide evidence for your critique of the strengths and weaknesses of a study.
7. *Provide a rationale for your critique.* Include justifications for your critique, and document your ideas with sources from the current literature. This strengthens the quality of your critique and documents the use of critical thinking skills.
8. *Suggest modifications for future studies.* Modifications in future studies will increase the strengths and decrease the weaknesses identified in the present study.
9. *Discuss the feasibility of replication of the study.* Is the study presented in enough detail to be replicated?
10. *Discuss the usefulness of the findings for practice.* The findings from the study need to be linked to the findings of previous studies. All these findings need to be examined for use in clinical practice.

All studies have both strengths and weaknesses. Recognizing these strengths is critical for generating scientific knowledge and using findings in practice. If only weaknesses are identified, nurses might discount the value of studies and refuse to invest time in examining research. The continued work of the researcher depends on the recognition of the study's strengths and weaknesses. If no study is good enough, why invest time conducting research? Adding together the strong points from multiple studies slowly builds a solid base of evidence for practice.

Two nursing research journals, *Scholarly Inquiry for Nursing Practice: An International Journal* and *Western Journal of Nursing Research,* include commentaries (partial critiques) after some of the published research reports. In these journals authors receive critiques of their work and have an opportunity to respond to the critiques. Published critiques usually increase the reader's understanding of the study and ability to critique other studies. Another more informal critique of a published study might appear in a letter to the editor. Readers have the opportunity to comment on the strengths and weaknesses of published studies by writing to the editors of journals.

ROLES OF NURSES IN CONDUCTING INTELLECTUAL RESEARCH CRITIQUES

Research is critiqued to broaden understanding, identify evidence for use in practice, and provide a background for conducting a study. All nurses, including students, practicing nurses, educators, administrators, and researchers, should critique studies. Basic knowledge of the research process and the critique process is often provided early in professional nursing education at the baccalaureate level. More advanced critique skills are taught at the master's and doctorate levels, with critique skills increasing as knowledge of the research process increases.

As a student, you are encouraged to critique published studies on relevant clinical topics, to increase your understanding of the research process, promote your interest in reading research articles, and improve your ability to determine how the accumulated research evidence can be used in practice. Critiques of studies by practicing nurses are essential for expanding understanding and making changes in practice. Nurses in practice should constantly update their nursing interventions in response to current research knowledge. In addition, accrediting agencies for health care facilities require that policy and procedure manuals used to direct nursing care be based on research.

Educators critique studies to update their knowledge of research findings. This knowledge provides a basis for developing and refining content taught in classroom and clinical settings. Instructors and textbooks often identify the nursing interventions that were tested through research. Many educators who conduct studies critique research as a basis for planning and implementing their studies. Researchers often focus on one area and update their knowledge base by critiquing new studies in this area. The outcome of the critique influences the selection of research problems, identification of frameworks, development of methodologies, and interpretation of findings in future studies.

UNDERSTANDING THE QUANTITATIVE RESEARCH CRITIQUE PROCESS

Critiquing research involves the use of a variety of critical thinking skills in the application of knowledge of the research process (Miller & Babcock, 1996). The research critique process includes four critical thinking phases: comprehension, comparison, analysis, and evaluation. These phases initially occur in sequence and presume accomplishment of the preceding steps. However, after you gain experience in the critique process, you will be able to perform several of these phases simultaneously. Conducting a critique is a complex mental process that is stimulated by raising questions. Thus relevant questions are provided for each phase of the critique process. The comprehension phase is covered separately because students who are new to critiquing should start with this phase. The comparison and analysis phases are covered together because they often occur simultaneously in the mind of the person conducting the critique. Evaluation is covered separately because of the increased expertise required to perform this phase. Each of the critical thinking phases involves examination of the steps of the quantitative research process and identification of the strengths and weaknesses of these steps.

Phase 1: Comprehension

The *comprehension phase* is the first step in the research critique process. This critique phase involves understanding the terms and concepts in the report and identifying the elements or steps of the research process, such as the problem, purpose, framework, and design. It is also necessary to grasp the nature, significance, and meaning of these steps in a research report.

Guidelines for comprehension of a research report

The first steps are reviewing the abstract, reading the entire study, and examining the references. Next, the following questions should be answered about the presentation of the study: Was the writing style clear and concise? Were the major sections of the research report, such as the literature review, framework, methods, results, and discussion, clearly identified? Were relevant terms clearly defined? (Burns & Grove, 2001). You are encouraged to underline terms you do not understand and look them up in the glossary at the back of this book. Next, it might help to read the article a second time and highlight or underline each step of the research process.

Comprehension Research Critique Guidelines

To write a beginning research critique that demonstrates comprehension of the study, concisely identify each step of the research process, and briefly respond to the following questions. Do not answer the questions with a *yes* or *no;* rather, provide a rationale or include examples or content from the study to address these questions.

1. What is the study problem?
2. What is the study purpose?
3. Is the literature review presented?
   a. Are relevant previous studies identified and described?
   b. Are relevant theories and models identified and described?
   c. Are the references current? Examine the number of sources in the last five years in the reference list.
   d. Are the studies critiqued by the author?
   e. Is a summary of the current knowledge provided? This summary needs to include what is known and not known about the research problem.

4. Is a study framework identified?
   a. Is the framework explicitly expressed or must it be extracted from the literature review?
   b. Is a particular theory or model identified as a framework for the study?
   c. Does the framework describe and define the concepts of interest?
   d. Does the framework present the relationships among the concepts and relate them to the variables of the study?
   e. Is a map or model of the framework provided for clarity?
   f. If a map or model is not presented, develop one that represents the study's framework and describe it.
   g. Is the framework related to nursing's body of knowledge?
5. Are research objectives, questions, or hypotheses used to direct the conduct of the study? Identify these.
6. Are the major variables or concepts identified and defined (conceptually and operationally)? Identify and define the appropriate variables included in the study:
   a. Independent variables
   b. Dependent variables
   c. Research variables or concepts
7. What attribute or demographic variables are examined in the study?
8. Is the research design clearly addressed?
   a. Identify the specific design of the study.
   b. Does the study include a treatment or intervention? If so, is the treatment clearly described and consistently implemented?
   c. Are the extraneous variables identified and controlled?
   d. Were pilot study findings used to design the major study? Briefly discuss the pilot study and the findings. Indicate the changes made in the major study based on the pilot.
9. Are the following elements of the sample described?
   a. Sample criteria
   b. Method used to obtain the sample
   c. Sample size (indicate if a power analysis was conducted to determine sample size)
   d. Characteristics of the sample
   e. Sample mortality
   f. Type of consent obtained
10. Are the measurement strategies described?
    a. Describe the methods of measurement, including the author of each instrument, how the instrument was developed, and how the instrument was used in the study.
    b. Identify the level of measurement achieved with each instrument.
    c. Describe the reliability of each instrument.
    d. Describe the validity of each instrument.
11. How were study procedures implemented and data collected during the study?
12. What statistical analyses are included in the research report?
    a. Identify the analysis techniques used to describe the sample.
    b. Identify the statistical procedures used to establish the reliability and validity of the measurement methods in the study.
    c. Was the level of significance or alpha identified? If so, indicate the level (0.05, 0.01, or 0.001).

Continued

    d. List the statistical procedures used and their outcomes for each research objective, question, or hypothesis. If objectives, questions, or hypotheses are not stated, link the analysis techniques to the study purpose.

13. What is the researcher's interpretation of the findings?

    a. Are the results related to the study framework? If so, do the findings support the study framework?

    b. Which findings are consistent with those expected?

    c. Which findings are unexpected?

    d. Are serendipitous findings described?

    e. Are the findings consistent with previous research findings?

14. What limitations of the study are identified by the researcher?

15. How does the researcher generalize the findings?

16. What implications do the findings have for nursing practice?

17. What suggestions are made for further studies?

18. What are the missing elements of the study?

19. Is the description of the study sufficiently clear to allow replication?

Phases 2 and 3: Comparison and Analysis

Critical thinking phases 2 and 3 (comparison and analysis) are frequently done simultaneously when critiquing a study. The *comparison phase* requires knowledge of what each step of the research process should be like, and then the ideal is compared to the real. During the comparison phase, you need to examine the extent to which the researcher followed the rules for an ideal study. Examine the steps of the study, such as the problem, purpose, framework, methodology, and results, based on the content presented in Chapters 2 through 10 of this book. Did the researcher rigorously develop and implement the study? What are the strengths of the study? What are the weaknesses of the study?

The *analysis phase* involves a critique of the logical links connecting one study element with another. For example, the presentation of the problem should provide background and direction for the statement of the purpose. In addition, the overall logical development of the study should be examined. The variables identified in the study purpose should be consistent with the variables identified in the research objectives, questions, or hypotheses. These variables should be conceptually defined in light of the study framework. The conceptual definitions provide the basis for the development of the operational definitions. The study design should be appropriate for the investigation of the purpose of the study and for the specific objectives, questions, or hypotheses. The instruments used in the study should adequately measure the variables. The sample selected should be representative of the population identified in the problem and purpose. Analysis techniques should provide results that address the purpose and the specific objectives, questions, or hypotheses. To determine the current knowledge of the study problem, the findings from a study should be linked to the framework and the findings from previous research. These findings are synthesized in the conclusions so that they can be generalized to individuals other than the study subjects. Depending on the quality of the findings, the researcher indicates the use of the findings in nursing practice. All steps of the research process provide a basis for the identification of future research projects. The steps of the research process need to be precisely developed and strongly linked to each other to conduct a quality study.

Guidelines for comparison and analysis of a research report

To conduct the comparison and analysis steps, review Chapters 2 through 10 of this text, as well as other references describing the steps of the research process (Burns & Grove, 2001; Mateo & Kirchhoff, 1999; Munro, 1997; Nieswiadomy, 1998; Polit, Beck, & Hungler, 2001). Then compare the steps in the study you are critiquing with the criteria established for each step in this textbook or other sources (Phase 2, comparison). Next analyze the logical links among the steps of the study (Phase 3, analysis). The guidelines in this section should assist you in implementing the phases of comparison and analysis for each step of the research process. Questions relevant to analysis are identified; all other questions direct the comparison of the steps of the study with the ideal. Use these questions to determine how rigorously the steps of the research process were implemented in published studies. Indicate which steps are strengths and which steps are weaknesses. When labeling a step as a strength or weakness, provide examples from the study and state a rationale, along with documentation to support your conclusions. In addition, identify the strengths in the logical way the steps of the study are linked together or any breaks or weaknesses in the links of a study's steps.

Comparison and Analysis Research Critique Guidelines

The written critique should be a narrative summary of the strengths and weaknesses that you note in the study. The guidelines below will assist you in examining the significance of the problem, fit of the framework, rigor of the methodology, and quality and relevance of the findings in published studies.

1. Research problem and purpose
   a. Is the problem sufficiently narrow in scope without being trivial?
   b. Is the problem significant and relevant to nursing?
   c. Does the purpose narrow and clarify the focus or aim of the study and identify the research variables, population, and setting?
   d. Was this study feasible to conduct in terms of money commitment; the researchers' expertise; availability of subjects, facility, and equipment; and ethical considerations?
2. Literature review
   a. Is the literature review organized to demonstrate the progressive development of ideas through previous research? *(Analysis)*
   b. Is a theoretical knowledge base developed for the problem and purpose? *(Analysis)*
   c. Does the literature review provide a rationale and direction for the study? *(Analysis)*

Continued

    d. Does the summary of the current empirical and theoretical knowledge provide a basis for the study?

3. Study framework
    a. Is the framework presented with clarity?
    b. Is the framework linked to the research purpose? *(Analysis)*
    c. Would another framework fit more logically with the study? *(Analysis)*
    d. Is the framework related to nursing's body of knowledge? *(Analysis)*
    e. If a proposition from a theory is to be tested, is the proposition clearly identified and linked to the study hypotheses? *(Analysis)*

4. Research objectives, questions, or hypotheses
    a. Are the objectives, questions, or hypotheses clearly and concisely expressed?
    b. Are the objectives, questions, or hypotheses logically linked to the research purpose? *(Analysis)*
    c. Are the research objectives, questions, or hypotheses linked to concepts and relationships (propositions) from the framework? *(Analysis)*

5. Variables
    a. Do the variables reflect the concepts identified in the framework? *(Analysis)*
    b. Are the variables clearly defined (conceptually and operationally) based on previous research and/or theories?
    c. Is the conceptual definition of a variable consistent with the operational definition? *(Analysis)*

6. Design
    a. Was the best design selected to direct this study?
    b. Does the design provide a means to examine all of the objectives, questions, or hypotheses? *(Analysis)*
    c. What are the threats to design validity? Were these threats identified by the researcher?
    d. Have the threats to design validity (statistical conclusion validity, internal validity, construct validity, and external validity) been minimized?
    e. Is the design logically linked to the sampling method and statistical analyses? *(Analysis)*
    f. If a treatment is implemented, is it clearly defined conceptually and operationally? Is the treatment appropriate for examining the study purpose and hypotheses? *(Analysis)*

7. Sample, population, and setting
    a. Is the target population to which the findings will be generalized defined?
    b. Is the sampling method adequate to produce a sample that is representative of the study population?
    c. What are the potential biases in the sampling method?
    d. Is the sample size sufficient to avoid a Type II error?
    e. If more than one group is used, do the groups appear equivalent?
    f. Are the rights of human subjects protected?
    g. Is the setting used in the study typical of clinical settings?

8. Measurements
    a. Do the instruments adequately measure the study variables? *(Analysis)*
    b. Are the instruments sufficiently sensitive to detect differences between subjects?
    c. Is the reliability of the instruments adequate for use in the study?
    d. Is the validity of the instruments adequate for use in the study?

e. Do the instruments need further research to evaluate validity and reliability?

f. Respond to the following questions that are relevant to the measurement approaches used in the study.

g. Scales and questionnaires

   (1) Are the instruments clearly described?

   (2) Are techniques to administer, complete, and score the instruments provided?

   (3) Is the reliability of the instruments described?

   (4) Is the validity of the instruments described?

   (5) Did the researcher examine the reliability and the validity of the instruments for the present sample?

   (6) If the instrument was developed for the study, is the instrument development process described?

h. Observation

   (1) Is what is to be observed clearly identified and defined?

   (2) Are interrater and intrarater reliability described?

   (3) Are the techniques for recording observations described?

i. Interviews

   (1) Do the interview questions address concerns expressed in the research problem? *(Analysis)*

   (2) Are the interview questions relevant for the research purpose and objectives, questions, or hypotheses? *(Analysis)*

   (3) Does the design of the questions tend to bias subjects' responses?

   (4) Does the sequence of questions tend to bias subjects' responses?

j. Physiological measures

   (1) Are the physiological measures or instruments clearly described? If appropriate, are the brand names (e.g., Space Labs or Hewlett-Packard) of the instruments identified?

   (2) Is the accuracy, selectivity, precision, sensitivity, and error of the physiological instruments discussed?

   (3) Are the methods for recording data from the physiological measures clearly described?

9. Data collection

a. Is the data collection process clearly described?

b. Is the training of data collectors clearly described and adequate?

c. Is the data collection process conducted in a consistent manner?

d. Are the data collection methods ethical?

e. Do the data collected address the research objectives, questions, or hypotheses? *(Analysis)*

10. Data analyses

a. Are data analysis procedures clearly described?

b. Do data analyses address each objective, question, or hypothesis?

c. Are data analysis procedures appropriate to the type of data collected?

d. Are the results presented in an understandable way?

e. Are tables and figures used to synthesize and emphasize certain findings?

f. Are the analyses interpreted appropriately?

g. If the results were nonsignificant, was the sample size sufficient to detect significant differences? Was a power analysis conducted to examine nonsignificant findings?

Continued

11. Interpretation of findings
    a. Are findings discussed in relation to each objective, question, or hypothesis? *(Analysis)*
    b. Are significant and nonsignificant findings explained?
    c. Were the statistically significant findings also examined for clinical significance?
    d. Does the interpretation of findings appear biased? Are the biases in the study identified?
    e. Are there uncontrolled extraneous variables that may have influenced the findings?
    f. Do the conclusions fit the results from the analyses? *(Analysis)*
    g. Are the conclusions based on statistically and clinically significant results? *(Analysis)*
    h. Did the researchers identify important study limitations?
    i. Are there inconsistencies in the report?

Phase 4: Evaluation

During the *evaluation phase* of a research critique, the meaning and significance of the study findings are examined. The evaluation becomes a summary of the study's quality that builds on conclusions reached during the first three phases (comprehension, comparison, and analysis) of the critique. This level of critique may or may not be conducted by a nursing student in a baccalaureate degree program. The level of critiquing attained during a student's educational program depends on when the research course is taken, during the junior or senior year of the curriculum, and how many credit hours are devoted to research. The guidelines for the evaluation phase are provided for those students who want to perform a more comprehensive critique of the literature to summarize findings for use in practice.

Guidelines for evaluation of a research report

The evaluation phase involves reexamining the findings, conclusions, limitations, implications for nursing, and suggestions for further study, which are usually presented in the discussion section of a research report. All nurses should be able to determine the value of research findings in the development of nursing knowledge and for use in practice.

 Evaluation Critique Guidelines

Using the following questions as a guide, summarize the quality of the study, the accuracy of the findings, and the usefulness of the findings for nursing practice. The evaluation phase involves developing a summary of the study's quality. This summary is a narrative that is usually the last paragraph of a critique.

1. How much confidence can be placed in the study findings? Are the findings an accurate reflection of reality?
2. Are the findings related to the framework?
3. Are the findings linked to those of previous studies?
4. What do the findings add to the current body of knowledge?

5. To what populations can the findings be generalized?
6. What research questions emerge from the findings? Are these questions identified by the researcher?
7. What is the overall quality of this study when the strengths and weaknesses are summarized? Could any of the weaknesses have been corrected?
8. Do the findings have potential for use in nursing practice?

EXAMPLE CRITIQUE OF A QUANTITATIVE STUDY

An example critique is presented in this section and includes the four phases of comprehension, comparison, analysis, and evaluation. The article critiqued, "Oxygen uptake and cardiovascular response in patients and normal adults during in-bed and out-of-bed toileting," by Winslow, Lane, and Gaffney (1984), precedes the example critique.

An initial critique might focus on comprehension and involve identification of the steps of the research process in the study. The comprehension critique might be written in outline format, with headings identifying the steps of the research process. A more in-depth critique includes not only the comprehension step but also the comparison, analysis, and evaluation phases. The example critique in this chapter includes all four phases; the comprehension, comparison, analysis, and evaluation steps are presented in narrative format. You might read the article and identify the steps of the research process, then try to list the strengths and weaknesses of the study, including the logical links among the study steps. You might want to use the questions in this chapter to develop a critique of this study that includes comprehension, comparison, and analysis. Then the example critique that follows the article can be compared with the critique that you have developed. Doing your own initial critique and then reading the example critique can help you expand your critique skills.

CRITIQUE ARTICLE

Oxygen Uptake and Cardiovascular Response in Patients and Normal Adults During In-Bed and Out-of-Bed Toileting

Elizabeth Hahn Winslow, PhD, RN, Lynda Denton Lane, BSN, RN, and F. Andrew Gaffney, MD

Patients dislike using the bedpan and urinal while in bed and often insist that it would be easier and better for them to get out of bed to toilet. Little data are available about the physiologic costs of toileting. Therefore, we measured oxygen uptake (VO_2), peak heart rate (HR_{peak}), peak rate-pressure product (RPP_{peak}), rating of per-

Continued

ceived exertion, and preference in 42 women who used the bedpan and bedside commode for urination and in 53 men who used the urinal while in bed and standing. The subjects included 26 healthy volunteers, 16 cardiac outpatients, 27 medical inpatients, and 26 acute post-myocardial infarction patients (two to 28 days postinfarction). No physiologically important differences were found between in-bed and out-of-bed toileting. Both in-bed and out-of-bed toileting produced small increases in energy cost and myocardial work over resting levels, with a mean $VO_2 < 1.6$ times resting VO_2, a mean $HR_{peak} < 100$ beats/min, and a mean $RPP_{peak} < 11,200$. The subjects clearly preferred getting out of bed to toilet. Out-of-bed toileting produces minimal energy expenditure and cardiac stress and can help reduce bed rest-induced orthostatic intolerance. In-bed toileting should be reserved for patients with specific contraindications to postural change.

Over 30 years ago Benton and co-workers[1] reported that using the bedpan required 50% greater energy cost above resting level than did using the bedside commode. Since then, many clinicians have recommended that the myocardial infarction (MI) patient use the bedside commode after hospital admission.[2-6] However, time-honored traditions change slowly, especially when only a single study of the topic is available. Many physicians still wait several days before permitting their acute MI patients to use the bedside commode or stand beside the bed to urinate. Patients often complain about this and insist that it would be easier and better for them to get out of bed to toilet.

To determine which toileting method is more appropriate for the acutely ill medical patient, one should consider both the total energy cost and also the approximate myocardial work of in-bed and out-of-bed toileting methods when performed by patients. Therefore, we measured oxygen uptake (VO_2), peak heart rate (HR_{peak}), peak rate-pressure product (RPP_{peak}) (systolic blood pressure x heart rate), rating of perceived exertion (RPE), and preference in 95 hospitalized and nonhospitalized adults during in-bed (bedpan and urinal) and out-of-bed (bedside commode and standing urinal) toileting. Data on which to base toilet method recommendations for the hospitalized patient are provided.

Materials and Methods

Subjects

The 42 women and 53 men (range 18-79 years) who volunteered for the study consisted of 26 healthy adults, 16 coronary artery disease patients who were participating in a supervised outpatient exercise program, 27 stable medical inpatients with a variety of cardiac and noncardiac disorders, and 26 stable acute MI inpatients who had their MI from 2 to 28 days earlier (8.81 ± 5 days [mean ± SD]) (Table I). Eight patients had their MI five days or less before the study began. Acute MI was established by history, clinical, electrocardiographic (ECG), and enzyme findings and by myocardial scintigraphy. Nineteen (73%) of the patients had transmural infarctions; seven (27%) had subendocardial infarctions. All medical and cardiac inpatients were ambulatory prior to hospitalization, and none had neural or musculoskeletal problems that would preclude standing unassisted. Six (37%) of the cardiac outpatients, seven (26%) of the medical inpatients, and five (19%) of the acute MI patients were receiving propranolol at the time of the study. The research protocol was approved by the Institutional Review Board, and informed written consent was obtained from all subjects prior to the study.

TABLE 1					

SUBJECT CHARACTERISTICS

SUBJECT GROUP	SEX	N	AGE (YRS ± SD)	WEIGHT (KG ± SD)	HEIGHT (CM ± SD)
Healthy volunteers	Female	11	38 ± 13	65 ± 8	168 ± 4
	Male	15	29 ± 7	77 ± 8	177 ± 4
Cardiac outpatients	Female	6	62 ± 4	58 ± 10	157 ± 6
	Male	10	58 ± 5	76 ± 8	173 ± 3
Medical inpatients	Female	14	57 ± 15	72 ± 16	161 ± 9
	Male	13	51 ± 10	84 ± 17	175 ± 7
Acute MI inpatients	Female	11	63 ± 11	76 ± 18	164 ± 6
	Male	15	61 ± 12	84 ± 17	172 ± 9

Methods

Oxygen uptake during rest and toileting was determined by open-circuit, indirect calorimetry. The subject had a nose clip and mouthpiece in place. During the timed period, expired air was collected via a one-way respiratory valve (Daniels) and 64-inch plastic tubing into a 30 L (rest) or 150 L (toileting) bag (Douglas). A standard adjustable helmet held the mouthpiece and valve in a comfortable, secure position; the Douglas bag was tied to a rolling intravenous pole. Expired air volume was measured by a Collins Chain Compensated Gasometer (Tissot), and air composition was analyzed by mass spectrometer (Perkin-Elmer Medical Gas Analyzer 1100). The mass spectrometer was calibrated electronically and checked against gases of known concentration. Standard equations were used to derive VO_2.

Gas collection was begun immediately before toileting when the subject was supine and was stopped when the subject had resumed the supine position. A continuous ECG (lead II) was recorded during toileting. Peak HR was the most rapid HR observed during any 15-second period. Blood pressure was measured by cuff sphygmomanometer immediately before and after toileting and after each position change. In the eight coronary care unit (CCU) patients, blood pressure was taken before and after toileting only. After each toileting method, the subject selected a number from the Borg scale of perceived exertion.[7] After both toileting methods, the subject completed a questionnaire wherein he ranked each method for comfort, pleasantness, and ease.

Protocol

Oxygen uptake, HR, and RPP were determined during a 3-minute supine rest period and during in-bed and out-of-bed toileting. A 10-minute rest period separated the randomly ordered toileting methods. Women used the bedpan and bedside commode for urinating; men used the urinal while lying in bed and while standing beside the bed. The subject simulated voiding if unable to void during the second toileting trial.

The toileting protocol simulated usual clinical conditions; therefore, toileting duration varied. The investigator assisted the women in lifting their hips for bedpan placement and removal, and placed the bedside commode in a standardized position beside the head of the bed. Subjects used their own techniques to get out of and back into bed and were not lifted by the investigator. The investigator left the room while the subject urinated and returned when given a signal from the subject. Subjects took as much time as they needed for urination.

Statistical Analysis

Oxygen uptake, HR, and RPP results were analyzed for each sex and group by repeated measures analysis of variance (ANOVA). Ratings of perceived exertion and preferences were analyzed by the Friedman two-way ANOVA by ranks. Spearman correlation coefficients were calculated for selected variables including VO_2, age, and toileting duration.

Results

Oxygen uptake, HR, and RPP results during rest and toileting are shown in Table II and Figures I, II, and III. During rest, VO_2 ranged from 2.15 to 4.52 ml/kg/min, HR from 44 to 104 beats/min, and RPP from 5,000 to 14,100. During toileting, VO_2 ranged from 2.77 to 5.84 ml/kg/min, HR_{peak} from 56 to 132 beats/min, and RPP_{peak} from 5,400 to 14,400.

During in-bed toileting, 14 subjects (15%) had an HR_{peak} of 100 beats/min or greater; during out-of-bed toileting, 19 subjects (21%) had an HR_{peak} of 100 beats/min or greater at some time during toileting. Only four subjects had an HR_{peak} over 108 beats/min. The subjects with the highest resting HRs had the highest HRs during toileting. The highest HRs observed during each study condition were 104, 120, and 132 beats/min during rest, bedpan use, and bedside commode use, respectively, in one elderly woman with atrial fibrillation and an uncontrolled ventricular response. None of the subjects experienced chest pain, shortness of breath, lightheadedness, palpitations, or other signs or symptoms of cardiovascular distress during toileting.

Statistically significant differences in VO_2, HR, and RPP between in-bed and out-of-bed toileting were found within some groups of subjects ($p < 0.05$). These differences represent mean differences of less than 1 ml/kg/min, 8 beats/min, and 1,300 units in VO_2, HR_{peak}, and RPP_{peak}, respectively.

TABLE 11

MEAN OXYGEN UPTAKE ($\dot{V}O_2$), HEART RATE (HR), AND RATE-PRESSURE PRODUCT (RPP) DURING REST AND MEAN $\dot{V}O_2$ PEAK HR, AND RPP$_{PEAK}$ DURING IN-BED AND OUT-OF-BED TOILETING

SUBJECT	ACTIVITY	WOMEN (W)			MEN (M)		
		$\dot{V}O_2$ (ml/kg/min ± SD)	HR (beats/min ± SD)	RPP (SBP × hr/100 ± SD)	$\dot{V}O_2$ (ml/kg/min ± SD)	HR (beats/min ± SD)	RPP (SBP × hr/100 ± SD)
Healthy volunteers (W = 11, M = 15)	Rest	3.43 ± 0.42	66 ± 10	79 ± 15	3.67 ± 0.41	60 ± 7	72 ± 12
	In-bed	4.84 ± 0.71	84 ± 10	92 ± 14	4.78 ± 0.46	87 ± 10	79 ± 12
	Out-of-bed	4.66 ± 0.63 (N = 11)	85 ± 9 (N = 10)	91 ± 15 (N = 11)	4.66 ± 0.52 (N = 15)	84 ± 8 (N = 12)	91 ± 14* (N = 15)
Cardiac outpatients (W = 6, M = 10)	Rest	3.20 ± 0.35	65 ± 12	89 ± 25	3.56 ± 0.36	59 ± 8	75 ± 17
	In-bed	4.43 ± 0.57	81 ± 16	104 ± 30	4.72 ± 0.59	77 ± 11	86 ± 20
	Out-of-bed	4.36 ± 0.61 (N = 5)	81 ± 17 (N = 6)	103 ± 24 (N = 6)	4.77 ± 0.47 (N = 9)	77 ± 12 (N = 10)	84 ± 15 (N = 10)
Medical inpatients (W = 14, M = 13)	Rest	3.14 ± 0.43	74 ± 14	97 ± 17	3.32 ± 0.37	73 ± 8	90 ± 13
	In-bed	3.91 ± 0.61	85 ± 15	111 ± 17	3.92 ± 0.53	89 ± 8	99 ± 18
	Out-of-bed	4.25 ± 0.79* (N = 11)	88 ± 16 (N = 14)	105 ± 19 (N = 14)	4.24 ± 0.42* (N = 12)	96 ± 9* (N = 13)	108 ± 21 (N = 13)
Acute MI inpatients† (W = 11, M = 15)	Rest	2.90 ± 0.65	77 ± 9	101 ± 26	3.22 ± 0.38	72 ± 7	89 ± 13
	In-bed	3.52 ± 0.59	89 ± 9	110 ± 22	3.78 ± 0.56	84 ± 12	94 ± 15
	Out-of-bed	3.84 ± 0.55 (N = 7)	94 ± 9 (N = 11)	109 ± 26 (N = 9)	4.21 ± 0.42* (N = 11)	91 ± 9* (N = 15)	102 ± 15 (N = 15)

*In-bed versus out-of-bed toileting ($p < .05$).

†Data from the eight coronary care unit patients (4W and 4M) are not included in $\dot{V}O_2$ results because a modified $\dot{V}O_2$ collection protocol was used (see text).

SD, Standard deviation; SBP, systolic blood pressure; N, number of subjects; MI, myocardial infarction.

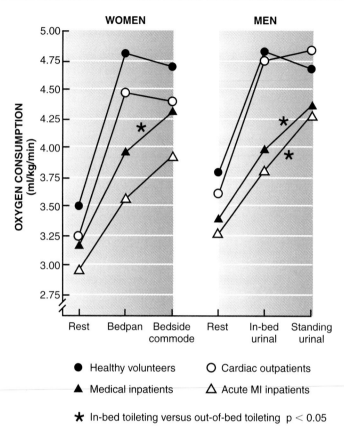

WOMEN   **MEN**

OXYGEN CONSUMPTION (ml/kg/min)

5.00
4.75
4.50
4.25
4.00
3.75
3.50
3.25
3.00
2.75

Rest   Bedpan   Bedside   Rest   In-bed   Standing
                 commode   urinal   urinal

● Healthy volunteers   ○ Cardiac outpatients

▲ Medical inpatients   △ Acute MI inpatients

★ In-bed toileting versus out-of-bed toileting $p < 0.05$

Figure I Mean oxygen uptake during rest, in-bed toileting, and out-of-bed toileting in four groups of subjects. *MI,* Myocardial infarction.

Analysis for differences among the four subject groups did not show any statistically significant differences in resting VO_2. However, during toileting, hospitalized patients generally had a significantly lower VO_2 value than did nonhospitalized subjects ($p < 0.05$). Heart rate and RPP responses during rest and toileting did not differ significantly among the four groups of female subjects; however, significant differences in cardiovascular response were found among some male groups. The hospitalized men generally had a significantly higher HR and RPP during rest and toileting than did nonhospitalized men ($p < 0.05$).

Mean duration for bedpan use (5.8 ± 1.5 min) did not differ significantly from that of bedside commode use (6.2 ± 1.4 min); however, duration for in-bed urinal use ($3.6 + 1.0$ min) was significantly shorter than that of out-of-bed urinal use (5.2 min $+ 0.9$ min) ($p < 0.05$). Analysis for group differences did not show a significant difference in duration among the four male groups; the healthy women, however, had a significantly shorter duration than did the other three groups of women ($p < 0.05$).

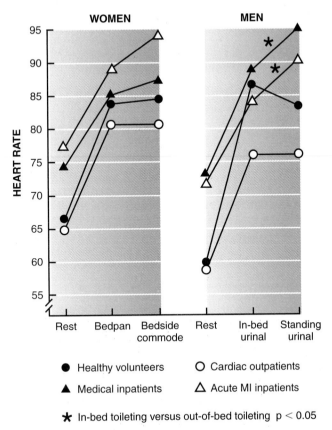

Mean heart rate during rest and mean peak heart rate during in-bed and out-of bed toileting in four groups of subjects. *MI,* Myocardial infarction.

The rating of perceived exertion (RPE) results showed that in-bed toileting was perceived to require significantly more exertion than out-of-bed toileting ($p < 0.05$). However, most subjects considered both in-bed and out-of-bed toileting light exertion. The mode RPE scores were 9 (very light) for bedpan, bedside commode, and out-of-bed urinal and 11 (fairly light) for in-bed urinal. The median RPE scores were 11 for bedpan, 10 for bedside commode, 11 for in-bed urinal, and 9 for out-of-bed urinal. Both men and women reported significantly higher comfort, pleasantness, and ease of ranking ($p < 0.0005$) for out-of-bed toileting compared with in-bed toileting.

Discussion

Both in-bed and out-of-bed toileting methods produced small increases in energy cost over resting levels. When the energy cost results are expressed as multiples of the subject's resting VO_2 (METs), the energy costs of using the bedpan and bedside commode were 1.3 and 1.4 METs, respectively; and the energy costs of using the uri-

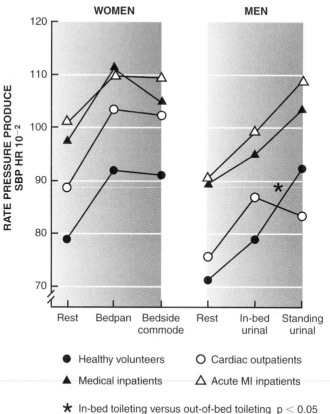

WOMEN   MEN

RATE PRESSURE PRODUCE SBP HR 10^{-2}

Rest   Bedpan   Bedside commode   Rest   In-bed urinal   Standing urinal

● Healthy volunteers   ○ Cardiac outpatients

▲ Medical inpatients   △ Acute MI inpatients

★ In-bed toileting versus out-of-bed toileting $p < 0.05$

Figure III   Mean rate-pressure product during rest and mean peak rate-pressure product during in-bed and out-of-bed toileting. *HR,* Heart rate; *MI,* myocardial infarction; *SBP,* systolic blood pressure.

nal while in bed and while standing were 1.2 and 1.3 METs, respectively. These results are comparable with those of Benton and co-workers,[1] who measured VO_2 in 15 cardiac subjects and 13 noncardiac subjects during simulated defecation in the bedpan and bedside commode and found that bedpan use required 1.6 METs and bedside commode use required 1.4 METs. The higher energy cost for bedpan use in the Benton study (1.6 METs) compared with that found in our study (1.3 METs) may be explained by differences in research protocol—the Benton subjects got on and off the bedpan unassisted, whereas our subjects received assistance.

The measured VO_2 values in Benton's study and ours are slightly lower than the actual VO_2 for toileting, because Benton measured VO_2 during toileting as well as during a recovery period following toileting, and we measured VO_2 during the entire toileting process, which included pauses for blood pressure measurement. When the blood pressure pauses were eliminated for the eight coronary care unit patients, the VO_2 values for in-bed and out-of-bed toileting were 4.3 and 4.6 ml/kg/min, respectively, for the women and 4.5 and 4.7 ml/kg/min, respectively, for the men. These results convert to 1.4 METs for bedpan use, 1.5 METs for bedside commode use, 1.3 METs for using the urinal while in bed, and 1.4 METs for using the urinal while standing. Therefore, toileting produces low energy costs, and the differences in energy cost between in-bed and out-of-bed toileting, though statistically significant in some groups of subjects, appear clinically and physiologically unimportant.

The findings of Benton and co-workers[1] have been misunderstood and misquoted in several publications. Gordon[8] erroneously stated that bedside commode use required 3.6 kcal/min (approximately 3 METs) and bedpan use required 4.6 kcal/min (approximately 4 METs). Zohman and Tobias,[9] Acker,[10] the editors of *Exercise Equivalents*,[11] and others quote Gordon's numbers and thus perpetuate Gordon's misinterpretation of the Benton data. In *Exercise Equivalents*,[11] the energy cost of using a bedside commode (3 METs) is shown to be equal to that of scrubbing a floor, and the energy cost of using a bedpan (4 METs) is shown to be equal to that of beating a carpet. Close examination of the Benton data, however, shows that use of the bedpan and bedside commode require only about 1.5 times resting energy cost and not the threefold to fourfold increase subsequently reported.

Our hospitalized patients generally had significantly lower VO_2 values during toileting than did the nonhospitalized subjects. Hospitalized patients also have been reported to have a significantly lower energy cost during bathing than did healthy volunteers.[12,13] Resting VO_2, adjusted for body weight, did not differ significantly among our four groups of subjects. Spearman rank correlation coefficients (r_s) were calculated to determine the relationship of toilet method VO_2 (ml/kg/min) to age and toileting duration. In nonhospitalized women, VO_2 during bedpan use correlated with toileting duration ($r_s = -0.60$, $p = 0.01$). In hospitalized men, age correlated with VO_2 during in-bed urinal use ($r_s = -0.60$, $p = 0.002$), and during standing urinal use ($r_s = -0.41$, $p = 0.05$). No other significant correlations were found. The meaning of the few significant correlations is unclear because of the lack of consistent trends. Conservation of effort may explain the hospitalized patients' lower energy expenditure, because in our study and in the bathing studies[12,13] the hospitalized patients appeared to move more slowly and deliberately than did the nonhospitalized subjects. However, none of the studies used matched groups; thus, other variables may also explain the VO_2 differences.

In addition to quantitating overall energy costs, we measured HR_{peak} and RPP_{peak} during toileting to estimate myocardial work.[14] The statistically significant differences in HR_{peak} and RPP_{peak} between in-bed and out-of-bed toileting in some groups of subjects represent increases of only 8% in HR and 15% in RPP. These differences are quite small and probably not of physiologic importance. The higher values in the hospitalized men can be explained by differences in conditioning, orthostatic tolerance, and the presence of arterial hypertension.

Benton and co-workers[1] recorded blood pressure, HR, and an ECG before, during, and after each toileting method but did not report the data because of their extreme variability. Singman and co-workers[15] recorded continuous ECGs during defecation in 51 CCU patients, including 23 with acute MI. Both bedpan (N = 15) and bedside commode (N = 48) were used. The ECGs were analyzed for ectopy and for changes in ST segments or of 10 beats/min or greater in HR. Only two patients had ECG changes other than an increased HR; the authors do not describe these changes. The finding that more patients increased HRs by 10 beats/min or more during bedside commode use than during bedpan use is an expected response to the upright posture. The virtual absence of ECG abnormalities supports our findings that the cardiovascular differences in bedpan and bedside commode use are physiologically insignificant.

Acute MI patients treated with strict bed rest for nine to 24 days have pronounced orthostatic intolerance during upright tilt or sitting posture; in contrast, orthostatic tolerance is not impaired in acute MI patients treated for seven to 18 days with modified bed rest—the patients performed active leg exercises, sat on the edge of the bed, and used the commode from the day of admission.[16] Signs of orthostatic intolerance develop after as little as six hours of bed rest[17] and progress as bed rest continues.[18] Orthostatic intolerance needs to be prevented in acute MI patients, because the postural changes in HR and blood pressure are potential causes of cerebral infarction and extension of MI.

Studies by Convertino and associates[19,20] show that orthostatic stress is the most important factor limiting exercise tolerance after bed rest and that exposure to gravitational stress for 3.5 hours daily may obviate much of the deterioration in cardiovascular performance resulting from bed rest. Getting the patient up for eating and toileting should provide the gravitational stress necessary to minimize bed rest-induced orthostatic intolerance.

The results of our study show that both in-bed and out-of-bed toileting methods produce minimal energy cost and cardiovascular stress for healthy volunteers, cardiac outpatients, stable medical inpatients, and stable inpatients who had an acute MI from 2 to 28 days earlier. Clinically or physiologically important differences were not found between staying in bed and getting out of bed to toilet. The subjects clearly preferred getting out of bed to toilet. Findings from other studies show that getting out of bed for short periods minimizes bed rest-induced orthostatic intolerance[16,20] and that the upright posture may even decrease myocardial oxygen demands.[21,22] In-bed toileting should be reserved for those patients with specific contraindications to postural changes. Thus, for medical patients without specific contraindications, we recommend out-of-bed toileting.

The authors thank Cathleen L. Michaels, MSN, PN, Ann McCash, BSN, RN, Jo Cole, MSN, RN, Robert Rude, MD, C. Gunnar Blomqvist, MD, and the nurses of the tenth floor, coronary care unit, and MILIS study at Parkland Memorial Hospital for assistance in the study; Kent Dana, MA, and Nancy Wilson, MS, at the University of Texas Health Science Center for statistical advice; and Carolyn Donahue for preparing the manuscript.

REFERENCES

1. Benton JG, Brown H, Rusk HA: Energy expanded by patients on the bedpan and bedside commode. *JAMA* 1950;144:1443-1447.
2. Gazes PC, Gaddy JE: Bedside management of acute myocardial infarction. *Am Heart J* 1979;97:782-796.
3. Levine SA, Lown B: Armchair treatment of acute coronary thrombosis. *JAMA* 1952;148:1365-1369.
4. Newman LB, Wasserman, RR, Borden G: Productive living for those with heart disease: The role of physical medicine and rehabilitation. *Arch Phys Med Rehabil* 1956;37:137-149.
5. Niccoli A, Brammell HL: A program for rehabilitation in coronary heart disease. *Nursing Clin North Am* 1976;11:237-250.
6. Wenger NK: Rehabilitation of the patient with myocardial infarction: Responsibility of the primary care physician. *Primary Care* 1981;8:491-507.
7. Borg G: Perceived exertion: A note on history and methods. *Med Sci Sports* 1973;5:90-93.
8. Gordon EE: Energy costs of activities in health and disease. *Arch Intern Med* 1958;101: 702-713.
9. Zohman LR, Tobis JS: *Cardiac Rehabilitation.* New York, Grune and Stratton, 1970.
10. Acker J: Early ambulation of post-myocardial infarction patients: Early activity after myocardial infarction, in Naughton JP, Hellerstein HK (eds): *Exercise testing and exercise training in coronary heart disease.* New York, Academic Press, 1973.
11. *Exercise Equivalents.* Denver Colorado Heart Association.
12. Gordon EE: Energy costs of various physical activities in relation to pulmonary tuberculosis. *Arch Phys Med* 1952;33:201-209.
13. Winslow EH, Gaffrey L: Oxygen consumption and cardiovascular responses in normal adults and acute myocardial infarction patients during basin bath, tub bath, and shower. *Nurs Res* (submitted for publication).
14. Kilamura K, Jorgensen CR, Gobel FL, Taylor HL, Wang Y: Hemodynamic correlates of myocardial oxygen consumption during upright exercise. *J Appl Physiol* 1972;32:516-522.
15. Singman H, Kinsella E, Goldberg E: Electrocardiographic changes in coronary care unit patients during defecation. *Vasc Surg* 1975;9:54-57.
16. Fareeduddin K, Abelmann WH: Impaired orthostatic tolerance after bed rest in patients with myocardial infarction. *N Engl J Med* 1969;280:345-350.
17. McCally M, Piemme TE, Murray RH: Tilt table responses of human subjects following application of lower body negative pressure. *Aerospace Med* 1966;37:1247-1249.
18. Chobanian AV, Lille RD, Tercyak A, Blevins P: The metabolic and hemodynamic effects of prolonged bed rest in normal subjects. *Circulation* 1974;49:551-559.
19. Convertino VA, Hung J, Goldwater D, DeBusk RF: Cardiovascular responses to exercise in middle-aged men after 10 days of bed rest. *Circulation* 1982;65:134-140.
20. Convertino VA, Sandler H, Webb P, Annis JF: Induced venous pooling and cardiorespiratory responses to exercise after bed rest. *J Appl Physiol* 1982;52:1342-1348.
21. Lecerof H: Influence of body position on exercise tolerance, heart rate, blood pressure, and respiration rate in coronary insufficiency. *Br Heart J* 1971;33:78-83.
22. Langou RA, Wolfson S, Olson EG, Cohen LS: Effects of orthostatic postural changes on myocardial oxygen demands. *Am J Cardiol* 1977;39:418-421.

Comprehension Phase

Example Critique

1. *Problem:* "Patients dislike using the bedpan and urinal while in bed and often insist that it would be easier and better for them to get out of bed to toilet. Little data are available about the physiologic costs of toileting" (Winslow et al., 1984, p. 409).*

---
*Page number refers to the version of the article reprinted in this text.

Continued

2. *Purpose:* The researchers "measured oxygen uptake (VO_2), peak heart rate (HR_{peak}), peak rate-pressure product (RPP_{peak}) (systolic blood pressure × heart rate), rating of perceived exertion (RPE), and preference in 95 hospitalized and nonhospitalized adults during in-bed (bedpan and urinal) and out-of-bed (bedside commode and standing urinal) toileting" (p. 410).

3. *Literature review:* A minimal review of literature is presented at the beginning of the article. However, many studies are cited in the discussion section, where the findings from this study are compared and contrasted with the findings from previous studies (see the research article, p. 410). Often in clinical specialty journals, such as the *Journal of Cardiac Rehabilitation* and *Heart & Lung*, studies are cited in the discussion section so that findings can be synthesized to indicate the current knowledge in a problem area. Therefore, when critiquing the review of literature for a study, examine both the beginning of the article and the discussion section.

   The researchers cited several studies, but few focused on the effects of in-bed and out-of-bed toileting (Benton, Brown, & Rusk, 1950; Singman, Kinsella, & Goldberg, 1975). Because limited research has been done in this area, additional study is needed. The references range from 1950 to 1982; most were published in the 1970s. These sources are considered current because the study being critiqued was published in 1984. The findings from studies are synthesized to indicate briefly what is known and not known about the study problem.

4. *Framework:* The framework is not identified by the researchers and must be extracted from the literature review. The key concepts of toileting, acutely ill adults, healthy adults, rehabilitating adults, and energy cost were identified but not defined in the article. The researchers indicate that Levine's Conservation Model, specifically the energy conservation principle and the overload and progression principle of exercise physiology, provided the framework for this study (Winslow, January 1994, personal communication). Based on the review of literature and personal communication with the primary researcher, we developed the following map to identify the relationships among the concepts relevant to this study.

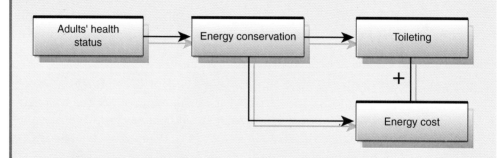

This map indicates that adults' health status (acutely ill, rehabilitating, or healthy) affects their use of energy conservation; their energy conservation affects their toileting and energy costs during toileting. Energy conservation involves the appropriate use of energy to prevent energy depletion and promote wholeness and integrity of the individual (Schaefer & Pond, 1991). Thus acutely ill adults with depleted energy conserve their energy more than do healthy adults. Toileting increases energy costs, but ill individuals conserve their energy more than do healthy individuals during toileting. The more they conserve their energy, the smaller their energy costs during activities such as toileting. When individuals are ill, they need to use the most appropriate toileting method to prevent excessive energy costs.

The adults in this study were male and female healthy volunteers, cardiac outpatients, medical inpatients, and acute myocardial infarction (MI) inpatients. The toileting methods examined were the in-bed methods of bedpan and urinal and the out-of-bed methods of bedside commode and standing urinal. The energy costs for different types of individuals during toileting were examined by measuring the variables of VO_2, HR_{peak}, RPP_{peak}, RPE, and *toileting preference*.

5. The researchers did not include objectives, questions, or hypotheses. The study purpose was used to direct the conduct of this study.

6. *Variables:* The researchers identified and operationally defined the variables but did not provide conceptual definitions. The operational definition and a possible conceptual definition follow for each variable.

Independent Variables

TOILETING METHODS

Conceptual definition. In-bed and out-of-bed toileting methods are actions performed by both ill and healthy adults that are influenced by the individual's level of energy conservation and require greater energy cost than a resting level.

Operational definition. In-bed toileting is the use of the bedpan by women and the urinal by men to urinate while lying in bed. Out-of-bed toileting is the use of the bedside commode by women and the standing urinal by men to urinate.

SUBJECTS' HEALTH STATUS

Conceptual definition. Adults with varying levels of health (acutely ill, rehabilitating, or healthy) conserve their energy appropriately during toileting to prevent energy depletion (Schaefer & Pond, 1991).

Operational definition. Subjects with four different health statuses were studied: healthy volunteers, cardiac outpatients, medical inpatients, and acute MI inpatients.

Dependent Variables

OXYGEN UPTAKE (VO_2)

Conceptual definition. The amount of oxygen used by the body during an activity that indicates energy cost or expenditure.

Operational definition. Oxygen uptake was "determined by open-circuit, indirect calorimetry.... Expired air volume was measured by a Collins chain compensated gasometer (Tissot), and air composition was analyzed by mass spectrometer (Perkin-Elmer Medical Gas Analyzer 1100).... Standard equations were used to derive VO_2" (Winslow et al., 1984, p. 411).

PEAK HEART RATE (HR_{PEAK})

Operational definition. The highest HR an adult reaches during an activity that indicates energy cost or expenditure.

Operational definition. "Peak HR was the most rapid HR observed during any 15-second period" (Winslow et al., 1984, p. 411).

PEAK RATE-PRESSURE PRODUCT (RPP_{PEAK})

Operational definition. The myocardial energy cost for an adult during an activity that indicates energy cost or expenditure.

Operational definition. A product of systolic blood pressure times HR. The highest RPP observed during toileting was defined as the RPP_{peak}.

PERCEIVED EXERTION

Operational definition. An individual's perception of the energy cost during an activity.

Operational definition. The subjects selected "a number from the Borg Scale of Perceived Exertion" to indicate their perceived level of exertion during toileting" (Winslow et al., 1984, p. 411).

PREFERRED TOILETING METHOD

Conceptual definition. The toileting method an individual liked best.

Operational definition. "After both toileting methods, the subject completed a questionnaire wherein he ranked each method for comfort, pleasantness, and ease" (Winslow et al., 1984, p. 465).

7. *Attribute variables:* The attribute variables were gender, age, weight, height, medical diagnosis, date and type of MI, and current medications.

8. *Research design:* The research design is not identified but appears to be a quasi-experimental repeated-measures design, in which each subject was exposed to both treatments (in-bed and out-of-bed toileting). The subjects were randomly assigned to an initial toileting method. The gas collections for VO_2 and HR were measured immediately before, during, and after each toileting method. Blood pressure for RPP was measured before and after each method of toileting (pretest and posttest). The Borg Scale of Perceived Exertion and the questionnaire for toileting preference were completed after each toileting method (posttest only).

   a. *Study procedures:* The following protocol was used to direct the study. "*Protocol:* Oxygen uptake, HR, and RPP were determined during a 3-minute supine rest period and during in-bed and out-of-bed toileting. A 10-minute rest period separated the randomly ordered toileting methods. Women used the bedpan and bedside commode for urinating; men used the urinal while lying in bed and while standing beside the bed. The subjects simulated voiding if unable to void during the second toileting trial" (Winslow et al., 1984, p. 412).

"The toileting protocol simulated usual clinical conditions; therefore, toileting duration varied. The investigator assisted the women in lifting their hips for bedpan placement and removal, and placed the bedside commode in a standardized position beside the head of the bed. Subjects used their own techniques to get out of and back into bed and were not lifted by the investigator. The investigator left the room while the subject urinated and returned when given a signal from the subject. Subjects took as much time as they needed for urination" (Winslow et al., 1984, p. 412).

b. *Extraneous variables* are not specifically identified, but the researchers structured the sample criteria, treatment protocols, and data collection process to eliminate extraneous variables. For example, the medical diagnoses of patients were clearly documented, and all patients were ambulatory and had no neural or musculoskeletal problems that might interfere with the toileting treatments. The treatments were randomly implemented, and the protocols for the treatments and measurements were highly structured and consistently implemented.

c. No *pilot study* was identified.

9. *Description of the sample*

a. *Sample criteria:* The subjects were adult male and female volunteers who were either healthy individuals, coronary artery disease patients who were participating in a supervised outpatient exercise program, stable medical inpatients with a variety of cardiac and noncardiac disorders, or stable acute MI inpatients whose MI had occurred at least 2 days earlier. "Acute MI was established by history, clinical, electrocardiographic (ECG), and enzyme findings and by myocardial scintigraphy.... All medical and cardiac inpatients were ambulatory prior to hospitalization, and none had neural or musculoskeletal problems that would preclude standing unassisted" (Winslow et al., 1984, pp. 410–411).

b. *Sample size:* There were 95 hospitalized and nonhospitalized adult subjects. The authors did not indicate that power analysis was used to determine sample size.

c. *Characteristics of the sample:* "The 42 women and 53 men (range 18-79 years) who volunteered for the study consisted of 26 healthy adults, 16 coronary artery disease patients.... 27 stable medical inpatients with a variety of cardiac and noncardiac disorders, and 26 stable acute MI inpatients who had their MI from 2 to 28 days earlier (8.81 ± 5 days [mean ± SD]) Eight patients had their MI five days or less before the study began.... Nineteen (73%) of the patients had transmural infarctions; seven (27%) had subendocardial infarctions.... Six (37%) of the cardiac outpatients, seven (26%) of the medical inpatients, and five (19%) of the acute MI patients were receiving propranolol at the time of the study" (Winslow et al., 1984, pp. 410–411). Some of the sample characteristics are also presented in a table (see Table I, p. 411).

   d. *Sample mortality:* No sample mortality was mentioned; data analyses included all 95 subjects.

   e. *Sampling method:* Nonprobability sample of convenience.

   f. *Type of consent:* "The research protocol was approved by the Institutional Review Board, and informed written consent was obtained from all subjects prior to the study" (Winslow et al., 1984, p. 411).

10. *Measurement strategies:* The researchers measured five variables—three (VO_2, HR_{peak}, and RPP_{peak}) with physiologic instruments, one (perceived exertion) with a self-report scale, and one (toileting preference) with a questionnaire.

   a. VO_2 was "determined by open-circuit, indirect calorimetry. The subject had a nose clip and mouth piece in place. During the timed period, expired air was collected via a one-way respiratory valve (Daniels) and 64-inch plastic tubing into a 30 L (rest) or 150 L (toileting) bag (Douglas).... Expired air volume was measured by a Collins Chain Compensated Gasometer (Tissot), and air composition was analyzed by mass spectrometer (Perkin-Elmer Medical Gas Analyzer 1100).... Standard equations were used to derive VO_2" (Winslow et al., 1984, p. 411).

   The measurement strategy produced ratio-level data. To demonstrate the precision and accuracy of the equipment, the "mass spectrometer was calibrated electronically and checked against gases of known concentration" (Winslow et al., 1984, p. 411).

   b. HR_{peak} was identified using a continuous ECG (lead II) that was recorded during toileting. "Peak HR was the most rapid HR observed during any 15-second period" (Winslow et al., 1984, p. 411). This measurement strategy produced ratio-level data. The brand name of the ECG equipment and the precision, sensitivity, accuracy, and error of the equipment were not addressed.

   c. RPP_{peak} was determined by multiplying systolic blood pressure times heart rate and selecting the highest RPP. "Blood pressure was measured by cuff sphygmomanometer immediately before and after toileting and after each position change" (Winslow et al., 1984, p. 411). This measurement strategy produced ratio-level data. The precision, sensitivity, selectivity, accuracy, and error of the blood pressure cuff and sphygmomanometer were not addressed. The manufacturer of this equipment was not identified.

   d. *Perceived exertion* was measured using the Borg Scale of Perceived Exertion. The level of data is unclear but was probably ordinal because nonparametric tests for ordinal data (Friedman two-way analysis of variance [ANOVA] by ranks and Spearman correlation coefficients) were used for analysis. The validity and reliability of the Borg Scale are not discussed, but a reference article is cited.

   e. *Preferred toileting method* was measured with a questionnaire that examined the comfort, pleasantness, and ease of each method. The data were probably ordinal because nonparametric tests were used to analyze the data. The development of this questionnaire was not discussed.

11. *Data collection procedures:* The data collection process was detailed in the methods and protocol sections of the article (pp. 411–412). Most of this content was presented in the measurement and design sections of this critique.

12. *Statistical analyses:* The analyses were descriptive and inferential. VO_2, HR, and RPP data were analyzed with descriptive statistics, including mean, range, and standard deviation. These results are presented in a table (see Table II, p. 413). Graphs are also presented, allowing the reader to visualize the differences among the four groups (healthy volunteers, medical inpatients, cardiac outpatients, and acute MI inpatients) in VO_2 (see Fig. I), HR (see Fig. II), and RPP (see Fig. III) during rest, in-bed toileting, and out-of-bed toileting.

The inferential statistical analyses were conducted primarily to examine differences between in-bed and out-of-bed toileting methods for four groups of subjects. "Oxygen uptake, HR, and RPP results were analyzed for each sex and group by repeated measures analysis of variance. Ratings of perceived exertion and preferences were analyzed by the Friedman two-way ANOVA by ranks. Spearman correlation coefficients were calculated for selected variables including VO_2, age, and toileting duration" (Winslow et al., 1984, p. 412). The repeated measures ANOVA results indicated that "no physiologically important differences were found between in-bed and out-of-bed toileting. Both in-bed and out-of-bed toileting produced small increases in energy cost and myocardial work over resting levels, with a mean $VO_2 < 1.6$ times resting VO_2, a mean HR_{peak} 100 beats/min, and a mean $RPP_{peak} < 11,200$" (Winslow et al., 1984, p. 410).

13. *Interpretation of findings:* The findings from the study "show that both in-bed and out-of-bed toileting methods produce minimal energy cost and cardiovascular stress for healthy volunteers, cardiac outpatients, stable medical inpatients, and stable inpatients who had an acute MI from two to 28 days earlier. Clinically or physiologically important differences were not found between staying in bed and getting out of bed to toilet. The subjects clearly preferred getting out of bed to toilet" (Winslow et al., 1984, p. 418). These findings were expected and were consistent with the findings from Benton et al. (1950) and Singman et al. (1975).

An unexpected finding was that hospitalized patients had significantly lower VO_2 values than nonhospitalized patients. The researchers hypothesized that hospitalized patients with depleted energy reduce their energy expenditure during toileting. No serendipitous findings were identified. Because the study has no clearly designated framework, the findings were not linked to a framework.

14. *Limitations of the study:* Limitations are not identified.

15. *Generalization of findings:* "In-bed toileting should be reserved for patients with specific contraindications to postural change.... For medical patients without specific contraindications, we recommend out-of-bed toileting" (Winslow et al., 1984, p. 418).

16. *Implications for nursing:* Nurses are encouraged to get stable medical inpatients and stable inpatients who have had an acute MI out of bed to toilet. This toileting method has minimal energy cost, is preferred by patients, and minimizes bed rest-induced orthostatic intolerance.

17. *Suggestions for further research:* The researchers provide no specific directions for further research.

18. *Missing elements of the study:* The study lacks a clearly expressed framework; reliability and validity information for one of the scales; precision, accuracy, and sensitivity information for some of the physiologic instruments; limitations; and recommendations for further research.

19. *Replication:* The study is sufficiently clear to replicate. Anyone planning replication should contact the researchers for clarification of parts of the data collection process and the research protocol and for more information regarding some of the measurement methods.

Comparison and Analysis Phases

This section discusses the strengths and weaknesses of the steps of the research process and the logical links among these steps. The title, abstract, problem, purpose, literature review, framework, methodology, results, and discussion elements of the article are critiqued.

Title and abstract. The title, although a little long, clearly indicates the focus of the study. The abstract includes the study problem, purpose, sample size, sample characteristics, significant results, relevant findings, and implications of the findings for nursing practice. This relevant information is presented in a way that captures the attention of the reader.

Problem and purpose. The problem is clearly identified in the abstract and in the first paragraph of the article. Determining the energy costs of different methods of toileting will provide direction in caring for hospitalized patients. Because toileting is the responsibility of nurses, this is a significant problem and requires investigation.

The purpose is expressed clearly in the abstract and in the second paragraph of the article. The purpose identifies the independent and dependent variables, the population, and the setting. The study was feasible to conduct because of (1) the clinical and research expertise of the investigators; (2) the financial support received for the study (see p. 411); (3) the availability of subjects, facilities, and equipment discussed in the methods section; (4) the cooperation of others (acknowledged at the end of the article); and (5) the ethical considerations given the subjects (informed consent) (Burns & Grove, 2001).

Literature review. The literature review is brief because of the limited number of studies conducted in this area. Additional related research and theoretical sources might have been cited to indicate the current knowledge of the problem. However, journals often limit the length of an article, and researchers must cut information from the literature review and other sections of their research reports to meet publication requirements. A final summary of what is known and not known about the problem studied would have added clarity to the literature review.

Framework. The study lacks a clearly identified framework. The concepts relevant to the study are identified but not defined, and the relationships among the concepts should have been clarified and documented. The variables are clearly defined operationally but are neither conceptually defined nor linked to the concepts identified. The study findings, if linked to Levine's conservation model, could have added support to this model and to the understanding of energy conservation in healthy and ill adults (Schaefer & Pond, 1991).

Methods. The methods section is a major strength of the study. The sample size was large (95 subjects) and included a variety of subjects (healthy volunteers, cardiac outpatients, medical inpatients, and acute MI inpatients). The heterogeneity of the subjects increases the generalizability of the findings (Burns & Grove, 2001). A limitation is that the study groups were of unequal size. The cardiac outpatient group had only 16 subjects, but the other three groups were fairly equal, with 26 to 27 subjects per group. The sampling method, sampling criteria, and sample characteristics are clearly presented. The study was ethical, since it was approved for conduct by an Institutional Review Board and informed written consent was obtained from the subjects.

The measurement methods seem appropriate for measuring energy cost, myocardial workload, perceived exertion, and preferred toileting method. The measurement of VO_2 is presented in detail, and the precision and accuracy of the equipment are described. The equipment (ECG, blood pressure cuff, and sphygmomanometer) for measuring HR and RPP are described, but the accuracy and precision of the equipment are not addressed (DeKeyser & Pugh, 1990). Discussion of the Borg Scale of Perceived Exertion and the questionnaire used to measure toileting preference is limited; discussing the reliability and validity of these instruments would have strengthened the study.

The design is not identified, and the threats to design validity are not discussed. However, the study protocol clearly describes the implementation of the independent variables and the measurement of the dependent variables. The toileting protocol simulated usual clinical conditions, which increases the ability to generalize the findings to patients in clinical practice. The researchers did not indicate who collected the data. If more than one person collected data, the reliability or consistency of the data collection process must be addressed (Burns & Grove, 2001).

Results. The statistical techniques used to analyze data from the measurement of the five dependent variables are clearly identified. The analysis techniques (descriptive and inferential) were appropriate for the level of measurement of the variables (Burns & Grove, 2001; Munro, 1997). The purpose of the study is clearly addressed in the results section. The results are presented in narrative form, tables, and graphs to facilitate understanding.

Discussion. The expected and unexpected findings are explained, and the statistical and clinical significance of the findings are addressed (Burns & Grove, 2001). The findings are consistent with previous research, and this is documented. The generalization of the findings and their implications for nursing are clearly presented. The researchers could have strengthened the report by identifying the study limitations and providing suggestions for further research.

Evaluation Phase

This study examines a significant nursing problem and provides important findings that can be used in nursing practice. The findings are consistent with those of previous research (Benton et al., 1950; Singman et al., 1975) and seem to describe accurately the energy costs of toileting for hospitalized and nonhospitalized patients. Out-of-bed toileting is recommended for medical patients without specific contraindications. These findings can be generalized to stable medical inpatients and stable inpatients who had an acute MI.

The following questions might generate further research: What additional dependent variables might be measured to determine the energy costs during toileting? How might these dependent variables be measured? What are the best toileting methods for other types of acutely and chronically ill patients? What are the energy costs for toileting in the bathroom? What are the energy costs for in-bed and out-of-bed toileting during defecation versus urination? Further research in these areas would strengthen the evidence-base related to toileting and enable nurses to provide evidence-based practice when assisting patients with toileting.

The strengths of this study greatly outweigh the weaknesses. The weaknesses regarding the framework, design, measurement methods, and suggestions for further research could easily be corrected in future studies. The findings support previous research and provide strong evidence to direct practice (Hamer & Collinson, 1999).

INTRODUCTION TO THE CRITIQUE PROCESS FOR QUALITATIVE RESEARCH

Qualitative studies are appearing more frequently in nursing journals and are providing relevant information for nursing practice. Therefore you need experience in critiquing both qualitative and quantitative studies. However, critiquing a qualitative study involves a different approach and guidelines to identify study strengths and weaknesses. You need to know the potential weaknesses of qualitative research and to be able to identify them in published studies.

A scholarly critique of qualitative studies includes a balanced evaluation of a study's strengths and weaknesses. Five standards have been proposed to evaluate qualitative studies: (1) descriptive vividness, (2) methodological congruence, (3) analytical preciseness, (4) theoretical connectedness, and (5) heuristic relevance (Burns, 1989; Burns & Grove, 2001). In the following sections, these standards and the threats to them are described.

Standard 1: Descriptive Vividness

To achieve *descriptive vividness*, the site, subjects (informants), experience of collecting data, and thinking of the researcher during the data collection process must be described so clearly that the reader has the sense of personally experiencing the event. For example, Glaser and Strauss (1965) believe that the social world studied should be described "so vividly that the reader can almost literally see and hear its people." (p. 9)

Threats to Descriptive Vividness

1. Failure to include essential descriptive information.
2. Lack of clarity in description.
3. Lack of credibility in description (Beck, 1993).
4. Inadequate length of time at the site to gain the familiarity necessary for vivid description.
5. Inadequate observational skills.
6. No indication that the researchers validated the findings with the subjects (Beck, 1993).
7. Inadequate skills in writing descriptive narrative.

Standard 2: Methodological Congruence

Evaluation of *methodological congruence* requires knowledge of the philosophy and the methodological approach the researcher used (see Chapter 11). Qualitative researchers should identify the philosophy and methodological approach they used and cite references for additional information (Munhall, 2001). Methodological excellence has four dimensions: documentation rigor, procedural rigor, ethical rigor, and auditability (Beck, 1993; Burns, 1989; Burns & Grove, 2001; Miles & Huberman, 1994).

Documentation rigor

Rigor in documentation requires clear, concise presentation of the following study elements: study subject, study significance, study purpose, research questions, assumptions, philosophy, researcher credentials, context, role of the researcher, ethical implications, sampling methods, subjects, data-gathering strategies, data analysis strategies, theoretical development, conclusions, implications for practice, suggestions for further study, and literature review. The study elements or steps are examined for completeness and clarity, and any threats to rigor in documentation are identified.

Threats to Documentation Rigor

1. Failure to present all elements or steps of the study.
2. Failure to present the elements of the study accurately or clearly.

Procedural rigor

Another dimension of methodological congruence is the rigor of the researcher in applying selected procedures for the study. To the extent possible, the researcher should clearly state the steps that were taken to ensure that data were accurately recorded and that the data obtained are representative of the data as a whole (Knafl & Howard, 1984).

When critiquing a qualitative study, you need to examine the description of the data collection process and the study findings for threats to procedural rigor.

Threats to Procedural Rigor

1. The researcher asked the wrong questions. The questions should tap the subjects' experiences, not their theoretical knowledge of the phenomenon (Kirk & Miller, 1986).
2. The subject (informant) might have misinformed the researcher; this can occur for several reasons. The informant might have had an ulterior motive for deceiving the researcher. Someone might have been present who inhibited free expression by the informant. The informant might have wanted to impress the researcher by giving the response that seemed most desirable (Dean & Whyte, 1958).
3. The informant did not observe the details requested or was not able to recall the event and substituted instead what he or she supposed happened (Dean & Whyte, 1958).
4. The researcher placed more weight on data obtained from well-informed, articulate, high-status informants (an "elite bias") than on data obtained from those who were less informed, less articulate, or low in status (Beck, 1993; Miles & Huberman, 1994).
5. The presence of the researcher distorted the event being observed (LeCompte & Goetz, 1982).
6. Insufficient data were gathered.
7. Insufficient time was spent gathering data.
8. The training of data collectors was insufficient.
9. The approaches for gaining access to the site or to subjects were inappropriate.
10. The selection of subjects was inappropriate (Miles & Huberman, 1994).

Ethical rigor

Ethical rigor requires recognition and discussion by the researcher of the ethical implications related to the study. Informed consent is obtained from subjects and documented. The report should indicate that the researcher took action to ensure that the rights of the subjects were protected during the study. As you critique the study, examine the data-gathering process, and identify potential threats to ethical rigor.

Threats to Ethical Rigor

1. Failure to inform the subjects of their rights.
2. Failure to obtain informed consent from the subjects.
3. Failure to ensure the protection of the subjects' rights.

Auditability

A fourth dimension of methodological congruence is the rigorous development of a decision trail (Miles & Huberman, 1994). Guba and Lincoln (1982) refer to this dimension as *auditability*. The research report should be sufficiently detailed to allow a second researcher, using the original data and the decision trail, to arrive at conclusions similar to those of the original researcher.

 Threats to Auditability

1. The description of the data collection process was inadequate.
2. The records of raw data were not sufficient to allow judgments to be made.
3. The researcher failed to develop or identify the decision rules for arriving at ratings or judgments.
4. Other researchers were unable to arrive at similar conclusions after applying the decision rules to the data (Beck, 1993).
5. The researcher failed to record the nature of the decisions, the data on which they were based, and the reasoning that entered into the decisions (Beck, 1993; Burns, 1989).

Standard 3: Analytical Preciseness

The analytical process in qualitative research involves a series of transformations during which concrete data are transformed across several levels of abstraction. The outcome of the analysis is a theory that imparts meaning to the phenomenon under study. The analytical process occurs primarily within the researcher's mind and is frequently poorly described in research reports. *Analytical preciseness* requires the researcher to make the intense effort needed to identify and record the decision-making processes through which the transformations are made.

 Threats to Analytical Preciseness

1. The interpretive theoretical statements developed do not correspond with the findings (Miles & Huberman, 1994).
2. The set of categories, themes, or theoretical statements fails to set forth a whole picture.
3. The hypotheses or propositions developed during the study cannot be verified by data.
4. Neither hypotheses nor propositions developed during the study are presented in the research report.
5. The study conclusions are not based on the data gathered (Burns, 1989).

Standard 4: Theoretical Connectedness

Theoretical connectedness requires that the theoretical schema developed from the study be clearly expressed, logically consistent, reflective of the data, and compatible with the knowledge base of nursing.

Threats to Theoretical Connectedness

1. The clarification of concepts is inadequate. For example, the concepts are inadequately identified and defined or the concepts are not validated by data.
2. The relationships among the concepts are not clearly expressed.
3. The proposed relationships among the concepts are not validated by data.
4. The theory developed during the study fails to yield a meaningful picture of the phenomenon under study.
5. A conceptual framework or map is not derived from the data.
6. No clear connection is made between the data and nursing frameworks.

Standard 5: Heuristic Relevance

To be of value, the results of a study should have *heuristic relevance* for the reader. This value is reflected in the reader's ability to recognize the phenomenon described in the study, its theoretical significance, its applicability to nursing practice, and its influence on future research. The dimensions of heuristic relevance include intuitive recognition, relationship to the existing body of knowledge, and applicability.

Intuitive recognition

Intuitive recognition indicates that when individuals are confronted with the theory derived from the data, it has meaning within their personal knowledge base. They immediately recognize the phenomenon and its relationship to a theoretical perspective in nursing.

Threats to Intuitive Recognition

1. The phenomenon is poorly described.
2. The reader lacks familiarity with the phenomenon.
3. The description is not consistent with common meanings or experiences.

Relationship to the existing body of knowledge

The existing body of knowledge, particularly the nursing theoretical perspective from which the phenomenon was approached, should be reviewed by the researcher and compared with the study findings. Similarities between the current knowledge base and the study findings add strength to the findings; reasons for differences should be explored by the researcher. When critiquing a study, you should examine the strength of the link between the study findings and the current knowledge base.

Threats to the Relationship to the Existing Body of Knowledge

1. The researcher failed to examine the existing body of knowledge.
2. The process studied is not related to nursing and health.

Applicability

Nurses should be able to integrate the research findings into their knowledge base and apply them in nursing practice. Also, the findings should contribute to theory development. You need to examine the discussion section of the research report for threats to applicability.

Threats to Applicability

1. The findings are not relevant to nursing practice.
2. The findings are not important for the discipline of nursing; for example, they do not contribute to theory development.

To determine the strengths and weaknesses of a study, the following five standards should be applied when critiquing a qualitative study: descriptive vividness, methodological congruence, analytical preciseness, theoretical connectedness, and heuristic relevance. The summary of strengths will indicate the researcher's adherence to the standards; the summary of weaknesses will indicate the potential threats to the integrity of the study.

SUMMARY

An intellectual critique of research requires careful examination of all aspects of a study to judge its strengths, weaknesses, meaning, and significance. The conduct of an intellectual critique involves the application of basic guidelines that stress the importance of critiquing the entire study and clearly, concisely, and objectively identifying the study's strengths and weaknesses. Research is critiqued to broaden understanding, improve practice, and provide a background for conducting a study. All nurses, including students, practicing nurses, nurse administrators, nurse educators, and nurse researchers, should critique research.

The critical thinking phases applied in the quantitative research critique process include comprehension, comparison, analysis, and evaluation. Phase 1, comprehension, involves understanding the terms and concepts in the report, as well as identifying and grasping the nature, significance, and meaning of the study elements. Phase 2, comparison, requires knowledge of what each step of the research process should be; the ideal is compared with the real. Phase 3, analysis, involves critiquing the logical links connecting one study element with another. Phase 4, evaluation, involves examining the meaning and significance of the study using certain criteria. Each step of the critique process is described, and questions are provided to direct the critique. A quantitative research report is provided with a critique that includes the four phases of: comprehension, comparison, analysis, and evaluation.

This chapter also provides an introduction to the critique process for qualitative research. The standards for critique of qualitative studies include descriptive vividness, methodological congruence, analytical preciseness, theoretical connectedness, and heuristic relevance. To achieve descriptive vividness, the site, subjects, data-collecting experience, and the researcher's thought processes should be pre-sented so clearly that the reader has the sense of personally experiencing the event. Methodological congruence has four dimensions: documentation rigor, procedural rigor, ethical rigor, and auditability. Analytical preciseness is essential for transforming concrete data across several levels of abstraction to develop a theory. The outcome of the analysis is a theory that imparts meaning to the phenomenon under study. Theoretical connectedness requires that the theory developed from the study be clearly expressed, logically consistent, reflective of the data, and compatible with the knowledge base of nursing. Heuristic relevance includes intuitive recognition, relationship to the existing body of knowledge, and applicability. These standards and the threats to them are presented to guide the critique of qualitative studies.

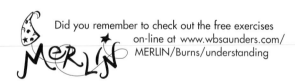

Did you remember to check out the free exercises on-line at www.wbsaunders.com/ MERLIN/Burns/understanding

REFERENCES

Beck, C. T. (1993). Technical Notes: Qualitative research: The evaluation of its credibility, fittingness, and auditability. *Western Journal of Nursing Research, 15*(2), 263–266.

Benton, J. G., Brown, H., & Rusk, H. A. (1950). Energy expended by patients on the bedpan and bedside commode. *Journal of the American Medical Association, 144*(17), 1443–1447.

Brown, S. J. (1999). *Knowledge for health care practice: A guide to using research evidence.* Philadelphia: Saunders.

Burns, N. (1989). Standards for qualitative research. *Nursing Science Quarterly, 2*(1), 44–52.

Burns, N., & Grove, S. K. (2001). *The practice of nursing research: Conduct, critique, and utilization* (4th ed.) Philadelphia: Saunders.

Dean, J. P., & Whyte, W. F. (1958). How do you know if the informant is telling the truth? *Human Organization, 17*(2), 34–38.

DeKeyser, F. G., & Pugh, L. C. (1990). Assessment of reliability and validity of biochemical measures. *Nursing Research, 39*(5), 314–317.

Glaser, B., & Strauss, A. L. (1965). Discovery of substantive theory: A basic strategy underlying qualitative research. *American Behavioral Scientist, 8*(1), 5–12.

Guba, E. G., & Lincoln, Y. S. (1982). *Effective evaluation.* Washington, DC: Jossey-Bass.

Hamer, S., & Collinson, G. (1999). *Achieving evidence-based practice: A handbook for practitioners.* Edinburgh: Baillière Tindal.

Kirk, J., & Miller, M. L. (1986). *Reliability and validity in qualitative research.* Beverly Hills, CA: Sage.

Knafl, K. A., & Howard, M. J. (1984). Interpreting and reporting qualitative research. *Research in Nursing & Health, 7*(1), 17–24.

LeCompte, M. D., & Goetz, J. P. (1982). Problems of reliability and validity in ethnographic research. *Review of Educational Research, 52*(1), 31–60.

Mateo, M. A., & Kirchhoff, K. T. (1999). *Using and conducting nursing research in the clinical setting* (2nd ed.). Philadelphia: Saunders.

Miles, M. B., & Huberman, A. M. (1994). *An expanded sourcebook: Qualitative data analysis* (2nd ed.). Beverly Hills, CA: Sage.

Miller, M. A., & Babcock, D. E. (1996). *Critical thinking applied to nursing.* St. Louis: Mosby.

Munhall, P. L. (2001). *Nursing research: A qualitative perspective.* Sudbury, MA: Jones & Bartlett.

Munro, B. H. (1997). *Statistical methods for health care research* (3rd ed.). Philadelphia: Lippincott.

Nieswiadomy, R. M. (1998). *Foundations of nursing research* (3rd ed.). Stamford, CT: Appleton & Lange.

Polit, D. F., Beck, C. T., & Hungler, B. P. (2001). *Essentials of nursing research: Methods, appraisal, and utilization* (5th ed.). Philadelphia: Lippincott.

Schaefer, K. M., & Pond, J. B. (1991). *Levine's Conservation Model: A framework for nursing practice.* Philadelphia: Davis.

Singman, H., Kinsella, E., & Goldberg, E. (1975). Electrocardiographic changes in coronary care unit patients during defecation. *Vascular Surgery, 9*(1), 54–57.

Winslow, E. H., Lane, L. D., & Gaffney, F. A. (1984). Oxygen uptake and cardiovascular response in patients and normal adults during in-bed and out-of-bed toileting. *Journal of Cardiac Rehabilitation, 4*(8), 348–354.

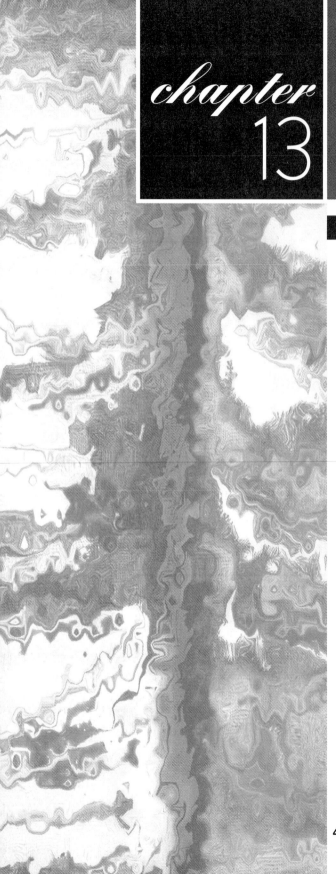

chapter 13

Using Research in Nursing Practice with a Goal of Evidence-Based Practice

Be sure to check out the free exercises on-line at
www.wbsaunders.com/MERLIN/Burns/understanding

MERLIN

Persuasion Stage
Decision Stage
Implementation Stage
Confirmation Stage
Evidence-Based Practice for Nursing
Algorithm to Facilitate Evidence-Based Practice in Nursing
Using Published Research-Based Protocols, Algorithms, or Clinical Pathways
in Nursing
Using Nationally Developed Clinical Practice Guidelines in Nursing

OBJECTIVES

Completing this chapter should enable you to:
1. Define research utilization.
2. Explore ways to communicate research findings in nursing.
3. Discuss the importance of the WICHE and CURN research utilization projects.
4. Identify barriers to using research in nursing practice.
5. Discuss strategies to promote the use of research in nursing practice.
6. Apply Rogers' theory of utilization of research knowledge in nursing.
7. Discuss the importance of an evidence-based practice for nursing.
8. Use published research-based protocols, algorithms, clinical pathways, and
national clinical guidelines in your clinical practice.

RELEVANT TERMS

Algorithm
Benchmark
Clinical pathway
Cognitive clustering
Communication of research findings
Current best evidence
Evidence-based health-care system
Evidence-based practice
Innovation
Innovators
Integrative review of research
Meta-analysis
Research-based protocol
Research utilization
Rogers's theory of research utilization
  Confirmation stage
    Continuance
    Discontinuance
      Disenchantment discontinuance
      Replacement discontinuance

Decision stage
  Adoption
  Rejection
    Active rejection
    Passive rejection
Implementation stage
  Direct application
  Indirect effects
  Reinvention
Knowledge stage
Persuasion stage
  Compatibility
  Complexity
  Observability
  Relative advantage
  Trialability
Social system

The expected outcome of nursing research is the use of the findings to improve practice. The preceding chapters of this text describe the steps of the research process, identify guidelines for critiquing studies, and present directions for summarizing research findings. Reading, critiquing, and summarizing research literature are essential steps in determining if the findings are ready for use in practice. During the last 20 years, many quality clinical studies have been conducted and replicated, providing research findings that are ready for use in practice. Thus the next step is the communication of these findings to nurses for use in their practice. Using research-based interventions, nurses can provide quality care, improve patient outcomes, and decrease health-care costs. Thus patients, nurses, and health-care agencies benefit from making changes based on research. The ultimate goal for professional nursing is an evidence-based practice.

Although extensive research knowledge has been generated in nursing, only a limited amount of this knowledge is being used in practice (Bueno, 1998; Coyle & Sokop, 1990; Michel & Sneed, 1995). Thus the purpose of this chapter is to assist you in using research findings to improve your practice. The concept of research utilization and the major nursing research utilization projects are introduced. The barriers to and the strategies for using research findings to improve practice are described, and a process for using research in your practice is provided. The chapter concludes with a discussion of evidence-based practice (EBP) and provides a model for facilitating EBP in nursing.

WHAT IS RESEARCH UTILIZATION?

Research utilization is the process of communicating and using knowledge generated through research to affect or change the existing practices in the health-care system. The main elements of research utilization include communicating or disseminating research findings to nurses, other health-care professionals, policy makers, and consumers of health care; summarizing research findings in a selected area; and using sound research knowledge in practice to achieve the desired outcomes for patients, nurses, and health-care agencies.

Communicating Research Findings

During the research utilization process, investigators communicate their study findings to other researchers and practicing nurses. *Communication of research findings* includes developing a research report and disseminating that report through presentations and publications to audiences of nurses, health-care professionals, policy makers, and health-care consumers. Research findings can be disseminated by one person communicating to another; by one individual communicating to several others; or by researchers using mass media such as journals, books, newspapers, television, and the Internet. Some strategies for communicating research findings to a variety of audiences are outlined in Table 13-1.

TABLE **13-1**

AUDIENCES AND STRATEGIES FOR COMMUNICATING RESEARCH

AUDIENCES	STRATEGIES FOR COMMUNICATION OF RESEARCH
Nurses	Presentations
	Nursing research conferences
	Clinical practice conferences and meeting
	Videotaped and audiotaped presentations from conferences and meetings
	In-service education programs
	Agency-based research committee
	Agency-based journal club
	Written reports
	Research publication in professional journals
	Research publications in books
	Monographs from research and clinical conferences and meetings
	Theses and dissertations
	Nursing research newsletter
	Electronic databases (WWW)
Other health-care providers	Presentations
	Professional conferences and meetings in other disciplines
	Interdisciplinary team meetings
	Written reports
	Research publications in professional journals and books in other disciplines
	Interdisciplinary research newsletter
Policymakers	Presentations
	Presentations on health problems to state and federal legislators
	Written reports
	Research reports developed for legislators
	Research reports published by funding agencies
	Electronic databases (WWW)
	Agency for Healthcare Research and Quality (AHRQ) clinical practice guidelines
Health-care consumers	Presentations
	Television and radio
	Community meetings
	Patient and family teaching
	Written reports
	Newspaper
	News and popular magazines
	Electronic databases (WWW)

Audiences of Nurses and Other Health-Care Professionals

Initially, nurse researchers usually communicate their study findings through presentations to nurses and other health-care professionals at conferences and meetings. An increasing number of nursing organizations and institutions are sponsoring research conferences. The American Nurses Association and many of its state associations sponsor annual nursing research conferences. The members of Sigma Theta Tau, the international honor society for nursing, sponsor international, national, regional, and local research conferences. Specialty organizations and associations, such as the Oncology Nurses Society and the American Heart Association, also sponsor research conferences. For a variety of reasons many practicing nurses and other health professionals are unable to attend research conferences. To increase the communication of research findings, conference sponsors provide audio-or videotapes of the research presentations. Some sponsors publish abstracts of studies with the conference proceedings or in specialty journals or make them available electronically on the World Wide Web (WWW).

Many nurse researchers not only present their studies at conferences but also publish their findings in nursing research journals, specialty practice journals, or other health professional journals. For example, Blegen, Goode, and Reed (1998) studied the relationships among the registered nurse (RN) skill mix and adverse patient outcomes of medication errors, patient falls, skin breakdown, patient and family complaints, infections, and deaths. These researchers found that the higher the RN skill mix, the lower the incidence of adverse occurrences in inpatient units, and the researchers published their findings in *Nursing Research.* This study documents the significance of RN care to patient outcomes and should be communicated to practicing nurses, other health-care professionals, policy makers, and consumers.

Practicing nurses often hear about research findings at conferences or read about them in journals and then communicate the findings to other nurses working in their clinical agencies. Research findings can be communicated in clinical agencies through e-mail, newsletters, in-service education programs, and interdisciplinary team meetings. For example, Bueno (1998) described the positive impact of a research newsletter in a clinical agency, which increased understanding of the research process and promoted communication of research findings.

Interpersonal communication involving face-to-face exchange has been extremely effective in making changes in nursing practice. The communication is most effective when the two interacting individuals have similar beliefs, values, education, social status, and professions (Rogers, 1995). For example, you might read the research findings of Blegen and colleagues (1998) about the effects of the RN skill mix on lowering the incidence of adverse occurrences for patients and communicate these findings to your closest co-workers. Together you and your colleagues might inform nursing administrators, physicians, and hospital administrators about the findings, so that the RN skill mix for hospital units might be increased to promote positive outcomes for patients and their families. This is extremely important research in this time of severe nursing shortage, where there are thoughts of decreasing the RN skill mix.

Audiences of Policy Makers and Consumers

Newspapers and television greatly increase the communication of research findings (see Table 13-1). Thus Blegen and colleagues (1998) could greatly expand the communication of their findings by developing a news release for their study. They might publish their research findings in an article in their state (Texas) newspaper, such as the *Dallas Morning News*. This article could then be picked up by other news services and published in papers across the country or presented on a local or national news program. Communicating research findings by mass media greatly increases the number of nurses, other health-care professionals, policy makers, and potential health-care consumers who are aware of the findings.

The federal government also strongly supports the conduct of research, the communication of research findings, and the use of findings to direct health care. The formation of the National Institute for Nursing Research (NINR) has significantly expanded the conduct of nursing research and the communication of findings. The Agency for Healthcare Research and Quality (AHRQ) was established to enhance the quality, appropriateness, and effectiveness of health-care services and access to these services. This agency has promoted research on patient outcomes and has facilitated the dissemination and use of research findings in practice. To promote the communication of research findings, AHRQ formed a work group for the dissemination of patient outcomes' research. This group included a variety of researchers and health practitioners, including nurses and physicians. The purpose of this group was to develop a plan for the dissemination of research findings, which identified the audiences and strategies for communication of research. The audiences included consumers, health-care practitioners, the health-care industry, policy makers, researchers, and journalists. Media for the dissemination of research included printed materials provided through direct mail, technical journals, health journals, the popular press, and electronic media, with communication by radio, television, and the WWW (http://www.ahrq.gov/).

Summarizing Research Findings

Research or empirical knowledge is generated through the conduct of a variety of quality studies (quantitative, qualitative, and outcomes). Often several studies on a specific topic are conducted, and these findings should be integrated in preparation for use in practice. The integration of findings from scientifically sound research to determine what is currently known is called *cognitive clustering*. Cognitive clustering is accomplished through integrative reviews and meta-analyses of nursing research. *Integrative reviews of research* are conducted to identify, analyze, and synthesize results from independent studies to determine the current knowledge (what is known and not known) of a particular topic. These reviews are published in a variety of research and clinical journals and in the *Annual Review of Nursing Research*. Chapter 4 provides guidelines for summarizing research findings and introduces the process for developing an integrative review of the research literature.

Some researchers have gone beyond critique and integration of research findings to analysis and synthesis of study findings through meta-analyses. *Meta-analysis* involves the use of statistical analyses to integrate and synthesize findings from completed studies to determine what is known and not known about a particular research area (Massey & Loomis, 1988). This approach allows the application of scientific criteria to such factors as sample size, level of significance, and variables examined. Through the use of meta-analysis, you can determine the following information (Burns & Grove, 2001; Smith & Stullenbarger, 1991).

1. Overall significance of pooled data from several studies
2. Average of the effect size, indicating the degree to which the null hypothesis is false or the degree to which the phenomenon is present in the population
3. Relationships among the variables studied

Meta-analyses make it possible to be objective rather than subjective in evaluating research findings. This objectivity makes it possible to determine accurately the usefulness of findings for practice. Published integrative reviews and meta-analyses of nursing research can assist you in summarizing the research literature in a selected area. These summaries of the research literature identify the changes or innovations that need to be implemented in practice. An *innovation* is an idea or nursing intervention that is perceived as new (although it may not be) by a nurse or the group of nurses adopting it. New interventions should be communicated in a clear, concise manner that will promote their use by practicing nurses.

Using Research Knowledge in Practice

The desired outcomes of research utilization are using research knowledge in practice to provide quality, cost-effective nursing care that will promote positive patient and family outcomes. Research knowledge is invaluable for expanding the assessment, diagnosis, and intervention expertise of practicing nurses. For example, the Braden Scale was developed through research to predict the risk of pressure ulcer development in patients. Using the Braden Scale, you might identify the patients at risk for developing a pressure ulcer and implement interventions to prevent ulcer development (Harrison, Wells, Fisher, & Prince, 1996). Preventing pressure ulcers promotes positive outcomes for patients and greatly reduces health-care costs.

Research utilization occurs within a specific social system. A *social system* is a set of interrelated individuals who engage in problem solving to accomplish a common goal (Rogers, 1995). Making a change in practice based on research might involve the nurses on a specific hospital unit, all the nurses in one hospital, or all the nurses in a corporation of hospitals. The larger social system requires more detailed communication and planning to use research knowledge to change practice. For example, the change might require review by several committees and approval by different administrators. Increasing the RN skill mix to decrease the incidence of adverse occurrences for patients might be started on a medical-surgical unit, then expanded to other units in the same hospital, and then implemented in other hospitals in a corporation (Blegen et al., 1998).

A social system has both a formal and an informal structure. The formal structure is related to authority and power. The informal structure is related to who interacts with whom under what circumstances. Health-care systems, such as hospitals and primary care clinics, have formal and informal leaders who are in favor of making changes *(innovators)* and those who are opposed. Some leaders are at the center of the system's interpersonal communication networks and tend to have extensive power in the system. When making research-based changes in nursing practice, you need the support of innovative nurses and of those who have power in the agency. The innovative nurses might be organized into a subcommittee whose purpose is to make a change in practice. They could verbalize the need for change and role-model the change for other nurses. The significance of research utilization for nursing practice is evident, but nurses need to be provided a background for using research findings in their practice.

RESEARCH UTILIZATION PROJECTS IN NURSING

The limited use of research findings in practice has been a problem in nursing for many years. To address this problem, some major research utilization projects were implemented. Two of these projects were the Western Interstate Commission for Higher Education (WICHE) regional nursing research development project and the Conduct and Utilization of Research in Nursing (CURN) project. These federally funded projects involved designing and implementing strategies to promote research use in practice. The outcomes of these projects and implications for nursing are discussed in this section.

Western Interstate Commission for Higher Education

The WICHE project, initiated in the mid-1970s, was the first major project to address research utilization in nursing. The 6-year project was directed by Krueger and colleagues (Krueger, 1978; Krueger, Nelson, & Wolanin, 1978) and was funded by the Division of Nursing of the National Institutes of Health (NIH). Members for this project were recruited from a variety of clinical agencies and educational institutions. The clinicians and educators were asked to participate in a workshop that focused on improving their skills in critiquing research. The participants selected research-based interventions that they were willing to implement in practice. These educators and clinicians developed detailed plans for using selected research findings in practice and functioned as change agents when the utilization projects were implemented in clinical agencies. At a second workshop, the participants reported the impact of using research findings in practice.

The WICHE project also included follow-up reports on the continuation of the research utilization activities at 3 and 6 months. These reports indicated that the WICHE project was successful in increasing the use of research findings in practice. Three reports from this project were published; the authors were Axford and Cutchen (1977), who developed a preoperative teaching program; Dracup and Breu

(1978), who devised a care plan for grieving spouses and tested its effectiveness; and Wichita (1977), who developed a program to treat and prevent constipation in nursing home residents by increasing the fiber in their diets. One of the outcomes of the WICHE project was the realization that only a limited number of quality clinical studies had been conducted and that most of the findings were not ready for use in practice.

Conduct and Utilization of Research in Nursing

The CURN project facilitated the development of clinical protocols to direct the use of selected research findings in practice. Many of these protocols (with modifications) are used in practice today. This project was directed by Horsley and funded by the Division of Nursing within the NIH (Horsley, Crane, & Bingle, 1978; Horsley, Crane, Crabtree, & Wood, 1983). The purpose of this 5-year (1975 to 1980) project was to increase the use of research findings in practice by communicating findings, facilitating organizational modifications necessary for implementation, and encouraging collaborative research that is directly useful in clinical practice. For this project, research utilization was viewed as a process to be implemented by an organization rather than by an individual nurse. From this perspective, research utilization required a decision by the clinical agency to implement research findings and the development of policies and procedures to guide the implementation process. The research utilization process included the following steps (Horsley et al., 1983).

1. Identification and synthesis of multiple studies on a selected topic (research base)
2. Organization of the research knowledge into a solution or clinical protocol for practice
3. Transformation of the clinical protocol into specific nursing actions (innovations) that are used with patients
4. Clinical evaluation of the new practice to determine whether it produced the desired outcome

During this project, published clinical studies were critiqued for scientific merit, replication, and relevance to practice. Determining the relevance of the research for practice involved examining its clinical merit or significance in addressing patient problems, the extent to which the clinical control belonged to nursing, the feasibility of implementing a change in an agency, and an analysis of the cost-benefit ratio. In 1975 the research findings in the following 10 areas were considered worthy of implementation in practice (CURN Project, 1981, 1982).

1. Structured preoperative teaching
2. Reducing diarrhea in tube-fed patients
3. Preoperative sensory preparation
4. Preventing decubitus ulcers
5. Intravenous cannula change
6. Closed urinary drainage systems

7. Distress reduction through sensory preparation
8. Mutual goal setting in patient care
9. Clean intermittent catheterization
10. Pain: deliberative nursing interventions (CURN Project, 1981, 1982).

The participants in the CURN project developed protocols based on research findings in 10 identified areas (Haller, Reynolds, & Horsley, 1979; Horsley et al., 1983). Each protocol detailed the implementation of a research-based nursing intervention. The protocols were implemented and evaluated in clinical trials. Based on the evaluations, a decision was made to reject, modify, or adopt the intervention. If the intervention was adopted, strategies were developed to extend this intervention to other appropriate nursing practice settings (Horsley et al., 1983).

Seventeen hospitals participated in the project. Each hospital identified a nursing unit as a site for the clinical trial and implemented one of the protocols. Data were collected before and after implementation of the protocols to determine the extent to which the findings were being used in practice. The effects of the protocols on patient outcomes were also evaluated. If the protocols produced positive patient outcomes, they were adopted in other units of the hospitals. Follow-up questionnaires were sent to the hospitals during the next 4 years, to determine the long-term effects of using the research-based protocols in the organization. Pelz and Horsley (1981) reported that, before the project, research utilization was low in all the hospitals. However, 4 years after the project concluded, most of the hospitals were still using the protocols. The clinical protocols developed during this project are available for use in your practice (CURN Project, 1981, 1982).

BARRIERS TO RESEARCH UTILIZATION

The WICHE and CURN projects were successful but limited in scope. Extensive additional research findings have been generated since the 1970s and 1980s; thus many more nurses in acute and primary care agencies should use current findings in their practice. This was evident in a study by Brett (1987), who examined the extent to which selected nursing research findings were being used by practicing nurses. One of the findings concerned the positioning of patients during intramuscular injection. Research demonstrated that "internal rotation of the femur during an injection into the dorsogluteal site, in either the prone or the side-lying position, results in reduced discomfort from the injection" (Brett, 1987, p. 346). Internal rotation of the femur is achieved by having the patient point the toes inward during an injection. Forty-four percent of the nurses were aware of this research finding, 34% were persuaded that it was useful for practice, and 29% were implementing it in practice sometimes, but only 10% were implementing it always.

Coyle and Sokop (1990) replicated Brett's (1987) study and found that 34% of the nurses surveyed were aware of the research finding about positioning during an injection and 21% were persuaded that the finding was useful for practice; however, only 4% used the intervention sometimes, and 22% used it always. Thus only a small percentage of these nurses were using the knowledge about positioning during intramuscular injections, even though it had been available for 15 years (Kruszewski, Lang, & Johnson, 1979).

The research finding about positioning patients during injections would be quite easy to implement in practice. The decision about positioning the patient during an injection could be made by the nurse alone; no physician's order would be needed. Administrative personnel would not have to give approval to make this change in practice. This nursing intervention would not increase costs or nursing time and would reduce the patient's discomfort during injections.

Why are many nurses not using research knowledge to improve their practice? The exact reasons are unknown, but several barriers to research utilization have been identified. They are related to the quality of the research findings, the characteristics of the nurses who should use the findings in practice, and the characteristics of the organizations where the findings should be used. The barriers to research utilization are discussed in this section, and some possible solutions are identified.

Barriers Related to Research Findings

As noted in the WICHE project, many of the early studies in nursing (those conducted from the 1930s to the 1970s) did not focus on clinical problems. Thus very little research knowledge was ready for use in practice before 1980. To overcome this barrier many researchers focused their studies on clinical problems during the 1980s and 1990s, and that focus continues in the twenty-first century. Thus the quantity and quality of clinical research studies are improving, and more findings are ready for use in practice.

Another barrier related to research findings is that many nursing studies have not been replicated. Two or three studies focused on the same problem do not provide sound research findings that can be used in a variety of practice settings. Thus studies need to be replicated in different settings with different populations to determine whether the findings are ready for use in practice. The different types of replication and their contribution to nursing knowledge are discussed in Chapter 4. The nursing profession now recognizes the significance of replication for the generation and refinement of nursing knowledge and supports the conduct of such studies. Replication studies are encouraged by the National Institute of Nursing Research (NINR), and funding is provided for replication research projects. More replication studies are presented at research conferences and published in research and clinical journals than in the 1980s.

Probably the most significant barrier to applying research results in nursing practice is that researchers often communicate their findings using words that are difficult for practicing nurses to understand (Bock, 1990; Liehr & Houston, 1993). In addition, some research reports do not indicate how the findings from a study are useful in nursing practice. Efforts are now being made to overcome this communication barrier. Clinical journals are including more studies written for nurses in practice; the journals *Applied Nursing Research* and *Clinical Nursing Research* were developed to communicate studies to practicing nurses. To increase the use of findings in practice, all researchers need to present their findings clearly and understandably, with an emphasis on how the findings can be used in practice.

Barriers Created by Practicing Nurses

Serious barriers to research utilization are created by nurses in practice, many of whom do not value research and are unaware of or unwilling to read research reports. Often these nurses lack the knowledge needed to read and critique studies and to use research findings in practice (MacGuire, 1990; Walczak, McGuire, Haisfield, & Beezley, 1994). To overcome these barriers, nursing students are being taught the steps of the research process, skills of research critique, and the process for using research findings in practice. Baccalaureate nursing programs have increased the focus on research, and educators often encourage students to make changes in practice based on research findings. Texts and lectures often include knowledge generated from research.

Through conferences and in-service programs, practicing nurses are being taught the skills to critique research and to use research findings in practice. Some agencies are hiring nurse researchers to increase practicing nurses' knowledge of research and to help them use research findings in practice. Nurse researchers are also conducting studies to address clinical problems and are encouraging practicing nurses to be involved in these studies. All these activities should expand a nurse's understanding of the research process and emphasize using research findings to make changes in practice.

Barriers Created by Organizations

Any organization has forces that promote stability and oppose change, as well as others that promote change. Generally organizations that have existed for a long time, value tradition, and have an authoritative management style oppose change. In this type of system, innovators are not valued and administrators support the institutional stance. These institutions often discourage making changes in practice by indicating that the changes are too time-consuming or costly, and those nurses proposing the changes are not rewarded for their innovativeness (Walczak et al., 1994). Practicing nurses as a group might need to identify a research-based change and then convince the administration that the change will improve patient outcomes with minimal or no cost to the institution. For example, Janken, Blythe, Campbell, and Carter (1999) wanted to implement a research-based change to support breast-feeding mothers. They conducted a research utilization project "to increase staff nurse support for four early postpartum breast-feeding practices: initiation in the delivery room, high frequency feedings, unlimited suckling time, and no supplementation" (Janken et al., 1999, p. 22). As a result of this research utilization project, the hospital administrators and the nurses valued research more and saw the importance of using research to make changes in practice.

Other organizations take pride in being innovative and actively encourage the use of new ideas. In these systems, management style and communication patterns facilitate the rapid spread of new ideas and support efforts to implement them. Resources needed for communicating and using research findings in practice are available, and innovators are nurtured in these systems.

Organizations in disarray also tend to be more receptive to change and to the adoption of innovations because the forces resisting change have weakened. Currently the entire health-care system is in disarray because of the changes in organization, settings, management styles, and mechanisms for health-care delivery. Economic constraints in the health-care system are greater now, but the potential for change has increased. Thus opportunities for practicing nurses to implement research findings in practice may be greater. Many changes have occurred in nursing, but the changes have often been imposed by external powers. Nursing has tended to be traditional and to rely on authorities; however, the values and norms of nursing as a social system are starting to change to support the use of research in practice. In addition, nurses are beginning to use research to shape health-care delivery (Fitzgerald, Hill, Santamaria, Howard, & Jadack, 1997).

STRATEGIES FOR USING RESEARCH FINDINGS IN PRACTICE

Most people believe that a good idea will sell itself; the word will spread rapidly, and the idea will quickly be used. Unfortunately, this is seldom true; several sound nursing research findings are not being widely used in practice. Research utilization is not a problem unique to nursing; many disciplines have experienced difficulties promoting change based on research knowledge. To address this problem, Rogers (1995) studied the processes for using research findings in society and developed a theory of research utilization. *Rogers's Theory of Research Utilization* included a five-stage process: (1) knowledge, (2) persuasion, (3) decision, (4) implementation, and (5) confirmation. The *knowledge stage* is the first awareness of the existence of an innovation or a new idea for use in practice. During the *persuasion stage,* nurses form an attitude toward the innovation. A decision is then made in the *decision stage* to adopt or reject the innovation. The *implementation stage* involves using the new idea to change practice. During the *confirmation stage,* nurses seek reinforcement of their decision and continue to adopt or reject the change in their practice. Fig. 13-1 presents a model of Rogers' innovation-decision process to promote the use of research findings. Rogers' model provided the basis for implementing the first nursing research utilization projects, WICHE and CURN. This model, including its five essential stages of research utilization, is presented to assist you in using research findings in your practice.

Knowledge Stage

Knowledge of research findings can be obtained by formal communication through conference presentations, publications in clinical and research journals, Internet sites, and news releases on television and in newspapers. In addition, informal communication within an agency from one nurse to another or among different health professionals can be effective in increasing awareness of research knowledge. Certain conditions influence the knowledge stage, such as previous practice, acknowledged needs and problems, innovativeness, and norms of the social system. Dissatisfaction with previous practice can lead to recognizing the needs or problems that require change. A need might create a search for an innovation to improve practice; knowl-

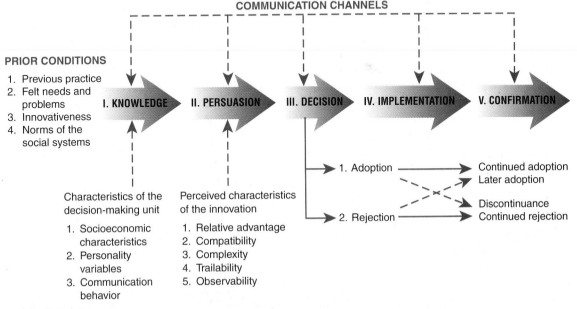

Fig. 13-1 A model of stages of the innovation-decision process. (Reprinted with the permission of *The Free Press*, an imprint of Simon & Schuster. Rogers, E. M. (1995). *Diffusion of innovation* (4th ed.). New York: Simon & Schuster.

edge of a new idea also might create a need for change. For example, knowledge of a new treatment for pressure ulcers might create the need to change the existing treatment protocol.

Innovativeness is the degree to which an individual or agency is willing to adopt new ideas and make changes in practice (Rogers, 1995). Those who read research and want to make changes in practice are innovators. They actively promote change and encourage others to change, but the degree and speed of change depend on the norms of the agency. Norms are the expected behavior patterns within an agency or social system. Norms can serve as barriers to change or can facilitate change. When the norms of the social system are oriented to change, the leaders in the agency tend to be innovative and facilitate change. When the norms are opposed to change, so are the agency leaders, thus creating barriers to change.

During the knowledge stage, it is necessary to examine the characteristics of the decision-making unit that is considering adoption of a research-based change. The decision-making unit might be an individual, a nursing unit, or the entire agency. The socioeconomic characteristics, personality variables, and communication behavior of the decision-making unit can support or interfere with the adoption of a new idea (see Fig. 13-1). Can the agency afford the change? Will the change save money? Examination of personality variables often indicates an individual's innovativeness and whether he or she will facilitate or resist change. Communication behavior, whether it is open and honest or closed and subversive, has a strong impact on the research utilization process.

Persuasion Stage

During the persuasion stage, an individual or agency develops either a favorable or unfavorable attitude toward the change or innovation (Rogers, 1995). Characteristics of an innovation that determine the probability and speed of its adoption include relative advantage, compatibility, complexity, trialability, and observability (see Fig. 13-1). *Relative advantage* is the extent to which the innovation is perceived to be better than current practice. *Compatibility* is the degree to which the innovation is perceived to be consistent with current values, past experience, and priority of needs. *Complexity* is the degree to which the innovation is perceived to be difficult to understand or use. If the innovation requires the development of new skills, complexity increases. *Trialability* is the extent to which an individual or agency can try out the idea on a limited basis with the option of returning to previous practices. *Observability* is the extent to which the results of an innovation are visible to others. An innovation with highly visible, beneficial results will probably be rapidly adopted. Innovations that have great relative advantage, are compatible within the agency, are not complex, have trialability, and are observable are usually adopted more quickly than those that do not meet these criteria.

In the persuasion stage the proposed change is best communicated in small groups or one-to-one interactions. You will be attempting to convince others that they need to make changes in their practice based on research. You will be asked many questions about the change, such as: Have you used this intervention in your practice? How do you feel about it? What are the consequences of using it? What are the advantages and disadvantages of using it in my situation? Would you advise me to use it? Will I still be approved of and accepted if I use it? Extensive, honest communication usually increases the likelihood of adoption.

Decision Stage

At the decision stage, the innovation is either adopted or rejected (see Fig. 13-1). *Adoption* involves full acceptance and the implementation of the innovation in practice. Adoption can be continued indefinitely or can be discontinued based on evaluation of the innovation's effectiveness for patients or the agency. *Rejection* of an innovation can be active or passive. *Active rejection* indicates that the innovation was examined and a decision was made not to adopt it. *Passive rejection* indicates that the innovation was never seriously considered. Over time, the agency might adhere to the decision to reject or might initiate adoption later.

Implementation Stage

In the implementation stage, the innovation is put to use by an individual, a unit, or an agency. A detailed plan for implementation that addresses the risks and benefits of the innovation will facilitate change. The types of implementation include direct application, reinvention, and indirect effects.

Direct application occurs when an innovation is used exactly as it was developed. In fact, some researchers would not consider an innovation to have been adopted unless its original form was kept intact. For example, if a study demonstrated that a particular intervention, conducted in specifically defined steps, was effective in achieving an outcome, adoption would require that the nurse perform the steps of the intervention in exactly the same way in which they were described in the study. This expectation reflects the narrow, precise definition of an innovation that is necessary to the scientific endeavor. However, this preciseness is not compatible with typical practice behavior, and research has indicated that maintenance of the original innovation does not always occur. A *research-based protocol* provides detailed guidelines that are documented with research sources for implementing an intervention in practice. These protocols promote direct application of an intervention in nursing practice (Haller et al., 1979). For example, the protocol in Fig. 13-2 provides direction for positioning a patient during an intramuscular (IM) injection to reduce the discomfort experienced by the patient. This protocol is brief and focuses on positioning during IM injections. Later in this chapter, a detailed research-based protocol is provided to direct you in selecting the best equipment to give an IM injection, identifying the IM injection site, positioning the patient to reduce discomfort with an injection, using appropriate techniques to give the injection, promoting absorption of the medication, and documenting the results.

---

1. Wash hands, gather necessary equipment for the injection, and put on gloves.
2. Explain to the patient that you will position him/her to decrease the discomfort of the injection.
3. Position the patient in the prone position or lying face down.
4. Identify the ventrogluteal (VG) site. (A picture of the site would be provided in the protocol.)
5. Have the patient turn his/her toes inward ("toe in"). This internal rotation of the femur causes relaxation of the gluteal muscle, which decreases the discomfort from the injection.
6. Give the injection, and reposition the patient for comfort after the injection.
7. Document how the injection was given and the patient's response or perceived level of comfort. (You might use the visual analogue scale presented in the section titled "Confirmation Stage" to document the discomfort experienced with the injection.

Beyea, S. C., & Nicoll, L. H. (1995). Administration of medications via the intramuscular route: An integrative review of the literature and research-based protocol for the procedure. *Applied Nursing Research, 8*(1), 23–33.

Keen, M. F. (1986). Comparison of intramuscular injection techniques to reduce site discomfort and lesions. *Nursing Research, 35*(4), 207–210.

Kruszewski, A., Lang, S., & Johnson, J. (1979). Effect of positioning on discomfort from intramuscular injections in dorsogluteal site. *Nursing Research, 28*(2), 103–105.

Rettig, F. M., & Southby, J. R. (1982). Using different body positions to reduce discomfort from dorsogluteal injection. *Nursing Research, 31*(4), 219–221.

Fig. 13-2 Protocol for positioning during IM injection.

Reinvention occurs when adopters modify the innovation to meet their own needs. Using this strategy, the steps of a procedure might be changed or deleted, or some of the steps might be combined with other care activities. Even with reinvention, nurses are using research findings to make changes in their practice. Nurses' use of research-based knowledge can also have *indirect effects*. For example, practicing nurses and researchers might discuss the findings, cite them in clinical papers and textbooks, and use them to strengthen arguments. Thus the knowledge would be incorporated into individuals' thinking and combined with their experience, education, and current values. In such instances determining that the research knowledge was being utilized would be more difficult; thus the use of certain nursing research findings may be underestimated.

Confirmation Stage

During the confirmation stage, nurses evaluate the effectiveness of the change in practice and decide to either continue or discontinue it. Using the example of the intervention to decrease patient discomfort during an IM injection, the nurse might evaluate the effectiveness of the injection technique by asking patients how much discomfort they felt during the injection or by having patients complete a visual analogue scale. On a 100-mm line like the one shown below, patients are asked to mark the level of discomfort they felt during the injection.

No   Extreme
Discomfort   Discomfort

After one month of using the intervention, the data obtained from the pain scale can be analyzed and shared with other staff members. If the results indicate that the injection technique causes minimal discomfort, the intervention would probably be continued *(continuance)* and the protocol included in the procedure manual. If the injection technique (the innovation or intervention) had been started on one unit, it might then be used on all units in the hospital. If the data analysis indicates that most patient's discomfort was still moderate to severe, the intervention would probably be discontinued.

Discontinuance can be of at least two types: replacement and disenchantment. With *replacement discontinuance*, the innovation is rejected to adopt a better idea. Thus innovations can occur in waves as new ideas replace outdated, impractical innovations. The computer is an excellent example; users can regularly upgrade their systems with new, more powerful interactive innovations in hardware and software. *Disenchantment discontinuance* occurs when an idea is rejected because the user is dissatisfied with its outcome.

EXAMPLE OF RESEARCH UTILIZATION IN PRACTICE

After examining research utilization projects, barriers, and theory, you should have some understanding of the research utilization process. Examining this information also raises questions. What research findings are ready for use in clinical practice? How can you use these findings to improve your nursing practice? What are the most effective strategies for implementing findings in practice? We suggest that effective strategies for using research findings require a multifaceted approach, taking into consideration research findings, practicing nurses, and the organizations within which nurses practice. In this section an example of research utilization is presented using Rogers' (1995) five-stage process: (1) knowledge, (2) persuasion, (3) decision, (4) implementation, and (5) confirmation (see Fig. 13-1). Research knowledge about the effects of heparin versus saline flush for irrigating intermittent intravenous devices (IID) is evaluated for use in nursing practice.

Knowledge Stage

The body of nursing research should be evaluated for scientific merit and clinical relevance; then the current findings are summarized in preparation for use in practice (Massey & Loomis, 1988; Tanner, 1987; Tanner & Lindeman, 1989).

Evaluation of Studies' Scientific Merit

The scientific merit of nursing studies is evaluated by criteria such as the following: (1) conceptualization and internal consistency, or logical links of a study; (2) methodological rigor, or the strength of the design, sample, instruments, and data collection and analysis processes; (3) generalizability of the findings, or the representativeness of the sample and setting; and (4) the number of replications of the study (Burns & Grove, 2001; Tanner & Lindeman, 1989). The critique steps discussed in Chapter 12 can be used to evaluate the scientific merit of studies. The research examining the efficacy of normal saline versus heparinized saline for the maintenance of IIDs has been extensive and conducted over several years (Epperson, 1984; Geritz, 1992; Shoaf & Oliver, 1992). In addition, two meta-analyses have been conducted to synthesize the findings from numerous studies (Goode et al., 1991; Peterson & Kirchhoff, 1991). The finding that normal saline is as effective as heparinized saline in maintaining an IID has been consistently supported by replication studies and the meta-analyses.

Evaluation of Studies' Clinical Relevance

Research-based knowledge can be used to solve practice problems, enhance clinical judgment, or measure phenomena in clinical practice. The scope of utilization might be a single patient-care unit, a hospital, or all hospitals in a corporation or community. For example, Shively Riegel, Waterhouse, Burns, Templin, and Thomason (1997) conducted a community-level research utilization project to promote the change from heparinized to saline flushes for IIDs of adult patients in three acute care facilities in one community. The change to saline flushes was successful in all three hospitals and has been maintained for 2 years. Research findings may also be used in primary care clinics and practitioners' offices. The nurse(s) desiring to implement a change in practice should be able to assure the agency that the cost in time, energy, and money and any real or potential risks are outweighed by the benefits of the change. The study by Shively et al. (1997) documented that heparinized saline flushes continue to be used in several clinical agencies despite the research support for the use of saline flushes for adult IIDs.

Summary of Research Knowledge

The research on a topic should be summarized to determine what is currently known and not known. Often you will have to review the literature in a selected area and summarize the findings for use in practice (see Chapter 4). In some areas researchers have conducted integrative reviews of the research literature or meta-analyses, which greatly facilitate the process of summarizing current knowledge in an area. For example, Goode et al. (1991) conducted a meta-analysis "to estimate the effects of heparin flush and saline flush solutions on maintaining patency, preventing phlebitis, and increasing duration of peripheral heparin locks or IIDs" (p. 324). The meta-analysis was conducted on 17 quality studies that are described in Table 13-2. The total sample size of the 17 studies was 4153; the settings were a variety of medical-surgical and critical care units. Goode et al. (1991) summarized the current knowledge as follows.

> "It can be concluded that saline is as effective as heparin in maintaining patency, preventing phlebitis, and increasing duration in peripheral intravenous locks. Quality of care can be enhanced by using saline as the flush solution, thereby eliminating problems associated with anticoagulant effects and drug incompatibilities. In addition, an estimated yearly savings of $109,100,000 to $218,200,000 U.S. health-care dollars could be attained." (p. 324)

The meta-analysis provides a sound scientific basis for making a change in practice. The clinical relevance is evident; the use of saline to flush IIDs promotes quality care and extensive cost savings.

If you are planning to make this change to your nursing practice, the following conditions need to be examined: previous practice, known needs or problems, innovativeness, and norms of the social system (Rogers, 1995). Does your institution currently use heparin, not saline, to irrigate IIDs? Do the nurses believe this is a problem? You need to highlight problems with heparin that have been identified in the research literature. Are the nurses innovative and willing to change or are they resistant to change? Which nurses might be most helpful in assisting with the change? You also need to talk with your administrator about the change. Is the administration in your agency open or resistant to change? What are the sources for resistance to the proposed change? How might the resistance be reduced?

Persuasion Stage

During the persuasion stage, you need to convince the administration and other nurses to change their current practice. Persuasion might be accomplished by demonstrating the relative advantage, compatibility, complexity, trialability, and observability of changing from heparin to saline as a flush solution (see Fig. 13-1). The relative advantages of using saline are the improved quality of care and cost savings that are clearly documented in the research literature (Geritz, 1992; Goode et al., 1991; Shoaf & Oliver, 1992). The cost savings for hospitals of different sizes are summarized in Table 13-3. The compatibility of the change can be determined by identifying the changes that will have to occur in your agency. What changes will the nurses have to make in irrigating IIDs with saline? What changes will have to occur in the pharmacy to provide the saline flush? Are the physicians aware of the research in this area? Are they willing to order the use of saline to flush the IIDs?

The change of peripheral IID irrigant from heparin flush to saline flush is not complex. Only the flush is changed, so no additional skill, expertise, or time is required by the nurse to make the change. Because saline flush, unlike heparin flush, is compatible with any drug that might be administered through the IID, potential complications are decreased. The change might be started on one unit as a clinical trial and then evaluated. Once the quality of care and the cost savings become observable to the nurses, physicians, and hospital administrators, the change will probably spread rapidly throughout the institution. Persuasion is likely to result in changing the irrigant from heparin flush to saline flush because the advantages are extensive and there are no identified disadvantages. The change is also compatible with existing nursing care and would be relatively simple to implement on a trial basis to demonstrate the positive outcomes for patients, nurses, and the health care agency.

Decision Stage

The decision to use saline flush rather than heparin flush as an irrigant requires approval by the institution, the physicians, and the nurses managing IIDs in their patients. When a change requires institutional approval, decision-making may be necessary at several levels of the organization. Thus a decision at one level may lead to contact with another official who must approve the action. In keeping with the guidelines of planned change, institutional changes are more likely to be effective if all those affected by the change have a voice in the decision. Who needs to approve the change in your institution? What steps do you need to take to get the change approved? Do the physicians support the change? Do the nurses on the units support the change? Who are the leaders in the institution? Can you get them to support the change? It may help to get the nurses to make a commitment and take a public stand to make the change; this should increase the likelihood that the change will occur. The appropriate administrators and physicians should be informed of the pros and cons of making the change to saline flush for irrigating IIDs. You need to indicate clearly to the physicians and administrators that the change is based on extensive research findings. Most physicians are positively influenced by research-based knowledge.

TABLE 13-2

STUDIES INCLUDED IN THE META-ANALYSIS

STUDY	N	SUBJECT	ASSIGNMENT	HEPARIN DOSE	CLOTTING EFFECT SIZE (d_c)	PHLEBITIS EFFECT SIZE (d_p)	DURATION EFFECT SIZE (d_d)
Ashton et al., 1990	16 exp_c 16 con_c 13 exp_p 14 con_p	Adult critical care	Random double blind	10/u/cc	0.3590	−0.1230	
Barrett et al., 1990	59 experimental 50 control	Adult med-surg patients	Nonrandom double blind	10/u/cc	−0.1068	−0.4718	
Craig & Anderson, 1991	129 exp 145 con	Adult med-surg patients	Random double blind crossover	10/u/cc	0.0095	−0.0586	
Cyganski et al., 1987	225 exp 196 con	Adult med-surg patients	Nonrandom	100/u/cc	0.2510		
Donham & Denning, 1987	8 exp_c 4 con_c 7 exp_p 5 con_p	Adult critical care	Random double blind	10/u/cc	0.0000	0.5480	
Dunn & Lenihan, 1987	61 experimental 51 control	Adult patients	Nonrandom	50/u/cc	−0.2057	−0.2258	
Epperson, 1984	138 exp 120 con 138 exp 154 con	Adult med-surg patients	Random double blind	10/u/cc 100/u/cc			−0.1176 −0.1232
Garrelts et al., 1989	131 exp 173 con	Adult med-surg patients	Random double blind	10/u/cc	−0.1773	−0.1057	−0.2753
Hamilton et al., 1988	137 exp 170 con	Adult patients	Random double blind	100/u/cc	−0.0850	−0.1819	−0.0604
Holford et al., 1977	39 experimental 140 control	Young adult volunteers	Nonrandom double blind	3.3, 10, 16.5, 100 132/u/cc	0.6545		

Study	Sample	Patient type	Design	Concentration			
Kasparek et al., 1988	49 exp 50 con	Adult medical patients	Random double blind	10/u/cc	0.3670	−0.5430	
Lombardi et al., 1988	34 experimental 40 control	Pediatric patients (4 wks–18 yrs)	Nonrandom sequential double blind	10/u/cc		−0.2324	0.0000
Miracle et al., 1989	167 exp 441 con	Adult med-surg patients	Nonrandom	100/u/cc	−0.0042		
Shearer, 1987	87 exp 73 con	Med-surg patients	Nonrandom	10/u/cc	−0.1170	−0.0977	
Spann, 1988	15 experimental 19 control	Adult telemetry step down	Nonrandom double blind	10/u/cc	−0.3163	−0.3252	
Taylor et al., 1989	369 exp 356 con	Adult med-surg patients	Nonrandom time series	10/u/cc	0.0308	0.0288	−0.1472
Tuten & Gueldner, 1991	42 exp 71 con	Adult med-surg patients	Nonrandom	100/u/cc	0.0000	0.1662	

From Goode, C. J., Titler, M., Rakel, B., Ones, D. S., Kleiber, C., Small, S., & Triolo, P. K. (1991). A meta-analysis of effects of heparin flush and saline flush: Quality and cost implications. *Nursing Research, 40*(6), p. 325. Copyright © 1991, The American Journal of Nursing Company. Used with permission.

TABLE 13-3

ANNUAL COST SAVINGS FROM CHANGING TO SALINE

STUDY	COST SAVING	HOSPITAL
Craig & Anderson, 1991	$40,000/yr	525-bed tertiary care hospital
Dunn & Lenihan, 1987	$19,000/yr	530-bed private hospital
Goode et al., 1991 (this study)	$38,000/yr	879-bed tertiary care hospital
Kasparek et al., 1988	$19,000/yr	350-bed private hospital
Lombardi et al., 1988	$20,000–$25,000/yr	52-bed pediatric unit
Schustek, 1984	$20,000/yr	391-bed private hospital
Taylor et al., 1989	$30,000–$40,000/yr	216-bed private hospital

From Goode, C. J., Titler, M., Rakel, B., Ones, D. S., Kleiber, C., Small, S., et al. (1991). A meta-analysis of effects of heparin flush and saline flush: Quality and cost implications. *Nursing Research, 40*(6), 325. Copyright © 1991, The American Journal of Nursing Company. Used with permission. All rights reserved.

Implementation Stage

Implementing a research-based change can be simple or complex, depending on the change. The change might be implemented as indicated in the research literature or may be modified to meet the agency's needs. In some cases a long time might be spent planning the implementation after the decision is made. In other cases, implementation can begin immediately. Usually a great deal of support is needed during initial implementation of a change. As with any new activity, unexpected events often occur, and the nurse adopter frequently does not know how to interpret them. Contact with a person experienced in the change can make the difference between continuation and rejection of the innovation.

The change from heparin flush to saline flush involves the physicians, who will have to order saline for flushing IIDs. You will need to speak with the physicians to gain their support for the change. You might convince some key physicians to support the change, and they are likely to convince other physicians. The pharmacy will have to package saline for use as an irrigant. The nurses should also be given information about the change and the rationale for it. It might be best to implement the change on one nursing unit and give the nurses on this unit an opportunity to design the protocol and plan for implementing the change. The nurses might develop a protocol similar to the one in Fig. 13-3. This protocol directs you in preparing to irrigate an IID, irrigating the IID, and documenting your actions.

Confirmation Stage

After a change has been implemented in practice, the nurses who implemented the change should confirm or document the effectiveness of the change. They should document whether the change improved quality of care, decreased the cost of care, and

1. Obtain the saline flush for irrigation from the pharmacy.
2. Wash hands, collect equipment for irrigating the IID, and put on gloves.
3. Cleanse the IID with alcohol prior to injecting with saline solution.
4. Flush the peripheral IID with 1 mL of normal saline every 8 hours.
5. If a patient is on IV medication, administer 1 mL of saline, administer the medication, and follow with 1 mL of saline.
6. Check the IID site for complications of phlebitis or loss of patency. The symptoms of phlebitis include erythema, tenderness, warmth, and a tender or palpable cord. Loss of patency is indicated by resistance to flushing, as evidenced by inability to administer 1 mL of flushing solution within 30 seconds.
7. Chart the time the IID was irrigated with saline and any complications of phlebitis or loss of patency.

Geritz, M. A. (1992). Saline versus heparin in intermittent infuser patency maintenance. *Western Journal of Nursing Research, 14*(2), 131–141.

Goode, C. J., Titler, M., Rakel, B., Ones, D. S. Kleiber, C., Small, S., et al. (1991). A meta-analysis of effects of heparin flush and saline flush: Quality and cost implications. *Nursing Research, 40*(6), 324–330.

Shoaf, J., & Oliver, S. (1992). Efficacy of normal saline injection with and without heparin for maintaining intermittent intravenous site. *Applied Nursing Research, 5*(1), 9–12.

Fig. 13-3   Protocol for irrigating IIDs.

saved nursing time. If the outcomes from the change in practice are positive, nurses, administrators, and physicians often want to continue the change. Nurses also usually seek feedback from those around them. The reactions of their peers to the change in nursing practice influence the continuation of the change. If peers approve, the nurses often adopt the change and even encourage others to do the same. If peers disapprove or provide negative feedback, the nurses often abandon the change.

You can confirm the effectiveness of the saline flush for irrigating IIDs by examining patient care outcomes and cost benefits. Patient care outcomes can be examined by determining the number of clotting and phlebitis complications with IIDs one month before and after the change is implemented. A finding of no significant difference supports the use of saline flush. The cost savings can be calculated for one month by determining the cost difference between heparin and saline flushes and multiplying by the number of saline flushes conducted in the month. This cost savings can then be multiplied by 12 months and compared with the cost savings summarized in Table 13-3. If positive patient outcomes and cost savings are demonstrated, the adoption of saline flush for irrigating peripheral IIDs will probably continue and be used by all nurses in the agency.

EVIDENCE-BASED PRACTICE FOR NURSING

A future goal for the United States is an evidence-based health-care system. An *evidence-based health-care system* incorporates health-care research evidence from a variety of disciplines, clinical expertise of the health-care providers, views of the patients and families, and the resources available to deliver health care (Cullum, 1998). EBP for medicine and nursing is essential in providing evidence-based heath care. EBP has been emphasized in medicine for years, and expert researchers, clinicians, and theorists have developed numerous evidence-based guidelines for the prevention of illness, and diagnosis and management of acute and chronic diseases (Friedland, 1998). Nurses are now faced with the challenge of developing EBP for nursing.

In some sources the terms research utilization and EBP are used synonymously, but they are different phenomena. Research utilization is a part of EBP and is a prescribed task of summarizing and using research findings to address a particular practice problem. In research utilization the research literature is analyzed, findings are synthesized, and a research-based protocol, algorithm, or clinical pathway is developed and used in practice to achieve specific patient and agency outcomes. EPB is *"the careful and practical use of current best evidence to guide health-care decisions"* (Omery & Williams, 1999, p. 51). *Current best evidence* includes clinical practice guidelines that are usually nationally developed by expert researchers, clinicians, and theorists in their areas of excellence. EBP involves the interpretation and implementation of these clinical guidelines by health-care providers based on their clinical expertise, the needs and the views of the patient and family, and the resources of the health-care system (Brown, 1999; Omery & Williams, 1999; Stetler, Brunell, Giuliano, Morsi, Prince, & Newell-Stokes, 1998). EBP in nursing would involve nurses making clinical decisions and delivering care based on the current best evidence and evaluating the outcomes from this evidence-based practice. The clinical guidelines used in nursing practice would be updated and revised by nurses as new empirical evidence became available. EBP is a complex phenomenon, so an algorithm was developed to facilitate the movement of nurses toward EBP.

Algorithm to Facilitate Evidence-Based Practice in Nursing

Nursing is in the initial stages of developing an EBP, and we can learn a great deal from medicine. In your role as a registered nurse, you will be applying clinical guidelines that were developed by nurses and physicians. An algorithm or diagram was developed for this text to facilitate your understanding the process for implementing an EBP in nursing (Fig. 13-4). We hope the algorithm will assist you in using current best evidence in your practice, with the goal of developing an EBP.

As shown in the algorithm, a practice problem stimulates nurses and other health-care providers to search for the current best evidence in making a health-care decision (Goode, 2000). The very strongest evidence to direct clinical practice is a nationally approved clinical practice guideline or standard that has been developed by a group of experts to manage a selected problem in clinical practice. The next best evidence nurses might have to use in providing care is a published research-based protocol, algorithm, or clinical pathway. This type of evidence is more commonly available to manage nursing problems than national clinical practice guidelines or standards. For some clinical problems the research findings have not been synthe-

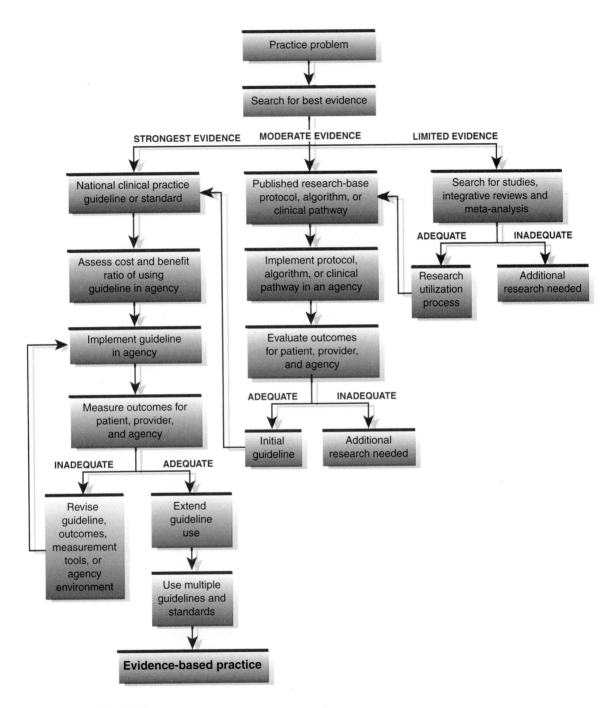

Fig. 13-4 Algorithm for facilitating evidence-based practice in nursing.

sized for use in practice in the form of protocols or clinical pathways. Thus you would need to conduct a literature search, synthesize the findings, and determine if the evidence is ready for use in practice (see Chapter 4). If the evidence is inadequate, then you recommend this as an area of research to other nurses and health-care providers. If the research evidence is adequate, then a research utilization project can be implemented. Hospitals sometimes develop their own clinical pathways and protocols to address clinical situations. These clinical pathways and protocols are often developed through committees and are based on a synthesis of the studies, integrative reviews, and meta-analyses in a selected area and are then used as a basis for current practice in that agency. Some of these pathways and protocols are published, but most are not, which limits the impact they have on nursing practice.

Using Published Research-Based Protocols, Algorithms, or Clinical Pathways in Nursing

As indicated in Fig. 13-3, using research findings in practice is facilitated by the publication of research-based protocols, algorithms, and clinical pathways in research and clinical journals. A *research-based protocol, algorithm, or clinical pathway* provides clearly developed steps for implementing a treatment or intervention in practice, and these steps are documented with research findings. These protocols are often developed by researchers who have conducted studies in a particular area where a change in practice is required. The researchers might develop an integrated review of the research literature or conduct a meta-analysis on studies in an area of interest. Integrative reviews and meta-analyses provide a synthesis of the research literature and a basis for the development of research-based protocols. Published research-based protocols, algorithms, and clinical pathways provide clear direction to nurses for making changes in their practice.

Beyea and Nicoll (1995) conducted an integrative review of the literature on the administration of medications via the IM route and then developed a detailed research-based protocol for this procedure. Table 13-4 includes a description of the different sites for an IM injection (Beyea & Nicoll, 1995). Table 13-5 provides a detailed research-based protocol for administration of IM injections that includes equipment to use, site, position, and injection techniques (Beyea & Nicoll, 1995). Each step of the protocol is documented with research sources. This protocol provides clear direction for giving IM injections to your patients. You could adopt this protocol individually and follow the procedures outlined in Table 13-5 when giving IM injections. This protocol might also be adopted by a clinical agency and published in the policy and procedure manual to provide guidelines for all nurses giving IM injections in an agency. As indicated in Fig. 13-4, the outcomes from implementing this research-based protocol should be examined within each clinical agency and health-care corporation implementing the protocol. The outcomes might include measurement of patient discomfort during an injection, number of complications from IM injections each month, and costs associated with IM injection complications. Based on these outcomes, the protocol might be revised as needed and benchmarks identified for clinical agencies. A *benchmark* is an identified standard an agency wants to achieve in patient care, such as having a 1% complication rate for IM injections.

As the number of studies of nursing interventions increases, more researchers and expert clinicians have the opportunity to summarize research knowledge with an integrative review or a meta-analysis and to use this knowledge to develop a research-based protocol, algorithm, or clinical pathway for practicing nurses. These protocols, algorithms, and clinical pathways should increase the use of research findings in practice, which should improve the quality of outcomes for patients, families, nurses, and health-care agencies. Ultimately, these protocols, algorithms, and clinical pathways might be developed into national clinical guidelines or standards for practice (see Fig. 13-4).

Using Nationally Developed Clinical Practice Guidelines in Nursing

The federal government, nursing, and medicine recognize the importance of evidence-based health-care practice. National guidelines and standards have been developed and implemented by expert practitioners and researchers in a effort to develop EBP. These national guidelines and standards have been developed by federal agencies and professional organizations and have been communicated at conferences, published in journals, and posted on web sites. The Agency for Health Care Policy and Research (AHCPR), within the U.S. Department of Health and Human Services (DHHS), convened panels of expert health-care providers and researchers to summarize research and develop clinical practice guidelines. These guidelines include a summary of the current research literature, mechanisms for assessing the clinical problem in practice, strategies for managing the clinical problem, and methods to evaluate patient and family outcomes. These panels summarized research findings and developed guidelines for practice in several areas. Many of these guidelines are extremely relevant to you in your nursing practice. The practice areas include the following: (1) management of acute pain in infants, children, and adolescents; (2) prediction and prevention of pressure ulcers in adults; (3) identification and treatment of urinary incontinence in adults; (4) treatment of cataracts in adults; (5) management of functional impairment; (6) treatment of depression in primary care; (7) screening, diagnosis, and management of sickle cell disease in newborns and infants; (8) management of cancer-related pain; (9) treatment of low back problems; (10) treatment of pressure ulcers in adults; (11) quality determinants of mammography; (12) treatment of otitis media in children; (13) screening for Alzheimer's and related dementias; and (14) availability of cardiac rehabilitation services. The AHCPR was renamed the Agency for Healthcare Research and Quality (AHRQ) in 1999. The AHRQ provides access to numerous clinical practice guidelines on their web site at: http://www.ahrq.gov/. Within AHRQ are EBP centers that synthesize scientific evidence to improve quality and effectiveness in clinical care (http://www.ahrq.gov/clinic/epc/).

Another source for practice guidelines is the National Guideline Clearinghouse (NGC), at http://www.guideline.gov/. The NGC provides more than 700 practice guidelines within two categories: (1) diseases and conditions and (2) treatments and

TABLE 13-4

WHAT'S IN A NAME?

SITE	LANDMARKS	ALSO DESCRIBED AS	TARGET MUSCLE	COMMENTS
Ventrogluteal (VG)	Place palm of hand against the greater trochanter and place the index finger on the anterosuperior iliac spine. Extend the middle finger along the iliac crest toward the iliac tubercle. (Right hand to left hip; left hand to right hip.)	Ventrolateral gluteal Anterior gluteal Hip	Gluteus medius	Although Zelman (1961) discussed the VG site, he called it the "anterior lateral site." This use of conflicting terms has confused the location and perhaps limited its usage.
Dorsogluteal	Draw an imaginary line between the superior iliac spine and the greater trochanter. Give the injection in an area above the imaginary line.	Upper outer quadrant of buttocks Inner aspect of the upper outer quadrant Buttocks Posterior gluteal muscle	Gluteus maximus May accidentally inject in the gluteus medius and/or gluteus minimus	This site was originally called "the buttocks." In the 1960s the description evolved to "the outer aspect of the upper quadrant." Previously, it had been described as "the upper outer quadrant." Confusion persists.

Site	Procedure	Landmarks		Rationale
Deltoid	Expose the entire shoulder and arm area. Administer injection 1 to 2 inches below the acromion.	Upper arm Fleshy muscle of the shoulder Outer aspect of the arm	Deltoid	Commonly referred to as the arm; identification of the deltoid site must be precise so as to avoid nerve and/or muscle injury.
Vastus lateralis	First locate the vastus lateralis muscle along the thigh. In infants and children, the site for injection lies below the greater trochanter of the femur and within the upper lateral quadrant of the thigh. For adults, the site is 4 inches below the greater trochanter and 4 inches above the knee laterally in middle third of the vastus lateralis muscle.	A hands breadth below the trochanter and a hands breadth above knee Thigh Front of the leg Anterolateral thigh	Vastus lateralis (part of the quadriceps muscle group)	In the past, many nurses were taught to use the rectus femoris muscle, which is associated with injury. The rectus femoris is part of the same muscle group as the vastus lateralis, but the rectus femoris is anterior and the vastus lateralis is lateral on the thigh.

From Beyea, S. C., & Nicoll, L. H. (1995). Administration of medications via the intramuscular route: An integrative review of the literature and research-based protocol for the procedure. *Applied Nursing Research, 8*(1), 25. Used with permission.

TABLE 13-5

PROCEDURE FOR ADMINISTRATION OF IM INJECTIONS

PROCEDURE	RATIONALE	REFERENCES
1. For adults, select a 1.5-inch needle. For children, select a 1-inch needle. Use a 21- to 23-gauge needle.	The needle must be long enough to reach the muscle. Injections into the subcutaneous tissue cause pain to the patient. The ventrogluteal (VG) site provides the most consistent depth of subcutaneous tissue; in adults, the adipose tissue layer over the VG muscle is less than 3.75 cm (1.47 in) in depth. Using a smaller gauge needle minimizes tissue injury and subcutaneous leakage.	Hick, Charboneau, Brakke, & Goergen, 1989; Johnson & Raptou, 1965; Michaels & Poole, 1970; Shaffer, 1929; Talbert, Haslam & Haller, 1967
2. The maximum volume to be administered in one injection should not exceed 4 ml in adults with well-developed muscles such as the ventrogluteal. Children and individuals with less well-developed muscles should receive no more than 1 to 2 ml. Children under the age of 2 years should not receive more than 1 ml. If using the deltoid, do not exceed a volume of 0.5 to 1.0 ml. The size of the syringe is determined by the volume to be administered, and the size of the syringe should correspond as closely as possible to the amount to be administered. Volumes less the 0.5 ml require a low-dose syringe such as a tuberculin syringe.	High-volume injections cause more pain. Finely graduated syringes such as tuberculin syringes ensure administration of the correct dose.	Farley, Joyce, Long, & Roberts, 1986; Losek & Gyuro, 1992; Zenk, 1982
3. Use a filter needle to draw up medication from a glass ampule or vial. Hold the vial or ampule down, and do not draw up the last drop in the container. After drawing the medication into the syringe, change the needle before administering. If using a prefilled syringe, such as Tubex® or Carpuject® and drawing from a vial or ampule, instill the medication into another syringe, and ensure the use of a clean needle before injection. If using a prefilled unit-dose medication, take caution to avoid dripping medication on the needle before injection. If this does occur, wipe the medication off the needle with a sterile gauze.	Glass and rubber particulate has been found in medications withdrawn with a regular needle. Holding the vial or ampule down will allow particulate matter to precipitate out of the solution, and leaving the last drops reduces the chance of withdrawing foreign particles. Changing the needle will prevent tracking the medication through the subcutaneous tissue during insertion of the needle, which can cause pain. Similarly, medication should be wiped from the needle, as this can also cause pain when it is tracked through the subcutaneous tissue.	Hahn, 1990; Keen, 1986; McConnell, 1982
4. Do not use an air bubble.	An air bubble affects the dose administered, causing an overdose of medication of at least 5% and as great as 100%, depending on the dose administered.	Chaplin, Shull, & Welk, 1985; Zenk, 1982, 1993
5. Select the VG muscle as the injection site for children over 7 months and adults unless there is a strict contraindication. Strict contraindications would include preexisting tissue injury and administration of hepatitis-B vaccine, which should only be administered in the deltoid. In infants less than 7 months, the vastus lateralis should be used for administering hepatitis-B vaccine.	The VG site is free of nerves and blood vessels. There are no documented reports of complications from IM injections administered at this site. The VG muscle is a well-developed muscle in infants, children, and adults.	Beecroft & Redick, 1990; Brandt, Smith, Ashburn, & Graves, 1972; Centers for Disease Control, 1990; Daly, Johnston, & Chung, 1992; Hochstetter, 1954, 1955, 1956

PROCEDURE	RATIONALE	REFERENCES
6. Before administering any IM injection, carefully assess the site for evidence of induration, abscesses, or other contra-indications for use of the site.	Injections are contraindicated in previously injured muscles or tissues.	Stokes, Beerman, & Ingraham, 1944
7. Position the patient to relax the muscle. Prone: Have the patient "toe in" to internally rotate the femur. Side-lying: Have the patient flex upper leg at 20 degrees. Supine: Have the patient flex both knees, if possible; if not possible, flex the knee on the side where the medication will be administered.	There is reduced pain with a relaxed muscle.	Keen, 1986; Kruszewski, Lang, & Johnson, 1979; Rettig & Southby, 1982
8. Identify the site by placing the palm of the hand on the greater trochanter with the index finger toward the antero-superior iliac spine and the middle finger spread away to form a "V." Use the right hand on the left VG site and the left hand on the right VG site.	The landmarks are described by Hochstetter.	Hochstetter, 1954, 1955, 1956; Zelman, 1961
9. Pull the skin down to administer the injection in a Z-track manner at a 90-degree angle to the iliac crest in the middle of the "V."	Z-track technique reduces discomfort and incidence of lesions.	Keen, 1983, 1986, 1990
10. Cleanse the skin in a circular fashion in an area of approximately 5 to 8 cm (2 to 3 in), and allow the alcohol to dry.	Deep tissues can be infected with skin contaminants injected via the needle; the skin is the first line of defense. Alcohol is irritating to the subcutaneous tissue and causes pain.	Berger & Williams, 1992; Murphy, 1991
11. Insert the needle with a steady pressure, and then aspirate for at least 5 to 10 seconds. Inject the medication slowly at a rate of approximately 10 sec/ml.	Aspirating for 1 to 10 seconds is adequate to ensure that the needle is not in a small, low-flow blood vessel. A slow, steady injection rate promotes comfort and minimizes tissue damage.	Stokes, Beerman, & Ingraham, 1944; Zelman, 1961
12. Wait 10 seconds after injecting the medication before withdrawing the needle.	Waiting 10 seconds allows the medication to be deposited in the muscle and to begin to diffuse through the muscle.	Belanger-Annable, 1985; Hahn, 1990, 1991; Keen, 1990
13. Smoothly and steadily withdraw the needle, and apply gentle pressure at the site with a dry sponge.	This minimizes tissue injury. Massaging the site can result in tissue irritation.	Newton, Newton, & Fudin, 1992
14. Encourage leg exercises.	Leg exercises will promote the absorption of the medication.	Stokes, Beerman, & Ingraham, 1944
15. Whenever possible, assess the site 2 to 4 hours after injection and as needed to identify any side effects.	Given the number of complications reported in the literature, it is important to assess the site for any signs of redness, swelling, pain, or other iatrogenic effects from the injection.	Beecroft & Redick, 1989, 1990

interventions. The AHRQ and the NGC provide a variety of guidelines that are used by physicians, advanced practice nurses, and registered nurses to implement EBP.

Fig. 13-4 shows that a quality national clinical guideline should be assessed for cost and benefits in your practice site. If the ratio is not adequate, what changes can be made in the guideline or the agency to facilitate the use of the guideline in your practice setting? If the cost-benefit ratio is adequate, nurses in your agency would implement the guideline in practice. Appropriate outcomes for patients, families, nurses, and the health-care agency would be measured and evaluated to determine the impact on practice. If the outcomes were not adequate, how should the guideline be revised? Which outcomes should be evaluated? What tools should be used to measure the outcomes? What changes should be made in the agency environment? The necessary revisions should be made, and the guideline should be implemented again. If the outcomes are adequate, use of the guideline can be extended from a single agency to several agencies in a city, state, or nationally. In this area, you and other nurses would be providing evidence-based care with progress toward an EBP. Additional guidelines and standards could then be implemented so the majority of care is evidence-based, resulting in EBP (Fields, 2000).

In the future, accrediting agencies for health-care organizations will require that protocols for nursing interventions be documented with research. The procedure manuals, standards of care, and nursing care plans should reflect current nursing research. Many progressive nurse executives realize the importance of research and are encouraging their nursing staffs to use research findings in practice. However, to improve nursing practice effectively with research knowledge, research utilization and EBP must become a priority for all nurses.

SUMMARY

The preceding chapters of this text describe the steps of the research process, present guidelines for critiquing studies, and provide direction for summarizing the research literature. Reading, critiquing, and summarizing research literature are essential steps for determining if findings are ready for use in practice. Many quality clinical studies were conducted and replicated in the 1980s and 1990s, providing research findings that are ready for use in practice. However, only a limited amount of this knowledge is being used to improve practice. Thus the purpose of this chapter is to assist you in using research findings in your practice.

Research utilization is the process of communicating and using research-generated knowledge to make an impact on or a change in the existing practices in the health-care system. The main elements of research utilization include summarizing knowledge generated through research; communicating the research knowledge to nurses, other health-care professionals, policy makers, and consumers; and achieving desired outcomes for patients, nurses, and health-care agencies. Research or empirical knowledge is generated through quality studies. Communication of research findings includes developing a research report and disseminating that report through presentations and publications to audiences of nurses, other health-care professionals, policy makers, and health-care consumers. The desired outcomes of research utilization include providing quality nursing care, increasing positive patient outcomes, and decreasing costs for health-care agencies.

Two major federally funded projects developed to increase utilization of nursing research findings are discussed: the WICHE project and the CURN project. The WICHE project focused on critiquing research and using research findings to improve practice. The CURN project was implemented to increase the utilization of research findings in the following ways: communicating findings, facilitating organizational modifications necessary for implementation, and encouraging collaborative research that is directly transferable to clinical practice. Clinical studies were critiqued, research-based protocols were developed from the findings, and implementation was initiated on test units within hospitals.

Many research findings are not being used in practice, and the barriers to research utilization are examined in this chapter. These barriers are related to the quality of the research findings, the characteristics of the nurses who should use the findings in practice, and the characteristics of the organizations in which the research should be utilized. The barriers related to the quality of the research findings include the following: studies are not focused on relevant clinical problems, the studies have not been replicated, and findings are not expressed in terms understood by practicing nurses. Some barriers are related to nurses; for example, many nurses do not value research, are unaware of or are unwilling to read research reports, have inadequate education related to the research process, and do not know how to apply research findings in practice. Some organizations create barriers to research utilization because they are traditional and oppose change.

Rogers' theory of research utilization is presented to direct your use of research findings in practice. Rogers proposes a five-stage process for research utilization: (1) knowledge, (2) persuasion, (3) decision, (4) implementation, and (5) confirmation. The knowledge stage is the first awareness of an innovation or new idea for practice. During the persuasion stage, nurses form an attitude toward the innovation. A decision is then made to adopt or reject the innovation. The implementation stage involves using the innovation to change practice. During the final stage, confirmation, nurses seek reinforcement of their decision and continue to adopt or reject the change in their practice. An example of research utilization is presented using Rogers' five stages. The research knowledge about the effects of heparin versus saline flush for irrigating IIDs is presented for use in practice.

A future goal for the United States is an evidence-based health-care system. An evidence-based health-care system incorporates health-care research from a variety of disciplines, clinical expertise of the health-care providers, views of the patients and families, and the resources available to deliver health care. EBP for medicine and nursing is essential in providing evidence-based heath care. EBP is the careful and practical use of current best evidence to guide health-care decisions. Current best evidence includes clinical practice guidelines that are usually nationally developed by expert researchers, clinicians, and theorists in their areas of excellence. EBP involves the interpretation and implementation of these clinical guidelines by health-care providers, based on the needs and the views of the patient and family and the resources of the health-care system. EBP in nursing would involve nurses making clinical decisions and delivering care based on the current best evidence and evaluating the outcomes from this evidence-based practice. EBP is a complex phenomenon, so an algorithm was developed to help facilitate the movement of nurses toward EBP. A research-based protocol, algorithm, or clinical pathway provides clearly developed steps for implementing a treatment or intervention in practice, and these steps are documented by findings from studies. Ultimately these protocols, algorithms, and clinical pathways might be developed into national clinical guidelines for practice. The AHRQ provides access to numerous clinical practice guidelines on their web site at: http://www.ahrq.gov/. Another source for practice guidelines is the National Guideline Clearinghouse (NGC) at http://www.

guideline.gov/. Recently, nursing has implemented an Academic Center for Evidence-Based Nursing with a web site at http://www.acestar.uthscsa.edu.

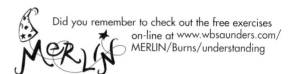

Did you remember to check out the free exercises on-line at www.wbsaunders.com/MERLIN/Burns/understanding

REFERENCES

Ashton, J., Gibson, V., & Summers, S. (1990). Effects of heparin versus saline solution on intermittent infusion device irrigations. *Heart & Lung, 19*(6), 608–612.

Axford, R., & Cutchen, L. (1977). Using nursing research to improve preoperative care. *Journal of Nursing Administration, 7*(10), 16–20.

Barrett, P. J., & Lester, R. L. (1990). Heparin versus saline flush solutions in a small community hospital. *Hospital Pharmacy, 25*(2), 115–118.

Beecroft, P. C., & Redick, S. A. (1989). Possible complications of intramuscular injections on the pediatric unit. *Pediatric Nursing, 15*(4), 333–336, 376.

Beecroft, P. C., & Redick, S. A. (1990). Intramuscular injection practices of pediatric nurses: Site selection. *Nurse Educator, 15*(4), 23–28.

Belanger-Annable, M. C. (1985). Long acting neuroleptics: Technique for intramuscular injection. *The Canadian Nurse, 81*(8), 41–44.

Berger, K. J., & Williams, M. B. (1992). *Fundamentals of nursing: Collaborating for optimal health.* Norwalk, CT: Appleton & Lange.

Beyea, S. C., & Nicoll, L. H. (1995). Administration of medications via the intramuscular route: An integrative review of the literature and research-based protocol for the procedure. *Applied Nursing Research, 8*(1), 23–33.

Blegen, M. A., Goode, C. J., & Reed, L. (1998). Nurse staffing and patient outcomes. *Nursing Research, 47*(1), 43–50.

Bock, L. R. (1990). From research to utilization: Bridging the gap. *Nursing Management, 21*(3), 50–51.

Brandt, P. A., Smith, M. E., Ashburn, S. S., & Graves, J. (1972). IM injections in children. *American Journal of Nursing, 72*(7), 1402–1406.

Brett, J. L. (1987). Use of nursing practice research findings. *Nursing Research, 36*(6), 344–349.

Brown, S. J. (1999). *Knowledge for health care practice: A guide to using research evidence.* Philadelphia: Saunders.

Bueno, M. M. (1998). Promoting nursing research through newsletters. *Applied Nursing Research, 11*(1), 41–44.

Burns, N., & Grove, S. K. (2001). *The practice of nursing research: Conduct, critique, and utilization* (4th ed.). Philadelphia: Saunders.

Centers for Disease Control. (1990). Recommendation of the Immunization Practices Advisory Committee. Diphtheria, tetanus, and pertussis: Guidelines for vaccine prophylaxis and other preventive measures. *Morbidity and Mortality Weekly Report, 34*(27), 405–426.

Chaplin, G., Shull, H., & Welk, P. C. (1985). How safe is the air-bubble technique for IM injections? *Nursing85, 15*(9), 59.

Coyle, L. A., & Sokop, A. G. (1990). Innovation adoption behavior among nurses. *Nursing Research, 39*(3), 176–180.

Craig, F. D., & Anderson, S. R. (1991). *A comparison of normal saline versus heparinized normal saline in the maintenance of intermittent infusion devices.* Unpublished manuscript submitted for publication.

Cullum, N. (1998). Evidence-based practice. *Nursing Management, 5*(3), 32–35.

CURN Project. *Using research to improve nursing practice.* Series of Clinical Protocols: *Clean intermittent catheterization* (1982), *Closed urinary drainage systems* (1981), *Distress reduction through sensory preparation* (1981), *Intravenous cannula change* (1981), *Mutual goal setting in patient care* (1982), *Pain: Deliberative nursing interventions* (1982), *Preventing decubitus ulcers* (1981), *Reducing diarrhea in tube-fed patients* (1981), *Structured preoperative teaching* (1981). New York: Grune & Stratton.

Cyganski, J. M., Donahue, J. M., & Heaton, J. S. (1987). The case for the heparin flush. *American Journal of Nursing, 87*(6), 796–797.

Daly, J. M., Johnston, W., & Chung, Y. (1992). Injection sites utilized for DPT immunizations in infants. *Journal of Community Health Nursing, 9*(2), 87–94.

Donham, J., & Denning, V. (1987). Heparin vs. saline in maintaining patency in intermittent infusion devices: Pilot study. *The Kansas Nurse, 62*(11), 6–7.

Dracup, K. A., & Breu, C. S. (1978). Using nursing research findings to meet the needs of grieving spouses. *Nursing Research, 27*(4), 212–216.

Dunn, D. L., & Lenihan, S. F. (1987). The case for the saline flush. *American Journal of Nursing, 87*(6), 798–799.

Epperson, E. L. (1984). Efficacy of 0.9% sodium chloride injection with and without heparin for maintaining indwelling intermittent injection sites. *Clinical Pharmacy, 3*(6), 626–629.

Farley, F., Joyce, N., Long, B., & Roberts, R. (1986). Will that IM needle reach the muscle? *American Journal of Nursing, 86*(12), 1327–1328.

Fields, S. D. (2000). Clinical practice guidelines: Finding and appraising useful, relevant recommendations for geriatric care. *Geriatrics, 55*(1), 59–64.

Fitzgerald, S. T., Hill, M. N., Santamaria, B., Howard, C., & Jadack, R. (1997). Nurses' perceptions of consensus reports containing recommendations for practice. *Nursing Outlook, 45*(5), 229–235.

Friedland, D. J. (1998). *Evidence-based medicine: A framework for clinic practice.* Stamford, Connecticut: Appleton & Lange.

Garrelts, J., LaRocca, J., Ast, D., Smith, D. F., & Sweet, D. E. (1989). Comparison of heparin and 0.9% sodium chloride injection in the maintenance of indwelling intermittent I.V. devices. *Clinical Pharmacy, 8*(1), 34–39.

Geritz, M. A. (1992). Saline versus heparin in intermittent infuser patency maintenance. *Western Journal of Nursing Research, 14*(2), 131–141.

Goode, C. J. (2000). What constitutes the "evidence" in evidence-based practice? *Applied Nursing Research, 13*(4), 222–225.

Goode, C. J., Titler, M., Rakel, B., Ones, D. S., Kleiber, C., Small, S., & Triolo, P. K. (1991). A meta-analysis of effects of heparin flush and saline flush: Quality and cost implications. *Nursing Research, 40*(6), 324–330.

Hahn, K. (1990). Brush up on your injection technique. *Nursing90, 20*(9), 54–58.

Hahn, K. (1991). Extra points on injections (letter). *Nursing91, 21*(1), 6.

Haller, K. B., Reynolds, M. A., & Horsley, J. A. (1979). Developing research-based innovation protocols: Process, criteria, and issues. *Research in Nursing & Health, 2*(1), 45–51.

Hamilton, R. A., Plis, J. M., Clay, C., & Sylvan, L. (1988). Heparin sodium versus 0.9% sodium chloride injection for maintaining patency of indwelling intermittent infusion devices. *Clinical Pharmacy, 7*(6), 439–443.

Harrison, M. B., Wells, G., Fisher, A., & Prince, M. (1996). Practice guidelines for the prediction and prevention of pressure ulcers: Evaluating the evidence. *Applied Nursing Research, 9*(1), 9–17.

Hick, J. F., Charboneau, J. W., Brakke, D. M., & Goergen, B. (1989). Optimum needle length for DPT inoculation of infants. *Pediatrics, 84*(1), 136–137.

Hochstetter, V. A. V. (1954). Über die intraglutäale Injektion, ihre Komplikationen und deren Verhütung. *Schweizerische Medizinische Wochenschrift, 84,* 1226–1227.

Hochstetter, V. A. V. (1955). Über Probleme und Technik der intraglutäalen injektion, Teil I. Der Einflu{{194}} des Medikamentes und der Individualität des Patienten auf die Entstehung von Spritzenschäden. *Schweizerische Medizinische Wochenschrift, 85,* 1138–1144.

Hochstetter, V. A. V. (1956). Über probleme und Technik der intraglutäalen Injektion, Teil II. Der Einflu{{194}} der Injektionstechnick auf die Entstehung von Spritzenschäden. *Schweizerische Medizinische Wochenschrift, 86,* 69–76.

Holford, N. H. G., Vozeh, S., Coates, P., Porvell, J. R., Thiercelin, J. F., & Upton, R. (1977). More on heparin lock. *New England Journal of Medicine, 296,* 1300–1301.

Horsley, J. A., Crane, J., & Bingle, J. D. (1978). Research utilization as an organizational process. *Journal of Nursing Administration, 8*(7), 4–6.

Horsley, J. A., Crane, J., Crabtree, M. K., & Wood, D. J. (1983). *Using research to improve nursing practice: A guide.* New York: Grune & Stratton.

Janken, J. K., Blythe, G., Campbell, P. T., & Carter, R. H. (1999). Changing nursing practice through research utilization: Consistent support for breast-feeding mothers. *Applied Nursing Research, 12*(1), 22–29.

Johnson, E. W., & Raptou, A. D. (1965). A study of intragluteal injections. *Archives of Physical Medicine and Rehabilitation, 46,* 167–177.

Kasparek, A., Wenger, J., & Feldt, R. (1988). *Comparison of normal versus heparinized saline for flushing of intermittent intravenous infusion devices.* Unpublished manuscript. Mercy Medical Center, Cedar Rapids, IA, pp. 1–18.

Keen, M. F. (1983). Adverse effects of frequent intramuscular injections. *Research Review, 10*(4), 15–16.

Keen, M. F. (1986). Comparison of intramuscular injection techniques to reduce site discomfort and lesions. *Nursing Research, 35*(4), 207–210.

Keen, M. F. (1990). Get on the right track with Z-track injections. *Nursing90, 20*(8), 59.

Krueger, J. C. (1978). Utilization of nursing research: The planning process. *Journal of Nursing Administration, 8*(1), 6–9.

Krueger, J. C., Nelson, A. H., & Wolanin, M. O. (1978). *Nursing research: Development, collaboration, and utilization.* Germantown, MD: Aspen.

Kruszewski, A., Lang, S., & Johnson, J. (1979). Effect of positioning on discomfort from intramuscular injections in the dorsogluteal site. *Nursing Research, 28*(2), 103–105.

Liehr, P., & Houston, S. (1993). Critiquing and using nursing research: Guidelines for the critical care nurse. *American Journal of Critical Care, 2*(5), 407–412.

Lombardi, T. P., Gunderson, B., Zammett, L. O., Walters, J. K., & Morris, B. A. (1988). Efficacy of 0.9% sodium chloride injection with or without heparin sodium for maintaining patency of intravenous catheters in children. *Children Pharmacy, 7*(11), 832–836.

Losek, J. D., & Gyuro, J. (1992). Pediatric intramuscular injections: Do you know the procedure and complications? *Pediatric Emergency Care, 8*(2), 79–81.

MacGuire, J. M. (1990). Putting nursing research findings into practice: Research utilization as an aspect of the management of change. *Journal of Advanced Nursing, 15*(5), 614–620.

Massey, J., & Loomis, M. (1988). When should nurses use research findings? *Applied Nursing Research, 1*(1), 32–40.

Mateo, M. A., & Kirchhoff, K. T. (1999). *Using and conducting nursing research in the clinical setting* (2nd ed.). Philadelphia: Saunders.

McConnell, E. A. (1982), The subtle art of really good injections. *RN, 45*(2), 25–35.

Michaels, L., & Poole, R. W. (1970). Injection granuloma of the buttock. *Canadian Medical Association Journal, 102*, 626–628.

Michel, Y., & Sneed, N. V. (1995). Dissemination and use of research findings in nursing practice. *Journal of Professional Nursing, 11*(5), 306–311.

Miracle, V., Fangman, B., Kayrouz, P., Kederis, K., & Pursell, L. (1989). Normal saline vs. heparin lock flush solution: One institution's findings. *The Kentucky Nurse, 37*(4), 1, 6–7.

Murphy, J. I. (1991). Reducing the pain of intramuscular (IM) injections. *Advancing Clinical Care, 6*(4), 35.

Newton, M., Newton, D., & Fudin, J. (1992). Reviewing the "big three" injection techniques. *Nursing92, 22*(2), 34–41.

Omery, A., & Williams, R. P. (1999). An appraisal of research utilization across the United States. *Journal of Nursing Administration, 29*(12), 50–56.

Pelz, D., & Horsley, J. (1981). Measuring utilization of nursing research. In J. Ciarlo (Ed.), *Utilizing evaluation.* Beverly Hills, CA: Sage.

Peterson, F. Y., & Kirchhoff, K. T. (1991). Analysis of the research about heparinized versus nonheparinized intravascular lines. *Heart & Lung, 20*(6), 631–642.

Rettig, F. M., & Southby, J. R. (1982). Using different body positions to reduce discomfort from dorsogluteal injection. *Nursing Research, 31*(4), 219–221.

Rogers, E. M. (1995). *Diffusion of innovations* (4th ed.). New York: Free Press.

Schustek, M. (1984). The cost effective approach to PRN device maintenance. *Journal of National Intravenous Therapy Associates, 7*, 527.

Shaffer, L. W. (1929). The fate in intragluteal injections. *Archives of Dermatology and Syphilology, 19*, 347–363.

Shearer, J. (1987). Normal saline flush versus dilute heparin flush patency in heparin locks. *National Intravenous Therapy Association, 10*(6), 425–427.

Shively, M., Riegel, B., Waterhouse, D., Burns, D., Templin, K., & Thomason, T. (1997). Testing a community level research utilization intervention. *Applied Nursing Research 10*(3), 121–127.

Shoaf, J., & Oliver, S. (1992). Efficacy of normal saline injection with and without heparin for maintaining intermittent intravenous site. *Applied Nursing Research, 5*(1), 9–12.

Smith, M. C., & Stullenbarger, E. (1991). A prototype for integrative review and meta-analysis of nursing research. *Journal of Advanced Nursing, 16*(11), 1272–1283.

Spann, J. M. (1988). Efficacy of two flush solutions to maintain catheter patency in heparin locks. *Dissertation Abstracts, 28*(01)1337125, 1–58.

Stetler, C. B., Brunell, M., Giuliano, K. K., Morsi, D., Prince, L., & Newell-Stokes, V. (1998). Evidence-based practice and the role of nursing leadership. *Journal of Nursing Administration, 28*(7/8), 45–53.

Stokes, J. H., Beerman, H., & Ingraham, N. R. (1944). *Modern clinical syphilology: Diagnosis, treatment, case study* (3rd ed.). Philadelphia: Saunders.

Talbert, J. L., Haslam, R. H. A., & Haller, J. A. (1967). Gangrene of the foot following intramuscular injection in the lateral thigh: A case report with recommendations for prevention. *Journal of Pediatrics, 70*(1), 110–117.

Tanner, C. A. (1987). Evaluating research for use in practice: Guidelines for the clinician. *Heart & Lung, 16*(4), 424–431.

Tanner, C. A., & Lindeman, C. A. (1989). *Using nursing research.* Pub. No. 15–2232. New York: National League for Nursing.

Taylor, N., Hutchinson, E., Milliken, W., & Larson, E. (1989). Comparison of normal versus heparinized saline for flushing infusion devices. *Journal of Nursing Quality Assurance, 3*(4), 49–55.

Tuten, S. H., & Gueldner, S. H. (1991). Efficacy of sodium chloride versus dilute heparin for maintenance of peripheral intermittent intravenous devices. *Applied Nursing Research, 4*(2), 63–71.

Walczak, J. R., McGuire, D. B., Haisfield, M. E., & Beezley, A. (1994). A survey of research-related activities and perceived barriers to research utilization among professional oncology nurses. *Oncology Nursing Forum, 21*(4), 710–715.

Wichita, C. (1977). Treating and preventing constipation in nursing home residents. *Journal of Gerontological Nursing, 3*(6), 35–39.

Zelman, S. (1961). Notes on the techniques of intramuscular injections. *The American Journal of Medical Science, 241*(5), 47–58.

Zenk, K. E. (1982). Improving the accuracy of mini-volume injections. *Infusion, 6*(1), 7–12.

Zenk, K. E. (1993). Beware of overdose. *Nursing93, 23*(3), 28–29.

Glossary

Abstract *(adjective)* Expressed without reference to any specific instance.

Abstract *(noun)* Clear, concise summary of a study, usually limited to 100 to 250 words.

Abstract thinking Thinking that is oriented toward the development of an idea, without application to or association with a particular instance; independent of time and space. Abstract thinkers tend to look for meaning, patterns, relationships, and philosophical implications.

Academic library Library located within an institution of higher learning; contains numerous research reports in journals and books.

Accessible population Portion of the target population to which the researcher has reasonable access.

Accidental sampling *See* convenience sampling.

Accuracy Addresses the extent to which a physiological instrument measures the concept defined in the study. Accuracy is comparable to validity.

Across-method triangulation Combining research methods or strategies from two or more research traditions in the same study.

Action application of research Using research findings as a driving force for change, as an impetus for evaluation of services, and as a model for practice.

Active rejection Decision to not adopt an innovation that was examined.

Adoption Full acceptance and implementation of an innovation in practice.

Algorithm Decision tree that provides a set of rules for solving a particular practice problem. Its development is usually based on research and theoretical knowledge.

Alpha (α) Cutoff point used to determine whether the samples being tested are members of the same population or of different populations; alpha is commonly set at 0.05, 0.01, or 0.001.

Alternate forms reliability Comparison of the equivalence of two versions of the same paper-and-pencil instrument.

Analysis of covariance (ANCOVA) Statistical procedure in which a regression analysis is carried out before performing ANOVA; designed to reduce the variance within groups by partialing out the variance due to a confounding variable.

Analysis of variance (ANOVA) Statistical test used to examine differences among two or more groups by comparing the variability between groups with the variability within each group.

Analysis phase Phase of a critique in which the reader determines the strengths and limitations of the logical links between study elements.

Analytic induction Qualitative research technique that includes enumerative induction, in which a variety of instances are collected that verify the model, and eliminative induction, in which the hypothesis is tested against alternatives.

Analytical preciseness Precision obtained by transforming concrete data across several levels of abstraction to develop a theoretical schema that explains the phenomenon under study.

Analyzing research reports Critical thinking skill that involves determining the value of a study by breaking the contents of a study report into parts and examining the parts for accuracy, completeness, uniqueness of information, and organization.

Anonymity Conditions in which the subject's identity cannot be linked, even by the researcher, with his or her individual responses.

Applied (practical) research Scientific investigations conducted to generate knowledge that will directly influence clinical practice.

Approximate replication Operational replication that involves repeating the original study under similar conditions, following the original methods as closely as possible.

Ascendance to an open context Ability to see depth and complexity within the phenomenon examined; a greater capacity for insight than is usually found with the sedimented view. Requires deconstructing sedimented views and reconstructing another view.

Associative hypothesis Hypothesis that identifies variables that occur or exist together in the real world, such that when one variable changes, the other changes.

Associative relationship Relationship in which variables or concepts that occur or exist together in the real world are identified; thus when one variable changes, the other changes. Hypotheses can be developed to identify associative relationships.

Assumptions Statements taken for granted or considered true, even though they have not been scientifically tested.

Asymmetrical relationship Relationship in which the following are true: if A occurs or changes, then B will occur or change; but if B occurs or changes, A will not necessarily occur or change (A → B).

Auditability Rigorous development of a decision trail that can be applied by a second researcher to the original data. This process is done to determine if the second researcher's conclusions are similar to those of the original researcher.

Authority Person with expertise and power who is able to influence the opinions and behavior of others.

Autonomous agents Prospective subjects who are informed about a proposed study and who can voluntarily choose whether to participate.

Basic (pure) research Scientific investigations for the pursuit of "knowledge for knowledge's sake" or for the pleasure of learning and finding truth.

Benchmark Identified standard an agency wants to achieve in the provision of health care, such as having a 1% complication rate for intramuscular injections.

Benchmarking Process of measuring outcomes from a health care agency for comparison with identified national standards.

Beneficence, principle of Principle that encourages the researcher to do good and "above all, do no harm."

Benefit-risk ratio Ratio considered by researchers and reviewers of research as they weigh potential benefits (positive outcomes) and risks (negative outcomes) of a study; used to promote the conduct of ethical research.

Between-group variance A source of variation of the group means around the grand mean.

Bias Influence or action in a study that distorts the findings or slants them away from the true or expected.

Bibliographical database Compilation of citations.

Bibliography List of publications for a specific topic or specialty area.

Bivariate analysis Statistical procedure in which the summary values from either two groups of the same variable or two variables within a group are compared.

Bivariate correlation Measure of the extent of the linear relationship between two variables.

Blocking System used in randomized block design in which subjects with various levels of an extraneous variable are included in the sample. The number of subjects are controlled at each level of the variable and are randomly assigned to groups within the study.

Body of knowledge Information, principles, and theories that are organized by the beliefs accepted in a discipline at a given time.

Borrowing Appropriation and use of knowledge from other disciplines to guide nursing practice.

Box-and-whisker plots Exploratory data analysis technique to provide fast visualization of some of the major characteristics of the data, such as the spread, symmetry, and identity of outliers.

Bracketing Qualitative research technique of suspending or setting aside what is known about an experience being studied.

Breach of confidentiality Accidental or direct action that allows an unauthorized person to have access to raw study data.

Byte Computer space for storing a single character, such as a number or a letter of the alphabet.

Canonical correlation Extension of multiple regression with more than one dependent variable.

Carryover effect Outcome observed when application of one treatment influences the response to subsequent treatments.

Case study In-depth analysis and systematic description of one patient or a group of similar patients to promote understanding of nursing interventions.

Case study design Intensive exploration of a single unit of study, such as a person, family, group, community, or institution.

Causal hypothesis Hypothesis that states the relationship between two variables, in which one variable (independent variable) is thought to cause or determine the presence of the other variable (dependent variable).

Causality Relationship that includes three conditions: (1) there must be a strong correlation between the proposed cause and effect, (2) the proposed cause must precede the effect in time, and (3) the cause must be present whenever the effect occurs.

Cell Intersection between the row and column in a table where a specific numerical value is inserted.

Central processing unit (CPU) Device that controls computer operations and includes the internal memory, control unit, and arithmetic and logic unit.

Centralized diffusion system System that involves group decision making within an organization; usually includes a change agent to promote utilization of research-based innovations.

Change agent A professional outside a social system who enters the system to promote adoption of a research-based innovation.

Chi-square test of independence Used to analyze nominal data to determine significant differences between observed frequencies within the data and frequencies that were expected.

Citation Information necessary to locate a reference. Citation for a journal article includes the author's name, year of publication, title, journal name, volume number, issue number, and page numbers.

Cleaning data Checking raw data to determine errors in data recording, coding, or entry.

Clinical pathway Method used in health care that organizes, implements, and evaluates a comprehensive plan of care for a patient. Agencies develop clinical pathways to facilitate the implementation of quality cost-effective care.

Clinical significance Importance (significance) of research findings in answering a clinical question or solving a clinical problem.

Cluster sampling Sampling in which a frame is developed that includes a list of all the states, cities, institutions, or organizations (clusters) that could be used in a study; a randomized sample is drawn from this list.

Cochran Q test Nonparametric test that is an extension of the McNemar test for two related samples.

Code Symbol or abbreviation used to classify words or phrases in qualitative data.

Codebook Record that documents the location or the column(s) that represent each variable and other information entered in a computer file.

Coding Way of indexing or identifying categories in qualitative data.

Coercion Overt threat of harm or excessive reward intentionally presented by one person to another in order to obtain compliance; an example is offering prospective subjects a large sum of money to participate in a dangerous research project.

Cognitive application of research Process in which research-based knowledge is used to affect a person's way of thinking, approaching, or observing situations.

Cognitive clustering Comprehensive, scholarly synthesis of scientifically sound research that is evident in integrative reviews of research and meta-analyses.

Cohorts Samples in time-dimensional studies within the field of epidemiology.

Coinvestigators Two or more professionals conducting a study, whose salaries may be paid partially or in full by grant funding.

Communication of research findings Developing a research report and disseminating it to a variety of audiences with presentations and publications.

Comparative descriptive design Design used to describe differences in variables in two or more groups in a natural setting.

Comparison group The group of subjects in a study not receiving a treatment when non-random methods are used for sample selection.

Comparison phase Phase or step of a critique in which the reader compares the ideal for each step of the research process with the real steps in a study.

Compatibility Degree to which an innovation is perceived to be consistent with current values, past experience, and priority of needs.

Complete observer Researcher who is passive and has no direct social interaction in the setting.

Complete participation Situation in which the researcher becomes a member of the group and conceals the researcher role.

Complete review Type of institutional review process for studies with risks that are greater than minimal. The review of a study is extensive or complete by an institutional review board.

Complex hypothesis Hypothesis that predicts the relationship (associative or causal) among three or more variables; thus the hypothesis can include two (or more) independent and/or two (or more) dependent variables.

Complex search Search that combines two or more concepts or synonyms in one search. The concepts selected for search may be based on the results of previous searches.

Complexity Degree to which an innovation is perceived to be difficult to understand or use.

Comprehending research reports Critical thinking process used in reading a research report, in which the focus is on understanding the major concepts and the logical flow of ideas within a study.

Comprehension phase Step of a critique during which the reader gains understanding of the terms in a research report; identifies the study elements; and grasps the nature, significance, and meaning of these elements.

Computer search Process of using computer databases to scan literature citations and identify sources relevant to a selected topic.

Computerized database Structured compilation of information that can be scanned, retrieved, and analyzed by computer and can be used for decisions, reports, and research.

Concept Term that abstractly describes and names an object or phenomenon, thus providing it with a separate identity or meaning.

Concept analysis Strategy used to identify a set of attributes or characteristics that are essential to the connotative meaning or conceptual definition of a concept.

Concept derivation Process of extracting and defining concepts from theories in other disciplines.

Concept synthesis Process of describing and naming a previously unrecognized concept.

Conceptual clustering step of critique Step in which current knowledge in an area of study is carefully analyzed, summarized, and organized theoretically to maximize the meaning attached to research findings, highlight gaps in the knowledge base, generate research questions, and provide knowledge for use in practice.

Conceptual definition Definition that provides a variable or concept with connotative (abstract, comprehensive, theoretical) meaning; established through concept analysis, concept derivation, or concept synthesis.

Conceptual map Strategy for expressing a framework of a study that diagrammatically shows the interrelationships of concepts and statements.

Conceptual model Set of highly abstract, related constructs that broadly explains phenomena of interest, expresses assumptions, and reflects a philosophical stance.

Conclusions Syntheses and clarifications of the meanings of study findings.

Concrete thinking Thinking that is oriented to and limited by tangible things or events observed and experienced in reality.

Concurrent relationship Relationship in which variables or concepts occur simultaneously.

Concurrent replication Simultaneous collection of data for both the original and replication study; the replication study provides a check of the reliability of the original study findings.

Confidence interval Range in which the value of the parameter is estimated to exist.

Confidentiality Management of private data in research in such a way that only the researcher knows the subjects' identities and can link them with their responses.

Confirmation stage Stage in Rogers's theory of research utilization in which nurses evaluate the effectiveness of the change in practice and decide whether to continue the change.

Confirmatory analysis Analysis performed to confirm expectations regarding data that are expressed as hypotheses, questions, or objectives.

Confounding variables Variables that cannot be controlled; they may be recognized before the study is initiated or not until the study is in process.

Consent form Written form, tape recording, or videotape used to document a subject's agreement to participate in a study.

Constant comparison Methodological technique in grounded theory research in which every piece of data is compared with every other piece.

Construct validity Measure of how well the conceptual and operational definitions of variables match each other; determine whether the instrument measures the theoretical construct it purports to measure.

Constructs Concepts at very high levels of abstraction that have general meanings.

Consultants People hired for specific tasks during a study.

Content analysis Qualitative analysis technique used to classify words in a text into a few categories that were chosen for their theoretical importance.

Content-related validity Extent to which the method of measurement includes all the major elements relevant to the construct being measured.

Contingency tables Cross-tabulation tables that allow visual comparison of summary data output related to two variables within a sample.

Contingent relationship Relationship that occurs only when a third variable or concept is present.

Continuance Decision to continue using an innovation and include the protocol in the procedure manual.

Control Writing of a prescription to produce the desired outcomes in practice. In research, the imposing of rules by the researcher to decrease the possibility of error and increase the probability that the study's findings are an accurate reflection of reality.

Control group The group of elements or subjects not exposed to the experimental treatment in a study where the sample is randomly selected.

Convenience sampling Including subjects in the study because they happened to be in the right place at the right time; entering available subjects into the study until the desired sample size is reached. Also referred to as accidental sampling.

Correlation matrix Correlational results for a number of variables that are presented in table form.

Correlational analysis Statistical procedure conducted to determine the direction (positive or negative) and magnitude or strength ($+1$ to -1) of the relationship between two variables.

Correlational design A study design for examining the relationships between or among two or more variables in a single group, which can occur at several levels.

Correlational coefficient Statistical term used to indicate the degree of relationship between two variables; the coefficients range in value from $+1.00$ (perfect positive relationship) to 0.00 (no relationship) to -1.00 (perfect negative or inverse relationship).

Correlational research Systematic investigation of relationships between two or more variables to explain the nature of relationships in the world; does not examine cause and effect.

Covert data collection Data collection that occurs without subjects' knowledge or awareness.

Cramer's V Analysis technique for nominal data; a modification of phi for contingency tables.

Criterion-referenced testing Comparison of a subject's score with a criterion of achievement that includes the definitions of target behaviors. When the behaviors are mastered, the subject is considered proficient in these behaviors.

Critical analysis of studies Examination of the strengths, weaknesses, meaning, and significance of nursing studies using four steps: comprehension, comparison, analysis, and evaluation.

Critique Careful examination of all aspects of a study to judge its strengths, limitations, meaning, and significance.

Cross-sectional designs Designs used to examine groups of subjects in various stages of development simultaneously, with the intent of inferring trends over time.

Cultural immersion Strategy used in ethnographic research for gaining increased familiarity with aspects of a culture, such as language, sociocultural norms, and traditions.

Culture Way of life belonging to a designated group of people.

Current best evidence Includes clinical practice guidelines that are usually nationally developed by expert researchers, clinicians, and theorists in their areas of excellence.

Curvilinear relationship Relationship between two variables that varies with the relative values of the variables.

Data Information that is collected during a study.

Data analysis Techniques used to reduce, organize, and give meaning to data.

Data coding sheet Sheet for organizing and recording data for rapid entry into a computer.

Data collection Identification of subjects and the precise, systematic gathering of information (data) relevant to the research purpose or the specific objectives, questions, or hypotheses of a study.

Data storage and retrieval Process in which vast amounts of data collected for a study are stored, usually in a computer, and later retrieved for examination and analyses.

Data triangulation Collection of data from multiple sources in the same study.

Database *See* Computerized database.

Debriefing Complete disclosure of the study purpose and results at the end of a study.

Debugging Identifying and replacing errors in a computer program with accurate information.

Decentralized diffusion system System involving one-to-one communication and individual decisions regarding the use of research-based innovations.

Deception Misinforming subjects for research purposes. After a study is completed, subjects must be debriefed or informed of the true purpose and outcomes of a study so that areas of deception are clarified.

Decision stage Stage in Rogers's theory of research utilization in which nurse(s) either adopt(s) or reject(s) an innovation or change in practice.

Decision theory Theory based on assumptions associated with the theoretical normal curve; used in testing for differences between groups, with the expectation that all of the groups are members of the same population. The expectation is expressed as a null hypothesis, and the level of significance (alpha) is set before data collection.

Decision trail *See* Auditability.

Declaration of Helsinki Ethical code that distinguishes therapeutic from nontherapeutic research; based on the Nuremberg Code.

Deductive reasoning Reasoning from the general to the specific or from a general premise to a particular situation.

Degrees of freedom (df) The freedom of a score's value to vary, given the values of other existing scores and the established sum of these scores ($df = N - 1$).

Delphi technique Method of measuring the judgments of a group of experts for assessing priorities or making forecasts.

Demographic variables Characteristics or attributes of subjects that are collected to describe the sample.

Dependent groups Subjects or observations selected for data collection that are in some way related to the selection of other subjects or observations. For example, when subjects in the control group are matched for age or gender with the subjects in the experimental group, these groups are dependent groups.

Dependent variable The response, behavior, or outcome that is predicted or explained in research; changes in the dependent variable are presumed to be caused by the independent variable.

Description Identification of the characteristics of nursing phenomena; may also identify the relationships among these phenomena.

Descriptive codes Terms used to organize and classify qualitative data.

Descriptive correlational design Design used to describe variables and examine relationships that exist in a situation.

Descriptive design Design used to identify a phenomenon of interest, identify variables within the phenomenon, develop conceptual and operational definitions of variables, and describe variables.

Descriptive research Research that provides an accurate portrayal or account of characteristics of a particular individual, event, or group in real-life situations; research that is conducted to discover new meaning, describe what exists, determine the frequency with which something occurs, and categorize information.

Descriptive statistics Statistics that allow the researcher to organize the data in ways that give meaning and facilitate insight; examples are frequency distributions and measures of central tendency and dispersion.

Descriptive time dimensional designs Designs for examining sequences and patterns of change, growth, or trends over time.

Descriptive vividness Description of the site, subjects, experience of collecting data, and the researcher's thoughts during the qualitative research process. Information is presented clearly enough for the reader to have a sense of personally experiencing the event.

Design Blueprint for conducting a study; maximizes control over factors that could interfere with the validity of the findings.

Design validity Quality of the study design and the ability of the design to generate accurate findings. Types of design validity include statistical conclusion validity, internal validity, construct validity, and external validity.

Deterministic relationships Statements of what always occurs in a particular situation, such as a scientific law.

Developmental grant proposals Proposals written to obtain funding for the development of a new program in a discipline.

Dialectic reasoning Reasoning that involves a holistic perspective, in which the whole is greater than the sum of the parts; examining factors that are opposites and making sense of them by merging them into a single unit or idea greater than either alone.

Diary Record of events kept by a subject over time that is collected and analyzed by a researcher.

Difference scores Deviation scores obtained by subtracting the mean from each raw score; measure of dispersion.

Diffusion Process of communicating research findings (innovations) through various channels over time to the members of a discipline.

Diminished autonomy Condition of subjects whose ability to give informed consent voluntarily is decreased because of legal or mental incompetence, terminal illness, or confinement to an institution.

Direct application Use of an innovation exactly as it was developed.

Direct measures Concrete variables that can be measured objectively with a specific measurement strategy, such as using a scale to measure weight.

Directional hypothesis Hypothesis stating the specific nature of the interaction or relationship between two or more variables.

Discomfort and harm Phrase used to describe the degree of risk for a subject participating in a study. These levels of risk include no anticipated effects, temporary discomfort, unusual levels of temporary discomfort, risk of permanent damage, or certainty of permanent damage.

Discontinuance Decision to stop or discontinue the use of an innovation. Two types of discontinuance are disenchantment and replacement discontinuance.

Discriminant analysis Analysis that allows the researcher to identify characteristics associated with group membership and to predict group membership.

Disenchantment discontinuance Decision to discontinue the use of an innovation because the user is dissatisfied with its outcome.

Dissemination of research findings The diffusion or communication of research findings.

Dissertation An extensive, usually original research project that is completed by a doctoral student as part of the requirements for a doctoral degree.

Distribution The spread of scores in a sample; includes the frequency and range of scores in the sample.

Effect size The degree to which the phenomenon studied is present in the population or to which the null hypothesis is false.

Electronic journals Journals that are published and available on the Internet.

Electronic mail (e-mail) Computer networking system that allows a user to rapidly exchange messages, files, data, and research reports using satellite networks.

Element A person (subject), event, behavior, or any other single unit of a study.

Eligibility criteria *See* Sampling criteria.

Embodied The belief that the person is a self within a body.

Emic approach Anthropological research approach to studying behaviors from within a culture.

Empirical generalizations Statements that have been repeatedly tested through research and have not been disproven (scientific theories have empirical generalizations).

Empirical literature Relevant studies published in journals and books; also includes unpublished studies such as masters theses and doctorate dissertations.

Empirical world The world we experience through our senses; the concrete portion of our existence.

Environmental variables Types of extraneous variables composing the setting in which a study is conducted.

Equivalence Comparison of measurements made by two or more observers measuring the same event; referred to as interrater reliability.

Error in physiological measures Errors caused by environmental factors, variations in operation of equipment, machine instability and calibration, and misinterpreted electrical signals.

Error score Amount of random error in the measurement process.

Ethical inquiry Intellectual analysis of ethical problems related to obligation, rights, duty, right and wrong, conscience, choice, intention, and responsibility to obtain desirable, rational ends.

Ethical principles Principles of respect for persons, beneficence, and justice that are relevant to the conduct of research.

Ethnographic research Qualitative research methodology for investigating cultures. The research involves collection, description, and analysis of data to develop a theory of cultural behavior.

Ethnonursing research Type of research that emerged from Leininger's Theory of Transcultural Nursing; focuses mainly on observing and documenting interactions with people to determine how daily life conditions and patterns influence human care, health, and nursing care practices.

Etic approach Anthropological research approach to studying behavior from outside the culture and examining similarities and differences across cultures.

Evaluation phase Step of a critique in which the reader examines the meaning and significance of a study according to set criteria and compares it with previous studies conducted in the area.

Event partitioning designs Merger of the longitudinal and trend designs to increase sample size and avoid the effects of history on the validity of findings.

Event-time matrix Qualitative analysis technique for comparing events that occurred in different sites during particular time periods.

Evidence-based health-care system Incorporates health-care research evidence from a variety of disciplines, clinical expertise of the health-care providers, views of the patients and families, and the resources available to deliver health care.

Evidence-based practice (EBP) Careful and practical use of current best evidence from quantitative, qualitative, and outcomes research to guide health-care decisions. EBP is used to promote understanding of patients' and families' experiences with health and illness; implement effective nursing interventions; and provide quality, cost-effective care within the health-care system.

Exact replication Precise or exact duplication of the initial researcher's study to confirm the original findings.

Exclusion criteria Sampling criteria or characteristics that can cause a person or element to be excluded from the target population.

Exempt from review Designation given to studies that have no apparent risks for the research subjects and thus are designated as exempt by an institutional review board.

Existence statement Declaration that a given concept or relationship exists.

Expedited review Institutional review process for studies that have some risks, but the risks are minimal or no greater than those ordinarily encountered in daily life or during the performance of routine physical or psychological examinations.

Experiment Procedure in which subjects are randomized into groups, data are collected, and statistical analyses are conducted to "support" a premise.

Experimental design Design that provides the greatest amount of control possible in order to examine causality more closely.

Experimental group Group of subjects receiving the experimental treatment.

Experimental research Objective, systematic, controlled investigation to examine probability and causality among selected variables for the purpose of predicting and controlling phenomena.

Explained variance Variation in values that is explained by the relationship between the two variables.

Explanation Clarification of relationships among variables and identification of reasons why certain events occur.

Explanatory codes Codes that are developed late in the data collection process after theoretical ideas from the qualitative study have begun to emerge.

Explanatory effects matrix Qualitative analysis technique that can assist in answering such questions as why an outcome was achieved or what caused the outcome.

Exploratory analysis Examining the data descriptively to become as familiar as possible with it.

External criticism Method for determining the validity of source materials in historical research; involves knowing where, when, why, and by whom a document was written.

External storage device Equipment for permanently storing data and programs outside a computer.

External validity Extent to which study findings can be generalized beyond the sample used in the study.

Extraneous variables Variables that exist in all studies and can affect the measurement of study variables and the relationships among these variables.

Fabrication Process of making up results and recording or reporting them.

Face validity Verification that the instrument measures the content desired.

Factor Closely related variables that are grouped together.

Factor analysis Analysis that examines interrelationships among large numbers of variables and disentangles those relationships to identify clusters of variables that are most closely linked. Two types of factor analysis are exploratory and confirmatory.

Factorial analysis of variance Analysis technique that is mathematically a specialized version of multiple regression; various types of factorial ANOVAs have been developed to analyze data from specific experimental designs.

Falsification Manipulating research materials, equipment, or processes, or changing or omitting data or results such that the research is not accurately represented in the research record.

Fatigue effect Effect that occurs when a subject becomes tired or bored with a study.

Feasibility of a study Suitability of a study; determined by examining the time and money commitment; the researcher's expertise; availability of subjects, facility, and equipment; cooperation of others; and the study's ethical considerations.

Findings The translated and interpreted results from a study.

Focus groups Measurement strategy designed to obtain the participants' perceptions in focused areas in settings that are permissive and non-threatening in a qualitative study.

Foundational inquiry Research on the foundations for a science, such as studies that analyze the structure of a science and the process of thinking about and valuing certain phenomena held in common by the science. Debates related to quantitative and qualitative research methods emerged from foundational inquiries.

Framework Abstract, logical structure of meaning, such as a portion of a theory, that guides the development of the study, is tested in the study, and enables the researcher to link the findings to nursing's body of knowledge.

Fraudulent publications Publications that do not reflect what was actually done; indicated by documentation or testimony from coauthors.

Frequency distribution Statistical procedure that lists all possible measures of a variable and tallies each datum on the listing.

Friedman two-way analysis of variance by ranks Nonparametric test used with matched samples or in repeated measures.

Full-text databases Internet resource that provides full text and list of citations of journal articles for a specific topic.

Generalization Extension of the implications of the findings from the sample or situation that was studied to a larger population or situation.

Gestalt Organization of knowledge about a particular phenomenon into a cluster of linked ideas; the clustering and interrelatedness enhance the meaning of the ideas.

Grant Proposal developed to seek research funding from private or public institutions.

Grounded Theory that has its roots in the qualitative data from which it was derived.

Grounded theory research Inductive research technique based on symbolic interaction theory; conducted to discover the problems that exist in a social scene and the process that persons involved use to handle them; involves formulation, testing, and redevelopment of propositions until a theory is developed.

Grouped frequency distribution Means of grouping continuous measures of data into categories.

Hawthorne effect Psychological response in which subjects change their behavior simply because they are subjects in a study, not because of the research treatment.

Heterogeneous sample Degree to which subjects have a wide variety of characteristics, thus reducing the risk of bias in studies not using random sampling.

Heuristic relevance Standard for evaluating a qualitative study, in which the study's intuitive recognition, relationship to the existing body of knowledge, and applicability are examined.

Hierarchical statement set Specific proposition and a hypothesis or research question. If a conceptual model is included in the framework, the set may also include a general proposition.

Highly controlled setting Artificially constructed environment that is developed for the sole purpose of conducting research, such as a laboratory, research or experimental center, or test unit.

Historical research Narrative description or analysis of events that occurred in the remote or recent past.

History effect Event that is not related to the planned study but occurs during the time of the study and could influence the responses of subjects to the treatment.

Homogeneity in design Degree to which objects are similar or share a form of equivalence, such as limiting subjects to only one level of an extraneous variable to reduce its impact on the study findings.

Homogeneity in instruments The correlation of various items within an instrument or multiple item scale that is calculated using the Cronbach alpha coefficient.

Homoscedastic Term describing data that are evenly dispersed above and below the regression line, indicating a linear relationship on a scatter diagram (plot).

Human rights Claims and demands that have been justified in the eyes of an individual or by the consensus of a group of individuals and are protected in research.

Hypothesis Formal statement of the expected relationship between two or more variables in a specified population.

Implementation stage Stage in Rogers' theory of research utilization in which an individual or agency adopts a research-based change. The types of implementation include direct application, reinvention, and indirect effects.

Implications The meaning of research conclusions for the body of knowledge, theory, and practice.

Implicit framework Rudimentary ideas for the framework of a theory or portions of a theory expressed in an introduction or in a literature review in which linkages among variables found in previous studies are discussed.

Inclusion criteria Those sampling criteria or characteristics that the subject or element must possess to be considered part of the target population.

Incomplete disclosure Failure to fully inform subjects about the purpose of a study because that knowledge might alter the subjects' actions; subjects should be debriefed when the study is finished.

Independent groups Study groups chosen so that the selection of one subject is unrelated to the selection of other subjects. For example, if subjects are randomly assigned to a treatment group or a control group, the groups are independent.

Independent (treatment or experimental) variable Treatment or experimental activity that is manipulated or varied by the researcher to cause an effect on the dependent variable.

Index Library resource that can be used to identify journal articles and other publications relevant to a topic.

Indirect effects Use of research findings by citing them in clinical papers and textbooks and incorporating them to strengthen arguments.

Indirect measures Methods used with abstract concepts that are not measured directly; rather, indicators or attributes of the concepts are used to represent the abstraction and are measured in the study.

Inductive reasoning Reasoning from the specific to the general, in which particular instances are observed and then combined into a larger whole or general statement.

Inference Generalization from a specific case to a general truth, from a part to the whole, from the concrete to the abstract, or from the known to the unknown.

Inferential statistics Statistics designed to allow inference from a sample statistic to a population parameter; commonly used to test hypotheses of similarities and differences in subsets of the sample under study.

Informed consent Agreement by a prospective subject to participate voluntarily in a study after he or she has assimilated essential information about the study.

Inherent variability Variability in which a few random observations can be naturally expected in the data in the extreme ends of the tail.

Innovation Idea, practice, or object that is perceived as new by an individual, a nursing unit, an entire agency, or another decision-making unit.

Innovation-decision process Process that includes the steps of knowledge, persuasion, decision, implementation, and confirmation to promote diffusion or communication of research findings to members of a discipline.

Innovators Individuals who actively seek out new ideas.

Input device Device that enables the user to enter data and instructions into the computer system.

Institutional review Process of examining studies for ethical concerns by a committee of peers.

Instrument validity Extent to which an instrument reflects the abstract construct being examined.

Instrumentation Component of measurement in which specific rules are applied to develop a measurement device or instrument.

Integrative review of research Review conducted to identify, analyze, and synthesize the results from independent studies to determine the current knowledge (what is known and not known) in a particular area.

Intellectual research critique Careful examination of all aspects of a study to judge the strengths, weaknesses, meaning, and significance of the study based on previous research experience and knowledge of the topic.

Interlibrary loan department Department that locates books and articles in other libraries and provides the sources within a designated time.

Internal criticism Criticism involving examination of the reliability of historical documents.

Internal validity Extent to which the effects detected in a study reflect reality rather than resulting from the effects of extraneous variables.

Internet Worldwide network that connects computers together.

Interpretation of research outcomes Process in which researchers examine the results from data analysis, form conclusions, consider the implications for nursing, explore the significance of the findings, generalize the findings, and suggest further studies.

Interpretive codes Organizational system developed late in the process of collecting and analyzing qualitative data, as the researcher gains insight into the existing processes.

Interpretive reliability Extent to which each judge assigns the same category to a given unit of data.

Interrater reliability Degree of consistency between two raters who are independently assigning ratings to a variable or attribute being investigated; also referred to as equivalence.

Interrupted time series designs Designs similar to descriptive time dimensional designs, except that a treatment is applied at some point in the observations.

Interval estimate Range of values (identified by the researcher) on a number line where the population parameter is thought to be.

Interval-scale measurement Use of interval scales or methods of measurement with equal numerical distances between intervals of the scale; follows the rules of mutually exclusive categories, exhaustive categories, and rank ordering, such as temperature.

Intervention Treatment or independent variable that is manipulated during the conduct of a study to produce an effect on the dependent or outcome variables.

Interview Structured or unstructured oral communication between the researcher and subject, during which information is obtained for a study.

Introspection Process of turning one's attention inward toward one's own thoughts, providing increased awareness and understanding of the flow and interplay of feelings and ideas.

Intuiting Process of looking at the phenomenon in qualitative research; all awareness and energy are focused on the subject of interest.

Intuition Insight or understanding of a situation or an event as a whole that usually cannot be logically explained.

Intuitive recognition Theoretical schema derived from the data of a qualitative study that has meaning within an individual's personal knowledge base.

Invasion of privacy Sharing private information with others without an individual's knowledge or against his or her will.

Investigator triangulation Phenomenon that occurs when two or more research-trained investigators with divergent backgrounds explore the same phenomenon.

Justice, principle of Principle stating that human subjects should be treated fairly.

Kendall's tau Nonparametric test used to determine correlations among variables that have been measured at the ordinal level.

Keywords Major concepts or variables of a research problem or topic that are used to begin a search of a database.

Knowledge Information that is acquired in a variety of ways, is expected to be an accurate reflection of reality, and is incorporated and used to direct a person's actions.

Knowledge stage Stage of Rogers's theory of research utilization in which nurses become aware of an innovation or new idea for use in practice.

Kolmogorov-Smirnov two-sample test Nonparametric test used to determine whether two independent samples have been drawn from the same population.

Kurtosis Degree of peakedness (platykurtic, mesokurtic, or leptokurtic) of the curve that is related to the spread or variance of scores.

Lambda Analysis technique that measures the degree of association (or relationship) between two nominal-level variables.

Landmark studies Major projects generating knowledge that influence a discipline and sometimes society in general.

Level of significance *See* Alpha.

Levels of measurement Organized set of rules for assigning numbers to objects so that a hierarchy in measurement from low to high is established. The levels of measurement are nominal, ordinal, interval, and ratio.

Library resources Library personnel, interlibrary loan department, circulation department, reference department, audiovisual department, computer search department, and photocopy services.

Library sources Sources for research, including journals, books, monographs, master's theses, dissertations, government documents, and other publications of research findings.

Likert scale Instrument designed to determine the opinion on or attitude toward a subject; contains a number of declarative statements with a scale after each statement.

Limitations Theoretical and methodological restrictions in a study that may decrease the generalizability of the findings.

Line of best fit Best reflection of the values on the scatterplot.

Linear relationship Relationship between two variables or concepts that remain consistent regardless of the values of each variable or concept.

Linking Activity on the World Wide Web that moves you from one web site to another.

Literature review Summary of theoretical and empirical sources to generate a picture of what is known and not known about a particular problem.

Logic A science in which valid ways of relating ideas are used to promote human understanding; includes abstract and concrete thinking and logistic, inductive, and deductive reasoning.

Logistic reasoning Reasoning used to break the whole into parts that can be carefully examined, as can the relationships among the parts.

Longitudinal designs Research designs used to examine changes in the same subjects over an extended time period.

Mainframe computer Computer with the largest memory and greatest speed; used in universities and large companies.

Manipulation Moving around or controlling the movement of, as in the manipulation of a treatment.

Mann-Whitney U test Test used to analyze ordinal data (with 95% of the power of the *t*-test) to detect differences between groups of normally distributed populations.

Manual search Examination of catalogs, indexes, abstracts, and bibliographies for relevant sources.

Map *See* Conceptual map.

Matching Selecting subjects in the control group who are equivalent to subjects in the experimental group in important extraneous variables.

Maturation effect Unplanned and unrecognized changes subjects experience during a study, such as growing older, wiser, stronger, hungrier, or more tired, that can influence the findings of the study.

McNemar test Nonparametric test used to analyze the changes that occur in dichotomous variables.

Mean The value obtained by summing all the scores and dividing the total by the number of scores being summed.

Measurement Process of assigning numbers to objects, events, or situations in accord with some rule.

Measurement error Difference between what exists in reality and what is measured by a research instrument.

Measures of dispersion Statistical procedures (range, difference scores, sum of squares, variance, and standard deviation) for examining how scores vary or are dispersed around the mean.

Measures of central tendency Statistical procedures (mode, median, and mean) for determining the center of a distribution of scores.

Median Score at the exact center of the ungrouped frequency distribution.

Memoing Method that is used by researchers to record insights or ideas related to notes, transcripts, or codes during qualitative data analysis.

Mentor Individual who provides information, advice, and emotional support to a protégé.

Mentorship Intense form of role modeling in which an expert nurse serves as a teacher, sponsor, guide, exemplar, and counselor for a novice nurse.

Meta-analysis Performing statistical analyses to integrate and synthesize findings from completed studies to determine what is known and not known about a particular research area.

Methodological congruence Standard for evaluating qualitative research, in which documentation rigor, procedural rigor, ethical rigor, and auditability of the study are examined.

Methodological designs Designs used to develop the validity and reliability of instruments to measure research concepts and variables.

Methodological limitations Restrictions in the study design that limit the credibility of the findings and the population to which the findings can be generalized.

Methodological triangulation The use of two or more research methods or procedures in a study (such as different designs, instruments, and data collection procedures).

Minimal risk Research subject's risk of harm anticipated in the proposed study that is not greater, considering probability and magnitude, than that ordinarily encountered in daily life or during the performance of routine physical or psychological examinations.

Mixed results Study results that included both significant and nonsignificant findings.

Modal percentage Percentage appropriate for nominal data; indicates the relationship of the number of data scores represented by the mode to the total number of data scores.

Modality Characteristic of distributions; symmetrical distributions are usually unimodal.

Mode Numerical value or score that occurs with the greatest frequency in a distribution but does not necessarily indicate the center of the data set.

Model testing designs Designs used to test the accuracy of a hypothesized causal model or map.

Monographs Sources that are usually written once, such as books, booklets of conference proceedings, or pamphlets, and may be updated with a new edition.

Mono-method bias Bias that occurs when more than one measure of a variable is used in a study, but all measures use the same method of recording.

Mono-operation bias Bias that occurs when only one method of measurement is used to measure a construct or concept.

Mortality The number of subjects who drop out of a study before its completion, creating a threat to the internal validity of the study.

Multicausality Recognition that a number of interrelated variables can cause a particular effect.

Multicollinearity Phenomenon that occurs when the independent variables in a regression equation are strongly correlated.

Multimethod-multitrait technique Technique in which a variety of data collection methods are used, such as interview and observation; the same measurement methods are used for each concept.

Multiple regression Extension of simple linear regression; more than one independent variable is analyzed.

Multiple triangulation Use of two or more types of triangulation (theoretical, data, methodological, investigator, and analysis) in a study.

Multistage sampling Randomized selection that continues through several stages.

Multivariate analysis techniques Techniques used to analyze data from complex, multivariate research projects; they include multiple regression, factorial analysis of variance, analysis of covariance, factor analysis, discriminant analysis, canonical correlation, structural equation modeling, time series analysis, and survival analysis.

Natural (field) setting Field setting or uncontrolled, real-life situation examined in research.

Necessary relationship Relationship in which one variable or concept must occur for the second variable or concept to occur.

Negative relationship Relationship in which one variable or concept changes (its value increases or decreases), and the other variable or concept changes in the opposite direction.

Network (or snowball) sampling Snowballing technique that takes advantage of social networks and the fact that friends tend to have characteristics in common; subjects meeting the sample criteria are asked to assist in locating others with similar characteristics.

Networking Process of developing channels of communication among people with common interests.

Nominal-scale measurement Lowest level of measurement used when data can be organized into categories that are exclusive and exhaustive, but the categories cannot be compared, such as gender, race, marital status, and nursing diagnoses.

Nondirectional hypothesis Hypothesis that states that a relationship exists but does not predict the exact nature of the relationship.

Nonequivalent control group designs Designs in which the control group is not selected by random means, such as the one-group posttest-only design, the posttest-only design with nonequivalent groups, and the one-group pretest-posttest design.

Nonparametric statistics Statistical techniques used when the assumptions of parametric statistics are not met; most commonly used to analyze nominal and ordinal data.

Nonprobability sampling Sampling in which not every element of the population has an opportunity for selection, such as convenience sampling, quota sampling, purposive sampling, and network sampling.

Nonsignificant results Results that are negative or contrary to the researcher's hypotheses; the results may accurately reflect reality or may be caused by study weaknesses.

Nontherapeutic research Research conducted to generate knowledge for a discipline; the results might benefit future patients but will probably not benefit the research subjects.

Norm-referenced Term describing test performance standards that have been carefully developed over years with large, representative samples, using standardized tests with extensive reliability and validity.

Normal curve Symmetrical, unimodal, bell-shaped curve that is a theoretical distribution of all possible scores; no real distribution exactly fits the normal curve.

Null (statistical) hypothesis Hypothesis stating that no relationship exists between the variables being studied; a hypothesis used for statistical testing and for interpreting statistical outcomes.

Nuremberg code Ethical code of conduct to guide investigators in conducting research ethically.

Nursing process Subset of the problem-solving process. Steps include assessment, diagnosis, plan, implementation, evaluation, and modification.

Nursing research Scientific process that validates and refines existing knowledge and generates knowledge that directly and indirectly influences clinical nursing practice.

Observability Extent to which the results of an innovation are visible to others.

Observational measurement Use of structured and unstructured observation to measure study variables.

Observed score Score or value obtained for a subject on a measurement tool.

Observer-as-participant Researcher whose time is spent observing and interviewing subjects, with less time spent in the participant role.

One-tailed test of significance Analysis used with directional hypotheses, in which extreme statistical values of interest are thought to occur in a single tail of the curve.

Open context Condition that requires deconstructing a sedimented view, allowing one to see the depth and complexity within the phenomenon being examined in qualitative research.

Operational definition Description of how variables or concepts will be measured or manipulated in a study.

Operational reasoning Identification and discrimination of many alternatives or viewpoints; focuses on the process of debating alternatives.

Ordinal-scale measurement Measurement yielding data that can be ranked, but the intervals between the ranked data are not necessarily equal, such as levels of coping.

Outcomes research Important scientific methodology that was developed to examine the end results of patient care. The strategies used in outcomes research are a departure from the traditional scientific endeavors and incorporate evaluation research, epidemiology, and economic theory perspectives.

Outliers Extreme scores or values that occur because of inherent variability, errors of measurement or execution, or error in identifying the variables important in explaining the nature of the phenomenon under study.

Output devices Devices used to display, print, or store information generated from a computer.

Parallel forms reliability *See* Alternate forms reliability.

Parameter Measure or numerical value of a population.

Parametric statistical analyses Statistical techniques used when three assumptions are met: (1) the sample was drawn from a population for which the variance can be calculated, and the distribution is expected to be normal or approximately normal; (2) the level of measurement should be at least interval, with an approximately normal distribution; and (3) the data can be treated as random samples.

Paraphrasing Clearly and concisely restating the ideas of an author using your own words.

Partially controlled setting Environment that is manipulated or modified in some way by the researcher.

Participant observation Special form of observation in which researchers immerse themselves in the setting so that they can hear, see, and experience what the participants do; the participants are aware of the dual role of the researcher (participant and observer).

Passive rejection Decision not to adopt an innovation that was never seriously considered.

Pearson's product-moment correlation Parametric test used to determine relationships among variables.

Percentage distributions Percentage of the sample whose scores fall into a specific group and the number of scores in that group.

Periodicals Literature sources such as journals that are published over time and are numbered sequentially for the years published.

Personal experience Knowledge gained through participation in rather than observation of an event, situation, or circumstance. Benner (1984) described five levels of experience in the development of clinical knowledge and expertise: (1) novice, (2) advanced beginner, (3) competent, (4) proficient, and (5) expert.

Persuasion stage Stage of Rogers's theory of research utilization in which an individual or agency develops a favorable or unfavorable attitude toward the change or innovation to be used in practice.

Phenomenological research Inductive, descriptive qualitative methodology developed from phenomenological philosophy for the purpose of describing experiences as they are lived by the study participants.

Phenomenon (*plural:* phenomena) An occurrence or a circumstance that is observed, something that impresses the observer as extraordinary, or a thing that appears to and is constructed by the mind.

Phi coefficient Analysis technique used to determine relationships in dichotomous, nominal data.

Philosophical analysis Use of concept or linguistic analyses to examine meaning and develop theories of meaning in philosophical inquiry.

Philosophical inquiry Research using intellectual analyses to clarify meanings, make values manifest, identify ethics, and study the nature of knowledge. Types of philosophical inquiry include foundational inquiry, philosophical analyses, and ethical analyses.

Philosophical stance Specific philosophical view held by a person or group of individuals.

Philosophies Rational, intellectual explorations of truths, principles of being, knowledge, or conduct.

Physiological measurement Techniques used to measure physiological variables either directly or indirectly; examples are techniques to measure heart rate or mean arterial pressure.

Pilot study Smaller version of a proposed study conducted to develop and refine the methodology, such as the treatment, instruments, or data collection process to be used in the larger study.

Pink sheet Letter rejecting a research grant proposal, with a critique by the scientific committee that reviewed the proposal.

Plagiarism Appropriation of another person's ideas, processes, results or words without giving appropriate credit, including those obtained through confidential review of others' research proposals and manuscripts.

Point estimate Single figure that estimates a related figure in the population of interest.

Population All elements (individuals, objects, events, or substances) that meet the sample criteria for inclusion in a study; sometimes referred to as a target population.

Positive relationship Relationship in which one variable changes (its value increases or decreases) and the second variable changes in the same direction.

Poster session Visual presentation of a study, with text, tables, and illustrations on a display board.

Posthoc analyses Statistical techniques performed in studies with more than two groups to determine which groups are significantly different. For example, ANOVA might indicate significant differences among three groups, but the post hoc analyses indicate specifically which groups are different.

Power Probability that a statistical test will detect a significant difference or relationship that exists; power analysis is used to determine the power of a study.

Power analysis Technique used to determine the risk of a Type II error so that the study can be modified to decrease the risk if necessary.

Practice effect Effect that occurs when subjects improve as they become more familiar with the experimental protocol.

Precision Accuracy with which the population parameters have been estimated within a study; also used to describe the degree of consistency or reproducibility of measurements with physiologic instruments.

Prediction Estimation of the probability of a specific outcome in a given situation that can be achieved through research.

Prediction equation Outcome of regression analysis.

Predictive correlational design Design developed to predict the value of one variable based on values obtained for other variables; an approach to examining causal relationships between variables.

Premise Proposition or statement of the proposed relationship between two or more concepts.

Preproposal Short document (generally four pages plus appendices) written to explore the funding possibilities for a research project.

Primary source Source whose author originated or is responsible for generating the ideas published.

Principal investigator Individual who will have primary responsibility for administering a research grant and interacting with the funding agency.

Privacy Freedom of an individual to determine the time, extent, and general circumstances under which private information will be shared with or withheld from others.

Probability Chance that a given event will occur in a situation; addresses the relative rather than the absolute causality of events.

Probability sampling Random sampling technique in which every member (element) of the population has a probability higher than zero of being selected for the sample; examples include simple random sampling, stratified random sampling, cluster sampling, and systematic sampling.

Probability statement Statement expressing the likelihood that something will happen in a given situation; addresses relative rather than absolute causality.

Probability theory Theory addressing statistical analysis from the perspective of the extent of a relationship or the probability of accurately predicting an event.

Problematic reasoning Reasoning that involves identifying a problem, selecting solutions to the problem, and resolving the problem.

Problem-solving process Systematic identification of a problem, determination of goals related to the problem, identification of possible approaches to achieve those goals, implementation of selected approaches, and evaluation of goal achievement.

Process Purpose, series of actions, and goal.

Process-outcome matrix Qualitative analysis technique that allows the researcher to trace the processes that led to differing outcomes.

Projective techniques Techniques for measuring individuals' responses to unstructured or ambiguous situations as a means of describing attitudes, personality characteristics, and motives of the individuals (e.g., the Rorschach inkblot test).

Proposition Abstract statement that further clarifies the relationship between two concepts.

Public library Library that serves the needs of the community in which it is located; usually contains few research reports.

Purposive sampling Judgmental or selective sampling that involves the conscious selection by the researcher of certain subjects or elements to include in a study. This sampling strategy is most frequently used in qualitative research.

Q-plots Exploratory data analysis technique in which the scores or data are displayed in a distribution by quartile.

Q-sort Technique for comparative rating, in which a subject sorts cards with statements into designated piles (usually 7 to 10 piles in the distribution of a normal curve) that might range from best to worst.

Qualitative research Systematic, subjective approach used to describe life experiences and give them meaning.

Quantitative research Formal, objective, systematic process used to describe, test relationships, and examine cause-and-effect interactions among variables.

Quantitative research process Conceptualizing, planning, implementing, and communicating the findings of a research project.

Quasi-experimental research Type of quantitative research conducted to explain relationships, clarify why certain events happen, and examine causality between selected independent and dependent variables.

Query letter Letter sent to a journal editor to determine interest in publishing an article or to a funding agency to determine interest in providing funds for a study.

Questionnaire Printed self-report form designed to elicit information that can be obtained through written or verbal responses of the subject.

Quota sampling Convenience sampling technique with an added strategy to ensure the inclusion of subjects who are likely to be underrepresented in the convenience sample, such as women, minority groups, and undereducated persons.

Random assignment Procedure used to assign subjects randomly to treatment or control groups; subjects have an equal probability of being assigned to either group.

Random error Error that causes individuals' observed scores to vary haphazardly around their true scores.

Random sampling Technique in which every member (element) of the population has a probability higher than zero for being selected for a sample, which increases the sample's representativeness of the target population.

Random variation The expected difference in values that occurs when one examines different subjects from the same sample.

Range Simplest measure of dispersion; obtained by subtracting the lowest score from the highest score.

Rating scale Scale that lists an ordered series of categories of a variable and is assumed to be based on an underlying continuum.

Ratio-scale measurement Highest measurement form; meets all the rules of other forms of measure: mutually exclusive categories, exhaustive categories, rank ordering, equal spacing between intervals, a continuum of values, and an absolute zero. An example is measurement of weight.

Reading research reports Process used to learn about research studies; skills used include skimming, comprehending, and analyzing the content of the report.

Reasoning Processing and organizing ideas to reach conclusions; types of reasoning include problematic, operational, dialectic, and logistic.

Refereed journal Journal that uses referees or expert reviewers to determine whether a manuscript will be accepted for publication.

Referencing Comparing a subject's score against a standard; used in norm-referenced and criterion-referenced testing.

Reflexive thought Process in which a qualitative researcher explores personal feelings and experiences that may influence the study and integrates this understanding into the study.

Refusal rate The percentage of subjects that declined to participate in the study. The study should include their rationale for not participating.

Regression analysis Statistical procedure used to predict the value of one variable using known values of one or more other variables.

Regression line The line that best represents the values of the raw scores plotted on a scatter diagram; the procedure for developing the line of best fit is the method of least squares.

Reinvention Modification of an innovation by its adopters to meet their own needs.

Rejection Decision not to use an innovation; can be active or passive. *See* Active rejection, Passive rejection.

Relational statement Declaration that a relationship of some kind exists between two or more concepts.

Relative advantage Extent to which an innovation is perceived to be better than current practice.

Relevant studies Sources that are pertinent or highly important in providing the in-depth knowledge needed to make changes in practice or to study a selected problem.

Reliability Extent to which an instrument consistently measures a concept; three types of reliability are stability, equivalence, and homogeneity.

Reliability testing Measure of the amount of random error in the measurement technique.

Replacement discontinuance Decision to discontinue the use of an innovation in order to adopt a better idea.

Replication studies Studies that are reproduced or repeated to determine whether similar findings will be obtained.

Representative sample Sample that is like the population it is supposed to represent in as many ways as possible.

Representativeness Degree to which the sample, accessible population, and target population are alike.

Research Diligent, systematic inquiry or investigation to validate and refine existing knowledge and generate new knowledge.

Research-based protocol Document providing clearly developed steps for implementing a treatment or intervention in practice that is based on findings from studies.

Research design Blueprint for conducting a study; maximizes control over factors that could interfere with the validity of the findings; guides the planning and implementation of a study in a way that is most likely to achieve the intended goal.

Research hypothesis Alternative hypothesis to the null hypothesis; states that a relationship exists between two or more variables.

Research misconduct Fabrication, falsification, or plagiarism in proposing, performing, or reviewing research, or in reporting research results.

Research objective Clear, concise, declarative statement expressed to direct a study; focuses on identifying and describing variables and relationships among variables.

Research outcomes Conclusions of findings, generalization of findings, implications of findings for nursing, and suggestions for further study presented in the discussion section of the research report.

Research problem An area of concern in which there is a gap in the knowledge base needed for nursing practice. Research is conducted to generate essential knowledge to address the practice concern, with the ultimate goal of providing evidence-based practice.

Research process Process that requires an understanding of a unique language and involves rigorous application of a variety of research methods.

Research proposal Written plan that identifies the major elements of a study, such as the problem, purpose, and framework, and outlines the methods that will be used to conduct the study.

Research purpose Concise, clear statement of the specific goal or aim of the study. The purpose is generated from the problem.

Research question Concise interrogative statement developed to direct a study; focuses on describing variables, examining relationships among variables, and determining the differences between two or more groups.

Research report Report summarizing the major elements of a study and identifying the contributions of that study to nursing knowledge.

Research topic Concept or broad problem area that provides the basis for generating numerous questions and research problems.

Research utilization Process of communicating and using empirical or research-generated knowledge to affect or change the existing practices in the health-care system.

Research variables or concepts The qualities, properties, or characteristics identified in the research purpose and objectives that are observed or measured in a study.

Researcher-participant relationships Relationships between the researcher and the individuals being studied in qualitative research.

Respect for persons, principle of Principle indicating that persons have the right to self-determination and the freedom to participate or not participate in research.

Results Outcomes from data analysis that are generated for each research objective, question, or hypothesis; results can be mixed, nonsignificant, significant and not predicted, significant and predicted, or unexpected.

Review of literature Summary of current theoretical and empirical sources to generate a picture of what is known and not known about a particular problem.

Review of relevant research literature Review of current studies conducted to generate what is known and not known about a problem and to determine whether the knowledge is ready for use in practice.

Rigor Excellence in research; attained through the use of discipline, scrupulous adherence to detail, and strict accuracy.

Robust Term describing an analysis procedure that will yield accurate results even if some of the assumptions are violated by the data being analyzed.

Rogers's Theory of Research Utilization Theory to direct the use of research findings in practice; includes the stages of knowledge, persuasion, decision, implementation, and confirmation.

Role modeling Process of teaching less-experienced professionals by demonstrating model behavior.

Sample Subset of the population that is selected for a study.

Sample characteristics Demographic data analyzed to provide a picture of the sample.

Sample mortality Number of subjects who withdrew from or who are lost during a study.

Sample size Number of subjects, events, behaviors, or situations that are examined in a study.

Sampling Process of selecting a group of people, events, behaviors, or other elements that are representative of the population being studied.

Sampling criteria List of the characteristics essential for inclusion or exclusion in the target population.

Sampling distribution Table of statistical values (such as the mean) of many samples obtained from the same population.

Sampling error Difference between a sample statistic used to estimate a parameter and the actual but unknown value of the parameter.

Sampling frame List of every member of the population; the sampling criteria are used to define membership in the population.

Sampling method Strategies used to obtain a sample, including probability and nonprobability sampling techniques; also called a sampling plan.

Sampling plan Process for making selections of subjects for inclusion in a study.

Saturation of data Phenomenon that occurs when additional sampling provides no new information, or there is redundancy of previously collected data. Sample size in a qualitative study is determined when saturation of data occurs.

Scale Self-report form of measurement composed of several items thought to measure the construct being studied; the subject responds to each item on the continuum or scale provided.

Scatterplot Diagram or figure used to illustrate the dispersion of scores on a variable or to illustrate the relationship of scores on one variable with scores on another variable. A scatterplot has two scales, horizontal (X-axis) and vertical (Y-axis).

Science Coherent body of knowledge composed of research findings, tested theories, scientific principles, and laws for a discipline.

Scientific community Cohesive group of scholars within a discipline who create new research ideas and develop innovative methodologies to conduct research.

Scientific method All procedures that scientists have used, currently use, or may use in the future to pursue knowledge; examples include quantitative research, qualitative research, outcomes research, and triangulation.

Scientific misconduct Practices such as fabrication, falsification, or forging of data; dishonest manipulation of the study design or methods; and plagiarism.

Scientific theory Theory that has been repeatedly tested through research with valid and reliable methods of measuring each concept and relational statement.

Search field Areas of research topics that are searched to identify relevant sources.

Secondary analysis design Design for studying data previously collected in another study; data are reexamined using different organizations of the data and different statistical analyses.

Secondary source Source whose author summarizes or quotes content from primary sources.

Sedimented view View from the perspective of a specific frame of reference, world view, or theory that gives a sense of certainty, security, and control.

Seeking approval to conduct a study Submitting a research proposal to a selected group for review and often verbally defending that proposal.

Selectivity of a physiological instrument Assessment of the accuracy of an instrument; the ability of the instrument to identify correctly the signal under study and to distinguish it from other signals.

Semantic differential scale Two opposite adjectives with a seven-point scale between them; the subject selects a point on the scale that best describes his or her view of the concept being examined.

Sensitivity of physiological measures Amount of change of a parameter that can be measured precisely.

Serendipity Accidental discovery of something valuable or useful during the conduct of a study.

Setting Location for conducting research; can be natural, partially controlled, or highly controlled.

Significant results Results that agree with those identified by the researcher.

Simple hypothesis Hypothesis stating the relationship (associative or causal) between two variables.

Simple linear regression Parametric analysis technique that estimates the value of a dependent variable based on the value of an independent variable.

Simple random sampling Random selection of elements from the sampling frame for inclusion in a study.

Situated Belief that the person is shaped by the language, culture, history, purposes, and values of his or her world and is constrained by that shaping in the ability to establish meanings.

Skewness Absence of symmetry in the curve formed by the distribution of scores; distribution can be positively or negatively skewed.

Skimming research reports Quickly reviewing a source to gain a broad overview of the content by reading the title, the author's name, the abstract or introduction, headings, one or two sentences under each heading, and the discussion section.

Social system Set of interrelated individuals (e.g., the nurses on a specific hospital unit, in one hospital, or in a corporation of hospitals) engaged in joint problem solving to accomplish a common goal or outcome.

Special library Library that contains a collection of material on a specific topic or specialty area.

Split-half reliability Technique used to determine the homogeneity of an instrument's items, in which the items are split in half and a correlational procedure is performed between the two halves.

Stability Type of measurement reliability that is concerned with the consistency of repeated measures; usually referred to as test-retest reliability.

Standard deviation Measure of dispersion that is calculated by taking the square root of the variance.

Standardized scores Scores used to express deviations from the mean (difference scores) in terms of standard deviation units, such as Z-scores, in which the mean is 0 and the standard deviation is 1.

Statements Express claims that are important to a theory; theories include existence and relational statements.

Statistic Numerical value obtained from a sample; it is used to estimate the parameters of a population.

Statistical conclusion validity Extent to which the conclusions about relationships and differences drawn from statistical analyses reflect reality.

Statistical regression Movement or regression of extreme scores toward the mean in studies using a pretest-posttest design.

Statistical significance Extent to which the results are probably not due to chance.

Stem-and-leaf displays Type of exploratory data analysis in which scores are visually presented to obtain insights.

Story Time-bound event shared orally with others.

Storytakers People who listen to a story.

Storytellers People who share a story.

Storytelling Process used to share stories.

Stratification Design strategy used to distribute subjects evenly throughout the sample.

Stratified random sampling Technique used when the researcher knows some of the variables in the population that are critical to achieving representativeness; the sample is divided into strata or groups using these identified variables.

Structural equation modeling Analysis technique designed to test theories.

Structured interview Interview in which strategies are used that give the researcher increasing control over the content. An example is a questionnaire with structured responses.

Structured observation Clear identification of what is to be observed and precise definition of how the observations are to be made, recorded, and coded.

Subjects Individuals participating in a study (those being studied).

Substantive theory Theory recognized within a discipline as useful for explaining important phenomena.

Substitutable relationship Relationship in which a similar concept can be substituted for the first concept and the second concept will occur.

Sufficient relationship Relationship in which, when the first variable or concept occurs, the second will occur, regardless of the presence or absence of other factors.

Summary statistics *See* Descriptive statistics.

Surfing the Web Following the links (underlined or highlighted name) on one Web site to reveal other Web sites.

Survey design Design used to describe a phenomenon by collecting data using questionnaires or personal interviews.

Survival analysis Set of techniques designed to analyze repeated measures from a given time (e.g., beginning of the study, onset of a disease, beginning of a treatment) until a certain attribute (e.g., death, treatment failure, recurrence of the phenomenon) occurs.

Symbolic interaction theory Explores how people define reality and how their beliefs are related to their actions.

Symmetrical relationship Relationship in which, if A occurs or changes, B will occur or change, and if B occurs or changes, A will occur or change (A ⟷ B).

Symmetry plot Exploratory data analysis technique designed to determine the presence of skewness in the data.

Synthesis of sources Clustering and interrelating ideas from several sources to form a gestalt or a new, complete picture of what is known and not known in an area.

Systematic bias Phenomenon that occurs when the selected subjects' measurement values vary in some way from those of the population.

Systematic error Measurement error that is not random but occurs consistently in the same direction, such as a scale that inaccurately weighs subjects 3 pounds heavier than their actual weight.

Systematic extension replication Constructive replication performed under distinctly new conditions, in which the researchers conducting the replication do not follow the design or methods of the original researchers; rather, the second investigative team begins with a similar problem statement but formulates new means to verify the first investigator's findings.

Systematic sampling Selecting every kth individual from an ordered list of all members of a population, using a randomly selected starting point.

Systematic variation *See* Systematic bias.

Tails Extremes of the normal curve, on which the significant statistical values fall.

Target population Population determined by the sampling criteria.

Tendency statement Deterministic relationship that describes what always happens if there are no interfering conditions.

Tentative theory Theory that is newly proposed, has had minimal exposure to critique by scholars in the discipline, and has had little testing.

Testable hypothesis Hypothesis containing variables that can be measured or manipulated in the real world.

Test-retest reliability Determination of the stability or consistency of a measurement technique by correlating the scores obtained from repeated measures.

Theoretical connectedness Theoretical schema developed from a qualitative study; is clearly expressed, logically consistent, reflective of the data, and compatible with nursing's knowledge base.

Theoretical limitations Weaknesses in the study framework and conceptual and operational definitions that restrict the abstract generalization of the findings.

Theoretical literature Concept analyses, maps, theories, and conceptual frameworks that support a selected research problem and purpose.

Theoretical triangulation Use of two or more frameworks or theoretical perspectives in the same study; the hypotheses are developed based on the different theoretical perspectives and are tested using the same data set.

Theory Integrated set of defined concepts, existence statements, and relational statements that present a view of a phenomenon and can be used to describe, explain, predict, and control that phenomenon.

Therapeutic research Research that provides a patient with an opportunity to receive an experimental treatment that might have beneficial results.

Thesis Research project completed by a student as part of the requirements for a master's degree

Time-dimensional designs Designs used to examine the sequence and patterns of change, growth, or trends across time.

Time lag Time span between the generation of new knowledge through research and the use of this knowledge in practice.

Time-series analysis Technique designed to analyze changes in a variable across time and thus uncover patterns in the data.

Traditions Truths or beliefs that are based on customs and past trends.

Trend designs Designs used to examine changes in the general population in relation to a particular phenomenon.

Trial and error Approach with unknown outcomes used in an uncertain situation when other sources of knowledge are unavailable.

Trialability Extent to which the results of an individual or agency allow an idea to be tried out on a limited basis, with the option of returning to previous practices.

Triangulation Use of two or more theories, methods, data sources, investigators, or analysis methods in a study.

True score Score that would be obtained if no measurement error occurred (but there is always some measurement error).

t-Test Parametric analysis technique used to determine significant differences between measures of two samples.

Two-tailed test of significance Analysis technique used for a nondirectional hypothesis when the researcher assumes that an extreme score can occur in either tail of the normal curve.

Type I error Error that occurs when the researcher concludes that the samples tested are from different populations (a significant difference exists between groups) when, in fact, the samples are from the same population (no significant difference exists between groups); the null hypothesis is rejected when it is true.

Type II error Error that occurs when the researcher concludes that no significant difference exists between the samples examined when, in fact, a difference exists; the null hypothesis is regarded as true when it is false.

Unexpected results Study results that indicate relationships between variables or differences among groups that were not hypothesized and not predicted from the framework being used.

Unexplained variance Part of the variation between or among two or more variables that is the result of things other than the relationship.

Ungrouped frequency distribution Means of identifying and displaying all numerical values obtained for a particular variable from the subjects studied.

Unitizing reliability Extent to which each judge (data collector, coder, researcher) consistently identifies the same units within the data as appropriate for coding.

Ungrouped frequency distribution Categorical data in the form of a table that is developed to display all numerical values obtained for a particular variable.

Unpredicted significant results Results opposite those predicted, which indicate flaws in the logic of both the researcher and the theory being tested. However, if results are accurate, they are an important addition to the body of knowledge.

Unstructured interview Interview that is initiated with a broad question; subjects are usually encouraged to elaborate further on particular dimensions of a topic and often control the content of the interview.

Unstructured observations Spontaneous observation and recording of what is seen; planning is minimal.

Utilization of research findings Use of knowledge generated through research to guide nursing practice.

Validity Extent to which an instrument accurately reflects the abstract construct (or concept) being examined.

Variables Qualities, properties, or characteristics of persons, things, or situations that change or vary and are manipulated or measured in research.

Variance Measure of dispersion, where the larger the variance, the larger the dispersion of scores. Variance is calculated as one of the steps in determining standard deviation.

Virus, computer Program developed to alter and destroy information stored in a computer.

Visual analogue scale A 100-mm line, with right angle stops at either end, on which subjects are asked to record their response to a study variable.

Voluntary consent Decision made by a prospective subject, of his or her own volition, without coercion or any undue influence, to participate in a research study.

Wald-Wolfowitz runs test Nonparametric analysis technique used to determine differences between two populations.

Wilcoxon matched-pairs signed-ranks test Nonparametric analysis of changes that occur in pretest-posttest measures or matched-pairs measures.

Within-group variance Source of variation that reflects the individual scores in a group that vary from the group mean.

World Wide Web (WWW) An information service for access to the Internet resources by content rather than file names.

Z-score Standardized score of the normal curve that is equivalent to the standard deviation of the normal curve.

Index

Page references followed by "f" denote figures;
those followed by "t" denote tables.

C

Care plans
and control, 6
Caring
defining concept of, 141
Case studies
definition of, 9
glossary definition of, 475
phenomenological research, 361-363
on quantitative research critique
process, 409-418
of quasi-experimental studies, 58-65
in research design, 204-206
Categories
of data, 268-269
Causal analyses, 332
Causal hypotheses
versus associative hypotheses, 89-92
definition of, 91-92, 475
Causality
definition of, 338, 475
in research design, 195-196
testing, 214
Cell, 475
Central processing unit (CPU), 475
Central tendency
in data analysis, 312-313
measures and discussion of, 324-325
Child abuse
and confidentiality, 173
Children
effects of long term abuse of, 39f
researching sexual abuse in, 37-47
rights of, 168
Chi-square tests
to examine variable differences, 328
of independence
definition and example of, 329-331,
332t, 475
interpreting statistical results of,
330-332
for posthoc analysis, 314
CINAHL, 121-124
Citations
within bibliographical databases, 118
definition of, 110, 475
Clinical Nursing Research, 446-447
Clinical pathways
publication of, 462-463
Clinical practice
benchmarks, 463
guidelines in nursing, 463, 464t-467t,
468
research, 360-363
Clinical significance, 350
Closed-ended questions, 289
Cluster sampling, 245-246, 476
Clustered sources, 127t, 128
Coding
of data, 381-382
glossary definition of, 476
Coefficient of multiple determination,
337

Coercion
glossary definition of, 476
violating self-determination rights,
167
Cognitive clustering, 441, 476
Communication
channels in innovation-decision
process, 449t
of research findings, 438, 439t,
440-441
strategies, 439t
Comparative descriptive design, 203,
476
Comparison phase
glossary definition of, 476
of quantitative study example
critique, 426-427
in research critique process, 404-408
Compatibility, 450, 476
Competence
and informed consent, 178-181
Competent
level of experience, 16
stage of nursing, 362
Complete review
glossary definition of, 476
by IRB, 184
Complex hypotheses
definition of, 93
glossary definition of, 476
Complex searches, 121-122, 476
Complexity, 450, 477
Comprehending
glossary definition of, 477
versus skimming or reading
of research reports, 53-54
Comprehension phase
glossary definition of, 477
of quantitative study example
critique, 418-421
in research critique process, 402-404
Concepts
critiquing, 153
defining in theory, 140-141
definition of, 40, 98, 477
example *versus* conceptual definition,
142-144
important to research design, 195-213
within research questions, 87-89
understanding when critiquing,
142-144
and validity, 274
Conceptual definition
definition and example of, 40
versus dictionary definition, 140
example *versus* concept, 142-144
glossary definition of, 477
of variables, 101-103
Conceptual framework
for nursing, 151f
Conceptual map
description and illustration of,
147-148

Conceptual map—cont'd
example of, 154f
glossary definition of, 477
Conceptual models, 138-139, 477
Conceptual nursing models
frameworks, 150-154
Conclusions
glossary definition of, 477
in statistical research, 348
Concurrent events
prediction of, 275
Concurrent replication, 227-228
Conduct and Utilization of Research in
Nursing (CURN), 443-445
Confidentiality
breaches of, 173
critiquing, 173
glossary definition of, 477
right to, 172-173
Confirmation stage
example of, 458-459
glossary definition of, 477
of research utilization process, 452
Confirmatory analyses, 314, 477
Confounding variables, 99, 477
Connotations, 140
Consent form, 179f, 477
Consistency
maintaining data collection, 299, 301
Construct validity, 199, 274-277, 478
Constructs
abstract, 274
critiquing, 153
defining in theory, 140
glossary definition of, 478
Consumers
as audience for research findings, 441
Content Validity Index (CVI), 274-275
Content-related validity, 274-275, 478
Continuance, 452, 478
Continuum of values, 269-270
Contrasting groups, 275
Control
glossary definition of, 478
maintaining research, 301
nursing research definition of, 6
in quantitative research process,
30-31
in research design, 197-198
Control groups
definition of, 214-218, 478
in samples, 313
Controlled extraneous variables, 98-99
Convenience sampling, 248-250, 478
Convergence, 275
Correlation matrix
discussion and example of, 334, 335t
Correlational analyses
glossary definition of, 478
in statistics, 332-336
Correlational design
algorithm for determining, 213f
glossary definition of, 478